Integrative Oncology

Integrative Oncology

EDITED BY

Donald I. Abrams, MD
Chief, Hematology-Oncology
San Francisco General Hospital
Osher Foundation Endowed Director of Clinical Programs
UCSF Osher Center for Integrative Medicine
Professor of Clinical Medicine
University of California San Francisco
San Francisco, California

Andrew T. Weil, MD
Director, Arizona Center for Integrative Medicine
Lovell-Jones Professor of Integrative Rheumatology
Clinical Professor of Medicine
Professor of Public Health
University of Arizona
Tucson, Arizona

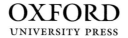

OXFORD
UNIVERSITY PRESS

2009

OXFORD
UNIVERSITY PRESS

Oxford University Press, Inc., publishes works that further
Oxford University's objective of excellence
in research, scholarship, and education.

Oxford New York
Auckland Cape Town Dar es Salaam Hong Kong Karachi
Kuala Lumpur Madrid Melbourne Mexico City Nairobi
New Delhi Shanghai Taipei Toronto

With offices in
Argentina Austria Brazil Chile Czech Republic France Greece
Guatemala Hungary Italy Japan Poland Portugal Singapore
South Korea Switzerland Thailand Turkey Ukraine Vietnam

Published by Oxford University Press, Inc.
198 Madison Avenue, New York, New York 10016
www.oup.com

Oxford is a registered trademark of Oxford University Press

Library of Congress Cataloging-in-Publication Data

Integrative oncology / edited by Donald I. Abrams, Andrew Weil.
p. ; cm.
Includes bibliographical references.
ISBN 978-0-19-530944-7
1. Oncology.   2. Cancer—Alternative treatment.   3. Cancer—Adjuvant
treatment.   4. Integrative medicine.
[DNLM: 1. Neoplasms—therapy. 2. Complementary Therapies.
QZ 266 I5687 2008] I. Abrams, Donald I. II. Weil, Andrew.
RC254.5.I52 2008
616.99'406—dc22   2008016137

1 3 5 7 9 8 6 4 2
Printed in the United States of America
on acid-free paper

To Clint for his nurturing, guidance, and inspiration

and

In memory of Sam for his friendship, wisdom, and good cheer

PREFACE TO THE SERIES

Integrative Medicine in Clinical Practice

ANDREW T. WEIL, MD

Integrative medicine (IM) is healing-oriented medicine that takes account of the whole person (body, mind, spirit), as well as all aspects of lifestyle. It emphasizes the therapeutic relationship and makes use of all appropriate therapies, both conventional and complementary. IM is not synonymous with alternative medicine or with CAM (complementary and alternative medicine). It neither rejects conventional medicine nor accepts alternative treatments uncritically.

Integrative medicine is a rapidly growing movement in North America. Consumer demand for it has increased steadily over the past decades. Now, as the conventional health-care system collapses because of out-of-control escalation of costs of high-tech medicine, medical institutions are finally taking IM seriously. The Consortium of Academic Health Centers for Integrative Medicine has 41 members; among them are many leading medical schools, whose deans and chancellors recognize the need to move medical education, research, and practice in this direction. A major reason for the new acceptance of IM is awareness that it can lower health-care costs in two ways: (1) by shifting the focus of health care from disease management to health promotion through its attention to lifestyle and the innate healing potentials of the human organism; and (2) by bringing lower-cost treatments into the mainstream that can give outcomes as good as or better than those of pharmaceutical drugs and other conventional therapies.

Practitioners are also increasingly drawn to IM because they recognize its potential to restore core values of medicine that have eroded in the era of profit-driven health care. Yet demand for clinicians trained to practice IM greatly exceeds supply. The Arizona Center for Integrative Medicine that I founded in 1994 has graduated more than 300 physicians (and some nurse practitioners) from comprehensive fellowships, mostly in distributed learning formats. Many of them now direct IM programs at other institutions, some are training others, and some have authored leading textbooks in the field. The Center also trains medical students, pharmacists, and medical residents. One of its major goals is to develop a core curriculum in IM that will become a required, accredited part of all residency training in all medical specialties.

In the meantime, there is an immediate need to organize and make accessible to many more clinicians the basic principles of IM in practical application to common health conditions. It is hoped that the present series of volumes will help fulfill that need. Each volume will cover the relevance of IM to a particular specialty, and each will draw on the editorial expertise of a specialist who is fully trained in IM as well as the advice of senior experts who are open to, but not directly involved with, the IM movement. Each volume will also give detailed protocols for the management of conditions that respond well to integrative treatment and will discuss areas of controversy and uncertainty where further research is needed.

Some physicians may find this information of use in meeting the needs of patients better. Some may use it to determine the best treatments for common conditions. Others may simply want to know more about CAM therapies their patients are using, if only to be able to discuss them intelligently and give advice about possible interactions between, say, conventional drugs and dietary supplements or botanical remedies.

Promoters of IM have been criticized for advocating unscientific or even antiscientific theories and practices. The commitment of all editors involved in this project is to present the evidence base for integrative treatment strategies. Readers should note, however, that IM teaches practitioners to use a sliding scale of evidence in making therapeutic choices: the greater the potential of a treatment to cause harm, the stricter the standard of evidence it should be held to for efficacy. We may recommend therapies that do not yet have a solid evidence base for efficacy if their potential for harm is low. Examples are suggesting therapeutic massage for persons with advanced forms of cancer as a means of improving quality of life or teaching hypertensive patients breathing techniques to increase the tone of the parasympathetic nervous system. All authors have been charged with the task of citing the best available evidence for both safety and efficacy of therapies discussed.

Although randomized controlled trials of specific interventions are helpful, what is most needed are outcome studies comparing integrative versus conventional management of common health problems, especially ones that absorb many of our health-care dollars. Because integrative protocols are complex—including, possibly, dietary change, dietary supplements, recommendations for physical activity and stress reduction, mind–body therapies, or use of a whole-system approach like Chinese medicine, in addition to selective use of conventional therapies—and because they are customized to address the problems of individual patients, studying them can be challenging. Nonetheless, it is outcomes data that we must have to evaluate the effectiveness and cost-effectiveness of IM relative to conventional medicine to advance the field and change reimbursement priorities that now fully cover costly conventional treatments but make it difficult for IM practitioners to get fair compensation for their time and effort.

I am grateful to Oxford University Press for having the vision to suggest this series of volumes, which I believe will be seen as a milestone in the development of integrative medicine. I am more than pleased with the outstanding work that the editors and coeditors have done in their selection of content and authors. I have learned a great deal in the course of acting as series editor, not the least from reading chapters as they came in. I hope you find these volumes as stimulating and refreshing as I do.

Tucson, Arizona

June 2008

PREFACE

Integrative oncology can be defined as the rational, evidence-based combination of conventional therapy with complementary interventions into an individualized therapeutic regimen that addresses the whole person living with and beyond cancer—body, mind, and spirit. The number of cancer patients and survivors incorporating complementary modalities into their treatment programs is difficult to estimate precisely but seems to be large and on the increase. Many choose not to disclose their use of complementary therapies to conventional oncologists for fear of being ridiculed, abandoned, or asked to stop. Others recognize that their oncology team has neither the time nor the information to answer their often complex questions, so they remain silent. Although there is little we can do to encourage patients living with or beyond cancer to discuss their integration of complementary therapies, we hope that this book will greatly assist all who care for them to become more familiar with and comfortable discussing the most widely utilized modalities.

This volume is targeted at health-care providers who seek an up-to-date, comprehensive, user-friendly source of information that will be relevant to the care of their cancer patients. We hope that it will quickly become the definitive resource in this emerging field. An outstanding group of renowned contributors has produced chapters discussing the latest information on the most widely used modalities employed in integrative oncology. We have attempted to provide a text that is as global and inclusive as possible. The presence of a chapter in the book does not necessarily indicate that we endorse a particular modality. Three chapters focus on the common cancers—breast, prostate, and colon—presenting rational integrative treatment plans that demonstrate how many of the individual modalities can be woven into a comprehensive therapeutic approach. We also include discussions on research challenges, communication issues, a patient perspective, and thoughts about the future of integrative oncology.

We know that this comprehensive book will serve as a valuable resource for all who provide care for patients living with cancer and cancer survivors. We hope that practitioners will be stimulated by these chapters to learn more and, begin to incorporate some of these modalities into their own treatment plans. Providing patients with other tools in addition to surgery, radiation, cytotoxic chemotherapy, hormonal manipulation, and targeted therapies is indeed a challenge, but one well worth the effort. Making a bit more time to inquire about nutrition, exercise, the use of supplements, mind–body interventions, and spirituality shows that we care about the whole person living with cancer, not just their malignancy. Providing patients with the opportunity to integrate these interventions with their conventional cancer care goes a long way in increasing the sense of empowerment and control that so many have lost at the time of diagnosis. Until that day when chapters like these are included in standard oncology textbooks, this book should be of value to those on the front lines of cancer care and their patients.

Donald I. Abrams

CONTENTS

CONTRIBUTORS

Donald I. Abrams, MD
Chief, Hematology-Oncology,
    San Francisco General Hospital
Osher Foundation Endowed Director
    of Clinical Programs
UCSF Osher Center for Integrative
    Medicine
Professor of Clinical Medicine,
    University of California
    San Francisco
San Francisco, CA

Lise N. Alschuler, ND, FABNO
Naturopathic Specialists, LLC.
Scottsdale, AZ

Sharyn D. Baker, PharmD PhD
Department of Pharmaceutical
    Sciences
St. Jude Children's Research Hospital
Memphis, TN

Aditya Bardia, MD, MPH
Resident, Department
    of Internal Medicine
Mayo Clinic College of Medicine
Rochester, MN

Debra L. Barton RN, PhD, AOCN
Associate Professor of Oncology
Department of Oncology
Mayo Clinic College of Medicine
Rochester, MN

Iris Bell, MD, PhD
Departments of Family and
    Community Medicine
Psychiatry, Psychology, Medicine
    (Program in Integrative Medicine),
    and Public Health, University
    of Arizona
Tucson, AZ

Keith I. Block, MD
Block Center for Integrative
    Cancer Treatment
Evanston, IL

Lisa W. Corbin, MD
Associate Professor,
Department of General Internal
    Medicine
University of Colorado Denver
    School of Medicine
Medical Director
The Center for Integrative Medicine,
    University of Colorado Hospital
Aurora, CO

Kerry S. Courneya, PhD
Faculty of Physical Education
University of Alberta
Edmonton, Alberta

Muriel Cuendet, PhD
Gerald P. Murphy Cancer Foundation
West Lafayette, IN

Anand Dhruva, MD
Hematology-Oncology, San Francisco
    General Hospital
Integrative Oncology, UCSF Osher
    Center for Integrative Medicine
Assistant Clinical Professor
University of California
    San Francisco, CA

Ann Marie Dose, PhD, RN, ACNS-BC
Clinical Nurse Researcher Nursing
    Research Division
Department of Nursing
Mayo Clinic
Rochester, MN

**Vinjar Fønnebø, MD, MSc
Epidemiology, PhD**
Professor in Preventive Medicine
Director of NAFKAM
Faculty of Medicine
University of Tromsø
Norway

**Heather Greenlee, ND, PhD
candidate**
Department of Epidemiology
Mailman School of Public Health
Columbia University
New York, NY

Manuel Guzman, Ph.D.
Professor of Biochemistry
    and Molecular Biology
School of Biology
Complutense University
Madrid, Spain

Peter Heusser, MD, MME
Professor of Anthroposophic Medicine
Institute of Complementary Medicine
    KIKOM, University of Bern
Switzerland

Judith S. Jacobson, DrPH, MBA
Department of Epidemiology,
    Mailman School of Public Health,
    and Herbert Irving Comprehensive
    Cancer Center, College of
    Physicians and Surgeons
Columbia University
New York, NY

Peter A.S. Johnstone, MD, FACR
Chair and William A. Mitchell
    Professor
Department of Radiation Oncology
Indiana University School
    of Medicine
Indianapolis, IN

Kara M. Kelly, MD
Columbia University Medical Center
Division of Pediatric Oncology
Morgan Stanley Children's Hospital
    of New York-Presbyterian
New York, NY

Gunver Sophia Kienle, MD
Senior Research Scientist
Institute for Applied
    Epistemology and Medical
    Methodology Freiburg
Bad Krozingen, Germany

Mary Jo Kreitzer, PhD, RN, FAAN
Director Center for Spirituality &
    Healing
Minneapolis, MN

Elena Ladas, MS RD
The Integrative Therapies Program
    for Children with Cancer
Columbia University
    Medical Center
Division of Pediatric Oncology
New York, NY

Brian D. Lawenda, MD
Assistant Professor of Radiology/
  Radiological Sciences
Uniformed Services University of the
  Health Sciences
Bethesda, MD
Adjunct Assistant Professor,
  Department of Radiation Oncology
Indiana University School of Medicine
Indianapolis, IN

Charles L. Loprinzi, MD
Professor of Oncology, Department
  of Oncology
Mayo Clinic College of Medicine
Rochester, MN

Susan K. Lutgendorf, PhD
Department of Psychology
Department of Obstetrics and
  Gynecology
Department of Urology
Holden Comprehensive Cancer
  Center, University of Iowa
Iowa City, IA

Mark A. Moyad, MD, MPH
Phil F. Jenkins Director of
  Preventive & Alternative
  Medicine
University of Michigan Medical
  Center-Department of Urology
Ann Arbor, MI

Elizabeth Mullen, MS
Department of Psychology
  University of Iowa
Iowa City, IA

Matthew P. Mumber, MD
Radiation Oncologist
Harbin Clinic Radiation Oncology
Rome, GA

Ramesh Nanal
Founder editor MadhuJeevana,
Mumbai, India

Vilas Nanal
Founder president Vaidya M. P. Nanal
  Foundation,
Pune, India

Alfred I. Neugut, MD, PhD
Department of Medicine and
  Herbert Irving Comprehensive
  Cancer Center, College of
  Physicians and Surgeons, and
Department of Epidemiology
Mailman School of Public
  Health
Columbia University
New York, NY

Menachem Oberbaum, MD
Director, Center for Integrative
  Complementary Medicine
Shaare Zedek Medical Center
Jerusalem, Israel

John M. Pezzuto, PhD
College of Pharmacy
University of Hawaii at Hilo
Hilo, HA

Ann B. Ready, ND, MPH
Bastyr University
Kenmore, WA

Rachel Naomi Remen, MD
Clinical Professor, Family and
  Community Medicine UCSF School
  of Medicine, San Francisco,
  California
Founder and Director The Institute for
  the Study of Health and Illness
  Commonweal Bolinas, CA

David S. Rosenthal, MD
Leonard P. Zakim Center for
    Integrative Therapies
Dana-Farber Cancer Institute
    Boston, MA

Martin L. Rossman, MD
Clinical Associate, Department
    of Medicine
University of California,
    San Francisco Medical School
Director of the Collaborative
    Medicine Center
Greenbrae, CA

**Stephen M. Sagar, BSc (Hons)
MB BS MRCP FRCR FRCPC**
Associate Professor
Departments of Oncology
    and Medicine
McMaster University, and Hamilton
    Health Sciences Cancer Program
Juravinski Cancer Centre
Hamilton, Ontario, Canada

**Manuchehr Shirmohamadi,
PhD, PE**
CTO, Power Transmission
    Solutions, Inc.
Berkeley, CA

Dean Shrock, PhD
Mind-Body Medicine Consultant
Triune Integrative Medicine
    Medford, OR

Shepherd Roee Singer, MD
Center for Integrative
    Complementary Medicine
Shaare Zedek Medical Center
Jerusalem, Israel

Gowsala Sivam, PhD
Bastyr University
Kenmore, WA

Amit Sood, MD, MSc
Assistant Professor of Medicine
Division of General Medicine
Department of Internal Medicine
Mayo Clinic College of Medicine
Rochester, MN

Alex Sparreboom, PhD
Department of Pharmaceutical
    Sciences
St. Jude Children's Research
    Hospital
Memphis, TN

**Leanna J. Standish, ND, PhD, Dipl.
Acup., FABNO**
Bastyr University Research Center
Kenmore, WA

Clare Stevinson, PhD
University of Alberta
Edmonton, Canada

Antonella Surbone, MD, PhD, FACP
Associate Professor of Medicine
New York University
    Medical School
Department of Medicine
Division of Medical Oncology
New York, NY
Lecturer in Bioethics
University of Rome, Italy

Cynthia A. Thomson
Department of Nutritional Sciences
Arizona Cancer Center
Tucson, AZ

Carolyn Torkelson, MD, MS
Assistant Professor
   Department of Family
   Medicine and Community
   Health
University of Minnesota
Minneapolis, MN

Debu Tripathy, MD
Professor of Internal Medicine
Director, Komen/UT Southwestern
   Breast Cancer Research
   Program
University of Texas Southwestern
   Medical Center
Dallas, TX

Dana Ullman, MPH
Homeopathic Educational Services
Berkeley, CA

Andrew T. Weil, MD
Director, Arizona Center
   for Integrative Medicine
Lovell-Jones Professor of
   Integrative Rheumatology
Clinical Professor of Medicine
Professor of Public Health
University of Arizona
Tucson, AZ

Cynthia A. Wenner, PhD
Research Associate Professor
Department of Basic Sciences
School of Natural Health Sciences
Bastyr University
Kenmore, WA

Qing Cai Zhang, MD, Lic. Ac.
SinoMed Research Institute
New York, NY

Integrative Oncology

1

Why Integrative Oncology?

ANDREW T. WEIL

I ntegrative medicine (IM) is an established movement in North America and China. It is a developing movement in parts of the Middle East and continental Europe, especially Scandinavia. I am confident that it is the direction medicine and health care must take to address demands from patients, dissatisfaction of practitioners, and the worsening economics of health care worldwide.

Many people consider IM and alternative medicine synonymous. This is not the case. Alternative medicine comprises all those therapies not taught in conventional (allopathic) medical schools, based on ideas that range from sensible and worth including in mainstream medicine to those that are foolish and a few that are dangerous.[1] The term *alternative medicine* has recently been incorporated into a broader term, *complementary and alternative medicine*, or "CAM," that is used by the federal government in the United States and other institutions; the National Institutes of Health now has a national CAM center (NCCAM).

Neither "alternative" nor "complementary" captures the essence of integrative medicine. The former suggests replacement of conventional therapies by others; the latter suggests adjunctive therapies, added as afterthoughts.

IM does include ideas and practices currently beyond the scope of the conventional, but it neither rejects conventional therapies nor accepts alternative ones uncritically. And it emphasizes principles that may or may not be associated with CAM:

- *The Natural Healing Power of the Organism*—IM assumes that the body has an innate capacity for healing, self-diagnosis, self-repair, regeneration, and adaptation to injury or loss. The primary goal of treatment should be to support, facilitate, and augment that innate capacity.

---

[1] Weil A. (1998). *Health and healing: The philosophy of integrative medicine.* Boston: Houghton Mifflin Co., rev. ed.

- *Whole Person Medicine*—IM views patients as more than physical bodies. They are also mental/emotional beings, spiritual entities, and members of particular communities and societies. These other dimensions of human life are relevant to health and to the accurate diagnosis and effective treatment of disease.
- *The Importance of Lifestyle*—Health and disease result from interactions between genes and all aspects of lifestyle, including diet, physical activity, rest and sleep, stress, the quality of relationships, work, and so forth. Lifestyle choices may influence disease risks more than genes and must be a focus of the medical history. Lifestyle medicine, which is one component of IM, gives physicians information and tools to enable them to prevent and treat disease more effectively.
- *The Critical Role of the Doctor–Patient Relationship*—Throughout history people have accorded the doctor–patient relationship special, even sacred, status. When a medically trained person sits with a patient and listens with full attention to his or her story, that alone can initiate healing before any treatment is offered. A great tragedy of contemporary medicine, especially in the United States, is that for profit, corporate systems have virtually destroyed this core aspect of practice. If practitioners have only a few minutes with each patient—the time limit set by the managed care systems they work for—it is very unlikely they will be able to form the kind of therapeutic relationships that foster health and healing.

Furthermore, this special form of human interaction has been the source of greatest emotional reward for the physician, and its disappearance in our time is a main reason for rising practitioner discontent. IM insists on the paramount importance of the therapeutic relationship and demands that health care systems support and honor it (e.g., by reimbursing physicians for time spent with patients rather than number of patients seen).

In essence, IM is conservative. It seeks to restore core values of the profession that have eroded in recent times. It honors such ancient precepts as Hippocrates' injunctions on physicians to "first do no harm" and "to value the healing power of nature." It is conservative in practice, favoring less invasive and drastic treatments over more invasive and drastic ones whenever possible, and it is fiscally conservative in relying less on expensive technology and more on simpler methods, *as appropriate to the circumstances of illness.*

The IM movement in North America is gathering momentum. Forty-one leading medical schools in the United States and Canada have now joined the Consortium of Academic Health Centers for Integrative Medicine (www.imconsortium.org), which seeks to advance the field on three fronts: education, research, and clinical practice. Textbooks of IM, written for clinicians, are appearing with increasing frequency.[2] And demand for training in the field is growing steadily.

To help answer that demand I founded the Program in Integrative Medicine (now the Arizona Center for Integrative Medicine or ACIM) at the University of Arizona in 1994 (www.integrativemedicine.arizona.edu) and continue to direct it. ACIM's focus has been the development of new educational models for training medical students, residents, physicians, nurse practitioners, pharmacists, and other health professionals. The Center has offered intensive fellowships to MDs and DOs, increasingly in distributed learning formats, mainly Internet based. The curriculum we have developed covers the philosophy of IM as well as broad subject areas currently slighted or omitted entirely from conventional medical education. These include nutritional medicine (e.g., designing an optimum diet for health and longevity; using dietary supplements appropriately; using dietary change as a primary therapeutic strategy, etc.), botanical medicine, mind–body medicine, manual medicine (such as osteopathic manipulative therapy), spirituality in health and illness, environmental medicine, and overviews of traditional systems of medicine (like Chinese medicine and Ayurveda) and CAM.

Our teaching about traditional medicine and CAM is intended to convey the philosophies behind these approaches, the evidence base for them, their strengths and weaknesses, and their appropriateness or inappropriateness in specific health conditions. We also cover the training and credentialing of CAM practitioners and information on how to find and refer to competent ones when appropriate.

Criticism of IM has mostly focused on perceived advocacy of ideas and practices not consistent with evidence-based medicine (EBM). Training at ACIM requires fellows to assess the evidence base for all recommended treatments, including conventional ones. The Center also trains future researchers, many of whom are working on new research designs to investigate complex systems and new outcome measures to assess the effectiveness and cost-effectiveness of integrative treatment plans (as opposed to single interventions). We also teach

---

[2] Some examples are Rakel D. (Ed.). (2007). *Integrative medicine.* Philadelphia: Saunders; Kligler B & Lee RA. (2004). *Integrative medicine.* New York: McGraw Hill; Audette JF & Bailey A. (2008). *Integrative pain medicine.* Totowa, New Jersey: Humana Press; Cohen MH, et al. (2006). *The practice of integrative medicine: A legal and operational guide.* New York: Springer; Low Dog T & Micozzi M. (2004). *Women's health in complementary and integrative medicine: A clinical guide.* Philadelphia: Churchill Livingstone.

practitioners to use a sliding scale of evidence in evaluating treatments: the greater the potential of an intervention to cause harm, the stricter the standard of evidence it should be held to for efficacy.

It has never been my wish or that of ACIM to see the field of IM evolve into a subspecialty of general medicine, family medicine, internal medicine, public health, or any other discipline. Rather, my colleagues and I consider training in IM to be foundational to the education and training of all physicians, as well as of nurses, pharmacists, and allied health professionals. Even a neurosurgeon or dermatologist should know the basics of nutrition and health, mind–body interactions, and botanical medicine. Every medical doctor should know the difference between an osteopathic physician and a chiropractor and have at least some sense of important traditional systems, like Chinese medicine and Ayurveda. Every medical professional should understand the influence of life-style on health.

For these reasons, the present focus of ACIM is development of a comprehensive curriculum of IM, consisting of several hundred hours of instruction that can be taught in a distributed learning format. Our goal is to have this become a required, accredited part of residency training in all medical specialties.

ACIM's graduates now include hundreds of physicians from many specialties, including, several oncologists. I am happy about this, because the demand for integrative oncology is overwhelming, but practitioners trained to practice it are very few. To cater to public demand, some leading cancer centers advertise that they offer integrative treatment, but I find the claims misleading. They offer selected CAM therapies, mostly the safest, least controversial ones, such as massage, stress reduction, and nutritional counseling but advise patients to shun botanical remedies that might ameliorate the toxic effects of chemotherapy and radiation as well as most dietary supplements and have no informed advice to give about more complex therapies, such as those from the Ayurvedic tradition of India. One chain of private cancer treatment centers that builds its reputation on an "integrative" philosophy employs conventional oncologists untrained in IM while using doctors of naturopathy (NDs) to supervise CAM therapies as adjuncts.

The first answer to "Why integrative oncology?" is that most patients with cancer want integrative care. The great majority—as many as 90% in some surveys—are using other therapies while receiving conventional treatment.[3]

---

[3] Deng G & Cassileth B. (2005). To what extent do cancer patients use complementary and alternative medicine? *Nature Clinical Practice Oncology*, 2, 496–497; Richardson MA, et al. (2000). Complementary/Alternative medicine use in a comprehensive cancer center and the implications for oncology. *Journal of Clinical Oncology*, 18, 2505–2514; see also http://nccam.nih. gov/health/camcancer/#use

Most of those do not tell their oncologists what else they are doing, because they expect to be criticized, ridiculed, or told to stop. In any medical situation, whatever the disease, the physician in charge ought to know all therapies that the patients are using, both to be able to avoid adverse interactions and to be able to assess outcomes. An integrative oncologist can elicit this information and give patients sound advice about CAM therapies.

Because nutrition, including the use of dietary supplements, is a core competency of IM education, integrative oncologists can answer some of the most common and urgent questions of cancer patients starting chemotherapy and radiotherapy, such as, "Are there any foods I should or shouldn't eat during treatment?" and "Can I continue to take my vitamins?"

Here is a glaring example of the present paucity of training about nutrition and cancer: the daughter of a woman undergoing chemotherapy for metastatic colon cancer consulted me in distress, because the medical oncologist told her mother to "eat only white foods" during the entire course of treatment. She wanted permission to encourage her mother to eat more wholesome meals. Numerous cancer patients tell me they are advised not to eat fruits and vegetables while receiving chemotherapy or radiotherapy, because the antioxidants in them would compromise the efficacy of those treatments. Countless others express dismay that their oncologists are unable to talk to them about best nutritional strategies for reducing risks of recurrence. "Just eat a balanced diet," or "Whatever you feel like eating," are common responses they get, leaving them frustrated and unsure about where to turn for better advice and information.

If a patient undergoing cancer treatment asks a conventionally trained oncologist about the value of the Chinese herb astragalus (from the root of *Astragalus membranceous*) to protect the bone marrow and white cell populations from some of the toxicity of some chemotherapeutic agents or the use of Asian mushrooms like maitake (*Grifola frondosa*) or enoki (*Flammulina velutipes*) to "boost immunity," it is unlikely the physician will know anything about these natural products. The reflexive response will be, "Do not take anything other than what we give you," again leaving patients frustrated and often angry about their doctors' limited knowledge. Hence the tendency to conceal the use of such products, which may have been recommended by friends, by books, by CAM providers, or by Internet sites. A major component of patients' frustration with these interactions is a strong sense of disempowerment and inability to have any partnership in shaping their medical destiny.

Given the fact that so few integrative oncologists exist and that cancer patients in our part of the world have such difficulty putting together sound and safe integrative treatment plans, it is surprising to learn that their counterparts in China are much luckier. At least in large Chinese cities, most cancer patients who undergo surgery, chemotherapy, and radiotherapy also get Chinese herbal therapy to increase efficacy and reduce toxicity of the conventional treatments, as well as acupuncture, massage, energy work (such as *Qigong*), and dietary recommendations to support general health and manage symptoms.[4]

Of the various specialties of medicine, oncology has been much slower to embrace IM than most. Family medicine, pediatrics, and psychiatry are quite open to IM philosophy and training, and there is receptivity in internal medicine as well, especially from cardiologists. Integrative oncology seems so sensible and so needed. What are the sources of resistance that have slowed its development?

One is surely the emotionalism that surrounds cancer—a frighteningly common, mysterious, and serious group of diseases. We can argue about whether the incidence of cancer is increasing or not, but most people I know feel that cancer now touches their lives more directly than it used to, affecting them, their immediate families, their friends, and neighbors. The possibility of developing cancer or having to care for or help someone who has it is very great. Moreover, conventional cancer treatments are also frightening, because they can be painful, debilitating, disfiguring, and not always as successful as those who perform them represent them to be. Many people have a strongly negative perception of chemotherapy and radiotherapy because of their obvious toxicity and known potential to cause mutations and malignant transformation.

Progress in the diagnosis and management of cancer has been significant. A dramatic example is that it is now possible to envision the management of metastatic breast cancer as a chronic disease, much like AIDS, rather than as an inevitable and premature death sentence. (At the same time, the incidence of breast cancer is at an all-time high.) The prospect of individualized and targeted therapies is already being realized, with significant reduction in toxicity. Still, I and many others look forward to the advent of new and better treatments—gene therapy, immunotherapy, antiangiogenesis therapy—that will render many of our current strategies obsolete and reduce some of the emotionalism that now fuels the debate about other ways of managing cancer.

Over the years I have looked at a number of *alternative* cancer treatments— those offered instead of surgery, chemotherapy, and radiotherapy. I have seen many patients who used them as primary therapies, others who tried them after recurrences or when they were terminal. I also served on a federal government advisory panel charged with evaluating alternative cancer treatments.

Although I have known individual patients who responded very well to one or another of these diverse therapies, none of them, in my experience, has produced reliably good outcomes in significant numbers of patients. Some of

---

[4] See the chapter by QC Zhang, MD, in this volume.

these therapies are based on utterly unsound ideas: that cancer is caused by infection with parasites or other germs that can be seen by developers of proprietary vaccines but not by mainstream microbiologists; that cancer results from nutritional deficiencies or excesses and can be cured by dietary change alone; and so forth. A prominent and disturbing message from the alternative cancer treatment community is that a conspiracy of pharmaceutical companies and medical organizations profits handsomely from conventional treatment and has suppressed effective natural and alternative therapies.

I will also say that I have come across elements of alternative cancer treatments that seemed to me possibly useful and worthy of investigation. A broad example is the repertory of Chinese herbal remedies used along with chemotherapy and radiotherapy to increase their efficacy and reduce toxicity. A narrow one is the use of a topical extract of bloodroot (*Sanguinaria canadensis*) to provoke an immune reaction against and kill some skin cancers. (This was a part of the notorious Hoxsey therapy, developed by a Texas chiropractor in the mid-20th century.)[5] Practitioners of integrative oncology should be informed about alternative cancer treatments and able to answer patients' questions about them factually. They should also encourage research on those that show any evidence of efficacy.

No integrative oncologist would ever advise a patient to forego evidence-based treatment in favor of unproved therapy of unknown safety and efficacy. But a major role for such a practitioner would be to help patients make difficult choices about standard therapeutic options. Often cancer patients must decide among different courses of treatment, such as whether or not to use chemotherapy after surgery or radiation, whether to submit to aggressive chemotherapy in the event of a recurrence, whether to try an experimental vaccine, or stem cell transplant. They must gamble—with their lives—on making the right choices.

In most medical situations that involve serious disease, both doctors and patients are forced to deal with uncertainty. Rarely do we have all the information we need to make decisions that will guarantee desired outcomes. Instead we must use incomplete information to estimate probabilities and place the wisest bets we can. Ultimately, patients must take responsibility for this, but doctors can and should help them understand the possible therapeutic options and their probable consequences.

Most of us, physicians and patients alike, have not been trained in the science of uncertainty and probability. There is such a science—gambling theory, a branch of mathematics—and I have long wanted to adapt it to a course on medical decision making. My intent is to include it in the comprehensive curriculum for IM in Residency under development at the University of Arizona.

[5] See www.drweil.com/drw/u/id/QAA361873.

Most of our cancer treatments have significant risks as well as benefits. Patients must understand the risk/benefit ratio for any treatment offered, especially impact on quality of life vs. quantity of life. If a patient opts to forego chemotherapy following surgical removal of a breast or lung tumor, choosing instead to make all the right lifestyle choices to reduce risk of recurrence and to use various herbs and dietary supplements as insurance, is this an informed and wise decision? It may be—if she has been able to estimate the probabilities of outcomes. She will be guessing in the midst of uncertainty, but if she can get and can understand the best available data on her particular type and stage of cancer and on the risks and benefits of the therapeutic options under consideration, she can bet wisely. As the provider and interpreter of medical information, the integrative oncologist is indispensable to this process.

I cannot overstress the urgency of need for this service. Most cancer patients I know are desperately seeking the advice and counsel of oncologists who are well trained and credentialed, up-to-date with the science of cancer and its treatment, open-minded and non judgmental, who are interested in the influence of all aspects of lifestyle on health and illness, understand the interactions of mind and body, and have at least basic knowledge of botanical remedies, dietary supplements, and commonly used CAM therapies. Most often patients (and their loved ones and friends) cannot find such practitioners.

In addition, because IM puts so much emphasis on total lifestyle, it is in a better position than conventional medicine to offer true preventive care. Preventive medicine as a field has accomplished much, but it has focused narrowly on public health measures like sanitation, eradication of insect vectors of disease, diagnostic screening, and immunization rather than on the choices people make about how to eat, get physical activity, play, and handle stress. Most of the chronic diseases that kill and disable people prematurely are diseases of lifestyle that could be avoided or postponed by making better choices and developing better habits of living. Because the treatment of cancer is difficult and costly, especially if it has spread from its primary site, cancer prevention must be a high priority—not only by means of diagnostic screenings but primarily by counseling patients and educating society about the details of lifestyles associated with lower risk.

In the case of the hormonally driven cancers, for example, of the breast and prostate, we know a great deal about dietary and other influences that both raise and lower risk, but much of this information is not yet common knowledge; neither are there societal incentives to encourage people to change behavior. For example, the chemistry of the formation of carcinogens as animal tissue cooks is well known: the higher the temperature and the longer the time of cooking, the higher the dose of carcinogens in the meat (or poultry or fish) that comes to the table. We also have clinical data indicating that a preference for meat cooked "well done" is a significant risk factor for breast cancer in women.[6] Most women I know, including some with family histories of breast cancer, are unaware of these facts; certainly, no physician has made them aware of the danger.

There is good evidence that moderate, regular consumption of whole soy foods, *beginning early in life*, affects the development of the female breast in ways that make it resistant to malignant growth.[7] I believe it also offers significant protection against prostate cancer in men. Integrative oncology should develop strategies for helping people, especially parents of young children, to access, understand, and implement this information.

Conversely, there is growing evidence that the hormonal content of cow's milk in North America (and products made from it) add to other hormonal pressures, both exogenous and endogenous, that increase the possibility of malignant growth in both the breast and the prostate. I refer to natural bovine hormones, not man-made ones. In our part of the world, dairy cows are maintained in almost continual states of pregnancy and lactation, an unnatural lifestyle that greatly increases levels of sex hormones in their milk.[8] Yet in the recent revision of the US government's Food Pyramid (www.mypyramid.gov), the medical community did not mount any counteroffensive, when, under pressure from the dairy industry, the Department of Agriculture increased the recommended daily servings of milk and milk products from two to three. Many similar situations exist where special-interest groups affect public policy in ways that promote rather than safeguard against the development of cancer. Integrative oncologists could take the lead in improving them.

A first generation of integrative oncologists will probably find themselves most in demand as consultants. These are the main areas in which their advisory role will be needed:

- Helping patients with difficult decisions about conventional treatment options.
- Helping patients put together integrative treatment plans that use dietary strategies, mind-body therapies, and selected CAM therapies during and after conventional cancer treatment.

---

[6] Steck SE, et al. (2007). Cooked meat risk of breast cancer—Lifetime versus recent dietary intake. *Epidemiology*, 18, 3, 373–382.

[7] Cabanes A, et al. (2004). Prepubertal estradiol and genistein exposures up-regulate BRCA1 mRNA and reduce mammary gland tumorigenesis. *Carcinogenesis*, 25, 5, 741–748.

[8] Rich-Edwards JW, et al. (2007). Milk consumption and the prepubertal somatotropic axis. *Nutrition Journal [Electronic Resource]*, 6, 28; see also www.news.harvard.edu/gazaette/2006/12.07/11-dairy.html

- Advising patients about possible risks and benefits of alternative cancer treatments
- Informing patients about strategies for increasing efficacy and reducing side effects of chemotherapy and radiotherapy
- Advising patients about nutritional and other lifestyle strategies for reducing risks of recurrence
- Teaching those at risk for cancer about lifestyle strategies for reducing risk
- Helping patients with incurable cancer to get the best palliative care, drawing on all therapeutic options
- Helping terminal patients and families with issues around death and dying.

Recently, a 64-year-old man with newly diagnosed bile duct carcinoma consulted both of the editors of this volume for help in several of these areas. All of the doctors involved with his case at a major academic health center agreed that a Whipple resection was indicated, but experts disagreed about follow-up treatment. Because this is a rare carcinoma, statistical evidence on outcomes is scant, and the conventional oncologists he talked with based their recommendations on experience with pancreatic cancer. He was strongly advised to do both a full course of radiotherapy followed by aggressive chemotherapy.

The patient was educated, health conscious, and most interested in other opinions from experts with a broader perspective. The conventional oncologists could not answer his questions about the wisdom of using the dietary supplements he was taking or about foods he should or shouldn't eat. They had nothing to say about physical activity, mental/emotional factors that might influence outcomes, or lifestyle factors that might have contributed to the development of his cancer or that might help his body contain any malignant tissue that might escape removal by surgery or destruction by radiation and chemotherapy.

I put him in touch with a practitioner of modern Chinese medicine—an MD trained in China with experience in the Chinese style of integrative cancer treatment—who recommended herbal products both to slow the growth of any cancer left behind by surgery and to protect his bone marrow and other immunologically active tissues from damage by radiation and chemotherapeutic drugs. He decided not to discuss these products with the surgical or medical oncologists with whom he finally partnered.

I also directed him to one of the few integrative oncologists in practice, who happened to work in a nearby city. The patient had two meetings with him prior to surgery and was able to get answers to his questions about nutrition and dietary supplements during treatment. He was also given recommendations for some additional ones.

The patient then had phone sessions with a hypnotherapist I referred him to in order to prepare for surgery, and he obtained from the therapist audio programs to use in the hospital. By the time he called Dr. Abrams for additional opinions, I felt he was in danger of getting too many points of view and too much information. I suggested he use the nearby integrative oncologist as his primary advisor in matters that his other physicians could not address. Dr. Abrams was able to put him in touch with a patient who had recently undergone a Whipple resection for pancreatic cancer and come through it very well. The two patients had a number of telephone conversations that proved very helpful, making the man facing surgery much more informed about what to expect and much more optimistic about recovery and outcome.

(In my own practice I have always tried to introduce patients with chronic diseases to others with the same or similar problems who have done well. There is no better way to convince a sick person that better health is possible. This may be especially important in people newly diagnosed with cancer.)

The surgical procedure went well. There was no evidence of spread of the tumor beyond the primary site, but because one margin was not clean, there was consensus that a course of radiotherapy was indicated. The question of concurrent chemotherapy, however, produced disagreement among experts.

The patient had a mostly smooth recovery, made sure he got good, healthful food, took the botanicals and dietary supplements, did his mind-body practice, and started walking every day as much as he could. His mental state was positive, but he wrestled with the decision about chemotherapy. His medical oncologist urged aggressive treatment, using cisplatin, but said she would be comfortable with giving a routine course of 5-FU, a much less toxic agent. Some of his consultants, including one surgical oncologist, advised against any chemotherapy, saying its benefits in bile duct carcinoma were negligible. After weighing all the opinions, he opted for 5-FU, and his integrative oncologist supported this choice, adjusting his dietary, herbal, and supplement regimen for the six-week course of concurrent radio- and chemotherapy.

According to the physicians directly involved in these treatments, the patient came through them with less difficulty, fewer side effects, and a better response than any comparable patient they had treated. The patient believes his good response to be due to all that he is doing to support his general health and body defenses, all of which he learned from his research into integrative cancer treatment. He feels confident about his future and motivated to be diligent about protecting his health by attending to all areas of his life under his control. He expresses willingness to act as a resource for other persons with cancer trying to find the information he sought and also to assist the development of the field of integrative oncology.

I wrote earlier that the ACIM is working toward the goal of making basic education in IM a required, accredited part of residency training in all specialties and subspecialties of medicine. When we achieve that, all clinicians, including oncologists, will have the perspective and information to practice IM. At that point also I hope we will be able to drop the word "integrative." This will just be good medicine, the kind that patients want, the kind that doctors find most rewarding to practice, the kind that produces the best outcomes. IM is not revolutionary, but it is *radical* in the literal sense of that word (from Latin *radix:* "root") in that it aims to reconnect medicine to its roots, to restore its core values.

Integrative oncology simply means doing the best we can to prevent and treat cancer and support those affected by it on all levels: body, mind, and spirit.

2

An Integrative Approach to Cancer Prevention

HEATHER GREENLEE

KEY CONCEPTS

- An individual's risk of developing cancer is determined in part by genetic predisposition and lifetime exposures. Information about these factors can be used to recommend an appropriate screening schedule.
- Conventional approaches to cancer prevention include behavioral modifications (such as dietary changes and physical activity), biological agents (such as antioxidants, multivitamins, minerals, hormone modulators, and anti-inflammatory agents), surgery, and vaccinations.
- Complementary and alternative medicine (CAM) approaches to cancer prevention include special diets, botanicals (for various properties including antioxidant, anti-inflammatory, immune modulating, hormone modulating, and adaptogenic effects, and the induction of biotransformation enzymes), vitamins and minerals, other dietary supplements, mind-body therapies, and energy therapies.
- Non-Western systems of healing such as Chinese medicine, Ayurvedic medicine, Tibetan medicine, and Native American medicine offer their own perspectives on what causes cancer and what can be done to prevent cancer.
- An integrative approach to cancer prevention encourages individuals to make healthy lifestyle choices, use appropriate cancer screening technologies, and maintain a sense of wellness and balance.

D isease prevention is generally viewed as encompassing three levels: primary, secondary, and tertiary. The goal of primary prevention is to reduce the risk of developing the disease. Primary cancer prevention measures include the use of chemopreventive agents, the avoidance of exposure to environmental carcinogens, and surgical removal of susceptible organs (e.g., prophylactic mastectomy) [1]. Secondary prevention involves screening and early detection methods, used among asymptomatic individuals to identify abnormal tissue changes or precancerous lesions before they become cancerous or detect them at an early stage when treatment is most likely to lead to a cure [1]. Tertiary prevention, often referred to as *cancer control*, involves preventing existing cancer from spreading, preventing recurrence, preventing second primary cancers, and preventing other cancer-related complications. Tertiary prevention includes a variety of aspects of patient care, including interventions to improve quality as well as duration of life, adjuvant therapies, surgical intervention and palliative care [1]. This chapter will focus on primary cancer prevention and will discuss what people without a cancer diagnosis can do to reduce the risk of developing cancer.

Current conventional cancer prevention approaches begin with risk assessment based on age, gender, genetics, personal and family medical history, and occupational and lifestyle exposures. Appropriate interventions are recommended based on the determination of individual risk. Everyone can benefit from a healthful diet and physical activity. Individuals at higher-than-average risk may want to consider pharmacological chemoprevention, surgery to remove the susceptible organ, and vaccinations. Complementary and alternative medicine (CAM) approaches include largely biologic therapies and behavioral modifications such as dietary modifications, botanicals (herbs), vitamins and minerals, other dietary supplements, mind-body therapies, energy medicine, and non-Western systems of healing.

Until recently, the mere concept of primary prevention of cancer was considered somewhat unconventional because there was little evidence to support the concept that carcinogenesis [1] could be reversed or halted, or that people could change their habits to prevent cancer. However, in the past two decades, clinical trials have shown both that cancer can be prevented (or postponed) and that people can modify their diet or stop smoking to reduce their cancer risk. The tamoxifen trial proved that a drug could reduce the risk of developing breast cancer among women at higher than average risk [2], and a low-fat diet was shown to reduce the likelihood of breast cancer recurrence [3]. These and other trials proved the principle that cancer can be prevented and provided support for the idea of a continuum between cancer prevention and cancer treatment.

Prevention and Risk

Some individuals without specific known risk factors for cancer are more focused on preventing cancer than on preventing other conditions, such as cardiovascular disease, for which their actual risk may be higher, or on maintaining their health and ability to enjoy life. The good news is that maintaining a heart-healthy lifestyle may also prevent cancer. For example, the impact of not smoking is greater on cardiovascular disease risk than on cancer risk.

Cancer prevention trials are generally conducted among individuals who are known to be at higher than average risk of developing cancer. The higher the cancer risk among the study subjects, the less person-time and cost required to observe the effects of the intervention, if any, and the greater the justification for exposing subjects to an intervention that may have adverse side effects. The risk reduction associated with a preventive intervention may not compensate for its effects on quality of life or its economic costs. For example, among women with a strong family history of breast cancer, prophylactic mastectomy has been shown to reduce breast cancer risk by 90% [4], and tamoxifen reduces risk by 50% [2]. But relatively few women, even with very high risk, have taken advantage of these options. Some are looking to CAM for less invasive and gentler alternatives.

Treatments that begin as CAM can become conventional, depending on research results and the ways in which both the therapy and the context for its use evolve. For example, green tea is now being studied for its chemopreventive potential [5]. Historically in many Asian cultures, green tea was an infusion prepared and sipped during important social interactions and considered part of the good life. Now, it is being studied as a pill or capsule that is swallowed quickly to prevent a disease. In the end, what we want to know is not whether a therapy is considered CAM or conventional but whether it is effective in preventing cancer.

This chapter discusses an integrated approach to cancer risk assessment and prevention therapeutics and provides an overview of conventional and CAM approaches commonly used in the United States.

Assessing Cancer Risk

A person's risk of developing cancer is based on several factors, including family medical history, genetic predisposition, and lifetime exposures. If a physician learns that a patient has a family history of cancer suggestive of genetic high risk, the patient may be referred to a genetic counselor who takes a detailed personal and family history and then makes a determination as to whether the individual should undergo DNA testing. Table 2.1 lists some mutations associated with cancer risk. Based on the risk assessment and possible genetic test results, individuals and their physicians can make joint decisions on what, if any, actions to take, including lifestyle modifications, increased screening, chemoprevention, and/or surgery [6]. The US National Cancer Institute (NCI) has regularly updated websites that explain the concept of risk to the public (http://understandingrisk.cancer.gov) and describe what is currently known about cancer causes and risk factors (http://www.cancer.gov/cancertopics/prevention-genetics-causes/causes).

New technologies are being developed and tested to provide biological assessments of cancer risk, including genetic profiles that determine how the body metabolizes endogenous and exogenous substances, that is, metabolomics and proteomics; thermography, which may detect areas of a breast that

Table 2.1. Examples of Genetic Testing for Inherited Cancer Syndromes.*

Cancer Syndrome	Gene(s)	Major Cancer Risks
Hereditary breast or ovarian cancer	*BRCA1, BRCA2*	Breast, ovarian
Li-Fraumeni syndrome	*P53*	Soft tissue sarcoma, osteosarcoma, breast, leukemia, adrenal cortex, brain
Cowden disease	*PTEN*	Breast, nonmedullary thyroid, endometrial
Multiple endocrine neoplasia type 2 (MEN2)	*RET*	Medullary thyroid
Familial adenomatous polyposis (FAP)	*APC, MYH*	Colorectal, other gastrointestinal
Hereditary nonpolyposis colon cancer (HNPCC)	*MLH1, MSH2, MSH6*	Colorectal, endometrial
Juvenile polyposis	*MADH4, BMPR1A*	Colorectal, other gastrointestinal
Peutz-Jeghers syndrome	*STK11*	Colorectal

* See GeneTests (www.genetests.org) for a comprehensive listing of currently available genetic tests.
Adapted from [7].

have increased metabolism; cytology sampling, such as ductal lavage and mammary aspiration for breast cancer; and blood-based biomarkers such as nuclear matrix proteins. The acceptance and uptake of new technologies for assessing cancer risk is generally based on results from clinical trial data, though there are no formal guidelines or governing bodies that regulate this area.

Some clinicians and laboratories offer alternative laboratory tests and in-office procedures that provide nonvalidated assessments of cancer risk. These may include urine analyses, blood analyses, genetic analyses, energy scans, electromagnetic scans, and so on. Many of these methods are based on epidemiological studies and/or theoretical assumptions, as opposed to clinical trials, and have not been validated as diagnostic of cancer risk. The tests are often co-marketed with neutraceutical products that will "correct" whatever imbalance is detected. Most of these tests and products have not been evaluated in cancer prevention clinical trials and their claims should be carefully scrutinized.

Cancer Prevention Modalities

Both conventional and CAM therapeutic modalities for primary cancer prevention involve lifestyle modifications, such as dietary changes, physical activity, behavioral modifications, and biological agents that may prevent or halt carcinogenesis. When considering any approach to cancer prevention, whether it be conventional, CAM, or integrative, it is important to determine the magnitude of expected benefit while accounting for safety, cost, and likelihood of adherence. Some prevention approaches are targeted to the population level, such as strengthening antismoking laws to prevent lung cancer. Other approaches are targeted to an individual, and have more predictably large effects, such as prophylactic mastectomy in a woman with a BRCA1 mutation. In addition, some cancer prevention strategies will also decrease the risk of other diseases, for example, increasing physical activity also decreases risk of cardiovascular disease.

It is important to acknowledge that it is often difficult to convince people to participate in cancer prevention interventions, whether conventional or CAM. Just because a conventional cancer prevention method is espoused by the conventional medical community, it is not necessarily widely in use or widely accepted by the general population. One of the biggest barriers to cancer prevention is convincing people that it is possible and beneficial to make changes in their lives, for example, quitting smoking. Sometimes, CAM approaches may be more appealing to individuals who are unwilling to tolerate some of the side effects of conventional therapies or who find that conventional therapies do not fit within their own personal or cultural system of beliefs and preferences.

CONVENTIONAL CANCER PREVENTION MODALITIES

Conventional recommendations on what people can do for cancer prevention are usually based on epidemiological and clinical trial evidence. These include dietary modifications, physical activity, behavioral modifications, biological agents, surgery, and vaccinations. Some of these cancer prevention approaches are believed to be important and safe enough to disseminate via public health messages and to make changes in public health policy, particularly pertaining to smoking cessation. Public smoking restrictions and tobacco taxation have both resulted in decreased smoking rates, even among youths [8]. Federal legislation has been proposed to reduce low-nutrition foods in public schools [9]. Grocery produce shoppers frequently see the "5 a day" message to encourage fruit and vegetable consumption [10]. New urban planning efforts and employer subsidies for health club memberships are beginning to promote increased opportunities for physical activity [11].

Diet and Physical Activity

It is generally accepted that high intake of fruits and vegetables is beneficial for cancer prevention [12]. The benefits are likely be due to the high concentrations of antioxidants, other phytonutrients, and fiber [12].

Cruciferous vegetables are one family of edible plants that may play a significant role in cancer prevention [13]. High intake of cruciferous vegetables, including broccoli, cauliflower, cabbage, kale, bok choy, Brussels sprouts, radish, and various mustards has been associated with decreased cancer risk. Crucifers have high content of glucosinolates and their hydrolysis products, isothiocyanates, protect against carcinogenesis. Crucifers also contain flavonoids, polyphenols, vitamins, fiber and pigments that may have anticancer activities. The most important chemoprevention mechanisms may be that crucifers inhibit phase I enzymes, for example, cytochrome P450s, which can activate carcinogen metabolites and they induce phase II enzymes, for example, glutathione transferase enzymes, which enhance carcinogen detoxification [13].

Epidemiological data has also suggested that a low-fat diet can help prevent cancer [12]; however, clinical trial data were lacking to support this. The recently published results from the WINS study showed that a low-fat diet was associated with a decreased breast cancer recurrence rate among women with hormone receptor-negative breast cancers [3]. Future clinical trials need to elucidate whether the type of fats consumed contributes to cancer risk.

It is generally accepted that maintaining a healthy body weight, which is defined as a body mass index (BMI) between 18 and 25 kg/m², can help prevent cancer. The mechanism here has not been fully elucidated but it is hypothesized that some of the endogenous hormones produced with increased body fat increase cancer risk. Maintaining a healthy body weight is best achieved by eating a balanced diet and engaging in regular physical activity.

There is also evidence to suggest that alcohol increases the risk of some cancers [12].

The American Institute of Cancer Research offers the following general diet and health guidelines [12]: (1) be as lean as possible within the normal range of body weight; (2) be physically active as part of everyday life; (3) limit consumption of energy-dense foods; avoid sugary drink; (4) eat mostly foods of plant origin; (5) limit intake of red meat and avoid processed meats; (6) limit alcoholic drinks; (7) limit consumption of salt; avoid mouldy cereals (grains) or pulse (legumes); (8) aim to meet nutritional needs through diet alone; (9) mothers to breastfeed; children to be breastfed; (10) cancer survivors to follow the recommendations for cancer prevention. See Table 2.2 for a cancer-site specific summary of risk factors and dietary and physical activity recommendations by the American Cancer Society.

Behavioral Modifications

A number of behavioral modifications beyond dietary and physical activity have been associated with decreased cancer risk. These include preventing tobacco use, ceasing tobacco use, decreasing sun exposure, and decreasing use of exogenous hormone therapy. Tobacco use, including smoking and chewing tobacco, has been strongly associated with cancers of the lung, lower urinary tract, upper aero-digestive tract, pancreas, stomach, liver, kidney, and uterine cervix, and causing myeloid leukemia [14]. Despite the fact that decreasing tobacco consumption by preventing initiation and promoting cessation would lead to preventing the largest numbers of cancers, this has been difficult to achieve and smoking rates are growing globally [15,16]. Regular sun exposure, especially at an early age, is associated with an increased risk of skin cancer. The regular use of sunblock and using sun-protective clothing have been associated with decreased risk of melanoma and nonmelanoma skin cancer [17]. The recently reported population level decrease in breast cancer incidence in 2003 is possibly associated with the decreased use of hormone replacement therapy after the results from the Women's Health Initiative were reported in 2002 [18];

Table 2.2. Cancer Site-Specific Risk Factors and Recommendations to Reduce Risk.

Cancer Site	Risk Factors	Strategies to Reduce Risk			
		Nutrition	Physical Activity	Body Size	Other
Bladder	Tobacco smoke Exposure to industrial chemicals	Drink more fluids Eat more vegetables			
Brain	No known nutritional risk factors				
Breast	First menstrual period before age 12 Not giving birth or first birth after age 30 Late age at menopause Family history of breast cancer Overweight or obese (among postmenopausal women) Weight gain during adulthood Alcohol consumption, especially if low folate intake Postmenopausal hormone replacement therapy	Eat a diet high in vegetables and fruits Lower fat intake greatly Avoid or limit intake of alcoholic beverages	Engage in moderate-to-vigorous physical activity 45 to 60 minutes per week	Avoid obesity Reduce lifetime weight gain through a combination of limiting your calories and regular physical activity	Limit the use of hormones, i.e., hormone replacement therapy

	Risk Factors	Dietary	Physical Activity	Weight	Other Prevention
Colorectal	Family history of colorectal cancer Long-term tobacco use Overweight or obese, especially obesity in men Lack of exercise and poor nutrition Diet high in processed and/or red meats Diet low in vegetables Excessive alcohol use	Eat a diet high in vegetables and fruits Limit intake of processed and red meats Avoid excess alcohol Calcium supplementation (men should limit to 1500 mg per day) Vitamin D supplementation	Moderate-to-vigorous physical activity	Avoid obesity	Finding and removing polyps through colorectal cancer screening Use of aspirin or other nonsteroidal anti-inflammatory drugs (NSAIDs) (currently not recommended because of potential side effects) Use of postmenopausal hormone replacement therapy (currently not recommended because of potential side effects)
Endometrium	Polycystic ovarian syndrome Overweight or obese Diet high in red meat, saturated fat, and animal fat Postmenopausal estrogen therapy Certain types of birth control pills	Eat a plant-based diet rich in vegetables, whole grains, and beans Decrease consumption of red meat, saturated fat, and animal fat	High physical activity	Maintain healthful weight through diet and regular physical activity	
Kidney	Tobacco smoke Overweight or obese			Avoid becoming overweight	Avoid tobacco use

(continued)

Table 2.2. (Continued)

Cancer Site	Risk Factors	Strategies to Reduce Risk			
		Nutrition	Physical Activity	Body Size	Other
Leukemias and Lymphomas	Obesity				
Lung	Tobacco smoke Chewing tobacco Snuff Radon exposure High doses of beta-carotene and/or vitamin A increased risk among smokers	Eat at least five servings of vegetables and fruits a day			Avoid tobacco use or exposure Avoid radon exposure
Oral and Esophageal	Tobacco (including cigarettes, chewing tobacco, and snuff) Alcohol A combination of tobacco and alcohol use Drinking very hot beverages Overweight or obese	Eat at least five servings of vegetables and fruits each day Restrict alcohol consumption		Avoid obesity	Avoid all forms of tobacco
Ovarian	Obesity No firmly established nutritional risks	Fruits and vegetables in the diet may lower risk Moderate alcohol consumption			

	Risk Factors	Diet	Physical Activity	Weight	Other
Pancreatic	Adult-onset diabetes Impaired glucose tolerance Tobacco smoke Obesity Physical inactivity Diets high in processed and red meats	Eat five or more servings of vegetables and fruits each day	Remain physically active	Maintain a healthful weight	Avoid tobacco use
Prostate	Overweight and obese Eating large amounts of red meat High intake of dairy products High calcium intake (primarily through supplements) increases risk for aggressive forms of prostate cancer	Eat five or more servings of vegetables and fruits each day, especially tomatoes, cruciferous vegetables, soy, beans and other legumes Eat foods and supplements containing antioxidant nutrients, such as vitamin E, selenium, beta-carotene, and lycopene Limit intake of red meat and dairy products	Vigorous exercise Active lifestyle	Maintain a healthy weight	
Stomach	Chronic stomach infections by bacterium Helicobacter pylori High intake of salt-preserved foods	Eat at least five servings of vegetables and fruits daily Reduce salt-preserved food consumption		Maintain a healthy weight	Eat fresh foods Refrigerate foods

Adapted from the American Cancer Society Prevention and Early Detection: The Complete Guide—Nutrition and Physical Activity [19,20].

however, this may also be due to a decrease in screening mammography. See Table 2.2 for a summary of behavior modification recommendations provided by the American Cancer Society.

Biologically Based Agents

Biological chemoprevention agents that can be taken as a drug in pill form are appealing because they are less laborious to administer and more easily standardized than lifestyle changes. Chemopreventive agents include vitamins, minerals, naturally occurring phytochemicals, and synthetic compounds. Currently, the most promising agents include biologicals that have antioxidant, hormone-modulating, or anti-inflammatory properties. Botanical agents have been shown to affect numerous molecular targets for chemoprevention, including protein kinases, antiapoptotic proteins, apoptotic proteins, growth factor pathways, transcription factors, cell cycle proteins, cell adhesion molecules, metastases, DNA methylation, and angiogenesis [21].

This is an active area of research involving pharmacological, biological, and nutritional interventions to prevent, reverse, or delay carcinogenesis. Currently, the only FDA-approved agents for cancer prevention are tamoxifen and raloxifene for breast cancer prevention among high-risk women [2,22]. However, the Division of Cancer Prevention of the US National Cancer Institute is actively pursuing new and novel compounds for cancer prevention. Some of these agents include NSAIDs, curcumin, indole-3-carbinol/DIM, deguelin, green tea (Polyphenon E), isoflavones in soy, lycopene, and resveratrol [5]. Many of these agents are used by CAM practitioners and some are discussed below under CAM therapies.

ANTIOXIDANTS Antioxidants include compounds such as vitamin E (α-tocopherol), vitamin C (ascorbic acid), β-carotene, selenium, and zinc. Many of these agents are found in foods and can also be taken as dietary supplements. Exogenous antioxidants ingested via foods or dietary supplements can quench procarcinogenic reactive oxygen species (ROS) and may halt carcinogenesis [23,24]. Many different kinds of exposures contribute to the carcinogenesis stages of initiation, promotion, and progression. An accumulation of reactive oxygen species may cause DNA mutations and cellular damage, which some authors suggest initiate most of carcinogenesis [23]. Reactive oxygen species can be byproducts of normal endogenous cellular metabolism; they may be produced during respiration, by neutrophils and macrophages during inflammation, or by mitochondria-catalyzed electron transport chain reactions [23,25]. Reactive oxygen species can also be produced by exogenous exposures, including nitrogen oxide pollutants, smoking, pharmaceuticals, and radiation. Reactive oxygen species cause oxidative stress, which can induce cancer-causing DNA mutations, damage cellular structures including lipids and membranes, oxidize proteins, and alter signal transduction pathways that enhance cancer risk [23,26,27].

Though this is a promising area of research, clinical trials that have used exogenous antioxidants or free-radical scavengers (such as vitamin E, vitamin C, or β-carotene) as chemopreventive agents have, on the whole, been markedly unsuccessful, and even harmful in some cases. Two trials testing β-carotene as a chemopreventive agent in male smokers and asbestos workers at high risk of developing lung cancer, the Alpha-Tocopherol, Beta-Carotene Cancer Prevention Trial (ATBC) and Carotene and Retinol Efficacy Trial (CARET) studies, showed that high doses of synthetic β-carotene actually increased risk of lung cancer [28,29]. It is unclear how to extrapolate these results to people of average risk using natural forms of the vitamins in low, normal, or high doses. The U.S. Preventive Services Task Force concluded that β-carotene supplementation is unlikely to provide important benefits and might cause harm in some groups [30]. A study of vitamin E supplementation for preventing second primary head and neck cancers showed that vitamin E supplementation was associated with increased risk of developing a second primary cancer and poorer survival [31]. In the Nutritional Prevention of Cancer Study, selenium supplementation did not decrease the incidence of basal cell or squamous cell skin cancer; however, secondary analyses suggested that selenium supplementation reduced the incidence of and mortality due to cancers in other sites, the most promising of which is prostate cancer prevention [32]. The Selenium and Vitamin E *Cancer* Prevention *Trial* (SELECT) for prostate cancer prevention is designed to test whether selenium and vitamin E supplementation can prevent prostate cancer [33] and another trial is testing the cancer prevention effect of selenium in men with high-grade prostatic intraepithelial neoplasia (PIN) [34].

MULTIVITAMIN AND MINERAL SUPPLEMENTS A recent synthesis of randomized, controlled trials assessed the efficacy of multivitamin and supplement use for cancer prevention [35]. The authors concluded that the evidence is currently insufficient to prove the presence or absence of benefits. However, two trials did show an effect. In poorly nourished Chinese living in Linxian, the combined supplementation of β-carotene, α-tocopherol, and selenium reduced gastric cancer incidence and mortality rates and reduced the overall mortality rate from cancer by 13% to 21% [36–38]. In the French Supplementation en Vitamines et Mineraux Antioxydants Study (SU.VI.MAX), combined supplementation of vitamin E, β-carotene, selenium, and zinc reduced the overall cancer rate by 31% in men, but not in women [39,40].

HORMONE MODULATORS Some cancers are hormone dependent, including hormone receptor–positive breast cancer, ovarian cancer, and prostate cancer.

Breast cancer prevention trials using selective estrogen receptor modulators (SERMs) to block estrogen receptors, Breast Cancer Prevention Trial (BCPT) and Study of Tamoxifen and Raloxifene (STAR), have been successful in decreasing breast cancer incidence in women at high breast cancer risk, though they had significant adverse effects including increased risks of endometrial cancer and osteoporosis [2,22]. Though the Women's Health Initiative study showed that estrogen plus progesterone therapy was protective against colon cancer, the increased risk of breast cancer and cardiovascular disease indicate that it is not an appropriate cancer prevention strategy [41]. The Prostate Cancer Prevention Trial (PCPT) tested the effects of finasteride, a 5-α-reductase inhibitor, on prostate cancer incidence and found that though it inhibited the formation of prostate cancer overall, it was associated with increased risk of high-grade prostate cancer and sexual side effects [42]. The ongoing Reduction by Dutasteride of Prostate Cancer Events (REDUCE) trial is testing the effects of dutasteride, a dual 5-α-reductase inhibitor, in men with an increased risk of developing prostate cancer [43]. In men with high-grade PIN, the SERM toremifene decreased the incidence of prostate cancer [44].

Vitamin D is involved in regulating bone metabolism. Vitamin D and its analogs have been receiving a considerable amount of attention for their possible antiproliferative roles in the prevention of cancer in many sites, including prostate, gastrointestinal, breast, endometrial, skin, and pancreatic cancers [45]. Clinical trials are underway to test these hypotheses.

ANTI-INFLAMMATORY AGENTS Observational studies have shown that non-steroidal anti-inflammatory drug (NSAID) use is associated with lower risk of breast and colon cancer occurrence [46,47]. Two clinical trials of COX-2 inhibitors, rofecoxib and celecoxib, to prevent colorectal cancer in high-risk individuals showed that they were effective; however, these drugs simultaneously increased risk of cardiovascular disease [48–50]. A recent risk:benefit analysis showed that in 1000 patients with colonic adenomas, celecoxib use would prevent 1.6 colorectal cancers but would cause 12.7 cardiovascular disease events [51]. Therefore, COX-2 inhibitors are not being recommended for cancer prevention.

Surgery

If an individual is considered to be at high risk for developing a specific cancer, he or she may be offered the option of surgically removing the organ or tissue. Women at high breast or ovarian cancer risk may have prophylactic mastectomies or oophorectomies. This approach is not without consequence, such as disfigurement and inability to conceive, and is not acceptable to many women [52,53]. Individuals with familial adenomatous polyposis or longstanding ulcerative colitis may choose to have colectomies, but morbidity, mortality, and quality of life issues should be considered [54].

Vaccinations

Vaccinations have also been successful in preventing some cancers. The hepatitis B vaccine has been shown to be effective in preventing chronic hepatitis, which often progresses to liver cancer [55]. More recently, the human papilloma virus (HPV) vaccine was shown to be effective at preventing HPV infection and precancerous lesions, which can cause cervical cancer [56]. The HPV vaccine is perhaps an unprecedented approach to cancer prevention in that it may be given to all sexually active females, regardless of their risk of cervical cancer. The feasibility and acceptability of implementing these strategies on a population-wide basis is under debate, especially in children [57]; however, the proof of principle has been established.

CAM CANCER PREVENTION THERAPEUTICS

As stated earlier, some conventional therapies used for cancer treatment, such as tamoxifen, are applied to high-risk individuals for cancer prevention. Likewise, many of the CAM therapies discussed elsewhere in this book that are used for cancer treatment are also used by cancer-free individuals for cancer prevention. The agents have varying levels of research evidence to support their use, and most of the evidence is from in vitro and animal studies, rather than clinical trials. Few clinical trials have been conducted in CAM cancer prevention; thus the use of these agents is primarily based on theoretical and hypothesized mechanisms. CAM cancer prevention therapeutics are presented in the following section under two broad categories: those that are biological agents and those that are behavior based.

BIOLOGICAL AGENTS

A wide variety of CAM biological agents have possible applications for cancer prevention. These include special diets, botanicals (also called herbs), vitamins, minerals, and other dietary supplements.

Special Diets

To date, an abundance of data is available to suggest that people who have high intake of fruits and vegetables are less likely to develop cancer than those with low intake [12]. The data are less clear regarding which specific vegetables should be consumed, during what phase of life, and for how long. Data on specific dietary patterns that are not considered CAM, such as the Mediterranean diet or eating a low-fat diet, suggest that eating in a specific pattern on a regular basis can have cancer prevention effects [12]. One dietary pattern that is gaining in popularity and that may be on the cusp between conventional medicine and CAM is a "whole foods" diet. A whole foods diet is one that emphasizes eating foods, especially grains, fruits, and vegetables, which are as close to their natural form as possible in order to benefit from the phytonutrients and fiber present, while avoiding additives that are in processed foods. However, it appears that only a small number of individuals have the inclination or ability to fully adopt this way of eating and preparing foods.

Other dietary patterns may be considered "CAM" because they are not followed by large numbers of individuals and are considered more out of the mainstream. These include vegan, raw foods, and macrobiotic diets. Vegan refers to not eating any animal products, usually for ethical and health reasons. A raw foods diet takes this one step further by eating a vegan diet and limiting the use of heat in order to preserve the naturally occurring plant enzymes and proteins and to prevent the formation of carcinogens, which occurs with heating proteins and carbohydrates [58]. A macrobiotic diet emphasizes locally grown, organically grown whole-grain cereals, legumes, vegetables, fruit, seaweed, and fermented soy products, combined into meals according to the principle of balance between yin and yang properties [59]. Although the epidemiological and clinical trial literature is sparse, the data suggest that adopting diets that promote increased fruit and vegetable consumption leads to commensurate reduction in fat and calorie intake, both of which have separately been associated with decreased cancer risk [12,60].

A diet which restricts caloric intake, also known as a hypocaloric diet, is hypothesized to reduce the occurrence of chronic disease, including cancer [61]. However, most of this evidence is based on animal studies and recent human data suggest that short-term caloric restriction may increase incidence of some cancers [62].

Some methods of producing and preparing food are hypothesized to prevent cancer by reducing exposure to carcinogens. This includes eating organically grown food to avoid pesticides and not cooking with or storing food in plastics to avoid chemicals that may leach into food.

Botanicals

Many plants contain phytochemicals that have potential anticancer proper-ties, including antioxidant, anti-inflammatory, immune modulation, modu-lation of detoxification enzymes, hormone modulation, and adaptogenic effects. Historically, these botanicals have often been used as foods, spices, and medicines [63]. Few of the agents have undergone phase III trials to demonstrate efficacy for cancer prevention; therefore, the data are insuffi-cient to derive specific recommendations on formulations, doses, and dura-tion of use.

ANTIOXIDANTS Most plants contain some form of antioxidants, typically found in their pigments and/or chemical defensive agents that are used to deter predators. As already stated, antioxidants are hypothesized to be beneficial for cancer prevention because they may prevent the formation of free radi-cals, which can lead to DNA damage and they may repair oxidative damage. Botanical compounds have been identified, which contain particularly high levels of antioxidants including curcumin in turmeric (*Curcuma longa*) [64], epigallocatechin-3-gallate (EGCG) in green tea (*Camellia sinensis*) [13,65], resveratrol in red grapes, peanuts, and berries [66], silymarin in milk thistle (*Silybum marianum*) [21], 6-gingerol in ginger (*Zingiber officinale*) [13,67], lycopene in tomatoes [12,68], and polyphenols in pomegranate juice [69].

ANTI-INFLAMMATORY AGENTS As stated earlier, inflammatory agents in the body, such as prostaglandins, are potentially carcinogenic. A number of botani-cal agents are known to have substantial anti-inflammatory effects by inhibiting cyclooxygenase (COX) or other part of the inflammation pathway. Curcumin [13,70,71] and ginger [12,67,72] are two of the most potent anti-inflammatory botanical agents. Preliminary in vitro and case report data suggest interesting anti-inflammatory effects of a combination herbal anti-inflammatory agent, Zyflamend®, on prostate cancer cells and in men with high-grade prostatic intraepithelial neoplasia (PIN) (without prostate cancer) [73,74].

IMMUNE FUNCTION MODULATORS A well-functioning immune system is hypothesized to be beneficial for cancer prevention because circulating immune cells can destroy nascent cancer cells. Some of the botanicals that have been identified for their effects on improving immune function include medicinal mushrooms, astragalus (*Astragalus membranaceus*), and ginseng (*Panax gin-seng*). Several varieties of immune-modulating mushrooms have been identi-fied, including *Ganoderma lucidum* (Reishi), *Coriolus versicolor*, and maitake

(*Grifola frondosa*) [75,76]. Astragalus, frequently used in Chinese medicine, is not as well studied but historically has been shown to improve immune function [77]. *Panax ginseng* has also demonstrated immune system–enhancing effects [77,78].

BIOTRANSFORMATION ENZYME MODULATORS Biotransformation enzymes modulate the effects of chemical carcinogens. Compounds in various botanical agents have been shown to induce or inhibit enzymes related to cancer risk. As discussed earlier, cruciferous vegetables can inhibit phase I enzymes and induce phase II enzymes. Indole-3-carbinol is a compound found in cruciferous vegetables. It has been shown to upregulate hepatic enzyme systems that metabolize endogenous carcinogens. Early-phase human trials have shown that it may have some applicability in lung, cervical, and breast cancer; however, liver toxicities may prevent its widespread use [79]. Curcumin has been shown to inhibit phase I enzymes and induce phase II enzymes, such as glutathione-S-transferase [80].

HORMONE REGULATORS Given that some cancers are hormone dependent, for example, some forms of breast cancer, ovarian cancer, prostate, and testicular cancer, botanicals that modulate endogenous hormone levels may be indicated for cancer prevention. There has been ongoing debate on the role of soy products in cancer prevention. Isoflavones are found in leguminous plants, such as soy. The most active isoflavones are diaidzein and genistein, both of which have been shown to possess both estrogenic and antiestrogenic activities. The current consensus is that there is insufficient evidence to recommend soy isoflavones as a cancer prevention tactic and therefore soy should be eaten in moderation [81].

Animal and observational data suggest that green tea consumption may lower blood estrogen levels, thus lowering breast cancer risk, while limited data suggest that black tea may increase breast cancer risk [82].

ADAPTOGENS Adaptogens are botanicals used to stimulate the central nervous system to decrease stress, decrease depression, eliminate fatigue, and enhance work performance. This may be of importance in psychoneuroimmunological models of cancer, which hypothesize that a positive neurological state leads to a well-functioning immune system. Botanicals used for this purpose include *Panax ginseng*, Siberian ginseng (*Eleutherococcos senticosus*), schisandra (*Schisandra chinensis*), and rhodiola (*Rhodiola rosea*) [78,83–85]. However, there is conflicting evidence whether *Panax ginseng* and rhodiola exert estrogenic effects, which would contraindicate their use in estrogen-dependent cancers [86–88].

COMBINATION FORMULAS Historically, botanical preparations have been used in combination to make use of synergistic properties between individual botanical agents. Traditional Chinese Medicine (TCM), Ayurvedic and Western botanical formulations operate on this principle. Two Western botanical formulations, Essiac tea and Hoxsey formula, have made claims to prevent and treat cancer. However, to date these claims have not been supported with scientific evidence [89,90].

Vitamins and Minerals

As discussed earlier, epidemiological studies suggest that vitamin and mineral intake can affect risk of developing specific cancers. Some people have interpreted this as evidence to support the use of mega doses of these agents. Taking doses of antioxidants, vitamins, and minerals above that which is found in a standard multivitamin may be considered CAM. Orthomolecular medicine, coined by Linus Pauling, PhD, refers to the practice of preventing and treating disease by providing the body with optimal amounts of substances which are natural to the body, which often results in the use of high doses of natural compounds [91]. Given the results from the ATBC and CARET trials discussed earlier, it is unclear how efficacious this high-dose approach may be. These studies were in high-risk populations and used high doses of synthetic forms of the vitamins. Coenzyme Q10 is a potent antioxidant but has limited clinical data to support its use specifically for cancer prevention [92].

Other Dietary Supplements

Other dietary supplements have been proposed as possible cancer prevention therapies. Some of the more promising dietary supplements include melatonin, omega-3 fatty acids, probiotics, and prebiotics.

Changes in circadian rhythm due to night shift work or increased ambient light dysregulates melatonin levels. Melatonin supplementation is hypothesized to have oncostatic, cytotoxic, and antiproliferative effects [93].

Omega-3 fatty acids, such as eicosapentaenoic acid (EPA) and docosahexaenoic acid (DHA) have several proposed mechanisms for lowering cancer risk. The most studied mechanism is inhibiting the formation of proinflammatory and procarcinogenic eicosanoids, such as prostaglandins [94,95].

Pro- and prebiotics may have chemopreventive roles in gastrointestinal cancer. Probiotics, such as *Lactobacillus sp.*, are hypothesized to confer chemopreventive benefits in gastrointestinal cancers by deactivating procarcinogenic cellular components of microorganisms, inhibiting and/or inducing colonic enzymes, controlling growth of harmful bacteria, stimulating the immune system, and producing physiologically active anticancer metabolites [96–98]. Prebiotics are short-chain carbohydrates, such as undigested polysaccharides, resistant starches and fiber, enhance the formation of beneficial bacteria and of short-chain fatty acids that can reduce oxidative stress and induce the chemo-preventive enzyme glutathione transferase [97,98].

BEHAVIORAL APPROACHES

One of the most basic differences between conventional and CAM approaches to cancer prevention is that a CAM approach often encourages people to do things beyond ingesting biological agents in order to reduce risk of developing cancer. These activities can be referred to as "mind-body" and "energy" medicine. Similar to many of the biological agents, these are lacking clinical trials to demonstrate efficacy, and are based on theoretical and hypothesized mechanisms.

Mind-Body Medicine

Available evidence links stress, behavioral response patterns and resultant neurohormonal and neurotransmitter changes to cancer development and progression [99]. Collectively this work suggests that stress management may modify neuroendocrine deregulation and immunological functions that potentially have implications for tumor initiation and progression [99]. Clinical studies indicate that stress, chronic depression, social support, and other psychological factors may influence cancer onset and progression [99]. This area of medicine is often called *mind-body medicine*, or *psychoneuro-immunology*.

There are a wide variety of types of therapies that fall under the rubric of mind-body medicine [99]. Sensory therapies include aromatherapy, massage, touch therapy, music therapy, and creating a calm and/or beautiful space such as a room with a view or a healing garden. Cognitive therapies include meditation, Mindfulness-Based Stress Reduction (MBSR), guided imagery, visualization, hypnosis, and humor therapy. Expressive therapies include writing, journaling, art therapy, support groups, individual counseling, and psychotherapy. Physical therapies include dancing, yoga, and tai chi. Though none of these approaches have been shown to prevent cancer per se, some of them have been shown to affect parameters associated with cancer development, such as improving immune function and decreasing circulating cortisol. It is of note that an early study showed that support groups increased survival in breast cancer patients [100]. However, these results have not been replicated and there is no evidence to date supporting the use of psychological interventions to prevent cancer [101].

Energy Medicine

Energy medicine refers to practices that use nonmaterial stimuli for the purposes of healing [102]. These stimuli may be via artificially generated electromagnetic fields, such as pulsed electromagnetic field therapy, or via human generated energies, such as reiki, Qigong, and healing touch. The hypothesized mechanism of action is that the applied energy causes a change in the human biomagnetic energy field which can affect a biochemical response in the body. In terms of cancer prevention, many of these energy medicines theorize that an early correction of stagnation or imbalances in energy patterns may lead to the prevention of cancer [103]. These theories are based on the concept that flows of energy or essence patterns in the body are dynamically balanced and must not be blocked. If blockages do occur, diseases can develop, including cancer. Energy medicine systems attempt to relieve these blockages via methods such as acupuncture, Reiki healing sessions, and qigong exercises. Some human studies have shown an effect of these energy therapies on parameters related to cancer incidence including increasing secretary immunoglobulin A [104], enhancing immune system response [105], and reducing stress [106]. A study in mice has shown a decrease in the growth of induced lymphoma via external Qigong [107].

Other Systems of Healing and Health

All cultures have systems to promote health and healing, many of which are highly developed and very different from the conventional medical model accepted in Western societies. The conventional medical model tends to be best at responding to and treating disease, and relatively ineffective at preventing disease. The goal of many of these other systems of healing is to promote health and wellness, thereby preventing disease. Some of these other systems include TCM, Ayurvedic medicine, Tibetan medicine, and Native American medicine. Each of these is briefly discussed in the following sections. It is important to note that though each tradition is a rich, complete system unto itself, practitioners within each tradition may be diverse in terms of their interpretations, approaches and therapeutics for preventing, diagnosing, and treating disease. The descriptions provided here are very basic. Even for clinicians practicing within the Western medical tradition, having a familiarity with other systems of healing and health may be a critical skill [108].

TRADITIONAL CHINESE MEDICINE

TCM is a medical system from China. TCM therapeutics aim to restore the body's balance and harmony between the natural opposing forces of yin and yang and the five elements (wood, earth, air, fire, water). An imbalance between any of these forces can block Qi, blood or phlegm which can result in disease, including cancer. Diagnostic techniques include tongue and pulse diagnosis. TCM therapeutic modalities include acupuncture, botanical formulations, Qigong, tui na (massage), moxibustion, and dietary modification [109]. TCM was popularized in the United States in the 1970s after the fall of the "bamboo curtain" [109]. Another form of Chinese medicine, Five Element acupuncture, focuses on the use of acupuncture to restore mental and spiritual balance [110].

AYURVEDIC MEDICINE

Ayurvedic medicine, Ayurveda, or "the science of life," comes from India. A central concept to Ayurveda is that the three doshas, or body constitutions, Kapha, Pitta and Vata, need to be kept in balance to maintain health. An imbalance results in disease, including cancer. Causative factors for these imbalances include eating unhealthy foods, poor hygiene, bad lifestyle habits and environmental exposures, which, if left uncorrected, lead to the accumulation of one or more doshas somewhere in the body [111]. Diagnostic techniques involve tongue and pulse diagnosis. Ayurvedic therapeutic modalities include dietary modifications, botanical formulations, massage, precious substances, yoga, and spiritual practice [112]. Ayurveda was popularized in the United States in the 1990s by Depak Chopra [113].

TIBETAN MEDICINE

Tibetan medicine comes from Tibet, and is based on Buddhist teachings. Here, the three humors, bile, phlegm and wind need to be kept in balance. Cancer is caused by an imbalance in one, two, or all three of the humors. In addition, cancer can arise due to contaminants that have been introduced into the atmosphere and the environment. Diagnostic techniques include examination of the tongue, pulse, and urine. Therapeutic modalities include diet therapy, botanical formulations, physical activity, precious metals, and meditation [114].

NATIVE AMERICAN MEDICINE

Each indigenous tribe in the Americas has a unique healing tradition and there is not a definition that can describe a single Native American medicine [103]. However, there are some common themes in these traditions. In Native American medicine, there is not a differentiation between medicine and religion. To heal, one must acknowledge an "Inner Healer." Many tribes teach that spirit is indivisible from mind and body and that a healthy balance, harmony and connection with spirit is vital for disease prevention [103]. Illness results when there is imbalance or disharmony and wellness occurs when balance is restored [115]. Ceremony is intrinsic to creating and maintaining harmony. It is important to note that cancer can also be caused by disturbing the sacred nature of the land [115].

Common to healing systems such as TCM, Ayurveda, Tibetan medicine, and Native American medicine is the recognition of a balance between an individual, their community, and their environment. Any disturbance in one of these areas can lead to disease, including cancer. Perhaps what we can learn from these systems of health and healing is that it behooves us to conceptualize a holistic approach to cancer prevention which incorporates body, mind, spirit, and environment.

A Vision for Future Clinical Services

Currently, in the United States there are few truly integrated medical centers providing cancer prevention care. Some cancer centers are beginning to offer risk assessment services; however, they are limited to genetic screening and medical history risk and do not have well-developed programs on prevention tactics. Two main factors that have limited the widespread provision of these services include a lack of research on efficacy of many cancer prevention approaches, and poor, if any, physician reimbursement for prevention care. In addition, patients are not reimbursed or rewarded for time and resources spent at being proactive about disease prevention. Unfortunately, all of these factors may make it confusing for individuals using conventional or CAM modalities for general health maintenance and for cancer prevention because they are without clear guidance.

In the future, it is possible that people will be able to visit specialized clinics to receive comprehensive assessments of their personal risk of developing cancer. These risk assessments will take into account the results of screening tests, personal disease history, family disease history, genetic tests, prior environmental exposures, dietary history, exercise history, and socio-economic status. New tools will be available to assess stress, immune function, and genetic risk including an individual's ability to metabolize various substances. Once this assessment is made, people will be offered and counseled on interventions to counter their risk, including pharmaceuticals, natural compounds, dietary changes, exercise programs, and mind-body interventions. The clinics will be staffed by people with varying areas of expertise, including genetics, medical oncology, radiation oncology, health psychology, nutrition, exercise, mind-body medicine, botanical medicine, and functional medicine.

Future Research Directions

Each of the cancer prevention approaches described would benefit from further investigation. Many of these approaches are promising, but few have enough evidence to promote large-scale implementation. The gold standard for determining whether a cancer prevention approach is effective is to use cancer incidence as the endpoint in large, randomized, phase III studies. Because these trials are expensive and can be difficult to implement, early-phase trials using intermediate or surrogate markers for predicting cancer occurrence may be warranted. These endpoints include clinical, histological, biochemical, and molecular biomarkers that can demonstrate responses to chemoprevention agents, behaviors, or healing modalities [116]. These studies will need to carefully screen potentially therapeutic strategies to identify which have the most promise, which target populations will benefit the most, and what the appropriate endpoints will be.

Most CAM practitioners are trained to tailor their therapies to an individual. Increasingly, conventional medical practitioners and researchers are acknowledging the benefit of individualizing health care delivery. This approach will be especially beneficial in the area of cancer prevention where it may be difficult to implement and sustain preventive measures in large numbers of individuals. Assuming that additional effective cancer prevention modalities will be identified in the future, individuals will be asked to regularly ingest substances, change their behaviors, and/or receive vaccinations. It will be important to tailor these recommendations to an individual to make them as effective and as acceptable as possible.

Conclusion

Cancer prevention is just one aspect of optimizing health. Average-risk individuals want to know what they can do to decrease their risk of developing any disease. Individuals at high cancer risk want to know their options for decreasing their specific cancer risk. Ideally, in the future people will have access to cancer prevention centers that offer an integrated team of clinicians to coordinate medical and lifestyle recommendations, with a focus on staying well, rather than on treating disease. Ideally, some of the CAM modalities that are proven efficacious for disease prevention and/or enhancing a sense of well-being will be offered at these centers. To be sustainable, this will need to be done in the context of a medical system that invests in prevention and pays and reimburses for prevention work.

In the meantime, we can consider advocating lifestyle changes that may prevent cancer initiation and/or progression, while simultaneously helping individuals increase their sense of wellness. We can eat a diet rich in fruits, vegetables and whole grains, stay physically active, maintain a BMI of less than 25, and keep stress at bay, possibly using one of the mind-body techniques described earlier. We can know our risk of developing cancer based on age, gender, family history, and exposures and be screened appropriately. Finally, we can live a full life, keeping in mind traditional systems of medicine that promote balance between body, mind, spirit and environment.

REFERENCES

1. Alberts DS & Hess LM. (2005). (Eds.). *Fundamentals of Cancer Prevention*. New York: Springer.
2. Fisher B, Costantino JP, Wickerham DL, Redmond CK, Kavanah M, Cronin WM, et al. (1998). Tamoxifen for prevention of breast cancer: Report of the National Surgical Adjuvant Breast and Bowel Project P-1 Study. *Journal of the National Cancer Institute*, 90, 1371–1388.
3. Chlebowski RT, Blackburn GL, Thomson CA, Nixon DW, Shapiro A, Hoy M, et al. (2006). Dietary fat reduction and breast cancer outcome: Interim efficacy results from the Women's Intervention Nutrition Study. *Journal of the National Cancer Institute*, 98, 1767–1776.
4. Hartmann LC, Schaid DJ, Woods JE, Crotty TP, Myers JL, Arnold PG, et al. (1999). Efficacy of bilateral prophylactic mastectomy in women with a family history of breast cancer. *The New England Journal of Medicine*, 340, 77–84.

5. Crowell JA. (2005). The chemopreventive agent development research program in the Division of Cancer Prevention of the US National Cancer Institute: An overview. *European Journal of Cancer*, 41, 1889–1910.

7. Burke W & Press N. (2006). Genetics as a tool to improve cancer outcomes: Ethics and policy. *Nature Reviews. Cancer*, 6, 476–482.

12. World Cancer Research Fund/American Institute for Cancer Research. (2007) *Food, Nutrition and the Prevention of Cancer: A global perspective.* Washington DC: American Institute for Cancer Research.

19. Kushi LH, Byers T, Doyle C, Bandera EV, McCullough M, Gansler T, et al. (2006). American Cancer Society Guidelines on Nutrition and Physical Activity for cancer prevention: Reducing the risk of cancer with healthy food choices and physical activity. CA Cancer *The Clinical Journal*, 56, 254–281; quiz 313–4.

20. American Cancer Society. (2006). *The Complete Guide—Nutrition and Physical Activity.*

100. Larkey LK, Greenlee H, & Mehl-Madrona LE. (2005). Complementary and alternative approaches to cancer prevention. *In:* DS Alberts & LM Hess (Eds.), *Fundamentals of Cancer Prevention.* New York: Springer.

(A complete reference list for this chapter is available online at http://www.oup.com/us/integrativemedicine).

3

Molecular Targets of Botanicals Used for Chemoprevention

MURIEL CUENDET AND JOHN M. PEZZUTO

KEY CONCEPTS

- The treatment of many diseases is dependent on natural products, and this is especially true for the treatment of cancer.
- Chemoprevention is the use of synthetic or natural agents to inhibit, retard, or reverse carcinogenesis, or prevent the development of invasive cancer.
- Dietary consumption of foods and herbal medicines is a convenient method of administrating potentially beneficial phytochemicals in a cost-effective manner.
- Extracts of plant or marine organisms can be evaluated for potential chemopreventive activity using a battery of in vitro bioassays developed to monitor inhibition of tumorigenesis at various stages.
- Resveratrol, curcumin, cruciferous vegetables, green tea, *Allium* vegetables, and tomatoes have shown cancer chemopreventive activities.
- Only a few compounds have been approved by the U.S. Food and Drug Administration (FDA) for use as chemopreventive agents.

The treatment of many diseases is highly dependent on natural products, and this is especially true for the treatment of cancer (Cragg, Newman, & Snader, 1997; Pezzuto, 1997). Several potent drugs have been isolated from plants. The *Vinca* alkaloids isolated from the Madagascar periwinkle, *Catharanthus roseus* G. Don, comprise a group of about 130 terpenoid indole alkaloids (Svoboda & Barnes, 1964). Their clinical value was clearly identified as early as 1965 and so this class of compounds has been used as anticancer agents for over 40 years and represent a true lead compound for drug development (Johnson, Armstrong, Gorman, & Burnett, 1963). Today, two natural compounds, vinblastine and vincristine, and two semisynthetic derivatives, vindesine and vinorelbine, have been registered. The antineoplastic activity of the *Vinca* alkaloids is usually attributed to disruption of microtubules, resulting in dissolution of mitotic spindles and metaphase arrest in dividing cells (Bruchovsky, Owen, Becker, & Till, 1965; George, Journey, & Goldstein, 1965; Krishan, 1968; Malawista, Sato, & Bensch, 1968; Lengsfeld, Schultze, & Maurer, 1981).

Over 60% of the approved drugs developed as anticancer or anti-infective agents are of natural origin.

In 1971, Wani et al. discovered the highly potent anticancer agent paclitaxel (Wani, Taylor, Wall, Coggon, & McPhail, 1971), which occurs widely in plants of *Taxus* species. Paclitaxel and an analog, docetaxel, are currently regarded as very useful anticancer chemotherapeutic agents. Among antineoplastic drugs that interfere with microtubules, paclitaxel exhibits a unique mechanism of action (Schiff, Fant, & Horwitz, 1979; Kumar, 1981; Thompson, Wilson, & Purich, 1981; Manfredi & Horwitz, 1984). Paclitaxel promotes assembly of microtubules by shifting the equilibrium between soluble tubulin and microtubules toward assembly, reducing the critical concentration of tubulin required for assembly. The result is stabilization of microtubules, which is damaging to cells because of the perturbation in the dynamics of various microtubule-dependent cytoplasmic structures that are required for such functions as mitosis, maintenance of cellular morphology, shape changes, neurite formation, locomotion, and secretion (Baum et al., 1981; Letourneau & Ressler, 1984; Roytta, Laine, & Harkonen, 1987; Rowinsky, Donehower, Jones, & Tucker, 1988).

Work on *Taxus brevifolia* leading to the discovery of paclitaxel (Taxol) started in 1962; Taxol did not reach the market until 1992.

In the early 1960s, the discovery of camptothecin (CPT) by Wall and Wani as an anticancer drug added an entirely new dimension to the field of chemotherapy (Wall, Wani, Cook, Palmer, McPhail, & Sim, 1966; Wall, 1998). CPT was first isolated from the Chinese ornamental tree *Camptotheca acuminate* Decne, also known as the "tree of joy" and "tree of love." Preliminary studies revealed a substantial antitumor activity in standard in vitro test system as well as in mouse leukemia cells. Interest in CPT and analogs remained at a low ebb until 1985 when it was discovered that CPT, by a unique mechanism, inhibited the enzyme topoisomerase I (Hsiang, Hertzberg, Hecht, & Liu, 1985; Redinbo, Stewart, Kuhn, Champoux, & Hol, 1998; Staker, Hjerrild, Feese, Behnke, Burgin, & Stewart, 2002). Topoisomerase I involves the transient single-strand cleavage of duplex DNA, followed by unwinding and relegation. These actions facilitate essential cellular processes such as DNA replication, recombination, and transcription (Gupta, Fujimori, & Pommier, 1995).

Cancer, however, is considered the end stage of a chronic disease process characterized by abnormal cell and tissue differentiation (Sporn & Suh, 2000). This process of carcinogenesis eventually leads to the final outcome of invasive and metastatic cancer. Recent advances in defining cellular and molecular levels of carcinogenesis, along with a growing body of experimental, epidemiological, and clinical trial data, have led to the development of cancer chemoprevention, a relatively new strategy in preventing cancer (Sporn, Dunlop, Newton, & Smith, 1976; Wattenberg, 1985). Cancer chemoprevention is defined as the use of synthetic or natural agents to inhibit, retard, or reverse carcinogenesis, or prevent the development of invasive cancer (Sporn, Dunlop, Newton, & Smith, 1976; Wattenberg, 1985; Kelloff, Sigman, & Greenwald, 1999).

Most human cancers seem to be potentially preventable because of controllable or removable causative exogenous factors, such as cigarette smoking, dietary factors, environmental and occupational chemicals, lifestyle and socioeconomic factors, radiation, and specific microorganisms (Greenwald, Kelloff, Burch-Whitman, & Kramer, 1995). These exogenous factors offer the most likely opportunities for interventions targeted to primary prevention—that is, elimination of or avoiding exposure to these factors (Fig. 3.1) (Surh, 1999). In addition, however, as a serious and practical approach to the control of cancer, cancer chemoprevention can play an integral role in the overall strategy geared toward reducing the incidence of cancer (Wattenberg, 1985; Sporn & Suh, 2000). Rational and successful implementation of chemopreventive strategies

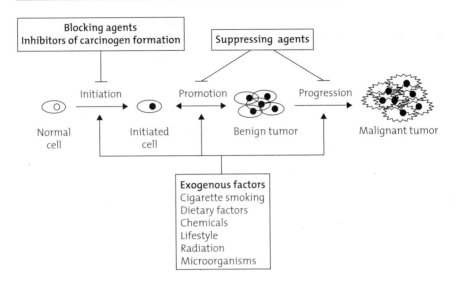

FIGURE 3.1. Schematic representation of multistage (initiation, promotion, progression) carcinogenesis. Exogenous factors act as tumor initiators, tumor promoters, or as complete carcinogens. These exogenous factors offer opportunities for intervention targeted to primary prevention. In addition, chemopreventive agents can play an integral role in the overall strategy geared toward reducing the incidence of cancer.

relies intrinsically on tests for efficacy and mechanistic assays, as well as availability of promising chemopreventive agents, reliable intermediate biomarkers, and appropriate clinical cohorts to discover safe and effective drugs for primary and secondary prevention of human cancers (Kelloff, et al., 1996). Dietary consumption of foods and herbal medicines is a convenient method of administrating potentially beneficial phytochemicals in a cost-effective manner.

Discovery of New Chemopreventive Agents from Natural Sources

In 1991, we instituted a multidisciplinary project supported by NCI wherein plant and (more recently) marine organism materials procured from throughout the world are used for activity-guided fractionation schemes that yield novel and otherwise unpredictable chemical entities with cancer chemoprevention activities. The overall aspects of this program have been summarized previously (Jensen & Fenical, 1994; Kinghorn, et al., 1998; Pezzuto, et al., 1999). Crude nonpolar and polar extracts, prepared from each plant or marine organism obtained, are evaluated for their potential chemopreventive activity using a battery of short-term in vitro bioassays developed to monitor inhibition of tumorigenesis at various stages (Fig. 3.1) (Pezzuto, Angerhofer, & Mehdi, 1998). For initiation, induction of NAD(P)H:quinone reductase (QR) activity (Song, et al., 1999), and antioxidant activity (Chung, et al., 1999) are assayed. For promotion, inhibition of activities such as cyclooxygenase (COX) activity (Cuendet & Pezzuto, 2000) and phorbol ester–induced ornithine decarboxylase (ODC) activity (Gerhauser, et al., 1997) are assayed. For progression, inhibition of aromatase activity (Jeong, Shin, Kim, & Pezzuto, 1999) and induction of human leukemia cell differentiation (Mata-Greenwood et al., 2001) are assayed. Over 20,000 tests have been performed, and the number of plants or marine organisms characterized as "active" is in the range of 5% of the total. In general, these "active" plant or marine organism extracts are tested in a secondary model of greater physiological complexity, such as the mouse mammary organ culture (MMOC) model. In this assay, test materials are evaluated for their ability to inhibit 7,12-dimethylbenz(a)anthracene (DMBA)-induced preneoplastic lesions (Mehta, Hawthorne, & Steele, 1997). Active leads in the secondary model are subjected to bioassay-guided fractionation using an in vitro system as a monitor to uncover their active principles. Active isolates are considered for evaluation in full-term animal studies, including the two-stage mouse skin model using DMBA as an initiator and 12-O-tetradecanoylphorbol-13-acetate (TPA) as a promoter, and the rat mammary carcinogenesis model with N-methyl-N-nitrosourea (MNU) or DMBA as a carcinogen (Jang, et al., 1997; Udeani, et al., 1997). Additional in vivo models are used as required. At present, isoliquiritigenin (QR inducer) (Cuendet, Oteham, Moon, & Pezzuto, 2006), abyssinone II (aromatase inhibitor) (Lee, Bhat, Fong, Farnsworth, Pezzuto, & Kinghorn, 2001), zapotin (HL-60 cell differentiation) (Mata-Greenwood et al., 2001), brusatol (HL-60 cell differentiation) (Luyengi, Suh, Fong, Pezzuto, & Kinghorn, 1996), and resveratrol (Bhat & Pezzuto, 2002) are undergoing further investigation in animal studies as lead compounds. Clinical trials are anticipated in due course.

Phase II Enzyme Induction

Carcinogenesis is a complex multistage process, yet the entire course can be initiated by a single event wherein a cellular macromolecule is damaged by an endogenous or exogenous agent.

Strategies for protecting cells from these initiating events include decreasing metabolic enzymes responsible for generating reactive species (phase I enzymes) while increasing phase II enzymes that can deactivate radicals and electrophiles known to intercede in normal cellular processes. Important defenses against electrophile toxicity are provided in the family of phase II enzymes, such as glutathione S-transferase (GST) and QR. Although phase I induction and functionalization of xenobiotics may be required for complete detoxification by the action of phase II enzymes, phase I enzyme elevation may also be considered a potential cancer risk factor for activation of procarcinogens to reactive species (Yang, Smith, & Hong, 1994). Therefore, an agent that induces phase II enzymes selectively would theoretically appear to be a better protector than selective induction of both phase I and II enzymes. QR elevation with in vitro and in vivo systems has been shown to correlate with induction of other protective phase II enzymes and provides a reasonable biomarker for the potential chemoprotective effect of test agents against cancer initiation (Talalay, 1992). In searching for novel cancer chemopreventive agents, we have utilized a rapid, sensitive QR assay to identify potential detoxification enzyme inducers (Talalay, Fahey, Holtzclaw, Prestera, & Zhang, 1995).

One of the most effective inducers of phase II enzymes is sulforaphane; high concentrations are found in broccoli sprouts.

Antioxidant Activity

Since reactive oxygen radicals play an important role in carcinogenesis and are involved in both initiation and promotion, antioxidants present in consumable fruits, vegetables, and beverages have received considerable attention as cancer chemopreventive agents (Mukhtar, Katiyar, & Agarwal, 1994).

Many antioxidants can also function as pro-oxidants. Paradoxically, pro-oxidants can have beneficial effects.

Several assay systems have been developed to discover potentially active compounds from synthetic and natural sources (Lee, Mbwambo, & Chung, 1998). It is important to note that a potential antioxidant lead must be evaluated in more than one antioxidant assay because of variability in the different test systems (Schlesier, Harwat, Bohm, & Bitsch, 2002). The presence of antioxidants in extracts has been assessed by determining scavenging activity with stable DPPH free radicals (Fujita, Uehara, Morimoto, Nakashima, Hatano, & Okuda, 1988), inhibition of TPA-induced free radical formation with cultured HL-60 cells (Sharma, Stutzman, Kelloff, & Steele, 1994), and inhibition of superoxide anion production in xanthine/xanthine oxidase systems (Sheu, Lai, & Chiang, 1998).

Cyclooxygenase Inhibition

Two COX isoforms, COX-1 and COX-2, are known. COX-1 is constitutively expressed in many tissues (Simmons, Xie, Chipman, & Evett, 1991; O'Neill & Ford-Hutchinson, 1993), and prostaglandins produced by COX-1 are thought to mediate "housekeeping" functions such as cytoprotection of the gastric mucosa, regulation of renal blood flow, and platelet aggregation (Merlie, Fagan, Mudd, & Needleman, 1988).

In contrast to COX-1, the more recently discovered isoform COX-2 is not generally detected in most tissues (Jouzeau, Terlain, Abid, Nedelec, & Netter, 1997). However, COX-2 is an inducible enzyme that is expressed in response to pro-inflammatory agents, including cytokines, endotoxins, growth factors, tumor promoters, and mitogens (O'Banion, Winn, & Young, 1992; Smith, Meade, & DeWitt, 1994). COX-2 is expressed in a few specialized tissues such as brain, testes, and macula densa of the kidney, in the apparent absence of any induction process.

Considerable evidence has accumulated to suggest that COX-2 is important for tumorigenesis. COX-2 expression is markedly increased in colorectal adenocarcinomas, as well as in other solid organ tumors, such as breast, lung, and prostate (Eberhart, Coffey, Radhika, Giardiello, Ferrenbach, & DuBois, 1994; Prescott & Fitzpatrick, 2000). As a result, COX-2 inhibitors have the potential of inhibiting tumor development, and many experimental studies using cell lines and animal models have demonstrated an ability to prevent tumor proliferation. Moreover, after performing a randomized study for polyp chemoprevention in patients with familial adenomatous polyposis (FAP), which showed that treatment with celecoxib significantly reduced the number of colorectal polyps, the U.S. Food and Drug Administration (FDA) quickly approved the clinical use of this drug for FAP patients (Steinbach, et al., 2000). It is important to note, however, that some COX-2 inhibitors were subsequently reported to increase the risk of serious cardiovascular events, including heart attack and stroke (Bombardier, et al., 2000).

Prostaglandins produced by COXs are represented by a large series of compounds that mainly enhance cancer development and progression, acting as carcinogens or tumor promoters with profound effects on carcinogenesis (Hong & Sporn, 1997). Thus, the ability to regulate the COX pathway provides a reasonable opportunity for cancer chemoprevention. The assay we use is based on measurement of PGE_2 produced in the COX reaction via an enzyme immunoassay (Cuendet & Pezzuto, 2000).

Selectivity of anti-inflammatory agents is important. Some may cause adverse side effects such as ulcers or cardiac problems.

Ornithine Decarboxylase Inhibition

ODC is the first and apparently the rate-limiting enzyme for the biosynthesis of polyamines in mammalian cells and is highly inducible by growth-promoting stimuli including growth factors, steroid hormones, cAMP-elevating agents, and tumor promoters (Pena, et al., 1993; Coffino, 2001). A number of factors finely tune ODC activity, including the expression, stability, and transcription rate of ODC messenger RNA; the stability and translation rate of the ODC enzyme; and also the posttranslational modification of the enzyme (van Daalen Wetters, Brabant, & Coffino, 1989). Further, ODC has been shown to play a role in transformation (Hurta, 2000) and to correlate with metastatic potential (Hardin, Mader, & Hurta, 2002). Since ODC activity is essential for proliferation of normal cells, and, on the other hand, is overexpressed in various cancer cell lines, it is now recognized that inhibition of ODC may be a good strategy for cancer chemoprevention and chemotherapy. To assess the inhibitory activity of extracts, we used TPA to induce ODC activity in T24 cells; enzyme activity is measured by quantifying CO_2 released from L-(1–14C) ornithine (Lee & Pezzuto, 1999).

NF-κB Inhibition

NF-κB is a ubiquitous transcription factor that is activated in a variety of cellular survival settings (Pahl, 1999). NF-κB is maintained in the cytoplasm in an inactivated or resting state by the chaperone molecule, inhibitory kappa B (IκB). Only after IκB is phosphorylated by inhibitor kappa kinase (IκK), is NF-κB liberated and free to translocate to the nucleus where it can perform its function (Zandi & Karin, 1999). Upon activation, NF-κB has been shown to transcriptionally upregulate many genes, most of which encode molecules involved in cellular survival pathways (Schwartz, Hernandez, & Mark Evers, 1999). The signaling pathways with which these molecules interface are diverse, and many are directly involved in subverting apoptosis. A wide range of drugs and molecules that activate NF-κB in tumor cells have been identified, including tumor necrosis factor-alpha (TNF-α) and chemotherapeutic agents (Das & White, 1997). The principle of the assay relies on the ability of the natural product to turn on a promoter, NF-κB, artificially constructed upstream of the luciferase gene. Once the promoter is triggered, it leads to transcription and eventually translation of the luciferase protein. Luciferase activity is easily measured using a luminometer.

Aromatase Inhibition

Estrogens are involved in the development of numerous hormone-related disorders, most notably carcinomas such as breast and endometrial cancers (Brodie & Njar, 1998). Estrogen deprivation is one strategy frequently used for treatment of hormone-dependent tumors. A decrease in estrogen levels can be achieved by blocking estrogen receptors with antiestrogens, also known as selective estrogen receptor modulators (SERMs), or by reducing estrogen production by inhibiting aromatase, the key enzyme in estrogen biosynthesis (Njar & Brodie, 1999). Aromatase is a reasonable target for inhibition since it catalyzes the last in a series of steps in steroid biosynthesis of estrone and estradiol. As a member of the P450 family, aromatase shares common features with other enzymes in the class. In this regard, the selectivity of aromatase inhibitors is an important issue because of the widespread presence of P450 systems in mammals; nonselective inhibition could cause serious side effects. Aromatase inhibitors have been developed primarily to treat breast cancer in postmenopausal women. However, three aromatase inhibitors, anastrozole, letrozole, and exemestane have been approved recently by the FDA for use as chemopreventive agents in the adjuvant treatment of postmenopausal women with hormone receptor–positive early breast cancer. To assess aromatase inhibition, a modified assay based on the fluorescence-based high-throughput screening system from BD Biosciences (San Jose, CA) is employed (Stresser, et al., 2000).

Differentiation-Inducing Agents

Differentiation-inducing agents have been shown to suppress cancer cell self-renewal selectively from normal stem cell renewal by inducing terminal differentiation followed by apoptosis. In addition, inducers of terminal differentiation, such as the retinoid and deltanoid (vitamin D_3 derivatives) class of compounds, have shown promising chemopreventive activity as suppressing agents that act during the promotion–progression stages of carcinogenesis (Kelloff, Boone, Crowell, Steele, Lubet, & Sigman, 1994). Although toxicity has hampered the development of these agents as primary chemopreventive agents, novel structural analogs with high affinity for specific nuclear receptors and high selective chemopreventive activity have been developed (Hong & Sporn, 1997). The HL-60 cell line is a valuable tool for research on myeloid maturation at the cellular and molecular level (Collins, 1987). This cell line can be induced to differentiate into the granulocytic, monocytic/macrophagic, or eosinophilic pathways of cellular development.

Active Compounds Isolated from Edible Plants

RESVERATROL

Resveratrol (3,4',5 trihydroxystilbene) is a phytoalexin produced in large amounts in grapevine skin in response to infection by *Bothrytis cinerea*. This production of resveratrol blocks the proliferation of the pathogen, thereby acting as a natural antibiotic. Numerous studies have reported interesting properties of *trans*-resveratrol as a preventive agent against various pathologies such as vascular diseases, cancers, viral infection, or neurodegenerative processes. Several epidemiological studies have revealed that resveratrol is probably one of the main microcomponents of wine responsible for its health benefits. Resveratrol acts on the process of carcinogenesis by affecting the three phases—tumor initiation, promotion, and progression—and suppresses the final steps of carcinogenesis, that is, angiogenesis and metastasis. It is also able to activate apoptosis, to arrest the cell cycle, or to inhibit kinase pathways (Signorelli & Ghidoni, 2005; Delmas, Lancon, Colin, Jannin, & Latruffe, 2006; Pezzuto, 2006) (Table 3.1). Moreover, concentrations of resveratrol in blood seem to be sufficient for anti-invasive activity. Interestingly, low doses of resveratrol can sensitize to low doses of cytotoxic drugs and provide a strategy to enhance the efficacy of anticancer therapy in various human cancers.

> Nearly 2000 manuscripts have appeared in the scientific literature describing the mode of action of resveratrol.

CURCUMIN

Curcumin, a yellow coloring ingredient present in turmeric (*Curcuma longa*), has emerged as one of the most powerful chemopreventive and anticancer

Table 3.1. Molecular Targets of Dietary Agents.*

Plant Name	Compound	Molecular Targets	References
Grapes (*Vitis vinifera*)	Resveratrol	Phase II enzymes COX, SIRT1, ODC MAPK, tyrosine kinases NF-κB, AP-1, Egr1 Cell cycle regulatory proteins Modulation of survival and apoptosis	Pezzuto, 2006
Turmeric (*Curcuma longa*)	Curcumin	ODC, ROS scavenger NF-κB, AP-1 Induction of apoptosis VEGF, Metalloproteins	Singh & Khar, 2006
Cruciferous vegetables (*Brassica* sp.)	Sulforaphane	Phase I and II enzymes NF-κB, induction of apoptosis	Keum, Jeong, & Wang, 2005
Green tea (*Camellia sinensis*)	EGCG	COX, iNOS Inhibition of DNA damage NF-κB, AP-1 Cell cycle regulatory proteins Metalloproteins	Hou, Lambert, Chin, & Yang, 2004
Allium vegetables (*Allium* sp.)	Organosulfur compounds	Phase II enzymes NF-κB, ODC Cell cycle regulatory proteins Induction of apoptosis	Singh, et al., 1998; Robert, Mouille, Mayeur, Michaud, & Blachier, 2001
Tomato (*Licopersicon esculentum*)	Lycopene	NF-κB, ROS scavenger Cell cycle regulatory proteins Induction of apoptosis	Bhuvaneswari & Nagini, 2005

*Also see reference Park & Pezzuto, 2002.

COX, cyclooxygenase; ODC, ornithine decarboxylase; MAPK, mitogen-activated protein kinases; SIRT1, silent mating-type information regulation 2 homolog; NF-κB, nuclear factor kappa B; AP-1, activator protein 1; Egr1, early growth response factor 1; ROS, reactive oxygen species; VEGF, vascular endothelial growth factor; EGCG, epigallocatechin gallate.

agents. This compound has been shown to exert anticarcinogenic effects in a diverse array of animal and cell culture models. It can act as a chemopreventive agent in cancers of colon, stomach, and skin by suppressing colonic aberrant crypt foci formation and DNA adduct formation (Singh & Khar, 2006). Also, curcumin has been shown to downregulate NF-κB thereby suppressing proliferation and inducing apoptosis, and to possess antiangiogenic properties by downregulating proangiogenic genes such as *VEGF* and decreasing migration and invasion of endothelial cells (Table 3.1). Cell lines that are resistant to certain apoptotic inducers and radiation become susceptible to apoptosis when treated in conjunction with curcumin.

CRUCIFEROUS VEGETABLES

Epidemiological evidence relating cancer risk reduction to the consumption of cruciferous vegetables such as broccoli, cauliflower, cabbage, kale, bok choy, Brussels sprouts, radish, or various mustards has been summarized in several comprehensive reports (Lin, et al., 1998; Michaud, Spiegelman, Clinton, Rimm, Willett, & Giovannucci, 1999; Cohen, Kristal, & Stanford, 2000; Spitz, et al., 2000; Zhang, et al., 2000; Zhao, et al., 2001). Highly significant cancer risk reduction with increasing crucifer intake was observed in cohorts that developed prostate (Cohen, et al., 2000), breast, bladder (Michaud, Spiegelman, Clinton, Rimm, Willett, & Giovannucci, 1999), and lung cancer (Spitz, et al., 2000; Zhao, et al., 2001), and non–Hodgkin lymphoma (Zhang, et al., 2000). A potential molecular mechanism of chemoprevention by cruciferous plants appears to be the induction of phase II enzymes and modulation of NF-κB and AP-1 (Keum, Jeong, & Kong, 2005) (Table 3.1). Some compounds are remarkably potent, such as sulforaphane and phenethyl isothiocyanate, components of broccoli and watercress, respectively (Hecht, 2000).

The American Cancer Society recommends at least five servings of cancer-fighting fruits and vegetables each day.

GREEN TEA

On a worldwide basis, the most popular chemopreventive drink is green tea. Green tea is the water extract of the dry leaves of *Camellia sinensis*. (–)-Epigallocatechin-3-gallate (EGCG), the most abundant catechin in green tea, is credited with the majority of health benefits associated with green tea consumption. The organ sites where tea or tea constituents are found to be effective include the skin, lung, oral cavity, esophagus, stomach, small intestine, colon, liver, prostate, and bladder. The mechanisms of carcinogenesis inhibition have also been investigated extensively, mostly in cell culture systems, but no clear conclusion can be reached concerning the in vivo cancer preventive mechanisms. Possible mechanisms include the inhibition of specific protein kinase activities, blocking of receptor-mediated functions, and inhibition of proteases (Table 3.1). These events may lead to cell cycle regulation, growth inhibition, enhanced apoptosis, inhibition of angiogenesis, and inhibition of invasion and metastases (Hou, Lambert, Chin, & Yang, 2004). The possible complications of translating results obtained in cell culture studies to animals and humans may come from possible artifacts due to the auto-oxidation of EGCG (Yang, Lambert, Hou, Ju, Lu, & Hao, 2006). Also, activities observed in cell culture with high concentrations of EGCG may not be relevant because of the limited systemic bioavailability of EGCG.

ALLIUM VEGETABLES

The large genus, *Allium*, includes onion, garlic, chive, leek, and shallot. Preclinical investigations demonstrate consistently that cancer chemoprevention by garlic and related sulfur compounds is clearly evident and appears to be independent of the organ site or the carcinogen employed (Milner, 1996; Knowles & Milner, 2001). The protection of tumor incidence by garlic may arise from several mechanisms, including blockage of *N*-nitro compound formation, suppression of the bioactivation of several carcinogens, enhanced DNA repair, reduced cell proliferation, and/or induction of apoptosis (Milner, 2001). Also, some studies showed that ODC was inhibited, QR was induced, and various genes related to cytochrome P450 isozymes were inhibited (Dion, Agler, & Milner, 1997; Singh, et al., 1998; Robert, Mouille, Mayeur, Michaud, & Blachier, 2001) (Table 3.1). Some organoselenium compounds are superior to the corresponding sulfur analogs in cancer prevention. Selenium-enriched garlic, selenium-enriched yeast, and selenium-enriched broccoli are more effective cancer chemopreventive agents in various animal models than regular garlic, yeast, and broccoli, respectively (Whanger, 2004). However, the active form or metabolite of selenium that is responsible for cancer prevention in epidemiological studies remains unknown. The selenium content of plants is dependent on the amount of selenium in the soil. Most of our common foods, including garlic, contain a very low level of selenium (Morris & Levander, 1970).

TOMATO

Epidemiological studies have provided evidence that high consumption of tomatoes effectively lowers the risk of reactive oxygen species (ROS)-mediated diseases such as cardiovascular disease and cancer by improving the antioxidant capacity. Tomatoes are rich sources of lycopene, an antioxidant carotenoid reported to be a more stable and potent singlet oxygen quenching agent compared to other carotenoids. In addition to its antioxidant properties, lycopene showed an array of biological effects including cardioprotective, anti-inflammatory, antimutagenic, and anticarcinogenic activities. The anticancer activity of lycopene has been demonstrated both in in vitro and in vivo tumor models. The mechanisms underlying the inhibitory effects of lycopene on carcinogenesis could involve ROS scavenging, interference with cell proliferation, inhibition of cell cycle progression, and modulation of signal transduction pathways (Bhuvaneswari & Nagini, 2005) (Table 3.1).

Consumption of pizza with red tomato sauce has been associated with reduced incidence of prostate cancer.

Conclusions

It is generally recognized that the lifetime probability for an individual to develop some form of cancer is in the range of 50% to 70%. In some of these cases, etiological factors are well established, such as overexposure to ultraviolet irradiation or cigarette smoking, so primary methods of prevention are obvious. Conversely, the etiology of major cancers, such as breast cancer and prostate cancer, remains largely unknown. In these situations, alternate methods of prevention are highly desirable. Similarly, in high-risk groups, such as individuals who have survived bouts with cancer, prevention strategies are of imminent importance. In many respects, dietary cancer chemoprevention is an ideal approach. A problem associated with this approach is that low levels of agents often occur in natural dietary materials, so actual effectiveness may be questionable. Natural selection of dietary components containing higher levels of chemopreventive agents may be one method to circumvent this problem, but bioengineering of plants would be more direct. In the past years, few compounds have been approved by the FDA for use as chemopreventive agents. They include the COX-2 specific inhibitor celecoxib to reduce the number of adenomatous colorectal polyps in familial adenomatous polyposis, as an adjunct to usual care, as well as tamoxifen and three aromatase inhibitors, anastrozole, letrozole, and exemestane, for the adjuvant treatment of postmenopausal women with hormone receptor–positive early breast cancer. These are tremendous breakthroughs. Nonetheless, a great deal of additional work is required. For example, dilemmas such as the near 100% probability of developing prostate cancer, given a sufficient lifespan, and the lack of effectiveness of agents such as tamoxifen against ER-negative breast cancer need to be recognized. Thus, new cancer chemopreventive agents are still required, and plant materials are a promising source for the identification of active lead compounds.

ACKNOWLEDGMENTS

The authors are grateful to the National Cancer Institute for support provided under the auspices of program project P01 CA48112 entitled "Natural Inhibitors of Carcinogenesis."

REFERENCES

Cragg GM, Newman DJ, & Snader KM. (1997). Natural products in drug discovery and development. *Journal of Natural Products*, 60, 52–60.

Jensen PR & Fenical W. (1994). Strategies for the discovery of secondary metabolites from marine bacteria: Ecological perspectives. *Annual Review of Microbiology*, 48, 559–584.

Kelloff GJ, Crowell JA, Hawk ET, Steele VE, Lubet RA, Boone CW et al. (1996). Strategy and planning for chemopreventive drug development: Clinical development plans II. *Journal of Cellular Biochemistry. Supplement*, 26, 54–71.

Kinghorn AD, Fong HHS, Farnsworth NR et al. (1998). Cancer chemoprevention agents discovered by activity-guided fractionation: A review. *Current Organic Chemistry*, 2, 597–612.

Park EJ & Pezzuto JM. (2002). Botanicals in cancer chemoprevention. *Cancer and Metastasis Reviews*, 21, 231–255.

Pezzuto JM, Angerhofer CK, & Mehdi H. (1998). In vitro models of human disease states. *Studies in Natural Products Chemistry*, 20, 507–560.

Pezzuto JM, Song LL, Lee SK, Shamon LA, Mata-Greenwood E, Jang M et al. (1999). Bioassay methods useful for activity-guided isolation of natural product cancer chemoprevention agents. In K. Hostettmann, MP Gupta, & A Marston (Eds.), *Chemistry, biological and pharmacological properties of medicinal plants from the Americas; Proceedings of the IOCD/CYTED Symposium, Panama City, Panama, 23–26 February 1997* (pp. 81–110). Harwood Academic Publishers, Chur, Switzerland.

Sporn MB, Dunlop NM, Newton DL, & Smith JM. (1976). Prevention of chemical carcinogenesis by vitamin A and its synthetic analogs (retinoids). *Federation Proceedings, 35,* 1332–1338.

Sporn MB & Suh N. (2000). Chemoprevention of cancer. *Carcinogenesis, 21,* 525–530.

Wattenberg LW. (1985). Chemoprevention of cancer. *Cancer Research, 45,* 1–8.

(A complete reference list for this chapter is available online at http://www.oup.com/us/ integrativemedicine).

4

Diet and Cancer:
Epidemiology and Prevention

CYNTHIA A. THOMSON

KEY CONCEPTS

- Cancer is a chronic disease that occurs through multiple insults to cells and tissue; therefore, it is most likely to be prevented by repeated exposures to sufficient amounts of cancer-preventive nutrients and bioactive food component consumed throughout the lifespan.
- Cancer-preventive bioactive compounds are found predominantly in foods of plant origin and most have several biological activities associated with reduced cancer risk.
- Diet alters carcinogenesis through a variety of molecular and cellular pathways including immune modulation, methylation, antioxidation, and anti-inflammatory effects.
- Specific dietary recommendations for cancer prevention are available from the American Cancer Society and the American Institute for Cancer Research/World Cancer Research Fund. These recommendations require significant behavioral change for most Americans and sufficient support for adopting healthier food choices should be provided.
- Cancer will be diagnosed in one in two males and one in three females in their lifetime; thus most Americans are "at-risk" for this disease and should be encouraged to adopt a cancer-preventive diet; select populations have even greater risk— cancer survivors, family members of cancer patients, smokers, those with high UV light or other environmental exposures and those with compromised immunity—these subgroups should be specifically targeted for cancer prevention education.

What one chooses to eat can have profound effects on his/her health, particularly when it comes to cancer prevention. In fact, food selections throughout the lifespan likely have relevance in terms of lifetime cancer risk. Cancer is a multi-stage, stepwise, and cumulative disease. It evolves from chronic damage to healthy cells and tissue in which both the localized tissue and the wider microenvironment demonstrate abnormalities ranging from genetic deletions, to p53 mutations, to cellular anoxia (Goldberg & Diamandis, 1993). The summative effects of multiple insults to tissue which escape repair by the immune system, over time, result in malignant transformations (Gatenby, 2003). Diet and the constitutive nutrients and bioactive food components (BAFC) play a vital role in enhancing the host response against cancer. Further, diet is a *modifiable* cancer risk factor. Unlike age or genetic predisposition, dietary choices can be changed by the individual with the goal of reducing cancer risk.

This chapter will provide an overview of the current recommendations for healthy eating associated with reduced cancer risk as well as practical information regarding how to implement healthy eating practices among patients. Cancer prevention strategies are appropriate for the population at large, but likely have greater relevance among cancer survivors and family members of those diagnosed with cancer. Individualizing diet therapy to meet the individual needs of a given patient is critical to long term adoption of healthy eating behaviors. In addition, changing eating behavior to promote health, does, for most Americans, propose significant challenges in terms of food knowledge, food purchasing, as well as food preparation. Support must be comprehensive and delivered incrementally to assure the long-term commitment to healthy eating.

Mechanisms of Anticancer Activity of Select Food Components

As with any research endeavor, efforts to elucidate more completely the anti-carcinogenic activity of the diet in relation to cancer risk has been fraught with roadblocks. At the most basic level, there has been significant research describing and targeting pathway-specific activity(ties) of food. These include bioactivity in relation to inflammation and immune modulation (Biesalski, 2007; Percival, Bukowski, & Milner, 2008; Federico, Morgillo, Tuccillo, Clardiello, & Loguercio, 2007), oxidative damage (Loft & Poulsen, 1996), methylation (Milner, 2006), nuclear factor-kappa B (NF-κB) inhibition and apoptosis (Ichikawa, Nakamura,

Kashiwada, & Aggarwal, 2007), promotion of cellular differentiation (Ovesna Vachalkova, & Horvathova, 2004), histone deacetylation (Dashwood & Ho, 2007; Moiseeva, Almeida, Jones, & Manson, 2007), cell cycle control (Meeran & Katiyar, 2008), hormonal regulation (Rock, 2004; Xu, Duncan, Merz, & Kurzer, 1998), and even inhibition of drug resistance in the therapeutic setting. Table 4.1 lists several biological targets for food/food components relevant to reducing cancer risk. Of importance, a recent analysis from the Women's Health Initiative (WHI) demonstrated that elevation in white blood cell count among post-menopausal women is associated with a significant increased risk for cancer (Margolis, Rodabough, Thomson, Lopez, & McTiernan, 2007).

Further, whole foods may act on a variety of molecular targets or biologically relevant pathways to reduce cancer risk while individual food components may have specific or broad anticancer effects. As an example, isothiocyanates

Table 4.1. Select Food Sources of Bioactive Food Components and Related Mechanisms of Cancer Prevention.

Bioactive Food Component	Mechanisms of Cancer Risk Reduction	References
Avocado	Cell cycle arrest, apoptosis	Ding, et al., 2007
Broccoli, broccoli sprouts	Histone deacetylation, hormone modulation, reduction in oxidative stress, carcinogen metabolism	Minich & Bland, 2007
Berries	Reduce malignant transformation, reduction in oxidative stress	Duthie, 2007
Curcumin	Anti-inflammatory apoptosis, cell cycle arrest	Ferguson & Philpott, 2007; Surh & Chun, 2007
Garlic/organosulfur compounds	Carcinogen detoxification, antimicrobial, DNA repair, cell cycle arrest	Moriarty, et al., 2007
Grapes (resveratrol)	Reduce oxidative stress, anti-inflammatory	Jang, et al., 1997
Green tea	Anti-inflammatory, reduce oxidative stress, inhibition of growth factor cell signaling	Chen & Zhang, 2007
Tomato products	Reduce oxidative stress, modulation of IGFs	Riso, et al., 2006

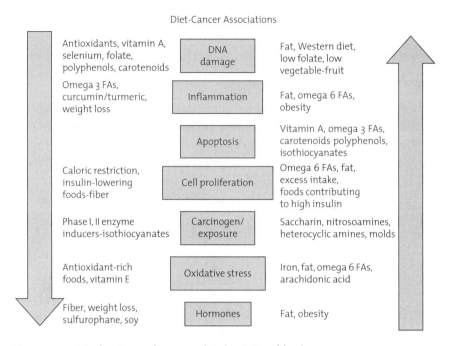

FIGURE 4.1. Mechanisms of cancer-related activity of food.

in cruciferous vegetables have been shown to reduce inflammatory response, repair oxidative damage, promote histone deacetylation, and upregulate estrogen receptor α, thus enhancing the antiestrogenic effects of tamoxifen (Higdon, Delage, Williams, & Dashwood, 2007). Several diet-derived compounds have been shown to modify T-cell function, including tannins in apples, dietary nucleotides, fatty acids, and alkylamines (Percival, Bukowski, & Milner, 2008) while others have broad anti-inflammatory effects (omega-3 fatty acids in fatty fish, curcumin/turmeric, carotenoids in vegetables and fruits, etc.) (Ferguson & Philpott, 2007).

To optimize these biologically based cancer preventive functions of foods, it is imperative that individuals consume a varied diet that provides some regular, repetitive, and sufficient exposure (intake and bioavailability) to cancer-preventive compounds to reduce cancer risk. Diets that only occasionally provide protective compounds or that limit exposure to low "dosage" levels are likely insufficient to reduce risk. On the other hand, variety in intake of protective foods will more likely result in consistent protective dietary effects that over time lower cancer risk.

It is also important to understand that dietary factors can modify cancer risk both in terms of reducing risk and, in relation to some components, increasing risk. Figure 4.1 summarizes these associations.

Dietary Recommendations

Periodically, most cancer-specific associations provide the public with updated guidelines with regards to healthy diet behaviors to reduce cancer risk. For the American Cancer Society (ACS) these guidelines were updated in 2006 and include the following recommendations (Kushi, 2006):

- **Maintain a healthy weight throughout life.**
  - Balance caloric intake with physical activity.
  - Avoid excessive weight gain throughout life.
  - Achieve and maintain a healthy weight if currently overweight or obese.

- **Eat a healthy diet, with an emphasis on plant sources.**
  - Choose food or beverages in amounts that help achieve and maintain a healthy weight.
  - Eat 5 or more servings of a variety of vegetables and fruits every day.
  - Choose whole grains in preference to processed (refined) grains.
  - Limit consumption of processed and red meats.

- **If you drink alcoholic beverages, limit consumption.**
  - Drink no more than 1 drink per day for women or 2 per day for men.

In addition to the aforementioned dietary recommendations, specific recommendations for physical activity were also provided. The ACS diet recommendations were developed by a "meeting of the minds" of leading researchers in cancer prevention research across North America who openly discussed the available peer-reviewed evidence to develop behavior-specific recommendations for both diet and physical activity to reduce cancer risk. These recommendations are updated approximately every 4 years.

The combined efforts of the American Institute for Cancer Research and the World Cancer Research Fund (AICR/WCRF) resulted in a recent update of recommendations for reducing cancer risk, recommendations that are supportive of the ACS recommendations (WCRF/AICR, 2007). The AICR/WCRF recommendations are based on over 20 comprehensive and systematic literature reviews of the available scientific evidence. The systematic reviews were then further discussed and reviewed by expert panels of academic researchers and clinical oncology practitioners. In the final step report development, the draft recommendations and supportive evidence were put through a secondary peer-review process by selected international reviewers before evidence-based recommendations were formulated for publication. Much of the evidence presented in the 2007 report, *Food, Nutrition, Physical Activity and the Prevention of Cancer: A Global Perspective,* has evolved from available epidemiological studies with greater weight given to randomized controlled intervention trials, followed by prospective cohort studies and lastly case-control study results. The recommendations state the following:

- Be as lean as possible within the normal range of body weight
- Limit consumption of energy-dense foods; avoid sugary drinks
- Eat mostly foods of plant origin
- Limit intake of red meat and avoid processed meat
- Limit alcoholic drinks
- Limit consumption of salt; avoid moldy cereals or pulses
- Aim to meet nutritional needs through diet alone
- Mothers to breastfeed; children to be breastfed
- Cancer survivors follow the recommendations for cancer prevention

The consistency of the recommendations in terms of the two organizations is clear. In fact, the current dietary recommendations to reduce cancer risk are consistent also with those for weight control, cardiovascular disease risk reduction, stroke prevention, and to a large extent diabetes control.

Expanding on Current Recommendations

PLANT FOODS

The recommendation that a diet rich in plant foods will reduce cancer risk has remained a primary focus of cancer prevention recommendations for the past several decades. This is despite what continues to be mixed epidemiological evidence to support this recommendation. One concern is that while case-control studies predominantly indicate a protective effect of plant foods, prospective cohort studies are less consistent in supporting statistically significant relationships. Unfortunately randomized controlled trials testing hypotheses using high plant diets versus usual diets have not been pursued due to the cost and longevity of such trials. Further, evidence from case-control trials is largely suspect when it comes to cancer outcomes in that people diagnosed with cancer commonly associate their disease with less healthy dietary choices, and thus misreporting of dietary intake based on recall of eating patterns before the cancer diagnosis is a real limitation to the interpretation of such research. Prospective cohort studies avoid the recall bias associated with case-control studies, but may be inaccurate due to the overall difficulty in estimating true dietary intake.

Table 4.2 provides a summary of select evidence from published meta-analyses by cancer site. As shown, inconsistencies in vegetable-fruit and cancer-associations exist. One explanation for the inconsistencies may be the fact that total vegetable and fruit intake would include both those rich in cancer-protective BAFC and nutrients (berries, spinach, carrots, tomato, broccoli, etc.) as well as those with relatively low health-promoting compounds (iceberg

Table 4.2. Association between Vegetable and Fruit Intake and Cancer Risk: Select Meta-analyses by Cancer Site.

Study	Sample Size	RR/OR (95% Confidence interval)	Clarifications
Steinhaus, et al., 2000	Bladder cancer	Low fruit and vegetables—1.40 (1.08–1.83)	Low intake increased risk; high intake was not evaluated in terms of protection
Smith-Warner, et al., 2001	200 breast cancer cases	Fruit/vegetables— RR 0.93(0.86–1.00)	No protective effect for sub-groups including green leafy vegetables
Koushik, et al., 2007	756,217/5838 colorectal cancer cases	OR 0.91(0.82–1.01)	Distal colon 0.74(0.57–0.95)
Bandera, et al., 2007	16 case-control studies in endometrial cancer	Vegetables—OR 0.71(0.55–0.91) Fruit—0.0(0.72–1.12)	Cruciferous vegetables—0.85 (0.74–0.97)
Lunet, et al., 2007	1434/305 cases gastric cancer	Fruit 0.58(0.38–0.89) Vegetables 0.63 (0.50–0.79)	Protective for cardia and noncardia sites
Pavia, et al., 2006	15 case-control studies; 1 cohort	Fruit 0.51(0.40–0.65) Vegetable 0.50(0.38–0.65)	

lettuce, cucumber, corn) (Russo, 2007). Thus, the total vegetable and fruit exposure variable used to evaluate protective effects of a high vegetable/fruit diet may or may not reflect exposure to a cancer-preventive diet. Further, there is evidence, albeit limited, that co-consumption of a mixture of plant foods rich in BAFC results in a synergistic response, particularly in terms of antioxidant response (Liu, 2004).

Generally the evidence suggests that diets higher in vegetables and fruit would reduce the risk of several cancers; however, the evidence is most substantial for cancers of the gastrointestinal tract including head and neck cancer (Lunet, 2005). Specific plant foods have also been suggested to reduce the risk of select cancers, as detailed in Table 4.3.

Clinicians must therefore rely on the overall trends in associations to formulate recommendations for the individual patient. The currently available evidence continues to support the recommendation that consuming a diet high in vegetables and other plant foods will reduce cancer risk.

DIETARY FAT

Historically, dietary fat has been suggested to be associated with increased risk of several cancers, particularly solid tumors such as breast, colorectal, ovarian,

Table 4.3. Studies Supporting a Reduced Risk for Site-specific Cancers in Relation to Intake of Select Vegetables and Fruit.

Cancer Type	Specific Vegetable and Fruit
Colorectal	Cruciferous vegetables, folate-rich vegetables and fruit (Larsson & Giovannucci, 2005)
Gastric/stomach	Garlic/allium (Nan & Park, 2005; Lissowska & Gail, 2004), green-yellow vegetables (De Stafani, et al., 2001; Ngoan & Mizoue, 2002)
Esophageal	Citrus and vegetables and fruit rich in vitamin C (De Stefani & Boffetta, 2005)
Lung	Carotenoid-rich (Wright, et al., 2003; Neuhouser, et al., 2003)
Pancreas	Folate-rich vegetables and fruit (Larsson, et al., 2006)
Prostate	Tomato, processed tomato products (Schuurman & Goldbohm, 2002)

gallbladder, and prostate cancers. However, as our understanding of the types of dietary fat has expanded, there is growing evidence that total fat may be a surrogate for other dietary factors that influence cancer risk more so than fat alone. Specifically, evidence that trans fats contribute to cancer risk was convincing enough (along with other deleterious effects on health, that is cardiovascular disease risk) to result in labeling regulation to reveal the trans fat content of foods on the label, although the recent AICR/WCRF report explains that trials assessing trans fat intake and cancer are limited and inconclusive (WCRF/AICR, 2007, p 137). In 2006, the results of the largest prospective randomized trial of dietary fat reduction in primary cancer prevention were published (Prentice, 2006). The Women's Health Initiative randomized trial of 48,835 post-menopausal women showed that a low fat diet, consisting of an average fat intake of 24.3% total energy (at year 1), for a period of 8.1 years did not demonstrate a significant reduction in breast and/or colorectal cancer as was hypothesized, HR = 0.91 (95% CI = 0.83–1.01). Of importance, among women who entered the study with a dietary pattern demonstrating fat intake within the highest quintile and who were able to achieve the greatest overall reduction in percent total energy intake as fat, breast cancer risk appeared to be significantly reduced. This suggests that small reductions in total fat intake after menopause are unlikely to reduce breast cancer risk in "healthy volunteers," but targeting women who demonstrate high fat intake can be advantageous. In terms of colorectal cancer for which 480 cases occurred over 8.1 years, no significant protective effects of the low-fat diet were shown, HR = 1.08 (95% CI = 0.90–1.29) (Beresford, 2006). Yet, a later analysis of ovarian cancer risk showed a protective effect of adopting the low fat diet (Prentice, 2007) with HR of 0.60 (95% CI = 0.38–0.96), an association which was not demonstrated for ovarian cancers diagnosed within 4 years of adopting the diet. These findings suggest that dietary efficacy in terms of reducing cancer risk is likely to require long-term changes in eating patterns and it is unlikely that shorter-term changes will modify risk.

Red meat intake has been associated with increased colorectal cancer risk, an association which has been hypothesized to be a result of higher iron intake, a known oxidant, as well as greater saturated fat exposure. The evidence suggesting that high intake of red meat is associated with greater colorectal cancer risk is more consistent from earlier epidemiological studies (Giovannucci & Willett, 1994; Willett, 1990), with associations somewhat less significant in more recent studies (Tiermersma, 2004; English, 2004) possibly related to the greater availability of lean cuts of red meat in the food supply. A prospective study of red meat and processed meat demonstrated an increased risk of esophageal, colorectal, liver, and lung cancers (Cross, 2007). The current recommendations, which consider dose-response, suggest that restriction in red meat intake is an appropriate behavior to reduce the risk for colorectal cancer.

Processed meats also have been associated with increased risk for colorectal cancer (English, 2004; Norat, 2005), although some inconsistencies in the evidence exist possibly related to the variability in defining processed meat for the analyses. Evidence is less consistent that processed meats increase risk of other cancers including prostate, lung, and stomach cancer (Breslow, 2000; Gonzalez & Riboli, 2006; Michaud, 2001). Recommending a reduction in processed meats, based on current evidence for cancer risk as well as association with other diet-related chronic diseases, such as cardiovascular disease and hypertension, is a prudent approach to improve health.

The Role of Body Weight in Cancer Prevention

When reviewing the recommendations, it is apparent that most recommendations are significantly influenced by the contribution of body weight on cancer risk. Increasingly there has been an emphasis on expanding assessment beyond weight and body mass index to include assessment of "healthy" percentage of body fat as a predictor of risk (Gallagher, 2000). Attaining and maintaining a healthy body weight is a central recommendation for reducing the risk of cancer, particularly the avoidance of adult weight gain. Increasing vegetable, fruit, and fiber intake is associated with reduced caloric intake and thus promotes weight control (Svendsen, Blomhoff, Holme, & Tonstad, 2007). Conversely, efforts to reduce intake of dietary fat and beverages high in simple sugars has similar effects on body weight. Overweight and obesity are thought to increase the overall risk for cancer by 14% to 20% (Calle, 2003) and overweight status plays an influential role in numerous cancers including post-menopausal breast, pancreatic, gallbladder, colorectal (males), ovary, cervical, endometrial, and esophageal cancers and multiple myeloma (AICR/WCRF, 2007). Evidence also suggests that being overweight contributes to a more advanced tumor type at the time of diagnosis, particularly in relation to prostate cancer (Amling, 2004).

Obesity may alter carcinogenesis through a variety of biological mechanisms including modulation of hormone levels, suppression of immune response, elevation in inflammatory cytokines, and growth factors (Insulin, insulin-like growth factors—IGFS) (Hursting, 2007), and contributing to physical inactivity. Obese individuals also demonstrate higher levels of oxidative stress (Vincent, Innes, & Vincent, 2007) that can lead to cellular damage resulting in both localized and systemic inflammatory response.

The current recommendations suggest that body mass index (BMI) should be maintained between 18.5 and 24.9 kg/m². While BMI represents one appropriate target, health care providers should also consider setting goals for waist circumference, as abdominal fatness appears to be of particular concern in relation to cancer risk (NHLBI, 1998).

Waist circumference goals (NHLBI, 1998)
 Males: ≤ 40 inches < 102 cm
 Females: ≤ 35 inches < 90 cm

Body fat percentage goals (Gallagher, 2000)
 Males: 13%–23%
 Females: 25%–35%

In addition, it is imperative that health care providers not only evaluate body weight at a specific point in time (individual provider visit), but also track trends in body weight over time, similar to the current practice of plotting growth curves in children or weight gain patterns through pregnancy. In this way, small elevations in body weight in adult life can be identified early and strategies can be implemented to reduce body weight before the problem accelerates in magnitude. Health care providers should also utilize dual X-ray absorptometry (DXA) scans to evaluate the individual's percentage body fat and lean mass over time. These assessments can be safely included in annual patient evaluations and provide accurate and detailed information regarding body composition along with bone biomarker data. In relation to body weight, the average adult in the U.S. gains approximately 14 kg between the ages of 18 and 50 years. Critical life events contributing to undesirable weight gain include marriage, pregnancy and childbirth, entrance into the workforce, menopause, divorce, and significant changes in job responsibilities. Thus, patients who have experienced any of these life events should be targeted for health promotion education. Further, body weight is tightly regulated in relation to diet and physical activity, making our ability to independently predict risk related to these factors difficult (Shin, 2008).

A summary of the current diet–cancer prevention recommendations by cancer site is presented in Table 4.4.

New Initiatives

Currently there are approximately 210 active research trials in the area of diet and cancer prevention funded by the National Cancer Institute. Access to the trial descriptions is available at: http://www.cancer.gov/clinicaltrials. Table 4.5 lists several trial titles of relevance to clinicians, which are likely to produce important data regarding approaches to cancer prevention and control

Table 4.4. Dietary Recommendations for Cancer Prevention by Cancer Site.

Cancer Site	Recommendation	Considerations
Breast	Avoid adult weight gain and abdominal fatness Avoid alcohol Breast feed	Even small unintentional increases in body weight should be addressed quickly and consistently Get active! Have body composition (fat) tested annually using dual X-ray absorptometry (DXA) Adequate folate intake reduces the detrimental effects of alcohol in terms of breast cancer risk Women should breast feed for a minimum of 6 months to reduce risk
Colorectal	Increase fiber intake to >25 grams/day Restrict intake of red meat and processed meat Avoid alcohol Avoid adult weight gain and abdominal fatness	Evidence from RCT does not support in terms of polyp prevention, but researchers/clinicians continue to support this recommendation based on multiple mechanisms for cancer risk reduction Lean cuts are likely less problematic; some menstruating females may need the iron provided by lean red meat Even small unintentional increases in body weight should be addressed quickly and consistently Get active!
Esophagus	Avoid alcohol Avoid excess body fat	Any amount is considered potentially harmful; drink green tea instead as it may reduce risk Even small unintentional increases in body weight should be addressed quickly and consistently Get active! Weight-bearing activity to promote increased lean mass in addition to weight control

(continued)

Table 4.4. (Continued)

Cancer Site	Recommendation	Considerations
Kidney	Avoid excess body fat	Even small unintentional increases in body weight should be addressed quickly and consistently Get active! Weight-bearing activity to promote increased lean mass in addition to weight control
Liver	Avoid aflatoxins Avoid alcohol	Any amount is considered potentially harmful; drink green tea instead as it may reduce risk
Lung	Consume fruits and vegetables rich in carotenoids Avoid arsenic in drinking water	Eat a variety of colored fruits and vegetables—several servings daily—9+; avoid supplements of individual carotenoids Check local water supply; also avoid fish from arsenic-containing waters
Mouth /oral	Avoid alcohol Consume vegetables and fruits rich in bioactive food compounds	Any amount is considered potentially harmful; drink green tea instead as it may reduce risk Eat a variety of colored fruits and vegetables—several servings daily—9+; avoid supplements of individual carotenoids
Ovary	Reduce dietary fat	Results from the Women's health Initiative trial suggest a diet low in fat <25% total energy—can reduce ovarian cancer risk
Pancreas	Consume vegetables and fruits rich in folate	Green leafy vegetables—broccoli, spinach, kale, salad greens— at least 1x/day
Prostate	Avoid adult weight gain and body fatness	Even small unintentional increases in body weight should be addressed quickly and consistently. Have body composition (fat) tested annually using dual X-ray absorptometry (DXA) Get active!

Adapted from AICR/WCRF, Food, Nutrition, Physical Activity and the Prevention of Cancer A Global Perspective, 2007.

that will influence clinical practice in this area. The studies are listed by three subgroups—those that are specific to the study of a specific nutrient, followed by those investigating BAFC and finally those addressing the area of body weight and cancer prevention. Several large clinical trials have been completed in diet and cancer prevention and provide on-going evidence for/against diet–cancer associations. These include, but are not limited to, the polyp prevention trial (low fat, high fiber, high fruit and vegetable, and polyp risk), the Women's Health Initiative (low fat diet and risk for breast or colorectal cancers as well as other cancer outcomes), Linxian trials of China (a randomized controlled trial of vitamin/mineral supplements), Women's Health Study (low-dose aspirin and vitamin E), Selenium and Vitamin E in Prostate Cancer (SELECT), and the Women's Healthy Eating and Living Study (WHEL) targeting a plant-based diet in women previously treated for breast cancer.

NUTRIGENOMICS

To better understand the role of diet in cancer prevention many investigators as well as the NIH have begun to more fully explore the interaction between nutrients, BAFC, proteins and the genetic code. Advancing our understanding in this area will not only afford us an opportunity to appreciate the interactive influences of diet and genes in carcinogenesis, but will also allow us to determine which of these interactions is of biological relevance in terms of protein function. This area of research may ultimately afford us information as to who demonstrates a genetic predisposition to be a "responder" versus a "nonresponder" to diet therapy designed to reduce cancer risk.

PRENATAL EXPOSURES

Currently the NIH is actively supporting research to better elucidate the role of prenatal dietary exposures and their role in cancer prevention. Data from the diethylstilbesterol cohort suggests that prenatal exposure to estrogen increases breast cancer risk (Palmer, 2006; Troisi, 2007) and several dietary constituents have been shown to modify estrogen exposure (cruciferous vegetables, soy, fiber, etc.). It has also been suggested that low birth weight infants may have an indirect but increased risk for obesity-related cancer related to excess body fat and insulin dysregulation in adult life, which is a result of an energy-deprived in utero experience (Xue & Michels, 2007). A better understanding of the role of maternal diet during both pregnancy and lactation on infant future cancer risk may provide for targeted diet counseling among pregnant and lactating women, a subgroup of the population that is likely to demonstrate high motivation for dietary improvement.

Table 4.5. Sample of Currently Funded NCI Diet–Cancer Research.

Study Title	Principal Investigator	Institution
Nutrient Related		
Antioxidants and inflammation in colorectal cancer	Ossowski L	Mount Sinai School of Medicine
Colorectal chemoprevention with calcium and vitamin D	Aron J	Dartmouth College
HPV clearance by folic acid supplementation	Piyathilake CJ	University of Alabama Birmingham
Prostate cancer prevention by N-3 fatty acids	Halperin J	Harvard University
Physician's health Study II: Prevention trial of vitamins	Gaziano J	Brigham and Women's Hospital
Bioactive Food Components (BAFC)		
Prevention of oral cancer by green tea: a mechanism study	Chung F-L	Georgetown University
Curcumin suppression of head and neck cancer	Wang M	Brentwood Biomedical Research Institute
Chemoprevention of green tea polyphenols on liver cancer	Wang J	Texas Tech University
Tomato-Soy juice for prostate cancer	Clinton S	Ohio State University
Breast cancer chemoprevention potential of common spices	Gupta RC	University of Louisville
Prevention of prostate cancer by sulfuraphane	Singh S	University of Pittsburg
Body weight		
Intermittent food restriction prevents mammary tumors	Cleary M	University of Minnesota
A Mediterranean diet in colon cancer prevention	Djuric Z	University of Michigan, Ann Arbor
Promoting healthy weight with "stability first"	Kiernan M	Stanford University

FOODS DEVELOPED FOR ENHANCED BIOACTIVE CONSTITUENTS

Efforts to enhance the cancer-protective properties of the food supply are also underway. Examples include tomato cultivars selected for higher lycopene content, garlic grown in selenium-rich soil to enhance selenium intake, or anthocyanin-rich purple carrots to provide not only a good source of carotenoids (α-and β-carotene) but also, anthocyanins known to reduce cancer risk in in vitro models through modulation of NF-κB (Kelley, 2006) and, indirectly, inflammatory response. In addition, efforts have focused on determining the appropriate dose, optimal processing and preparation method (Shi, 2000) food matrix (Parada, 2007) and meal composition as well as dietary fat source to optimize bioavailability of select BAFC for humans (Hedren, 2002).

Patient Counseling and Resources

Despite the wealth of information regarding the role of diet in cancer prevention, little effort is placed on counseling patients in this area. While one in two males and one in three females will be diagnosed with cancer in their lifetime (ACS, 2007) most patients do not see themselves at risk. Clinicians and public health advisors will need to enhance efforts in this area, particularly as our population ages and the overall rates of cancer are likely to rise. To meet this demand the following guidelines should be considered:

1. Identify high-risk patients—not only related to germline genetic mutations, but also those with a family history of cancer, obese patients, smokers, and those with known environmental exposures.
2. As part of the patient's health risk assessment routinely evaluate cancer risk behaviors such as smoking, high alcohol consumption, obesity, and in particular longitudinal increases in body weight over adult life, low physical activity, low vegetable and fruit intake, high intake of processed foods, high-fat foods, particularly meals eaten away from home.
3. Prioritize desired behavior change, approach it incrementally and involve the patient in setting measureable goals—walk 30 minutes/day, drink green tea each morning, eat a green vegetable every day—add an orange vegetable as well, limit television and/or computer time, evaluate local restaurant menus to identify healthy selections, count fat grams—set a goal of 40 g to 60 g/day, count fiber grams—set a goal of 20 increasing to 30 g/day, and so on.

4. Reevaluate—ensure all patients get feedback on their efforts. Without feedback the behavior improvements will not be maintained.
5. Avoid prejudices—offer support to obese patients, smokers, or others you may be inclined to characterize as noncompliant.

A list of valuable resources is presented in Table 4.6. In addition to providing patients with reliable written and online information regarding the role of diet in cancer prevention, it is also imperative to establish a clinical practice approach that exemplifies and reinforces these positive healthy messages. For example, food available in the clinic or surrounding area should always support the patient's efforts. Vending machines should only dispense cancer-preventive foods; fresh fruit might be available in the waiting area. Instead of candy dishes on staff desks, sugar-free mints, or dried fruit could be on hand. Magazines on display should also reflect the healthy eating message. The balance scale should

Table 4.6. Web-Based Diet–Cancer Resources.

Organization	Website	Content
American Cancer Society	www.cancer.org	Dietary recommendations, eating tips, recipes,
American Institute of Cancer Research	www.aicr.org	Dietary recommendations, eating tips, recipes, ask the dietitian
Physicians' Committee for Responsible Medicine	www.cancerproject.org	Variety of resources from books to podcasts to videostreams
University Of Minnesota Cancer Center	http://www.cancer.umn.edu/ cancerinfo/prevention-diet.html	Wide variety of cancer prevention-diet resources; diet–cancer prevention guidelines
American Association for Cancer Research	www.aacr.org	Professional organization for cancer researchers from basic science to bedside. Updates on cancer prevention research
YouTube	www.youtube.com/ watch?v=yp6yy03GZ-Y&feature=related	Diet and cancer prevention video by registered dietitian Bonnie Taub-Dix, RD

provide immediate feedback regarding a healthy weight by placing a target weight poster above the scale along with a reminder that even small, incremental reductions in body weight for overweight people can have significant health benefits. The exam rooms could also be stocked with recipe booklets and/or pamphlets for increasing activity. Hand weights could be provided for clients to expend a few calories lifting while waiting for their physician visit. While behavior change is challenging, no behavior change can be expected if the message is not delivered. Further, small behavioral changes are more likely to be sustained and it is long-term behavior change that is necessary to reduce cancer risk.

REFERENCES

Calle EE, Rodriguez C, et al. (2003). Overweight, obesity, and mortality from cancer in a prospectively studied cohort of U.S. adults. *Neuroreport, 348*(17), 1625–1638.

Ferguson LR & Philpott M. (2007). Cancer prevention by dietary bioactive components that target the immune response. *Current Cancer Drug Targets, 7*(5), 459–464.

Hursting SD, Lashinger LM, Colbert LH, Rogers CJ, Wheatley KW, Nunez NP, et al. (2007). Energy balance and carcinogenesis: Underlying pathways and targets for intervention. *Current Cancer Drug Targets, 7*(5), 484–489.

Kushi LH, Byers T, et al. (2006). American cancer society guidelines on nutrition and physical activity for cancer prevention: Reducing the risk of cancer with healthy food choices and physical activity. *CA: A Cancer Journal for Clinicians, 56*, 254–281.

Liu RH. (2004). Potential synergy of photochemicals in cancer prevention: Mechanisms of action. *The Journal of Nutrition, 134*, 3479S–3485S.

Margolis KL, Rodabough RJ, Thomson CA, Lopez AM, & McTiernan A. (2007). Prospective study of leukocyte count as a predictor of incident breast, colorectal, endometrial and lung cancer and mortality in postmenopausal women. (For the WHI Research Group). *Archives of Internal Medicine, 167*(17), 1837–1844.

Milner JA. (2006). Diet and cancer: Facts and Controversies. *Nutrition and Cancer, 56*, 216–224.

Prentice R, Thomson CA, Caan B, Hubbell FA, Anderson GL, Beresford SA, et al. (2007). Low fat dietary pattern and cancer incidence in the women's health initiative dietary modification randomized controlled trial. *Journal of the National Cancer Institute, 99*(20), 1534–1543.

World Cancer Research Fund/American Institute for Cancer Research. (2007). Food, Nutrition, and the Prevention of Cancer: A Global Perspective, World Cancer Research Fund.

Xue F & Michels KB. (2007). Intrauterine factors and risk of breast cancer: A systematic review and meta-analysis of current evidence. *The Lancet Oncology, 8*(12), 1088–1100.

(A complete reference list for this chapter is available online at http://www.oup.com/us/integrativemedicine).

5

Nutritional Interventions in Cancer

KEITH I. BLOCK

KEY CONCEPTS

- Single vitamins, minerals, or antioxidants, in the absence of a comprehensive diet intervention, have very limited ability to prevent cancer or retard its progression.
- To control cancer-promoting inflammation, intake of animal fat and omega-6 fatty acids should be limited, while intake of omega-3 fatty acids and monounsaturated fats should be emphasized.
- To control insulin levels, carbohydrates should come from whole grain products, vegetables, and fruits, while refined flours and added sugars should be limited or eliminated.
- Plant proteins, egg whites, and fish are the safest protein sources for cancer patients.
- Soy isoflavone supplements, with possible estrogenic effects, should be avoided by patients with estrogen receptor positive breast cancer; a moderate intake of soy foods is unlikely to be problematic, especially if they are substituted for meats.
- Obesity worsens prognosis in several common cancers. Nutritional counseling should be provided to adjust caloric intake and physical activity levels to help patients achieve healthy weights.
- Several small studies indicate that specific foods or phytochemicals may improve specific cancer markers in patients with early stage cancers.
- Several alternative diets are of interest to cancer patients, some of which promote vegetable and fruit intake and plant-based diets. Dietary counseling is often needed with patients on these diets to optimize food choices and caloric intake.

- Nutritional counseling should routinely be provided to cancer patients to promote integrative dietary and physical activity goals. Patients with obesity or cachexia present special problems.

■

I n the conventional cancer treatment setting, nutrition has long been recognized to be of paramount importance in combating the malnutrition and wasting among patients in later stages of disease. In the integrative setting, however, nutrition plays a central role as part of a comprehensive approach addressing all stages of disease. It is considered essential in addressing not only malnutrition and ensuring adequate caloric intake but also for transforming the biological, molecular, and treatment environment needed to improve quality of life and survival. It should be noted at the outset, though, that nutritional therapy alone is not sufficient to optimize outcomes in cancer patients in the integrative care setting.

Integrative diets, which have been implemented clinically for over two decades at the author's clinical facility, the Block Center for Integrative Cancer Treatment, are typically based on whole food interventions, and aim to lower inflammatory potential, decrease insulin resistance, and promote high intake of vegetables and fruits rich in phytochemicals and antioxidants. Inflammation is now thought to play a major role in cancer, but anti-inflammatory diets (AID) may need to be supplemented and individualized with natural anti-inflammatory agents (Block, 2005) or prescription drugs to impact a given patient's cytokine environment. Dietary supplements may be needed to compensate for past and current nutritional deficits or the nutritional impacts of chemotherapy. Supplements need to be individualized to the patient's disease, stage, treatment history, and comorbidities. Supplementation may include selected botanicals in addition to nutrients and food concentrates. Comprehensive nutritional assessment and testing can provide critical information defining a patient's unique biochemical disruptions and imbalances. Such results, along with matching supplements to conventional therapies, symptoms and side effects, can help to optimize supplement use.

With the emerging recognition of the role of obesity in cancer has come the realization that physical activity and strength training must be incorporated to help patients achieve appropriate caloric balance for weight loss, gain, or maintenance. Systematic monitoring of weight and strength assessments must parallel physical activity interventions. Because of the major stresses of cancer, a mind–body program for stress management is also fundamental in integrative care. The isolation and life disruption of cancer warrants an emphasis on this mode of healing, as well as therapeutic bodywork that both relieves stress and facilitates physical activity. Developing a clinical intervention that incorporates all these approaches and applies them systematically to each patient's personal and biological needs is a scientific, therapeutic, and administrative challenge (Block, Block, & Gyllenhaal, 2004).

This chapter focuses on the nutritional intervention itself, with the understanding that good patient care necessitates a comprehensive approach with a full range of relevant treatment strategies. Scientific literature on the role of nutrition after the diagnosis of cancer is reviewed, and the potential mechanisms and effects of fats, proteins, carbohydrates, micronutrients, calories, and phytochemicals are then presented, with a short summary at the end of each section. We then briefly review the clinical approach used for nutritional counseling in our integrative cancer center. The outcomes that this chapter discusses are those related to countering disease progression, recurrence, and mortality, but readers should be aware that diet also has substantial potential to contribute to improving quality of life, especially during cancer treatment.

Integrative Diets, Reductionistic Research

Integrative, complementary, and alternative medical practices are commonly based on a holistic approach not only to patients but also to interventions. The integrative view of cancer is that while it arises out of a discrete set of genetic events, its progress is affected by systemic imbalances in multiple physiological systems. Cancers are known to comprise multiple, genetically diverse cellular clones that frequently develop resistance to treatments, resulting in recurrence. Integrative cancer interventions are therefore multifocal in nature rather than directed at single molecular targets (Block, 2003). Comprehensive lifestyle changes, major or even radical dietary adjustments, and frequently the use of natural compounds are enlisted to block potential pathways of cancer progression. These are considered justified both because of clinical studies and mechanistic analyses that indicate potential synergy of different dietary elements and because the epidemiological evidence relating nutrition and cancer outcomes is actually based on populations that eat whole foods in dietary patterns that are often correlated with other lifestyle characteristics.

In contrast, research in cancer-directed nutritional interventions has overwhelmingly been concentrated on single micro- or macronutrients. This focus arises in part because of the evolution of the scientific debates on diet and cancer: Does fat cause breast cancer? Can β-carotene prevent cancer? The reductionistic strategy arises also because of the relative ease of designing intervention studies that manipulate a single variable, preferably with a single pill. Interventions that simultaneously manipulate exercise, supplementation, and stress management patterns along with major dietary changes (e.g., eliminating meat and refined sugar consumption) in the context of medical treatment raise many questions. Little is known about reliable means to implement them, and researchers may question the wisdom of subjecting patients to such complicated regimens, even though these are exactly the regimens that are used by integrative practitioners. Research studies thus typically manipulate only one or a few nutritional variables. Synergies, whole foods, and effects of dietary patterns—the basis of integrative interventions—have thus scarcely even been addressed in the current evidence base for cancer nutrition. To provide an adequate scientific rationale for integrative nutrition, therefore, this chapter not only discusses recent reviews of clinical studies in cancer nutrition that generally focus on single nutrients but also surveys results of cohort studies of nutritional variables in cancer patients. Recent clinical trials of integrative-type diets and phytochemicals are also reviewed.

Current Status of Evidence for Nutritional Interventions in Cancer

A recent meta-analysis summarizes nutritional intervention studies in cancer and precancerous lesions (Davies, et al., 2006). Interventions in this review included overall dietary advice and a variety of single nutrient therapies such as vitamins, minerals, or antioxidants published before late 2003. Mortality and disease recurrence were assessed separately. Among the 19 trials conducted in patients with cancer, "healthy-diet" studies did not decrease mortality, although the three breast cancer trials in the study did suggest decreases in all-cause mortality (OR = 0.70, i.e., the diet group had only 70% of the mortality rate of the control group) and cancer-specific mortality (OR = 0.53). Antioxidant supplements did not decrease mortality. Thirteen trials reported effects on cancer recurrence or second cancers. The "healthy-diet" studies overall did not decrease recurrences, although the largest diet study (Sopotsinskaia, et al., 1992) reported an OR of 0.20 for recurrences for a low-fat diet group. Trials of retinol and antioxidants did not reduce recurrences overall, although results were variable. Coulter et al. (2006) analyzed the effects of vitamins E and C on cancer prevention, development of new tumors, and mortality. Significant benefits were found only in a study in which vitamin C was combined with other vitamins in a study of bladder cancer recurrence (in addition to BCG), a study in which vitamin E was combined with omega-3 fatty acids in advanced cancers, and one in which vitamin E was found to reduce new tumors in prostate cancer, without any effect on mortality.

The nutritional strategies of the studies included in these analyses differ substantially from contemporary integrative cancer care as previously presented by the author (Block, et al., 2004). The "healthy-diet" studies generally focused on low-calorie diets without specific changes to diet composition (although the study by Sopotsinskaia et al. counseled subjects to reduce fats and carbohydrate intake). Interventions in other studies were based simply on counseling patients to increase calories during cachexia or periods of nutritional risk. Use of single nutrients or antioxidants, as much as it may simplify experimental design, is not how most patients use supplements, and would not be considered by contemporary practitioners to be an integrative intervention. Some patients may indeed undertake supplementation with a single nutrient. They should be advised that such supplementation is unlikely to be productive.

To supplement the reductionistic experimental models used in the analyses of Davies et al. and Coulter et al., the results of cohort studies of diet in cancer patients can be examined. Table 5.1 lists studies published since 2000 that examined cancer mortality or recurrence in cohorts of patients with established cancers, in relationship to dietary variables. Vegetables, fruits, and phytochemicals in nearly all cases are associated with lower rates of cancer-related events, while higher fat intake usually increases rates of cancer-related events. Goodwin et al. (2003) reported a U-shaped survival curve, in which those with both the highest and the lowest intakes of carbohydrates had lowered survival, suggesting that both a high sugar/low protein diet pattern and a high-protein/high-fat pattern might reduce survival. Goodwin et al. (2002) and Borugian et al. (2004) observed that elevated fasting insulin (associated with insulin resistance and high body mass index (BMI)) doubled mortality, an observation possibly related to the poor survival of patients who ate large amounts of carbohydrates (most likely refined carbohydrates). Kroenke et al. (2005) assessed consumption of a "prudent" versus a Western diet, and observed that the healthy "prudent" dietary pattern appeared to reduce noncancer mortality but not cancer-specific mortality. This suggests some caution in interpreting results, although the "prudent" diets followed by the population observed may not approach integrative dietary recommendations.

Relevant clinical studies of integrative-type diets were published after the end of data collection for the reviews of Davies et al. and Coulter et al., or had alternative outcome variables or research designs, and were thus not included in their analyses. These trials indicate that manipulation of dietary patterns may indeed have positive effects in cancer. A trial of "watchful waiting" in prostate cancer patients randomized to a low-fat vegetarian diet and lifestyle program versus conventional care found reduced prostate-specific antigen (PSA) levels in the vegetarian group, but increased levels in the usual care group (Ornish, et al., 2005). A recent pilot study of a plant-based diet in men with rising PSA

Table 5.1. Cohort Studies Published in 2000 or Later Measuring Correlations of Nutritional Values with Cancer-related Outcomes in Patients with Established Cancers (Nonsignificant Values Noted).*

Cancer/Country	n	Outcome Variable	Nutritional Variable	Hazard/Risk Ratio*	Comments	References
Breast/USA	516	Mortality	Total fat	3.12	Postmenopausal, premorbid diet	Jaiswal McEligot, et al., 2006
			Fiber	0.48		
			Vegetables	0.57		
			Fruit	0.63, ns		
			α-carotene, dietary	0.77, ns		
			β-carotene, dietary	0.50		
			β-cryptoxanthin, dietary	0.54		
			Lutein, dietary	0.54		
			Lycopene, dietary	0.76, ns		
Breast/USA	1235	Mortality	Any fruit, fruit juice, or vegetable	0.68, ns	Postmenopausal only	Fink, et al., 2006
			Same	0.54, ns	ER + subjects	
			Same	0.66, ns	PR + subjects	
Breast/USA	1551	New breast cancer event	Plasma carotenoids	0.57	Control arm of diet intervention trial	Rock, et al., 2005
Breast/USA	2619	Nonbreast cancer mortality	Prudent diet	0.54	Diet pattern was not correlated with cancer-specific mortality	Kroenke, et al., 2005
		All-cause mortality	Western diet	1.53		

Breast/USA	177	Mortality	Dietary folate	0.88	Patients treated with antifolate chemotherapy	Sellers, et al., 2002
Breast/China	1459	Disease-free survival	Usual soy intake	0.99, ns		Boyapati, et al., 2005
Breast/Canada	520	Recurrence	Total cholesterol, serum	1.62	Early breast cancer, no hyperlipidemia or diabetes	Bahl, et al., 2005
Breast/Canada	603	Mortality	Fat Protein Insulin	4.8 0.40 1.9	Premenopausal Pre- and post menopausal Plasma level, post-menopausal	Borugian, et al., 2004
Breast/Canada	512	Distant recurrence	Insulin Insulin	2.0 3.1	Plasma level	Goodwin, et al., 2002
Breast/Canada	477	Mortality	% Protein % Fat % Carbohydrate Oleic acid PUFA/MUFA Cholesterol	1.9 (for lowest intake) 1.7 (for lowest intake) 1.3, 1.7 1.7 (for lowest intake) 1.6, 1.4 4.2 (for lowest intake)	Variables adjusted for BMI U-shaped curve, higher mortality for lowest and highest % U-shaped curve	Goodwin, et al., 2003

(continued)

Table 5.1. (Continued)

Cancer/Country	n	Outcome Variable	Nutritional Variable	Hazard/Risk Ratio*	Comments	References
Colorectal	511	Mortality	Meat (proxy for arginine intake)	2.24	Familial colorectal cancer	Zell, et al., 2007
				No association	Sporadic colorectal cancer	
Gastric/Italy	382	Mortality	Animal protein	2.07	Have first-degree relatives with gastric cancer	Palli, et al., 2000
			Animal fat	1.96	Have first-degree relatives with gastric cancer	
			Animal protein, fat	No association	No first-degree relatives with gastric cancer	
Prostate/US	1202	Progression	Fish	0.73		Chan, et al., 2006
			Tomato sauce	0.56		
			Milk	1.3 ns		
			Fresh tomatoes	1.58		
Prostate/Canada	408	Mortality	MUFA	0.3	All patients, premorbid diet	Kim, et al., 2000
			Energy intake	0.1	Toronto patients	
			Energy intake	2.6	Vancouver patients	

Cancer/Location	Number	Outcome	Dietary element	Ratio	Notes	Reference
Lung/Denmark	353	Mortality	All vegetables	0.84	Smokers	Skuladottir, et al., 2006
			Fruit	0.81		
			Potatoes	1.51		
Lung/USA	1129	Mortality	Multi-vitamin/ mineral use	0.74	Self-prescribed supplements	Jatoi, et al., 2005
Ovarian/Australia	609	Mortality	Vegetables	0.75	Protein, red and white meat had nonsignificant inverse correlation	Nagle, et al., 2003
			Crucifers	0.75		
			Lactose	1.32	Dairy products had nonsignificant positive correlation	
Laryngeal/ hypo-pharyngeal cancer, Southern Europe	876 males only	Second primary tumor incidence	Citrus	0.40	Lung tumors	Dikshit, et al., 2005
			Butter	10.7	Upper aero-digestive tract tumors	
Oral, pharyngeal or laryngeal	259	Mortality	Lycopene	0.53	Plasma values. All patients	Mayne, et al., 2004
			Lycopene	0.08	Nonsmokers	
			α-Carotene	0.25		
			Total carotenoids	0.22		

* Highest versus Lowest Comparison Group. Ratios geater than 1.0 indicate that larger amounts of relevant dietary element increase mortality or recurrence rates while ratios less than 1.0 indicate that larger amounts decrease mortality or recurrence.

ER, estrogen receptor; MUFA, monounsaturated fatty acids; PUFA, polyunsaturated fatty acids.

levels after conventional treatment observed significant reductions in the time it took PSA levels to double after 3–6 months on the diet (Saxe, et al., 2006). A randomized trial of a low-fat diet in early stage breast cancer patients resulted in a significantly lower risk of recurrence (HR = 0.76), especially among estrogen receptor negative patients (HR = 0.58) (Chlebowski, et al. 2006). These positive results, and the cohort studies listed in Table 5.1, suggest that there may be benefits to the typical integrative cancer diet that were missed in the recent systematic reviews.

Fats

Fats contribute to inflammatory potential in the diet (n-6 fats) and modulate the hormonal milieu (saturated fats). The role of nutrition and supplements in modulating the inflammatory cascade, including eicosanoids synthesized by cyclooxygenases and lipoxygenases is reviewed by Wallace (2002). Cyclooxygenase-2 (COX-2) is upregulated in and impacts the growth of most solid tumors. Through its product prostaglandin E2 (PGE2), it promotes cell proliferation, inhibits apoptosis, increases angiogenesis, and invasiveness and suppresses immune function. Nutritional modification of eicosanoids is accomplished by changing the composition of cyclooxygenase and lipoxygenase substrates—the dietary n-3 and n-6 essential fatty acids. Metabolism of the n-6 fatty acids linoleic acid (LA) and arachidonic acid (AA) results in the production of inflammatory eicosanoids. Metabolism of the n-3 fatty acids, such as α-linolenic acid (ALA) and eicosapentaenoic acid (EPA) results in anti-inflammatory, cancer-inhibiting eicosanoids. Because the n-3 and n-6 fatty acids are metabolized by the same enzymes, they act competitively in eicosanoid production. The primary nutritional intervention for decreasing the cancer-promoting eicosanoids is, therefore, lowering dietary intake of n-6 fatty acids, which predominate in the meats, poultry, and dairy components of the Western diet as well as several widely used vegetable oils (e.g., corn, soy, safflower). Integrative nutritional programs, such as that used at the Block Center, typically accomplish this by counseling patients with prescriptive dietary and supplement advice. Patients are counseled to increase consumption of cold-water fish, fish oil, and plant oils such as walnut and flax oil. To favorably affect clinical parameters, fish oil usually must be supplied in supplemental amounts.

Inflammation affects various aspects of cancer. Elevated inflammatory cytokines appear, for instance, to be a factor in post-chemotherapy fatigue in breast cancer survivors (Bower, et al., 2002; Collado-Hidalgo, Bower, Ganz, Cole, & Irwin, 2006). Jho et al. (2004) review studies of fish oil supplementation in various inflammatory diseases and conclude that there is evidence that supplementation improves clinical parameters related to inflammation. Specifically, studies in cancer cachexia (n = 5) and perioperative nutrition (n = 13) for gastrointestinal cancers in which n-3 fats were given, usually as liquid enterals, observed various improved clinical parameters. Other studies (Fearon, et al., 2006), however, did not reproduce these effects. Further, a meta-analysis of cohort studies and randomized trials of n-3 intake found that supplementation or n-3 intake did not result in lower cancer incidence or mortality (Hooper, et al., 2006). However, a critical problem with these studies is that none assessed or implemented the combined reduction of n-6 fats with n-3 supplementation, which may be needed to obtain clinically relevant effects.

As stressed by Simpoulos (2002) as well as in the nutritional programs of our Center, the n-6/n-3 ratio may need to be altered rather precisely. A study in which this ratio was adjusted to 2.5/1 resulted in reduced rectal cell proliferation in colorectal cancer patients, while a ratio of 4/1 did not, even though the absolute amount of n-3 fats was the same. Adam et al. (2003) observed this synergistic effect in a study of rheumatoid arthritis patients supplemented with fish oil and taking either a Western or an AID (only plant-derived oils, no egg yolks, only reduced-fat dairy products, meat only twice weekly). Patients on the Western diet experienced a 17% improvement in joint pain parameters, while those on the AID experienced a 31% improvement.

Saturated fats. Meat and poultry are major sources of AA in the Western diet, and low-fat diets commonly restrict animal fat intake. Studies of animal fats also suggest a potential adverse impact of saturated fat on cancer outcomes. Men with prostate cancer who had the highest intakes of saturated fat had a mortality rate three times higher than those whose diets were lowest in saturated fat (Meyer, Bairati, Shadmani, Fradet, & Moore, 1999). In the Iowa Women's Health Study, breast cancer patients with the highest consumption of saturated fat were twice as likely to die from their disease as women with the lowest intakes (Zhang, Folsom, Sellers, Kushi, & Potters, 1995). Breast cancer patients with the highest levels of serum cholesterol have a higher risk of recurrence than those in lower quartiles (Bahl, et al., 2005).

> Breast cancer patients who gain weight after diagnosis, including during chemotherapy treatment, have worsened prognoses.

Saturated fats may affect cancer in several ways, including reduction of natural killer cell activity (Barone, Hebert, & Reddy, 1989). An estrogen-lowering effect of low saturated-fat diets has been hypothesized to be relevant in breast cancer. A low-fat, high-fiber diet decreased serum estradiol in breast cancer patients (Rock, et al., 2004), although a low-fat, soy-supplemented diet given for 2 months did not (Wu, et al., 2005). A very low-fat diet combined with exercise, however, reduced serum estradiol after 2 weeks (Barnard, Gonazalez, Liva, & Ngo, 2006). Pre- and post-intervention serum samples from this study population were subjected to in vitro studies. Post-intervention serum decreased proliferation of breast cancer cell lines and increased apoptosis relative to preintervention samples.

Summary.   What level of dietary fat would be appropriate for cancer patients? Given the limitations of the current evidence, a dietary fat content of between 10% and 12% (goal of the Ornish study) and 20% (the goal of the Chlebowski study) may be appropriate. Our approach at the Block Center is to aim for a 14% to 18% fat diet for patients with cancers such as breast and prostate cancer (cachectic patients will be prescribed diets higher in specific fats to provide the caloric density needed in the situation of uncontrolled weight loss). Optimal fat sources are oils high in n-3 or monounsaturated fats, and fish oil supplementation to modify n-3/n-6 ratios should be instituted. Laboratory testing of nutritionally-related parameters (e.g., C-reactive protein, interleukin-6 and others) is used to tailor diet and supplement recommendations for patients' individual needs.

Carbohydrates

Carbohydrate intake became a focus of major interest in cancer with the realization of the relationships between type 2 diabetes and cancer occurrence. Obesity, type 2 diabetes, and the metabolic syndrome can result in insulin resistance, which leads to hyperinsulinemia, as well as an associated chronic inflammation (Bastard, et al., 2006). Cytokine abnormalities and elevated levels of insulin-like growth factor-1 (IGF-1), both known to promote cancer growth, also are correlated with hyperinsulinemia. Insulin and insulin-like growth factors were recently reviewed by Boyd (2003) and Kaaks (2004). Insulin increases the synthesis of IGF-1 and decreases its binding proteins (IGFBP-1 and-2). Both insulin and IGF-1 promote an anabolic state, stimulating tumor development and cell proliferation while inhibiting apoptosis. Several cancers are related to elevated levels of one or both, including colon, pancreas, endometrial, breast, and prostate cancers. This suggests that attention to factors that aggravate synthesis of insulin and IGF-1, including weight management and diet composition, may have a positive impact on these cancers.

Diet and the insulin-IGF-1 axis: carbohydrates and fats.   Whole grain intake has a significant inverse association with the metabolic syndrome and blood glucose (Sahyoun, Jacques, Zhang, Juan, & McKeown, 2006). Diets high in fiber are usually recommended in insulin resistance (McAuley & Mann,

2006), since fiber slows the absorption of dietary carbohydrates. A higher ratio of fiber to energy intake, for instance, was recently observed to be associated with lower insulin levels in postmenopausal women; high waist–hip ratio ("apple" body shape) and BMI predicted elevated insulin levels (Bhargava, 2006). Thus to minimize the likelihood of persistently elevated insulin levels in cancer patients, carbohydrates should come from whole grains or fiber-rich vegetables, and not from refined flours or sugar.

Low-carbohydrate diets, a recent weight loss fad, represent an error in thinking based on a lack of differentiation between complex and simple carbohydrates. Complex carbohydrates have advantages over simple carbohydrates in possessing lower glycemic index values. They should thus be encouraged, while simple carbohydrates should be discouraged or used sparingly. The potential seriousness of including high levels of simple sugars in the diet is shown in the finding of Goodwin et al. (2003) that elevated insulin levels predicted higher rates of distant metastasis and mortality in breast cancer patients. Simple sugar consumption is especially likely to raise insulin levels in patients with insulin resistance.

Another treatment for insulin resistance is low-fat diets, since lowering fat content may reduce the energy density and thus caloric content of the diet (depending upon what replaces the fat and whether food intake increases). Additionally, insulin resistance is shown in both epidemiological and intervention studies to be aggravated by saturated fat, while monounsaturated fats improve it (Riccardi, Giacco, & Rivellese, 2004). Animal studies have shown n-3 fats to enhance insulin sensitivity.

Summary.   Our approach at the Block Center to the problem of insulin resistance and cancer is to counsel patients to restrict or completely avoid refined flours and sugars, replacing them with whole grain products, to promote normal insulin levels. Further counseling on carbohydrate intake is necessary for overweight patients who are likely to be insulin resistant.

Protein

Consumption of red meat, liver, and bacon resulted in a doubling in the risk of breast cancer recurrence for each time that these were consumed on a daily basis in an observational study (Hebert, Hurley, & Ma, 1998). Red meats contain high amounts of iron, an oxidant that may drive malignancies.

Although large prospective studies of breast cancer do not suggest that animal fat consumption elevates breast cancer incidence (Kim, et al., 2006), a recent study indicated higher risk of estrogen receptor positive/progesterone receptor positive breast cancer among premenopausal women with high red meat intake (Cho, et al., 2006).

Soy products. The potential impact of soy on breast cancer prognosis was recently summarized by Messina et al. (2006). Soy isoflavones have a molecular structure similar to estrogens, and bind to estrogen receptors. They exert estrogen-like effects in some experimental conditions, and genistein, a major isoflavone, also stimulates growth of some estrogen-sensitive tumor cell lines in laboratory studies. However, genistein and other isoflavones also have non-estrogenic activities that inhibit cancer cell growth, making them potentially useful in a variety of cancers. A recent meta-analysis of 18 epidemiological studies that examined soy and breast cancer risk concluded that soy intake is associated with a modestly reduced risk of breast cancer (OR = 0.86); this relationship was stronger in premenopausal women (Trock, Hilakivi-Clarke, & Clarke, 2006). While a definitive statement on soy and breast cancer is not possible at this time, most experts feel that modest intake of soy foods as part of the diet is reasonable for breast cancer patients (Block, et al., 2002), but that soy isoflavone supplements need further evaluation in high-risk women (Messina, McCaskill-Stevens, & Lampe, 2006) and are questionable for estrogen receptor positive breast cancer patients. Soy foods as part of the diet may be helpful since many meat substitutes are made from soy, and these are generally lower in calories and fat than the meats they replace.

Use of soy products in prostate cancer is less controversial, and randomized trials of soy and prostate-related variables have been conducted. A recent cross-over trial of a high-soy (2 servings daily) versus a low-soy diet in healthy men with normal PSA levels found that PSA levels declined by 14% ($P = 0.10$) while serum testosterone did not change (Maskarinec, et al., 2006). A 2-step study in asymptomatic, hormonally naïve prostate cancer patients of a low-fat diet, with soy protein supplementation added in case of PSA progression, observed a trend toward longer PSA doubling time and prolongation of time to progression during the soy phase versus the low-fat phase. IGF-1 levels also increased during the soy phase, a potentially undesirable effect (Spentzos, et al., 2003). A slight increase in IGF-1 was also observed in a study by Maskarinec et al. (2005) of premenopausal women, and was attributed to higher protein intake. A study of low-soy, high-soy, and milk protein diets in young men observed a greater reduction of dihydrotestosterone on the high- than the low-soy diet (Dillingham, McVeigh, Lampe, & Duncan, 2005). Both soy diets were lower than the milk diet. Testosterone was decreased during the low-soy diet relative to the other two diets; there were also minor effects on other hormones. These effects may be positive for prostate cancer but need more investigation.

Dairy products. IGF-1, a tumor growth factor, is found in cow's milk, and long-term consumption of milk may increase levels of IGF-1 in humans (Hoppe,

Molgaard, & Michaelsen, 2006). Epidemiological studies have observed higher levels of IGF-1 in Western than non-Western populations (Larsson, Wolk, Brismar, & Wolk, 2005; Morimoto, Newcomb, White, Bigler, & Potter, 2005; Norat, et al., 2007). British women who never drank milk had a lower risk of insulin resistance (OR = 0.55) than milk drinkers (Lawlor, Ebrahim, Timpson, & Davey Smith, 2005). Epidemiological evidence suggests a moderate association of IGF-1 with breast cancer in premenopausal women (Rinaldi, et al., 2005; Schernhammer, Holly, Pollak, & Hankinson, 2005), although overall dairy consumption has not been related to breast cancer risk (Parodi, 2005). High calcium and dairy intake have been positively associated with prostate cancer risk (Giovannucci, Liu, Stampfer, & Willett, 2006; Tseng, Breslow, Graubard, & Zieler, 2005), through a calcium- or vitamin D-related pathway. A meta-analysis of 12 cohort studies of dairy consumption indicates a modest elevation of ovarian cancer risk at high levels of lactose consumption (Genkinger, et al., 2006). These observations suggest caution about the role of milk products in cancer, as well as awareness of the potential need for vitamin D supplementation, especially in patients consuming high levels of dietary calcium.

Few intervention studies have examined the effects of milk on insulin, insulin resistance, or IGF-1. High intakes of milk, but not meat, (53 g protein/day, 7 days) increased serum insulin and insulin resistance in children (Hoppe, Molgaard, Vaag, Barkholt, & Michaelsen, 2005). Increasing soy consumption alone did not decrease IGF-1 level in premenopausal women, but may slightly increase the level because of greater protein intake (Maskarinec, et al., 2005). However, prostate cancer patients who consumed the highest levels of milk had a small elevation of risk of recurrence or mortality, while fish and tomato sauce were associated with lower risk (Chan, et al., 2006). The whey protein fraction of milk has been associated with increased glutathione in laboratory studies and is considered potentially beneficial in cancer, while the casein fraction is commonly used as a tumor stimulant in animals.

Summary.   Proteins most suitable for cancer patients include vegetable proteins, fish and moderate amounts of soy foods. High levels of dairy products should not be encouraged.

Micronutrients

Micronutrients include vitamins and minerals. As discussed earlier, randomized trials of supplementation with single vitamins have not been found to be effective in suppressing cancers. Some controlled trials have shown increased mortality or higher cancer rates with vitamin supplementation, casting even the common multivitamin supplement into a controversial position. Bairati et al., (2006), for instance, showed increased mortality in a study of vitamin E supplementation for head and neck cancer patients who were given radiation therapy. β-Carotene was also given early in this study but was discontinued following reports of increased lung cancer incidence with supplementation in the Alpha-Tocopherol, Beta-Carotene (ATBC) study in Finland.

A more recent analysis of a cohort from the ATBC study showed that higher baseline levels of serum vitamin E were associated with lower total, cancer, and cardiovascular mortality (Wright, et al., 2006). This suggests that vitamin E derived from diet may be protective whereas that from supplements is not (only 10% of ATBC subjects used supplements at baseline). Baseline data from the ATBC study were also subjected to principal components analysis (PCA) to determine a comprehensive dietary antioxidant index (Wright, et al., 2006) based on carotenoids, flavonoids, vitamins E and C, and selenium. This index was then tested against lung cancer incidence in the ATBC cohort. Relative risk calculation showed a highly significant inverse relationship between dietary antioxidants and lung cancer. Both of Wright's studies suggest that specific vitamins or minerals that predict cancer mortality in an epidemiological study may be more productively viewed as markers for dietary intake of certain food classes or complex mixtures, rather than as single compounds to be extracted and given as supplements.

With this interpretation in mind, Table 5.2 was assembled to show the effects of micronutrient levels on mortality or recurrence in cohort studies of cancer patients. Supplemental use of vitamins C and E had contradictory data on cancer events in different studies, although both studies of multiple-antioxidant users found reduced risks with use [supplement users also have higher fiber, fruit, and vegetable intake, are less likely to smoke or drink alcohol, and are more physically active than nonusers (Touvier, Kesse, Volatier, Clavel-Chapelon, & Boutron-Ruault, 2006)]. A larger number of studies observed intake of vitamins contained in foods. Three studies of dietary vitamin C, likely a marker of fruit and vegetable intake, found reduced risk with higher vitamin C intake, while three found no association. Two studies of vitamin E found no association with risk, two found inverse associations, and three observed positive associations. Two studies of vitamin A found no association and one a positive association with risk. It should be noted that dietary vitamin E is likely associated with fat intake, and preformed vitamin A with animal products. More studies of dietary intake thus found reduced risks of cancer events with vitamins E and C than studies of supplementation. This suggests that whole foods or food extracts may be a more reliable means of reducing risks than single nutrient supplementation. Supplements given to patients with inadequate diets should be as close to whole foods as possible, for example, mixed tocopherols and mixed carotenoids.

Other micronutrients have also recently attracted attention. In two meta-analyses, calcium supplementation has been determined to reduce adenoma recurrence as well as colorectal cancer in patients with previous adenomas (Shaukat, Scouras, & Schunemann, 2005; Weingarten, et al., 2005). Men with low selenium levels appear to be at increased risk of prostate cancer (Brinkman, Reulen, Kellen, Buntinx, & Zeegers, 2006), and a trial of selenium supplementation in patients with skin cancers found reduced overall cancer mortality and reduced incidence of prostate, lung, and colorectal cancers—although no reduction of skin cancer recurrences (Combs, Clark, & Turnbull, 1997). A trial of selenium and vitamin E in prostate cancer prevention has consequently been initiated, the SELECT trial. Dietary heme iron in red meat catalyzes oxidative damage and may be involved in initiating cancers (Tappel, 2007), suggesting that iron supplementation and red meat should be avoided in cancer (iron supplementation may be necessary when iron-deficiency anemia is confirmed by lab testing). Copper is involved in multiple pathways of angiogenesis, suggesting that copper supplementation should be avoided (Brewer & Merajver, 2002). Magnesium may play both promoting and inhibiting roles in cancer growth (Wolf, et al., 2007). More important clinically, however, is the magnesium depletion that may accompany treatment with cisplatin or cetuximab. Low magnesium levels may increase the cardiotoxicity of anthracyclines as well. Supplementation with magnesium is thus undertaken with patients in treatment, and supplementation with other micronutrients may also be needed.

Vitamin D and sunlight have recently taken on a new importance in cancer. While sunlight has for a decade or more been avoided as a cause of skin cancers, several studies have recently shown a dependence of cancer survival on season of diagnosis. Norwegian breast cancer patients diagnosed in the summer, for example, have better prognosis than those diagnosed in the winter (Porojnicu, et al., 2007). Patients from southern Norway diagnosed in summer had a relatively better prognosis than those from the north, where summer sun exposure is lower. The differential was not found for patients diagnosed in winter, when sun exposure is similar in both regions, even though dietary vitamin D is 17% higher in the north. Similar findings are seen in the study of Zhou et al. (2005) summarized in Table 5.2. Preliminary studies of both cholecalciferol and calcitriol supplementation in prostate cancer have observed promising results (Gross, Stamey, Hancock, & Feldman, 1998; Woo, Choo, Jamieson, Chander, & Vieth, 2005).

Summary.   Specific micronutrient supplementation may be needed for patients in treatment or those with inadequate food intake. General micronutrient supplementation should be as close to dietary forms as possible, emphasizing food extracts, concentrates, and micronutrient mixtures.

Table 5.2. Cohort Studies Measuring Correlations of Nutritional Values with Cancer-Related Outcomes in Patients with Established Cancers (Nonsignificant Values Noted). Studies Published before 2000 Are Included.

Cancer/Country	n	Outcome Variable	Nutritional Variable, Type of Intake	Hazard/Risk Ratio*	Comments	References
Breast/USA	99	Recurrence	Vitamin C supplements, >500 mg/day	0.11	Patients receiving stem cell transplants, self-prescribed supplements	Bruemmer, et al., 2003
Breast/USA	385	Mortality or recurrence	Antioxidant supplements	0.54	Supplement users vs. nonusers, after diagnosis	Fleischauer, et al., 2003
			Vitamin E supplements	0.33	Used supplements 3 years or more, after diagnosis	
			Premorbid dietary vitamins E and C	No association		
Breast/USA	516	Mortality	Folate, dietary	0.34	Postmenopausal, premorbid diet	Jaiswal McEligot, et al., 2006
			Vitamin C, dietary	0.45		
Breast/Australia	412	Mortality	Vitamin C, dietary	0.76		Rohan, et al., 1993
Breast/Canada	641	Mortality	Vitamin C, dietary	0.48		Jain, et al., 1994
Breast/USA	698	Mortality	Vitamin A, dietary	No association		Zhang, et al., 1995
			Vitamin C, dietary	No association		
			Vitamin E, dietary	No association		
Breast/France			Vitamin E, plasma level over 22 μmol/L	1.7	Value adjusted for TNM status	Saintot, et al., 2002

Site/Country	N	Outcome	Dietary element	Ratio	Comments	Reference
Breast/Sweden	240	Treatment failure in 1st 2 years of followup	Vitamin E, 1-mg increase in intake per 10 megajoules energy	1.19	Fat intake as percentage of total energy intake also predicts failure	Holm, et al., 1993
Gastric/Italy	382	Mortality	Vitamin E, dietary Vitamin C, dietary Retinol	0.75 1.02, ns 1.13, ns		Jain, et al., 1994
Leukemia/USA	321	Nonrelapse mortality Mortality or relapse	Vitamin C supplements, >500 mg/day Vitamin E supplements, >400 IU/day	2.25 1.77	Patients receiving stem cell transplants, self-prescribed supplements Patients receiving stem cell transplants, self-prescribed supplements	Bruemmer, et al., 2003 Bruemmer, et al., 2003
Lung/USA	1129	Mortality	Multi-vitamin/mineral use	0.74	Self-prescribed supplements	Jatoi, et al., 2005
Lung (NSCLC)/USA	456	Recurrence-free survival	Vitamin D, dietary	No association	Pts with high vitamin D blood levels and surgery in summer had HR of 0.32 vs. patients with low vitamin D and surgery in winter	Zhou, et al., 2005
Ovarian/Australia	609	Mortality	Vitamin E, dietary	0.75	Calcium had a positive, nonsignificant association	Nagle, et al., 2003
Oral, pharyngeal or laryngeal	259	Mortality	Retinol, plasma Alpha-tocopherol, plasma	3.56 2.47	Smokers only	Mayne, et al., 2004

*Highest versus Lowest Comparison Group. Ratios geater than 1.0 indicate that larger amounts of relevant dietary element increase mortality or recurrence rates while ratios less than 1.0 indicate that larger amounts decrease mortality or recurrence.

Caloric Balance

Weight management in cancer is critical in two situations: counteracting the uncontrolled weight loss of cancer cachexia in lung and gastrointestinal cancers, and reducing risk of recurrence or progression in breast, prostate, and ovarian cancer. Cancer cachexia is now felt to be associated with high levels of pro-inflammatory cytokines (Argiles, 2005). Dietary interventions for cachexia typically involve elevating caloric intake. Enteral formulas that contain high levels of n-3 fatty acids have been developed (Jho, Cole, Lee, & Espat, 2004) and are now being tested along with various supplements (e.g., green tea polyphenols) and prescribed medications (megestrol acetate, Celebrex) (Mantovani, et al., 2006). A combination of fish oil and melatonin stabilized weight in a small trial (Persson, et al., 2005). Careful food choices are necessary for cachectic patients to favorably adjust caloric intake without increasing intake of LA or AA.

> For patients with cachexia, increased caloric intake is crucial. To ensure adequate calories, an increased amount of dietary fats is appropriate, but healthy fats should be used, including omega-3 fatty acids and monounsaturated fats. Medium chain triglycerides are also useful.

Excess body weight was recently estimated to account for 14% of cancer deaths in men, and 20% of cancer deaths in women in the United States (Calle, Rodriguez, Walker-Thurmond, & Thun, 2003). Excess body weight appears to increase risk of tumor recurrences. Obese and overweight breast cancer patients are more likely to have disease recurrences or to die of breast cancer (Loi, et al., 2005; Whiteman, et al., 2005). Increased BMI is associated with higher recurrence rates after radical prostatectomy, and with the development and progression of renal cancer (Amling, 2004). Both obese and underweight (possibly cachectic) women with colon cancer are at increased risk of death (Doria-Rose, et al., 2006). Among ovarian cancer patients with advanced disease (FIGO Stages 3–4), obesity was associated with shorter time to recurrence and overall survival (Pavelka, et al., 2006). Obesity also increases complications after cancer surgery, predisposes patients to second cancers, complicates chemotherapy dosing and reduces immune functioning (McTiernan, 2005).

These studies suggest that avoiding weight gain, and in fact, achieving weight loss to normalize BMI may be a strategy to reduce recurrence or mortality risks in certain cancers. Low-fat diets have been advocated for weight loss and cancer risk reduction. However, in the Women's Health Initiative, counseling subjects to a low-fat diet alone did not result in as high a difference in dietary fat as originally planned, much less caloric intake (Kim, et al., 2006). This suggests that weight control will need a more comprehensive approach to dietary change: addition of strong patient education and training along with exercise counseling may be needed to achieve a negative caloric balance.

Summary.   Specific counseling and psychological support regarding both food intake and exercise patterns, including proper choices of foods, will likely be necessary to intervene with overweight cancer patients. Patients with cachexia, however, need to be counseled in high-calorie food choices that do not promote inflammation, and may need specially developed protein-calorie supplements.

Fruits, Vegetables, and Phytochemicals

While the guideline of five servings daily of fruits and vegetables has been widely accepted in nutritional circles, seven servings daily are actually recommended for cancer prevention (World Cancer Research Fund, 1997). The Block Center program recommends a dozen or more servings, particularly in patients whose lab assessments indicated moderate to marked oxidative stress. Fruits and vegetables may contribute to cancer prevention either through decreasing the caloric density of the diet or through the additive and synergistic activities of phytochemicals (Liu, 2004). Aggarwal & Shishodia (2006) point out that common processes underlie the prevention of cancer and its treatment, specifically molecularly targeted cell-signaling pathways. Numerous agents identified in fruits and vegetables and dietary condiments may interfere with multiple signaling pathways that have therapeutic relevance in cancer. Curcumin (from turmeric) alone targets NF-κB, AP-1, COX-2, 5-LOX, IKK, HER-2, JNK and others. Green tea and resveratrol (grape) also target multiple signaling pathways. Other phytochemicals including lycopene (tomato), ellagic acid (pomegranate, berries), indole-3-carbinol (crucifers) also show inhibition of signaling pathways. NF-κB, for instance, is inhibited by phytochemicals found in many foods, including blueberries, raspberries, grapes, chili peppers, tea, tomato, citrus, licorice, oranges, and broccoli. These foods are being investigated as concentrates and extracts in addition to dietary elements. We will examine both the overall roles of high fruit and vegetable diets and a few phytochemical sources of interest.

High fruit and vegetable diets.   Fruits and vegetables are low in fat and caloric density, and may replace fatty foods in the diet, resulting in weight loss in addition to increases in phytochemicals. The Women's Healthy Eating and Living Study has shown that it is possible to increase the intake of phytochemical-rich fruits and vegetables in cancer survivors, in addition to lowering dietary fats (Pierce, et al., 2004). Fruit and vegetable intake can also be increased in head and neck cancer (Cartmel, Bowen, Ross, Johnson, & Mayne, 2005) and Barrett esophagus (Kristal, et al., 2005). However, increases in fruit and vegetable content, and lowering of dietary fat did not change weight or body composition in breast cancer patients after 6 months (Thomson, et al., 2005), and did not inhibit biomarkers of cellular proliferation in Barrett esophagus (Kristal, et al., 2005). A small trial of low-fat versus high fruit/vegetable diets found that the oxidative stress marker 8-isoprostane-F2α did not change in high fruit/vegetable diets, but only in low-fat diets, which resulted in weight loss in this study. Changes in BMI were associated with changes in the marker levels (Chen, et al., 2004).

Observational studies, however, indicate that there is more to be explored in this area, as can be seen in some studies in Table 5.1. Among 353 lung cancer patients in a prospective study, for instance, a reduced risk of mortality was found in those with high consumption of vegetables (HR 0.81) and fruits (HR 0.84) (Skuladottir, Tjonneland, Overvad, Stripp, & Olsen, 2006). In the Polyp Prevention Trial those in the highest quartile of increase in dry bean intake— an increase of 370% over baseline—had a significantly reduced (OR = 0.35) risk of advanced adenoma recurrence (Lanza, et al., 2006).

Phytochemicals and cancer. Table 5.3 shows results of recent experimental studies of food extracts/phytochemicals in cancer, with studies of prostate cancer predominating. Epidemiological studies have detected a strong inverse relationship between prostate cancer risk and tomato consumption. As lycopene was the most active carotenoid in laboratory testing, intervention trials were begun using lycopene-rich tomato concentrates as well as tomato diets. One model that was examined was the pre-prostatectomy intervention. In a study by Bowen et al. (2002) patients with localized prostate adenocarcinoma diagnosed by biopsy were given tomato sauce–enriched pasta dishes for 3 weeks before radical prostatectomy. Prostatic lycopene levels tripled compared to biopsy levels. Compared to biopsy specimens, the prostatectomy specimens had lower levels of 8-hydroxydeoxyguanosine (8-OHdG) in prostate cells, as well as lower leukocyte 8-OHdG in serum. Apoptotic index was also higher in these lycopene-rich prostatectomy samples than in biopsy samples.

A second model for assessing effects of supplements on prostate cancer is the post-prostatectomy rising PSA (biochemical recurrence) model used by Saxe et al. (2006). In these studies, rising PSA demonstrates disease recurrence, but no visible metastases are present. Stabilization or lowering of the rising PSA, or an increase in the PSA doubling time (the time before PSA levels double), indicate an antineoplastic effect. This model was used in the studies of Pantuck et al. (2006) and Schroder et al. (2005). Of the studies in Table 5.2, those that used models such as PSA doubling time, indicating slowing of disease progression, were more successful than those that used standard measures such as disease regression. Two phase I studies of green tea in advanced cancers showed small rates of disease stability. A study of flaxseed in breast cancer patients, however, showed substantial lowering of Ki-67 and c-erB2 expression, and higher levels of apoptosis in cells of patients receiving flax supplements before definitive surgery (Thompson, Chen, Strasser-Weippl, & Goss, 2005). Flax is high in lignans that have cancer-suppressive potential.

Summary. Phytochemically rich foods show promise in limiting particular cancers. Diets high in fruits and vegetables can decrease caloric density of the overall diet while providing fiber and exposure to a wide variety of phytochemicals.

Clinical Application of Integrative Diets

Epidemiological and mechanistic perspectives on the role of diet in cancer suggest far more potential for improvement of cancer outcomes than has so far been determined in reductionistic experimental models. It is the whole pattern of combined food choices, exercise, and supplements that may be the "active constituent" in integrative care. Synergisms, such as that demonstrated by Adam et al. (2003) in the AID and fish oil, may be much more critical, and widespread, than has been acknowledged to date. It is clear from the discussions of obesity and insulin resistance that inflammation, fat, and carbohydrate choices, and caloric balance may all be involved in the maintenance of a cancer-promoting or cancer-resisting environment. Combinations of fruits and vegetables may be more effective than the single nutrients used in most experiments: A recent in vivo study of lycopene, tomato, and broccoli found that the vegetables given alone reduced implanted tumor growth by 34% and 42% respectively, while lycopene alone reduced growth by only 7% to 18%. Giving both vegetables together reduced growth by 52% (Canene-Adams, et al., 2007). Nutritional research has barely scratched the surface of the provocative findings on the epidemiology of cancer and diet. Patients and integrative practitioners, however, find the mechanistic and epidemiological arguments compelling, and the risks of eating fruits, vegetables, whole grains, and legumes small. Given the disappointing results of many areas of conventional cancer treatment, the most rational path appears to many practitioners to be the adoption of the integrative nutritional strategies.

Food choices, caloric intake, and individualization by type and stage of cancer are all of potential relevance in cancer therapy. In addition, patients seeking consultation on integrative diets may already have adopted one of the alternative diet therapies, and may need to be counseled with sensitivity to the benefits and drawbacks of such diets. This section will review these alternative

Table 5.3. Experimental Studies of Phytochemicals/Foods/Food Extracts in Established Cancers with Variables Related to Disease Progression or Response.

Disease	Model	n	Supplement	Outcome Variable	Results	Reference
Breast	Post biopsy, before definitive surgery	32	Flaxseed	Ki-67 labeling c-erB2 expression Apoptosis	34.2% decrease 71% decrease 30.7% increase No change in placebo group	Thompson, et al., 2005
Lung	Advanced cancers, Phase I	17	Green tea extract	Disease progression	7 with stable disease up to 16 weeks; no CR or PR	Laurie, et al., 2005
Prostate	Hormone refractory	19	Green tea extract	PSA or measurable disease progression	9 patients had progression after 2 months	Choan, et al., 2005
Prostate	Hormone refractory	42	Green tea	PSA decline $>/=$ 50%	2% response	Jatoi, et al., 2003
Prostate	Preprostatectomy	26	Lycopene	% with tumor volume $<$ 4 mL Organ-confined disease (lycopene versus placebo group)	80% vs.45% 72% vs. 18%	Kucuk, et al., 2002
Prostate	Biochemical relapse	36	Lycopene	PSA response	0 PSA decrease 63% SD	Clark, et al., 2006
Prostate	Metastatic cancer	20	Lycopene	PSA normalization and disappearance of disease	5% CR 30% PR 50% SD	Ansari, et al., 2004

Prostate	Metastatic cancer	54	Lycopene + orchiectomy	PSA response Mortality (lycopene versus placebo group)	3.01 vs 9.02 ng/mL 7% vs. 22%	Ansari, et al., 2003
Prostate	Preprostatectomy	29	Soy grits versus wheat control	Total PSA (pre- versus post-prostatectomy)	−12% vs +40%	Dalais, et al., 2004
Prostate	Preprostatectomy	32	Tomato sauce	Serum PSA Apoptotic index (pre- versus post-prostatectomy)	17.5% decrease Increase	Bowen, et al., 2002
Prostate	Biochemical relapse	48	Pomegranate juice	PSA doubling time (pre-versus post-juice)	15 m to 54 m	Pantuck, et al., 2006
Prostate	Preprostatectomy	13 (11 assessable)	Soy isoflavone supplement	Serum testosterone decrease Serum estrogen decrease ERα decreased AR expression	9 of 11 subjects 8 of 10 subjects Highest dose level No effect	van Veldhuizen, et al., 2006
Prostate	Biochemical relapse	49	Soy isoflavones, lycopene, silymarin, antioxidants	PSA doubling time (pre- versus post-supplementation)	445 d to 1150 d	Schroeder, et al., 2005
Prostate	Biochemical relapse	80	Vitamin E, selenium, vitamin C, Co-Q10	Serum PSA, testosterone, dihydrotestosterone, luteinizing hormone, sex-hormone binding globulin	No differences versus control group	Hoenjet, et al., 2005
Solid tumors	Phase I	49	Green tea	Tumor response	10 SD	Pisters, et al., 2001

AR, androgen receptor; CR, complete response; PR, partial response; SD, stable disease.

diets and then briefly discuss the assessments, food recommendations, and counseling strategies implemented at the Block Center for Integrative Cancer Treatment.

Alternative cancer diets.   Most "alternative" diets used by cancer patients follow rather closely the low-fat, plant-based pattern described above. However the diets are potentially problematic for cancer patients in certain situations and generally lack the quantitation of food intake necessary for optimal diet therapy. Five such diets are commonly used.

Macrobiotic Diet.   The macrobiotic diet is an adaptation of the traditional Japanese diet. It comprises 50% to 70% whole grains, 20% to 25% vegetables, 5% to 10% beans and sea vegetables and 5% vegetable soups. Nuts, seeds, fruits, and fish are consumed occasionally, but red meat, dairy, and sugar are avoided. Macrobiotic counselors adapt the diet according to personal conditions, season, climate, and other factors. Difficulties can arise for patients with cachexia due to the low caloric density of this diet.

Gerson Diet.   Max Gerson developed this diet in the early 1900s. It emphasizes a vegetarian diet, raw vegetables, and fruit juices. Fasting and coffee enemas are included in the protocol, which can be very rigorous and sometimes difficult to follow. Monitoring for adequate protein intake in patients with cachexia is necessary, and the intake of fruit juice may compromise blood sugar control.

Kelly Diet (Metabolic types).   Developed by dentist William Kelly, this diet is similar to the Gerson diet but includes more cooked foods and animal proteins, pancreatic enzymes, fasting, colonic irrigation, and coffee enemas. Diets are tailored to the type of cancer and aspects of the patient's condition, classified as metabolic types. Diets high in vegetables and fruits are recommended for some cancers, but other cancers require high-meat diets, which are questionable on epidemiologic grounds. A variant used by Nicholas Gonzalez adds supplementation with micronutrients, amino acids, glandular substances, and digestive enzymes. The very large number of supplements can be problematic for some patients.

Living Foods Diet.   Ann Wigmore of the Hippocrates Institute developed a diet based on only raw foods, fermented vegetables, sprouted grains, and juices such as wheatgrass juice. Inadequate protein and n-3 fatty acid intakes have been raised as potential problems with long-term use of this diet.

Atkins Diet.   This diet, developed by Robert Atkins, is based on a marked reduction in carbohydrate consumption, emphasizing fats and proteins to promote weight loss. A supplementation program includes multivitamins and essential fatty acids. The low intake of fiber from limited grain intake, general lack of emphasis on fruits and vegetables, and high animal protein levels of this diet are not consistent with the studies reviewed above.

Nutritional assessments and individualizing the integrative diet.   The Block Center for Integrative Cancer Treatment serves a patient population with a high diversity of cancer types, generally concentrated in more advanced disease stages. A majority of patients attending the outpatient chemotherapy unit, in fact, have recurrent or Stage IV disease and many have recurred following multiple prior chemotherapies. With a high proportion of patients thus at increased risk for nutritional complications, the Center has developed a strong nutritional counseling protocol. Diet recommendations are individualized for cancer type, stage of disease, nutritional status at intake and underlying biochemical and metabolic predispositions of the patient. All nutritional counseling at the Center is provided by registered dietitians, and supervised by staff physicians. Nutritional counseling begins with traditional dietetic assessment of patients as to current intake (1- to 3-day food records and food frequency questionnaire); assessment of BMI, recent weight gain, or loss along with physical signs of cachexia; and discussion of potential nutritional risk factors such as overweight and obesity, current conventional treatments, or weight loss induced by cancer or cancer treatment. Body composition is also assessed. Specific recommendations for caloric intake are based on height and weight using the Harris-Benedict equation. These recommendations are modified based on the need to gain or lose weight depending on nutritional risk factors. The Center uses recognized nutritional standards for calculating grams of protein per kg body weight for patients with cachexia as well as patients of normal weight.

The Center uses laboratory tests to determine aspects of nutritional risk that may dictate food choices and dietary supplement use. The internal biochemical environment of each patient is assessed to determine the presence of factors such as inflammation, insulin resistance, oxidation, immunological deficits or other conditions that could promote cancer progression or recurrence. Tests used for these conditions include C-reactive protein, fibrinogen, blood sugar, and insulin levels, oxidized LDL, levels of specific phytochemicals such as tocopherols and carotenoids, CBC and natural killer cell cytotoxicity. In addition, whenever possible a variety of tumor markers are assessed in tumor tissue in addition to commonly reported markers. If assessing the biochemical environment indicates excessive inflammation, oxidation, or other abnormal values, specific food choice and supplement recommendations are made. If the tests indicate pathological levels of these factors, prescription drugs may be used to normalize these values. Patients who have low levels of phytochemicals are given recommendations for food choices (Mayland, Bennett, & Allan 2005). If levels are particularly low and do not recover, specific dietary supplements (e.g., mixed tocopherols, mixed carotenoids, vitamin C) are advised. If tumor markers indicate that molecular target drugs (e.g., trastuzumab) will be useful, they are prescribed. However, if molecular targets that lack current drug recommendations are present, we recommend selected nutraceuticals that are supported by experimental or early clinical trial evidence.

Food choices for patients are summarized in a series of seven recommendations, as follows:

1. Eat large amounts of vegetables and fruits, emphasizing diversity by using different plant families (e.g., crucifers, onions) and phytochemical content as shown in bright colors.
2. Consume plentiful whole grains and whole grain products.
3. Consume an adequate amount of calories and protein to maintain or attain healthy body weight, emphasizing proteins from legumes, soyfoods, fish, and n-3 rich eggs.
4. Limit total fat intake, shifting towards n-3 fats and monounsaturated fats.
5. Substitute milk, cheese, and ice cream with nondairy alternatives based on soy, rice, oat, almond, or related products.
6. Use fruits and small amounts of healthful sweeteners (e.g., rice syrup, barley malt, agave, kiwi, stevia) to reduce sweet cravings.
7. Drink adequate, healthful fluids including safe water, herb teas, green tea, and diluted fruit juice to maintain hydration.

Patients are given specific recommendations for quantifying the amounts of vegetables, fruits, grains, proteins, nuts and oils, and other foods, based on calculations of caloric totals and protein content. Specific foods are given ratings based on one to three stars, and patients are given lists of foods to emphasize and others to avoid. Dietitians instruct patients on portion sizes and practicalities such as shopping; a support group is available for patients working on diet change. With patients who are overweight or suffering muscle loss due to cachexia, dietitians work with the staff physicians on countering underlying physiological imbalances and with our physical therapist on exercise recommendations. Dietitians provide ongoing nutritional consultation based on four-day food records submitted by patients. They also recommend supplements, with consultation by physicians as needed.

Nutritional consultation with patients at the Block Center is begun soon after initial medical evaluation and in consultation with medical staff. Since nutritional therapy is regarded as foundational to the entire integrative system, it is provided to every patient. Patients who are receiving their medical care at other centers may come to the Center for integrative care and may have nutritional consultations with the Block dietitians. Dietitians are commonly scheduled to meet with patients as they undergo chemotherapy treatments, along with other integrative practitioners, despite the administrative burden of scheduling multiple practitioner visits.

The policy of dietetic care for every patient certainly poses a logistic challenge. However, the potential benefits of nutrition as the foundation of integrative care are, as outlined in this paper, sufficiently powerful that every effort should be made to ensure that patients have constant access to nutritional care as their battle with cancer proceeds. Future studies should further explore the application of whole foods regimens that are tailored to the specific needs of cancer patients, emphasizing the use of macronutrients, micronutrients, botanicals, and phytochemicals in restraining cancer growth and recurrence, improving treatment response and tolerance, and optimizing patients' quality of life. Despite the challenges posed by research on entire nutritional and integrative care systems, such research may offer a more direct pathway to improvements in the care of cancer patients than the reductionistic approaches of the past.

REFERENCES

Aggarwal BB & Shishodia S. (2006). Molecular targets of dietary agents for prevention and therapy of cancer. *Biochemical Pharmacology*, 71(10), 1397–1421.

Block KI. (2003). Multiple molecular targets in oncology and integrative care. *Integrative Cancer Therapies*, 2(3), 209–211.

Block KI, Block P, & Gyllenhaal C. (2004). The role of optimal healing environments in patients undergoing cancer treatment: Clinical research protocol guidelines. *Journal of Alternative and Complementary Medicine*, 10 Suppl 1, S157–S170.

Block KI, Constantinou A, Hilakivi-Clarke L, Hughes C, Tripathy D, & Tice JA. (2002). Point-counterpoint: Soy intake for breast cancer patients. *Integrative Cancer Therapies*, 1(1), 90–100.

Boyd DB. (2003). Insulin and cancer. *Integrative Cancer Therapies*, 2(4), 315–329.

Jho DH, Cole SM, Lee EM, & Espat J. (2004). Role of omega-3 fatty acid supplementation in inflammation and malignancy. *Integrative Cancer Therapies*, 3(4), 98–111.

McTiernan A. (2005). Obesity and cancer: The risks, science and potential management strategies. *Oncology (Williston Park)*, 19(7), 871–881.

Messina M, McCaskill-Stevens W, & Lampe JW. (2006). Addressing the soy and breast cancer relationship: Review, commentary and workshop proceedings. *Journal of the National Cancer Institute*, 98(18), 1275–1284.

Ornish D, Weidner G, Fair WR, Marlin R, Pettengill EB, Raisin CJ, et al. (2005). Intensive lifestyle changes may affect the progression of prostate cancer. *Journal of Urology*, 174(3), 1065–1069.

Saxe GA, Major JM, Nguyen JY, Freeman KL, Downs TM, & Salem CE. (2006). Potential attenuation of disease progression in recurrent prostate cancer with plant-based diet and stress reduction. *Integrative Cancer Therapies*, 5(3), 206–213.

(A complete reference list for this chapter is available online at http://www.oup.com/us/ integrativemedicine).

6

Botanical Medicine in Integrative Oncology*

LEANNA J. STANDISH, LISE N. ALSCHULER, ANN B. READY,
CAROLYN TORKELSON, GOWSALA SIVAM,
AND CYNTHIA WENNER

KEY CONCEPTS

- Many of our best chemotherapy drugs originally came from plants (e.g., paclitaxel from the yew tree, vincristine, vinblastine, vinorelbine from the red periwinkle plant, camptothecin from the Chinese tree *Camptotheca accuminata*, podophyllin from mayapple).
- It is likely that there are still antineoplastic and immunomodulatory plant medicines to be discovered.
- The use of botanicals in oncology is based on the synergistic hypothesis—that combinations of well-selected active constituents from one or more botanical species will together have a synergistic anticancer effect. Some ancient Traditional Chinese Medicine combination therapies have been shown to improve efficacy of chemotherapy in pancreatic and colon cancer patients.
- Botanicals are used in naturopathic oncology in several ways: to prevent cancer and metastasis in high-risk patients, to manage side effects of conventional cancer therapy, as adjuvants to improve efficacy and safety of chemotherapy agents, and as immunomodulators to prevent cancer relapse after treatment.
- At this time, the botanicals with the highest level of preclinical and clinical evidence as anticancer or immunomodulatory agents include: garlic, curcumin, green tea, mistletoe, quercetin, bromelain, milk thistle, astragalus, ashwagandha, and the medicinal mushrooms (Turkey Tail, Reishi, Shiitake, and Maitake).
- As the use of botanicals by cancer patients and their integrated oncologists increases there is a critical need for clinical research trials of single botanical agents as well as combination botanical

* Editing and bibliography by Ana Nelson, ND candidate.

treatments, in both the adjuvant setting and in prevention of tumor relapse after standard treatment.

■

P lant medicines, or herbal therapies, often called phytopharmaceuticals, are used by integrative oncologists and self-prescribed by cancer
patients to treat cancer. Botanical medicines are used in cancer chemoprevention, as adjunctive therapy to chemo- and radiotherapy to mitigate
side effects, and in secondary prevention. There is evidence that specific phy-
topharmaceutical agents as well as whole herbal preparations can both harm
and benefit cancer patients who are undergoing primary conventional cancer
treatment. The integrative oncologist must be informed on drug–herb interactions and the growing body of literature regarding the potential benefits and
risks of concurrent antioxidant therapy during radiation treatment (Lamson &
Brignall, 1999; Lamson & Brignall, 2000a; Lamson & Brignall, 2000b) as well
as the growing body of literature showing improved outcomes from chemotherapy when specific herbal medicines are used (Chu, 2006).

Botanical medicines have been hypothesized to play a significant role in
secondary chemoprevention in reducing risk of recurrence of disease locally or
metastases following primary conventional treatment. The clinical application
of herbal therapies in secondary prevention is growing within the most progressive integrated oncology clinics. It is here that botanicals may have their greatest role.

The search for natural products as potential anticancer agents dates back to
Papyrus Ebers, an Egyptian physician who listed more than 700 drugs, mostly
from plants, during the middle of the second millennium BC (Subbaraju, 2005).
In the 21st century plant medicines are used by integrative oncologists in six ways:

- In primary prevention of cancer in patients at high risk for malignancy (antioxidants and immunomodulators)
- As phytopharmaceuticals with direct tumoricidal and apoptotic effects
- As adjuvants to improve the cytotoxic activity of cancer drugs
- As immunomodulators to enhance endogenous immunological tumori-cidal activity
- To treat radiation-related reactions and fatigue
- To mitigate the hematological, neurological, and gastroenterological toxicities of U.S. Food and Drug Administration (FDA)-approved chemo-therapy pharmaceuticals.

This chapter is written and designed for the clinician who seeks the current state of the preclinical and clinical science for botanical therapy in cancer treatment, from diagnosis, through conventional primary treatment, in secondary prevention and "wellness" care, in management of metastatic stage IV patients, and in palliative oncologic care.

Rationale for Botanical Oncology Research in the 21st Century

The foundations and principles of botanical oncology are sound, but the science is far behind the theoretical uses of plant medicines in cancer patients. Evidence for even some of the most popular herbal medicines used by cancer patients has only been sketchy, often only level I in vitro evidence. Nevertheless, the long traditional uses of these herbs, many of which are available over-the-counter, indicates that some may be relatively harmless, some harmful as chemotherapy adjuvants, and some helpful, appearing to have a wide therapeutic window. In the last 60 years researchers have applied Western methods of science to botanical formulas of ancient Chinese and Ayurvedic medicine, as well as the indigenous plant medicines from ancient peoples all over the globe. We have been impressed time and again by the power of some of these plant medicines.

If we, in the Western world, have not found effective plant medical treatments for cancer, it is, in our opinion, because we have not tried hard enough. From the indigenous Amazonian entheogenic plant medicine perspective, we lack a plant medicine cure for cancer because we have not listened to or learned from the plants. The concept of plant intelligence is just beginning to be explored by ethnopharmacologists. We anticipate an exciting future in the clinical study of indigenous plant medicines, including psychoactive plant medicines, used in traditional healing. We have much to learn from our plants and from indigenous peoples who know their plants.

Plants Are the Original Source of Many FDA-Approved Cytotoxic Chemotherapy

Botanical medicines are the original source of some of our most powerful U.S. Food and Drug Administration (FDA)-approved cytotoxic chemotherapy agents. In the West, drug-based chemotherapy is more than 50 years old. Natural products have been major molecular structural resources for drug discovery. Among the 520 new drugs approved in the United Sates between

1983 and 1994, 157 were natural products or derived from natural products and more than 60% of antibacterials and anticancer drugs have originated from natural products (Zaidman, Yassin, Mahajna, & Wasser, 2005). There are now more than 100 FDA-approved anticancer agents. Many of our most powerful chemotherapy drugs are synthetic analogs of molecules first discovered in natural products, including bacteria, animals, and especially plants. For example, the microtubulin-disrupting taxane chemotherapy drugs (paclitaxel, docetaxel, albumin-bound paclitaxel) were developed from the Pacific Yew tree (*Taxus brevifolia*). Originally vincristine and vinblastine, chemotherapeutic agents with microtubulin-disrupting activity used in leukemias and lymphomas, were developed from the vinca alkaloids found in the pink or red periwinkle plant (*Catharanthus roseus*). Vinorelbine is another vinca alkaloid with anticancer activity used in several adenocarcinomas, including breast and ovarian cancer. The topoisomerase-targeting camptothecin (derived from an alkaloid produced by the Chinese tree *Camptotheca acuminata*) was identified by Western scientists as an antineoplastic agent in the 1960s. The mayapple (*Podophyllum peltatum*) is Minnesota's native plant and has a long history of use in treating cancer by Native Americans. Podophyllin, the active constituent, is an alcohol extract of the roots and rhizomes of the tree. Inspired by mayapple's traditional use and activity against warts, the NCI explored its potential as an anticancer drug in animal and human trials in the 1950s. However, because it was too toxic, clinical trials were abandoned. Later, in the 1960s, Sandoz Ltd resumed research on podophyllotoxin, leading to the development of semisynthetic analogs that later became the FDA-approved drugs, teniposide and etoposide, that are widely used in treating non–small cell lung carcinoma, lymphomas, and leukemias.

Triterpenoid acids such as oleanolic and ursolic acid, which are common plants constituents, are known to have anti-inflammatory and antitumor activities. Attempts to synthesize new analogs have led to in vitro and in vivo studies, especially in ovarian cancer (Melichar, et al., 2004). β-Lapachol is a simple napthoquinone extracted from the bark of the lapacho tree, *Tabebuia avellanedae*, found in South America. It has a long history of ethnobotanical use in the Amazonian basin. However, the isolated compound β-lapachol showed unacceptable levels of toxicity, and further investigation was dropped by the NCI (Cragg & Newman, 2005). Many plant cytotoxic molecules have been abandoned for further development by the NCI because isolated single constituents have unacceptable toxicities.

Unfortunately, but not surprisingly, the use of whole plants or combination plant constituents has not been pursued by mainstream oncology researchers. Even those who have pursued whole plant botanical oncology research have been stymied by the absence of adequate taxonomic, chemical, and bioassay validation of the natural products used in research. Botanical oncology research can succeed only with knowledge-based consensus on the plants, the parts of plants, and the active constituents that should be studied and the bioassays that should be used to confirm activity. With leadership and support from the National Center for Complementary and Alternative Medicine (NCCAM) and the NIH Office of Dietary Supplements, this work is moving forward.

Chemotherapy for many types of cancer relies on well-selected combinations of agents. Conventional combination chemotherapy utilizes multiple single molecular agents that have additive or synergistic activity. FDA-approved cancer medicines are single molecules, many of which have been modified to increase cytotoxic activity and reduce toxicities. The most compelling rationale for combination chemotherapy is twofold: (1) tumor cell heterogeneity and its associated drug resistance and (2) the success of combination chemotherapy in the clinic (Henderson, et al., 2003). Primary treatment for breast cancer, ovarian cancer, colorectal cancer, pediatric lymphoblastic leukemia, acute myeloblastic leukemia, Hodgkin's disease, and small and non–small cell lung carcinomas involve two to seven agents (Frei & Joseph Paul, 2003). Study medication development, quality assurance, and quality control in clinical research of natural products is far more complex than single molecule drug trials. Nevertheless, the potential of combination plant therapy in cancer treatment warrants the extra effort required to conduct high-quality clinical trials using complex plant mixtures.

Botanicals in Oncologic Practice: Which Plants Show the Greatest Potential?

The use of botanical medicines by integrative oncologists in the West is largely evidence based. The peer review literature is rich with in vitro studies of plant constituents for their cytotoxic, apoptotic, anti-inflammatory, gene stabilization, and antiangiogenic effects. Many herbs in common use also have supporting animal studies using murine models of specific tumor types. However, it was not until John Boik's 2001 publication of *Natural Compounds in Cancer Therapy* (Boik, 2001) that integrative oncologists had an evidence-based systematized list of most promising botanicals. On the basis of in vitro, animal, and human data, Boik identified 21 higher fungi and vascular plants on which significant anticancer data was available to warrant further clinical trials. They are listed here ranked by level of evidence from the highest to the lowest level: *Trametes versicolor*, genistein and daidzein, ginseng, bromelain, astragalus, quercetin, Eleutherococcus, green tea, boswellic acid, ganoderma (Reishi), shiitake, curcumin, garlic, resveratrol, Flax seed, anthocyanins from berries, hypericin, parthenolide (Fever Few), centella, butcher's broom, and horse chestnut. Many of these botanical therapies are prescribed by naturopathic physicians who specialize in the treatment of cancer patients. The most commonly used botanical medicines for each cancer type are listed below.

Breast cancer—*T. versicolor*, garlic, quercetin, bromelain, curcumin, green tea, flax seeds, 3,3'-diindolylmethane (DIM) extracted from cruciferous vegetables
Prostate cancer—garlic, green tea, soy, pomegranate, silymarin, curcumin
Lung cancer—astragalus, green tea, curcumin, silymarin, bromelain
Colorectal and gastric cancer—*T. versicolor*, garlic, astragalus, green tea, mushrooms, flax seeds
Head and neck cancer—curcumin, green tea
Glioblastoma multiforme—resveratrol from grape seeds, curcumin
Melanoma—green tea, curcumin, flavonoids, mistletoe (*Viscum alba*)
Ovarian cancer—ginkgo biloba, soy, green tea, curcumin
Hepatocellular carcinoma—green tea, ginseng, AHCC, milk thistle
Lymphoma—green tea, astragalus, soy
Leukemia—green tea, astragalus, soy
Multiple myeloma—Curcumin, green tea, astragalus, soy

Evidence for Botanical Therapies in Primary Treatment and Secondary Prevention of Cancer

In this section we review the current state of the preclinical and clinical science for eight of the most commonly used botanicals in integrative oncology by naturopathic physicians who are board certified in naturopathic oncology. Mistletoe cancer treatment is widely used in Europe. A review of the literature on the use of alternative cancer therapies reports that mistletoe preparations are listed among 11 of the most commonly used CAM methods in Europe (Hauser, 1991). Please see Chapter 16 for further details.

GARLIC (*ALLIUM SATIVUM*)

Garlic and related vegetables of the *Allium* genus have an especially wide variety of beneficial effects on human health. Among the potential effects are prevention and amelioration of certain cancers. When garlic is cut or crushed, enzymes are activated to produce several organosulfur compounds, including the volatile substances that give garlic its odor. These sulfur-containing chemicals are implicated in the beneficial dietary effects of garlic. Although these volatile and unstable molecules are difficult to study, the understanding of their chemistry is far ahead of an understanding of their biology. In fact, very little is known about the mechanisms by which garlic constituents affect human cancer cells. We have shown that garlic extract induces apoptosis of several breast cancer cell lines, but not normal fibroblast cells.

High consumption of fruits and vegetables is associated with decreased risk of cancer at many sites. *Allium* vegetables, particularly garlic (*Allium sativum*) have had an important dietary and medicinal role for centuries. Several lines of investigation have demonstrated anticancer effects of garlic (Lea, 1996). Epidemiologic studies have indicated decreased site-specific cancer incidence associated with fresh garlic consumption.

For example, Steinmetz et al. conducted a large prospective cohort study of colorectal cancer among women in Iowa (Steinmetz, et al., 1994). They analyzed intake of 15 vegetable and fruit groups and dietary fiber. The strongest inverse association found in the study was for garlic consumption with an adjusted relative risk of 0.68. A Swiss study reported a substantially greater protective effect (0.32) for colorectal cancer in the upper tertile of garlic consumption (Levi, et al., 1999). Studies in China and Italy have observed similar results for gastric and laryngeal cancer (Buiatti, et al., 1989; Cipriani, et al., 1991; Zheng, et al., 1992). Case–control studies of dietary factors have also shown inverse associations with breast and prostate carcinomas (Challier, Perarnau, & Viel, 1998; Key, Silcocks, Davey, Appleby, & Bishop, 1997). Table 6.1 lists the results for published epidemiological studies related to fresh garlic consumption.

Several biologic activities have been identified for garlic extracts that may be relevant to cancer, including lipid-lowering effects, antiplatelet, immunomodulatory, and antioxidant properties (Agarwal, 1996). There are also reports of direct action of garlic extracts on tumor cells. Antiproliferative effects of garlic extract have been reported for human colon carcinoma, hepatoma and leukemia cell lines at IC_{50} concentrations from 30 to 480 µg/mL (Siegers, et al., 1999). Various single components in fresh or aged garlic extracts, including diallylsulfenic acid (allicin), diallyl di- and tri-sulfides, ajoene, and S-allylcysteine, and S-allylmercaptocysteine have also been demonstrated to have antiproliferative, and in some cases, apoptotic effects on cancer cell lines (Dirsch, Gerbes, & Vollmar, 1998; Pinto, et al., 1997; Sakamoto, et al., 1997; Scharfenberg, et al., 1994; Sigounas, et al., 1997a; Sigounas, et al., 1997b; Sundaram & Milner, 1996; Zheng, et al., 1997). Nonmalignant cells were reported to be less sensitive to these organosulfur compounds (Sakamoto,

Table 6.1. Epidemiological Studies on Cancer and Garlic Consumption.[*]

Country	Reference	Cancer Type	Food	Cancer Association (Odds Ratio)[†]
Argentina	Iscovich, et al., 1992	Colon	Garlic	0.2–0.4
China	Mei, et al., 1982	Stomach	Raw garlic (20 g/day)	0.08 [‡]
China	You, et al., 1989	Stomach	Garlic (>4 g/day) Garlic (0.3–4 g/day) All *Allium* species (44–64 g/day)	0.7 0.8 0.5
China	Zheng, et al., 1992	Larynx	Garlic	0.5–0.6
Italy	Buiatti, et al., 1989	Stomach	Cooked garlic	0.4–0.6
Italy	Cipriani, et al., 1991	Stomach	Garlic and onion	0.8
Iran	Cook-Mozafari, et al., 1979	Esophagus, men	Raw garlic (≥1 serving/month) Pickled garlic (ever)	1.1 [§] 0.6
Switzerland	Levi, et al., 1993	Breast Endometrium	Garlic Garlic	0.6–0.7 0.6
USA	Steinmetz & Potter, 1994	Colon Colon (distal)	Garlic (>1 serving/week) Garlic (≥1 serving/week)	0.7 0.5

[*] Taken from Lawson, 1996 with the permission of the author.

[†] Values below 1 indicate decreased risk of cancer.

[‡] Cancer incidence was only 8% of those consuming less than 1 g/day.

[§] Not statistically significant, but all other studies are.

et al., 1997). Several biochemical mechanisms have been proposed, including reduction in polyamine levels, oxidative stress, and activation of the transcription factor nuclear factor kappa-B (NF-κB) (Dirsch, et al., 1998; Pinto, et al., 1997).

The organosulfur compounds of garlic are secondary metabolites and are responsible for the characteristic odor of crushed garlic (Lawson, 1996). The organosulfur compounds of intact garlic cloves contain mainly the amino acid cysteine, and include approximately equal amounts of *S*-alkylcysteine sulfoxides and α-glutamyl-S-alkylcysteines, the alkyl groups being strictly allyl, methyl, and trans-1-propenyl (Table 6.2). When garlic cloves are crushed, chewed, or cut (or when dehydrated, powdered garlic is exposed to water), the vacuolar enzyme, alliinase or alliin lyase rapidly lyses the cytosolic cysteine sulfoxides (Lawson, 1996) to form sulfenic acids, which immediately condense to form the alkyl alkanethiosulfinates, the compounds that are responsible for the odor of fresh cut or crushed garlic. At room temperature, this process is complete in a few minutes.

Aged garlic (Kyolic) contains S-allylcysteine and S-allylmercaptocysteine, both of which have demonstrated anticancer activity. A study of 51 patients with colorectal precancerous adenomas seen on screening colonoscopy and removed surgically were randomized to garlic or placebo. Aged garlic significantly suppressed both the size and number of colon adenomas after 12 months of treatment (Tanaka, et al., 2006). Aged garlic extract was shown to prevent decline in natural killer (NK) cell number and activity in patients with advanced

Table 6.2. Principal Organosulfur Compounds in Whole and Crushed Garlic Cloves.*

Compound	Whole Garlic (mg/g)	Crushed Garlic (mg/g)
S-(+)-Alkyl-L-cysteine sulfoxides		
Allylcysteine sulfoxide (aliin)	7.0–14	Not detectable
Methylcysteine sulfoxide	0.5–2	‹›
trans-1-Propenylcysteine sulfoxide	0.1–2	‹›
g-L-Glutamyl-S-alkyl-L-cysteines		
g-Glutamyl-S-trans-1-propenyl-cysteine	3–9	3–9
g-Glutamyl-S-allylcysteine	2–6	2–6
g-Glutamyl-S-methylcysteine	0.1–0.4	0.1–0.4
Alkyl alkanethiosulfinates		
Allyl 2-propenethiosulfinate (allicin)	Nd	2.5–4.5
Allyl methyl thiosulfinates	Nd	0.3–1.2
Allyl trans-1-propenyl thiosulfinates	Nd	0.05–1.0
Methyl trans-propenyl thiosulfinates	Nd	0.05–0.15
Methyl methanethiosulfinate	Nd	0.05–0.15

* Taken from Lawson, 1996, with the permission of the author.

colorectal, liver or pancreatic cancer (Ishikawa, et al., 2006). Another garlic-derived organosulfur component called ajoene was shown to decrease basal cell carcinoma tumor size after topical application in 21 patients (Tilli, et al., 2003). On the basis of in vitro experiments, the authors speculate that ajoene reduces basal cell carcinoma by inducing a mitochondrial-dependent apoptotic mechanism.

Garlic Summary

Several garlic constituents have apoptotic and immune modulating activity with strong preclinical evidence. Sadly, as yet there have been no cancer clinical trials of garlic in the United States. A phase I/II clinical trial of allicin in breast cancer is a high-priority study.

CURCUMA LONGA: CURCUMIN IN CANCER PREVENTION AND THERAPY

Curcumin (diferuloylmethane) is a polyphenol derived from the rhizome of the plant curcuma longa, a member of the ginger (*Zingiberaceae*) family. Also known as turmeric, Indian yellow root or Indian saffron, curcuma longa is cultivated throughout Asia and used extensively as a culinary spice and is a principal ingredient in curry. Curcumin also has a long history of use as a botanical medicine in both traditional Chinese and Indian (Ayurvedic) medicines to treat a wide variety of conditions. Current research has focused on curcumin as an anti-inflammatory, anti-oxidant, hepatoprotective, anti-microbial, and anti-carcinogenic agent.

There is an impressive amount of peer-reviewed literature on curcumin. A Pubmed search in late 2006 yielded more than 1700 articles on curcumin, over 600 of which are specifically related to its impact on carcinogenesis. Curcumin has been shown to exhibit multiple anticancer effects in a wide variety of cancer types. The mechanisms through which curcumin is believed to interfere with carcinogenesis are many. They include inhibition of inflammation, promotion of programmed cell death (apoptosis), interference with new blood vessel growth to tumors (angiogenesis), reduction in cancer cell motility and possibly synergistic effects with some chemotherapeutic agents and radiotherapy. Oral administration of curcumin in doses up to 8 to 10 g per day without dose-limiting toxicity further marks curcumin as a promising therapy for both the prevention and treatment of cancer (Aggarwal, et al., 2005).

A key mediator in all stages of carcinogenesis is the transcription factor NF-κB, which is involved in pro-inflammatory pathways at all stages of carcinogenesis, including initiation, promotion, and progression (Thangapazham, Sharma, & Maheshwari, 2006). In experimental models, curcumin has been shown to block recruitment of leukocytes, a source of inflammatory cytokines linked to carcinogenesis via inhibition of NF-κB (Kumar, Dhawan, Hardegen, & Aggarwal, 1998). In colon cancer cell lines, Su and colleagues reported that curcumin decreased not only levels of NF-κB, but also levels of other inflammatory mediators, including COX-2 and matrix metalloproteinase (MMP)-2, at both protein and mRNA levels. Plummer and colleagues also found a reduction in COX-2 levels in tumor necrosis factor (TNF)-induced colon cancer cells by curcumin and traced this reduction to mediators in the NF κB pathway (Plummer, et al., 1999). Animal studies have shown that curcumin is effective in reducing experimentally induced colitis via inhibition of NF-κB (Jian, et al., 2005) and COX-2 (Zhang, et al., 2006). Curcumin has also been shown to suppress cyclin D1, COX-2 and MMP-9 as well as block the activation of NF-κB in lung cancer cells exposed to NF-κB activating free radicals from cigarette smoke (Shishodia, et al., 2003).

DNA adducts, which form as a result of oxidative damage, can result in mutagenesis and can therefore promote carcinogenesis (Phillips, 2005). Curcumin has been shown to act as an antioxidant and reduce DNA adduct formation in experimental models. Animal studies have suggested that curcumin reduces DNA adduct formation in oral cancers and reduces the number, size and grade of oral lesions (Krishnaswamy, Goud, Sesikeran B, Mukundan MA, & Krishna, 1998).

Curcumin has been shown to induce apoptosis in a wide variety of cancer cell types by interacting with many of these ligands and receptors. Numerous studies have shown that curcumin promotes cell cycle arrest at the G(2) phase by increasing p53/BAX expression (Choudhuri, Pal, Das, & Sa, 2005; Liontas & Yeger, 2004; Shi, et al., 2006), inhibiting NF-κB (Aggarwal, Takada, Singh, Myers, & Aggarwal, 2004; Han, Chung, Robertson, Ranjan, & Bondada, 1999; Li, et al., 2005; Mukhopadhyay, et al., 2001; Zheng, et al., 2004), altering Bcl2 and caspase expression (Mukhopadhyay, et al., 2001; Shi, et al., 2006; Woo, et al., 2003), down-regulating IAPs (Woo, et al., 2003) and other mechanisms.

Through these mechanisms, curcumin has been shown to induce apoptosis in a wide variety of cancer cell lines, including breast (Choudhuri, et al., 2005; Ramachandran & You, 1999), prostate (Mukhopadhyay, et al., 2001), ovarian (Shi, et al., 2006), lung (Radhakrishna Pillai, et al., 2004), pancreas (Li), head and neck (Aggarwal, et al., 2004), melanoma (Zheng, et al., 2004), renal (Woo, et al., 2003), B cell lymphoma (Han, et al., 1999), acute myelo-blastic leukemia (Mukherjee Nee Chakraborty, et al., 2006), neuroblas-toma (Liontas & Yeger, 2004), glioblastoma (Karmakar, et al., 2006), gastric (Moragoda, et al., 2001), endometrial (Hu & Kavanagh, 2003), and colon cell lines (Jaiswal, Marlow, Gupta, & Narayan, 2002). In comparing the effects of anti-inflammatory medicines on apoptosis, Wei and colleagues found that curcumin induced a more potent apoptotic response than celecoxib, nife-dipine, or sundilac in colon cancer cells with defects in mismatch repair (MMR) genes (Wei, et al., 2004).

Using animal models, researchers have demonstrated that curcumin interferes with angiogenesis via several mechanisms. Arbiser and col-leagues demonstrated that curcumin effectively inhibited basic fibroblast growth factor (FGF)-mediated corneal neovasculariztion in the mouse model (Arbiser, et al., 1998). Yoysungnoen and colleagues demonstrated reduced neovascularization in mice inoculated with hepatocellular carci-noma cells treated with curcumin and found that treated mice had sig-nificant reductions in COX-2 over-expression and decreased serum levels of VEGF (Yoysungnoen, et al., 2006). Gururaj and colleagues also found that curcumin reduced neovascularization in two in vivo angiogenesis systems with concomitant reduction in pro-angiogenic gene expression (VEGF, angiopoietin-1 and 2) (Gururaj, et al., 2002). Curcumin has also been reported to inhibit angiogenesis via the FGF and MMP signaling path-ways (Mohan, et al., 2000) and to inhibit endothelial sprout formation via lipoxygenase inhibition (Jankun, et al., 2006).

Experimental and animal data support the hypothesis that curcumin inhibits the process of metastasis by reducing motility of cancer cells or their invasive potential. Reductions in the invasive capacity of curcumin-treated cancer cell lines have been demonstrated in colon (Su, et al., 2006), liver (Ohashi, et al., 2003), and prostate cancer (Hong, Ahn, Bae, Jeon, & Choi, 2006). Suppression of transcription of several genes involved in inva-sion has also been observed in lung cancer cell lines, including suppression of MMP 14, cell adhesion molecules, integrins, and heat shock proteins (Chen, et al., 2004). In prostate cancer cell lines, curcumin has been shown to arrest cell movements by altering microfilament organization and function (Holy, 2004).

In animal models of prostate cancer, treatment with curcumin not only reduced tumor size in the primary site but was also found to decrease the number of metastatic nodules possibly through inhibition of MMPs (Hong, et al., 2006). Ohashi and colleagues demonstrated that oral curcumin altered formation of actin stress fibers resulting in functional alterations in the organization of the cytoskeleton and suppression of intrahepatic metastasis (Ohashi, et al., 2003).

There are currently limited data on the effects of curcumin in combination with conventional chemotherapy and radiotherapy. However, initial reports suggest that this may be an area worthy of exploration. Experimental data supports a role for curcumin along with another polyphenol, quercetin, in sensitizing ovarian cancer cells to cisplatin-mediated killing, possibly through reduction in autologous IL-6 production and other mechanisms (Chan, Fong, Soprano, Holmes, & Heverling, 2003). Curcumin has also demonstrated potential in cell culture in reducing resistance of cancer cells to chemotherapy by inhibiting drug efflux pumps such as multi-drug resistance protein 1 (MRP1) (Chearwae, et al., 2006). Aggarwal and colleagues found curcumin effective at interfering with the paclitaxel (Taxol)-induced expression of antiapoptotic, proliferative and metastatic proteins. Also in experimental models, researchers have found curcumin capable of decreasing post-radiation colony counts significantly in models of squamous cell carcinoma, likely through its effects in cell cycle arrest at stages of the cell cycle in which radiotherapy is the most effective (Khafif, et al., 2005).

The bulk of the experimental data suggests that curcumin favorably affects several key processes in carcinogenesis including promotion of apoptosis and inhibition of inflammation, angiogenesis, cell motility and metastasis. Curcumin may therefore be an effective medicine in both chemoprevention and treatment of many different types of cancer. Some clinical data have been generated to evaluate how well curcumin performs as an anticancer therapy in humans. A phase I dose-escalation study of curcumin in patients with advanced colorectal cancer found that curcumin and its metabolites are evident in serum and urine, suggesting bioavailability, at doses of 3.6 g per day with no dose limiting toxicities. Although abundant amounts of curcumin can be recovered from the feces at this dose and dosages as low as 450 mg daily, curcumin appears to have a short half-life with serum retention times of 37 minutes or less (Sharma, et al., 2004). Other investigators found no evidence of serum curcumin at levels up to 8 g daily, when tested 1 hour after administration, but did at levels up to 12 g with excellent tolerability and minimal side effects such as diarrhea, yellow stool, headache and rash (Lao, et al., 2006). Owing to the rapid clearance of curcumin, it may be appropriate to test for serum curcumin and its metabolites within 30 minutes of oral administration.

Curcumin has been evaluated in combination with quercetin (a bioflavonoid) in five patients with familial adenomatous polyposis (FAP), an autosomal dominant disorder notable for the development of hundreds of polyps and the greatly increased risk of developing colon cancer. After 6 months of treatment with curcumin 480 mg plus 20 mg of quercetin three times daily, all five patients had a decrease in both number (mean reduction 60.4%) and size of polyps (mean reduction 50.9%), and both findings were statistically significant (Cruz-Correa, et al., 2006).

It appears from the phase I studies that doses between 3.6 to 8 g daily are well tolerated and demonstrate serum bioavailability when accessed within 30 minutes after administration. Future investigation may benefit from using this dosage range, particularly for sites outside the gastrointestinal system.

With a wealth of experimental, safety and bioavailability data behind it, curcumin is clearly ready for clinical trails in a multitude of cancer types, and these investigations are beginning to get underway. Researchers at the University of Pennsylvania are currently conducting a Phase II study to evaluate the effects of curcumin on cellular proliferation, apoptosis, and COX-2 expression in patients with previously resected adenomatous polyps. The National Cancer Institute is sponsoring a Phase II trial evaluating the effects of curcumin on multiple biomarkers in current smokers with aberrant crypt foci.

Investigators at MD Anderson Cancer Center are conducting a Phase II trial evaluating the effects of curcumin on response rates and survival of patients with adenocarcinomas of the pancreas and a Phase I trial assessing safety and tolerability of curcumin in patients with multiple myeloma. Preliminary data was presented at the Society for Integrative Oncology meeting in November 2006 by Dhillon (Dhillon, 2006). Twenty-five patients with advanced pancreatic cancer received 8000 mg of curcumin (Sabinsa Corp, Piscataway, NJ) by mouth daily for 2 months. Two patients had stable disease for over 6 months (8 and 10+ months) and one patient had a brief partial remission (73% reduction in tumor size) that lasted for 1 month. No toxicities were observed.

Curcumin Summary

Curcumin is emerging as a promising anti-cancer agent and may prove to be a powerful intervention in the chemoprevention and treatment of a wide variety of cancer types. The experimental data suggest that curcumin acts through a diverse array of mechanisms. Safe and well tolerated at doses up to 8 g daily, curcumin is clinical trial-ready. Phase I/II and III studies are needed to further evaluate safety; impact on appropriate surrogate biomarkers; efficacy of curcumin as a chemopreventive agent in patients with pre-cancerous lesions and other high-risk groups; and as a treatment for those with established cancers, either alone or in combination with conventional therapies.

CAMELLIA SINENSIS

Green tea has been consumed throughout Asia since at least 3000 BC to promote longevity, improve mental functions, and prevent disease. *Camellia sinsensis*, the common tea plant, remains the most widely consumed hot beverage on the planet. *Camellia sinensis* is cultivated in Indonesia and China, India, Japan, and Sri Lanka. The plant grows to fifteen meters and bears oblong-ovate, dark green, shiny leaves. Research on *Camellia sinsensis* over the past several decades has marked this plant as one of the most indicated and potent botanical chemopreventive and antineoplastic agents. Admittedly, the vast and growing body of research on green tea is mostly preclinical research. Additional clinical trials should seal the fate of this botanical as a mainstay in an integrated oncology prevention and treatment plan.

The young shoots are picked and to make green tea, the young leaves are allowed to wilt and then rolled. This rolling exudes some of the cell sap, and the leaf structure is partly broken down. To make black tea, the leaves are then fermented to convert the polyphenols to phlobaphenes and for aromatic substances to be formed. The fermentation occurs as a result of the leaf enzymes, particularly polyphenol oxidase, on tannins and catechins. To make green tea, fermentation is omitted and instead the leaves are steamed ("roasting" in the Chinese method and "sweating" in the Japanese method), which inactivates the enzymes and thus preserves the polyphenols. Red tea (oolong) and yellow tea are partially fermented tea. The leaves are then dried by hot air. Green tea contains several compounds including polyphenols— catechins (30%–42% of the extractable solids) and gallocatechins (including epigallocatechin gallate); flavonols 5%–10%; theogallin 2%–3%; quinic acids 2%; methylxanthines—caffeine 3%–5%, theophylline 0.02%, theobromine 0.1%; theanine 4%–6%; carotenoids; trigalloylglucose; minerals 6%–8%, depending on soil content of aluminum and maganese.

Green tea interferes with the majority of the steps of carcinogenesis (Lin, Liang, et al., 1999) and metastasis. The multiple points of interference lend broad applicability to green tea as an agent of chemoprevention. These actions are summarized in Figure 6.1. Tea extract inhibits mutagens and carcinogens extracellularly and intracellularly. Green tea catechins, namely, epicatechin (EC), epicatechin-3-gallate (ECG), epigallocatechin-3-gallate (EGCG), and gallocatechin (GC) inhibit cytochrome P450-dependent metabolic activation of promutagens and induce detoxification of mutagens via induction of glutathione and other phase II enzymes. Additionally, these same catechins scavenge free radicals, thereby inhibiting free radical–induced oncogene mutations, or

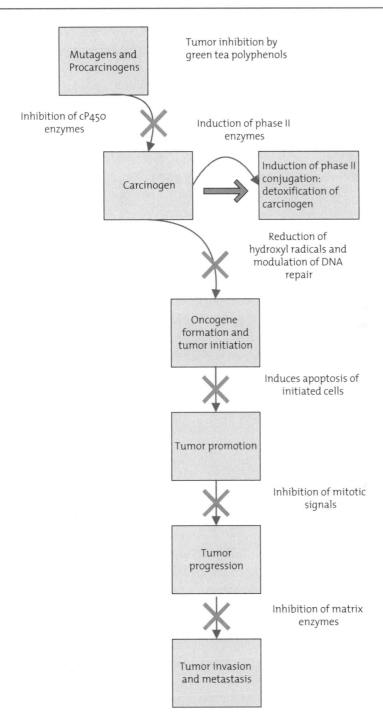

FIGURE 6.1. Chemoprevention by *Camellia sinensis*.

tumor initiation. The catechins EGCG and ECG increase DNA repair and support DNA replication of healthy cells while inhibiting the replication of neoplastic cells.

Green tea catechins have been found to inhibit colonic aberrant crypt formation in rats, evidencing their genomic reparative actions (Franke, et al., 2002). Epigallocatechin gallate and EGCG induce apoptosis in a variety of ways. Ironically enough, one major apoptogenic mechanism is the induction of reactive oxygen species with high electron transfer properties. Green tea catechins exert significant interference with promotion. This effect is, in part, due to EGC, EGCG, and GC inhibition of tumor necrosis factor (TNF)-α release from neoplastic cells (Fujiki, Suganuma, et al., 2000). TNFα is an endogenous tumor promoter and a central mediator of cancer development. The ability to inhibit TNF-α release is considered to be one of the most important mechanisms of the antipromotion activity of green tea (Fujiki, 1999). Furthermore, green tea catechins and EGCG inhibit matrix enzymes (urokinase), thus inhibiting tumor invasion and metastasis (Kuroda & Hara, 1999).

The apoptogenic effect of green tea extracts and EGCG in particular has been demonstrated in a variety of studies. EGCG and ECG induce apoptosis by inhibition of telomerase (Kuroda & Hara, 1999) and via downregulation of cyclin D1 and cyclin-dependent kinase (bladder tumor cells) (Chen, Ye, & Koo, 2004). In vitro and in vivo models have elucidated the molecular targets of green tea polyphenols in prostate carcinoma cells. The experimental administration of epigallocatechin gallate (EGCG) from green tea to androgen-dependent and androgen-independent human prostate cancer cells (LNCaP, DU145, and PC-3 cells) results in apoptosis. EGCG inhibits 5α-reductase, thus inhibiting the conversion of testosterone to its activated form, dihydrotestosterone, resulting in decreased hyperplasia (Adhami, Ahmad, & Mukhtar, 2003).

Green tea has also demonstrated antipromotional and antimetastatic activities (Annabi, et al., 2002). Additionally, EGCG inhibits proteasome, which results in tumor-growth arrest. Green tea extract and EGCG also suppress mRNA protein expression, resulting in a significant decrease in vascular endothelial growth factor (VEGF) and associated angiogenesis and tumor growth (Zhang, et al., 2006).

Several animal studies have confirmed the in vitro anticarcinogenic actions of green tea. The chemopreventative effects of green tea have been demonstrated in a rat model of bladder cancer. The growth of N-butyl-N-(4-hydroxybutyl)-nitrosamine–induced bladder cancers was prevented in rats that were prefed with green tea leaves (Sato & Matsushima, 2003). The antitumorigenic effects of tea extracts have been demonstrated for prostate cancer in several animal models. One such study implanted athymic nude mice with androgen-sensitive human prostate carcinoma cells (CWR22Rnul) and then gave the mice water extracts of green tea polyphenols, black tea, EGCG, and theaflavins. All tea extracts, given at humanly achievable concentrations, caused significant inhibition of tumor growth, reduction in PSA, induction of apoptosis, and decreases in VEGF (Siddiqui, et al., 2006).

Inhibition of lung carcinoma has been shown in mice with experimentally caused lung tumors. Out of several concentrations of oral green tea solution, the highest concentration, 0.6%, significantly reduced the number of lung tumors, inhibited angiogenesis, and resulted in a higher apoptotic index (Liao, et al., 2004). This concentration corresponds to approximately five cups of green tea for humans.

The cancer chemopreventive actions of green tea have been demonstrated in epidemiological studies. A 1988 review of the epidemiological studies (Bushman, 1998) concluded that, in the majority of studies, green tea consumption was inversely correlated with pancreatic cancer, colorectal cancer, gastric cancer, and urinary bladder cancer. In these studies, consumption of at least 5 cups of green tea daily was required for a preventive effect to be noted. Epidemiological studies also suggest a chemopreventive effect of tea against prostate cancer in humans (Jain, Hislop, Howe GR, Burch JD, & Ghadirian, 1998). More recent epidemiological studies clarify the chemopreventive potential of green tea and elucidate the importance of dosing. One such prospective study (Nagano, et al., 2001) followed 58,540 people for 15 years. A self-administered questionnaire ascertained the consumption of green tea (never, once daily, 2–4 times daily, and 5 or more times daily). The incidence of solid cancers, hematopoietic cancers and cancers of all sites combined were noted. The study concluded that green tea consumption was unrelated to incidence of cancers under study. However, the authors of this study note that this study may not have evaluated a minimum effective dose. The maximum studied dose in this study was 5 cups daily, a dose below the concentration of green tea extract used in the majority of in vivo studies that demonstrate benefit—an amount equivalent to 10 cups of green tea per day in humans.

To this point, another large prospective cohort study (Imai, Suga, & Nakachi, 1997) followed Japanese individuals living in Japan who consumed 10 cups of green tea daily for 10 years. This study did show a chemopreventive effect. The study included 8552 male and female participants, all of whom were above the age of 40. During the study, 153 men and 109 women died of cancer. Male participants who consumed over 10 cups of green tea daily survived 3.6 years longer than did their male counterparts who drank less than 3 cups daily. Female participants who consumed over 10 cups of green tea daily lived 7.8 years longer than did their female counterparts who drank less than 3 cups daily. In addition, the age at onset of cancer was 3.0 years later in men and 8.7 years later among women who drank over 10 cups of green tea daily than in those drinking less than three cups of green tea daily. The difference between men and women was explained by the higher tobacco use by men. Finally, in an extension of the same study, the researchers determined that women who drank over 10 cups of green tea daily showed a lower relative risk of cancers of the lung, colon, and liver. While this quantity of green tea may seem to be high, it should be noted that the "cups" referred to in these studies are Japanese tea cups, which hold approximately 6 oz. of tea. Additionally, this quantity of tea appears to be well-tolerated.

In contrast with the favorable data trends regarding the chemoprevention properties of green tea against the development of most solid tumors, there appears to be no chemoprevention of gastric cancer. In a population-based, prospective cohort study in Japan, 26,311 volunteers completed a self-administered questionnaire that included questions about the frequency of consumption of green tea. During 199,748 person-years of follow-up (over a period of 8 years), Cox regression was used to estimate the relative risk of gastric cancer according to consumption of green tea and no association was found. The study controlled for co-variables, but did not assess for the impact of dose on the chemopreventive effect (Tsubono, et al., 2001).

Green tea has been studied for its secondary and tertiary chemoprevention effects in women with breast cancer. In a prospective cohort study (Nakachi, et al., 1998) of 472 Japanese women with histologically confirmed invasive breast carcinomas (stage I, II and III), the subjects were assessed for axillary lymph node metastases and progesterone and estrogen receptor expression at the time of partial or total mastectomy. These women were then followed up for 7 years for recurrence in relation to green tea consumption. This study found that the premenopausal women who drank more than 5 cups of green tea daily had a lower mean number of metastasized lymph nodes. Subsequent to surgery, among the women with stage I and II breast cancer, green tea drinkers of greater than five cups daily experienced a 16.7% recurrence rate, while consumers of less than four cups per day experienced a 24.3% recurrence rate ($P < 0.05$). In addition, those who drank over five cups per day of green tea had a longer disease-free period by 3.6 years compared with those who drank fewer than four cups each day.

Inoue et al. (2001) also looked at the impact of regular green tea consumption on the risk of breast cancer recurrence (Inoue, et al., 2001). This study was conducted over a 9-year period from 1990 to 1999. In 1990, 1160 new surgical cases of invasive breast cancer in female patients at a Japanese cancer center were enrolled in the study. These women were monitored for recurrence and daily green tea consumption over a 9-year period. The average age was 51.5 years.

During 5264 person-years of follow-up (average 4.5 years per subject), 133 subjects (12%) experienced recurrence. A 31% decrease in risk of recurrence, as measured by hazard ratio, adjusted for stage, was observed with consumption of three or more daily cups of green tea (HR = 0.69). This risk reduction was particularly statistically significant in stage I patients with an observed risk reduction of 57%. The risk reduction was present, but was less significant, in stage II and not present among patients with more advanced stages.

Additional epidemiologic evidence is available to support the benefits of green tea as in chemopreventative agent in ovarian, oropharyngeal, colon, lung, prostate, and cancers of the hepatobiliary tree. No apparent chemoprotective effect, however, has been seen in gastric cancer.

Green tea may have synergistic actions with chemotherapeutic antineoplastic agents. Green tea extracts have been studied with doxorubicin (Adriamycin). Although there are no human trials, the preliminary in vitro and animal data is consistent with a beneficial relationship between these two agents. When doxorubicin was administered intraperitoneally to mice with implanted Ehrlich ascites carcinoma, a 25% reduction in tumor weight was observed. When mice ingested green tea during the time of *DOX* administration, a decrease of 37% in tumor weight was observed. The ingestion of green tea enhanced the doxorubicin tumor inhibition by 2.5-fold. The tumors of the green tea-fed mice demonstrated an increase in doxorubicin concentration by 1.7-fold compared to the doxorubicin-alone group. Additionally, the doxorubicin concentrations in the heart and liver did not increase with ingestion of green tea; in fact the doxorubicin concentration in the heart was less than the doxorubicin-alone group (Sadzuka, Sugiyama, et al., 1998). These results suggest that the addition of green tea to doxorubicin may intensify the antitumor action of doxorubicin while protecting healthy tissue against doxorubicin-induced toxicity.

State of the Evidence: Green Tea

The body of evidence clearly supports a role for green tea and its catechins in a cancer prevention and treatment program. Green tea appears to be most effective in preventing cancer and has promise as a treatment in early stage cancers. The selectivity of the antineoplastic effect of green tea on malignant tissue combined with the protective and reparative effect on cardiac, renal, and myeloplastic cells is a powerful combination. The question that remains unanswered is optimal concentration and length of administration of green tea extracts in people with active malignancies.

Flavonoid Plant Compounds

Flavonoid compounds are ubiquitous in the plant kingdom. Plants rely on flavonoids to survive the ultraviolet energy of the sun. Flavonoids protect plants by absorbing reactive oxygen species generated in the course of photosynthesis. Flavonoids are responsible for the colors of flowers and fruits and darker colored fruit skins and flower petals represent a high density of flavonoids. There are many types of flavonoids such as quercetin, hesperidin, and anthocyanidins (cyanidin, delphinidin, malvidin, pelargonidin, peonidin, and petunidin). While not all flavonoids have been studied for their cancer chemoprevention or antineoplastic activities, there are a few flavonoids that are emerging as promising agents in this regard.

Flavonoids, as a group of compounds interfere with inflammation and carcinogenesis in a variety of ways. Several flavonoids quench reactive oxygen species (Huang, Wu, & Yen, 2006). Ingested fruit juices concentrated in anthocyanin/polyphenol flavonoids exert significant antioxidative actions. An intervention study compared a red mixed berry juice to a polyphenol-depleted juice (Weisel, et al., 2006). After a 3-week run-in period, 18 male subjects consumed 700 mL juice, and 9 consumed control juice for 4 weeks, followed by a 3-week wash-out. During the intervention with polyphenol-rich juice, biomarkers of DNA oxidative damage decreased and reduced glutathione and glutathione status increased. These values returned to run-in levels in the subsequent wash-out phase. In addition to the reduction of oxidative damage, flavonoids enhance cellular detoxification and antioxidation enzymes via activation of Nrf-2. Other flavonoids suppress the proinflammatory and growth promoting gene expression mediated by NF-κB (Surh, et al., 2005).

Flavonoids also interfere with signal transduction pathways, thereby reducing tumor initiation and promotion. Tyrosine kinases are key regulators of intracellular signaling and when overexpressed or mutated, contribute to the development and progression of tumors. This makes the tyrosine kinase pathway and, in particular, its receptors, such as epidermal growth factor receptor (EGFR), excellent targets for antineoplastic effects. An example of this inhibition is ellagic acid, a polyphenol present in fruits and nuts. Ellagic acid inhibits VEGF receptors (Labrecque, et al., 2005).

Quercetin, a bioflavonoid found in high concentrations in onions, has been demonstrated in vitro to interfere with signal transduction pathways in ovarian epithelial cancer cells (Nicosia, et al., 2003). Quercetin inhibits protein kinase and thus may reduce ovarian tumor cell growth, survival and progression. Quercetin has also been shown to block epidermal growth factor receptor-signaling pathway in MiaPaCa-2 human pancreatic cells (Lee, et al., 2002). This disruption results in significant growth inhibition of these cells and the induction of apoptosis.

Delphinidin, an anthocyandin flavonoid found in berries, red grapes, purple sweet potatoes, red cabbages, and other pigmented fruits and vegetables, interferes with signal transduction pathways. In vitro, low concentrations of delphinidin inhibit vascular endothelial growth factor (VEGF)-induced tyrosine phosphorylation of VEGFR-2, leading to the inhibition of downstream signaling and VEGF-induced activation of ERK-1/2 signaling. In vivo, delphinidin is able to suppress basic FGF-induced vessel formation in the mouse Matrigel plug assay. This VEGF inhibition by delphinidin holds promise as a naturally occurring antiangiogenesis agent (Lamy, et al., 2006).

The polyphenol bioflavonoids derived from pomegranates (*Punica granatum*) possess anticarcinogenic actions, albeit derived from a different mechanism. Pomegranate polyphenols interfere with estrogen biosynthesis from androstenedione and testosterone by inhibiting aromatase enzyme. Additionally, fermented pomegranate juice polyphenols exert significant inhibitory effects on 17-β-estradiol resulting in reduced proliferation especially of estrogen-dependent MCF-7 breast cancer cells (Kim, et al., 2002). Pomegranate polyphenols also suppress human prostate cancer cell growth (Albrecht, et al., 2004).

State of the Evidence: Flavonoids

Data regarding the anticancer potential of flavonoids is just emerging. Flavonoids are potent antioxidants, appear to stimulate apoptosis, exert antiangiogenesis actions, and inhibit metastasis. These effects have been aptly demonstrated in vitro. Several critical questions remain unanswered, the most critical of which is to determine how much of the preclinical data translates into clinical effects.

Plant Enzyme Therapies

Enzymes from plant sources have long played a role in traditional and complementary cancer therapy. Enzymes are believed to be both anti-inflammatory and catalytic to tumors. Bromelain is the most commonly used plant enzyme in cancer therapy.

Bromelain is a water extract from pineapple stem that contains cysteine proteinases that have several purported therapeutic effects, including antimetastatic, antithrombotic (Eckert, et al., 1999; Glaser & Hilberg, 2006), antiedematous, fibrolytic, and immunomodulatory actions. In vitro studies have shown that bromelain inhibits the metastatic invasion of glioma cells (Tysnes, et al., 2001), and alters cell adhesion cell surface molecules in leukocytes (Hale, et al., 2002). Bromelain has been shown to stimulate both innate and adaptive aspects of immune function both in vitro to activate murine macrophages and NK cells (Engwerda, Andrew, Murphy M, & Mynott, 2001b) and in murine in vivo experiments (Engwerda, Andrew, Ladhams A, & Mynott, 2001a). Oral doses of bromelain reduced inflammatory cytokine release in rats injected intraperitoneally with lipopolysaccharide (Hou, Chen, Huang, & Jeng, 2006). Bromelain inhibited growth of lung tumors in mice inoculated with tumor cells (Beuth & Braun, 2005).

Bromelain is routinely used in naturopathic oncology to prevent post-radiation fibrosis and to reduce the risk of lymphedema. This practice is based on a small number of clinical studies in post-traumatic and postsurgical edema using Phlogenzym, a mucos proteolytic combination enzyme formula containing bromelain from a Germany pharmaceutical company (Kamenicek, Holan, & Franĕk, 2001). It is also used for prevention and treatment of post-operative ileus although this has only been demonstrated thus far in a rodent study (Wen, et al., 2006). The use of bromelain in prevention of post-radiotherapy fibrosis is supported by a Ukranian paper (Hubarieva, et al., 2000) reporting on the use of bromelain in preventing lymphogranulomatosis in cancer patients receiving radiation therapy. Doses are often expressed in terms of milk clotting units (MCU) or F.I.P. or sometimes in simple milligram weights. Adult oral doses range from 400 to 4000 mg/day.

State of the Evidence: Bromelain

Because bromelain has been shown to be generally safe in oral doses, integrative oncologists should feel comfortable prescribing it to cancer patients for short-term therapeutic trials for a variety of cancer-related conditions including postradiotherapy fibrosis, postsurgical edema, ileus, lymphedema, immunomodulation, and inflammatory bowel disorders.

SILYMARIN OFFICINALIS

Silymarin officinalis or milk thistle is a herb with significant experimental evidence as a general chemopreventive agent. European herbalists have used milk thistle for hundreds of years for the treatment of liver diseases, specifically alcoholic liver disease. Milk thistle contains a polyphenoloic flavonoid antioxidant, silymarin. Silymarin is composed of silybin, dehydrosilybin, silydianin, and silycristin. Of these, silybin has been most well studied. Silybinin inhibits the conversion of initiated cells to dormant tumor cells. This growth inhibition has been noted in human prostate, breast, and cervical carcinoma cells (Bhatia, Zhao, Wolf, & Agarwal, 1999). This effect is mediated via impairment of receptor and non receptor tyrosine kinase signaling pathways (Ahmad, Gali, Javed, & Agarwal, 1998) along with inhibition of TNF-α release and associated changes in cell cycle progression (Zi, Mukhtar, et al., 1997). This effect has been confirmed in vivo. In vitro and animal studies suggest that silymarin may exert significant chemopreventive effects against prostate, breast, oral, and hepatocellular cancers. Of concern, however, was the finding that in cell culture, treatment of human MCF-7 breast cancer cells with serum-achievable concentrations of silymarin in the rodent models stimulated their growth, in part through an estrogen-like activity. It would appear that the estrogenic activity of silibinin outweighs the antiproliferative actions in estrogen-dependent cancers.

Silybin, a constituent of *Silybum marianum* (milk thistle), has also been studied for its protective activity against cisplatin toxicity in an animal model of testicular cancer. In an in vitro study, silybin exerted a dose-dependent growth inhibitory effect to drug-resistant ovarian cancer cells. Additionally, silybin potentiated the cytotoxic effect of cisplatin on these cells (Scambia, et al., 1996). Orally delivered silibinin suppresses human non–small cell lung carcinoma A549 xenograft growth and enhances the therapeutic response of doxorubicin in athymic BALB/c nu/nu mice while simultaneously preventing doxorubicin-caused adverse health effects (Singh, et al., 2004).

State of the Evidence: Milk Thistle

The data on milk thistle as a chemopreventative agent is almost entirely preclinical. The preclinical data paints a convincing case for the apoptogenic, antiproliferative, and antiangiogenic actions of milk thistle extracts in a variety of cancers. While the estrogenic characteristics of milk thistle flavonoids may preclude its use in breast carcinomas, there is great potential for milk thistle in other cancers. Of particular value is the indication of a synergistic effect of milk thistle extracts with various chemotherapy agents.

ASTRAGALUS MEMBRANACEUS

Astragalus membranaceus (astragalus) has been used in Chinese herbal medicine as a Qi tonic. In Chinese herbal medicine, Qi tonics are used to strengthen parenchymal tissue and bodily processes that are weak to help build defenses against disease. Tonic herbs tend to strengthen and penetrate deep into the body tissue and structures. Astragalus has been used in Chinese herbal medicine for wasting/thirsting syndrome, to stabilize the exterior to stop sweating, to promote urination and reduce edema, to promote healing, particularly in diabetic ulcerations, and to help rebuild Qi and blood postpartum, or after significant loss of blood.

Astragalus has been widely studied for its immune-potentiating activity in the context of malignancy. One study looked at the effects of various fractions of astragalus on mononuclear cells derived from healthy normal donors and from colon cancer patients using the local xenogeneic graft-versus-host reaction. The astragalus extracts exhibited remarkable immunopotentiating activity and one fraction was capable of fully correcting in vitro T-cell function deficiency (Chu, Wong, & Mavligit, 1988).

Tolerance to cyclophosphamide can be limited by the immunosuppression that this drug may cause. Cyclophosphamide reduces leukocyte counts and suppresses both humoral and cellular immune responses. An aqueous extract of an isolated fraction from *Astragalus membranaceus* was given intravenously to rats for 8 days. The study rats that received astragalus in addition to the immunosuppressive CPA, experienced almost complete restoration of immune function, as evidenced by their increasing ability to reject grafted human tissue (Chu, et al., 1988).

A meta-analysis of astragalus-based Chinese herbs and platinum-based chemotherapy for advanced non–small cell lung cancer concluded that astragalus may increase the effectiveness of platinum-based chemotherapy (McCulloch, et al., 2006). Thirty-four randomized studies representing 2,815 patients met the inclusion criteria of the study. Combined results from the meta-analysis demonstrate overall benefit. Twelve studies reported reduced risk of death at 12 months. Thirty studies reported improved tumor response. Performance status in most studies was stable or improved. Among the studies reporting median survival, none included confidence intervals or *P* values of variance. Therefore, a meta-analysis of median survival could not be done. Despite this, the authors of the analysis conclude that combining astragalus with platinum-based chemotherapy in the treatment of non–small cell lung cancer may increase survival, tumor response, performance status, and reduce chemotherapy toxicity when compared to platinum-based chemotherapy alone.

State of the Evidence: Astragalus

Astragalus has been used for immune stimulation for centuries and modern research is uncovering the nature of these effects. The strongest indication for astragalus in the context of oncology care is to help prevent the immunosuppression caused by chemotherapy agents. Additionally, there is some indication that astragalus may also potentiate the cytotoxic effects of certain chemotherapy agents.

WITHANIA SOMNIFERA (ASHWAGANDHA)

Withania somnifera (Ashwagandha) has historically been used as a strengthening herb. One of the common names for *W. somnifera* is Indian ginseng. This name hints at its restorative properties. In fact, ashwagandha has historically been used in individuals who are debilitated and who suffer from nervous exhaustion, emaciation and anemia. In these individuals, ashwagandha is helpful in convalescence after acute illness or stress, impotence, chronic disease with inflammation and bony degeneration, and as a general tonic, for hypertension and high cholesterol. One important characteristic of ashwagandha is that it exerts a sedative effect and thereby rests and restores the health of the nervous system and person overall.

Ashwagandha has demonstrated immunostimulatory effects in chemotherapy-induced immunosuppression. Ashwagandha was fed to mice at a dose that corresponds to 4 to 6 g per day in humans. When ashwagandha was combined with cyclophosphamide, it prevented myelosuppression, resulted in a significant increase in hemoglobin concentration, red blood cell count, white blood cell count, platelet count and body weight as compared with mice treated with cyclophosphamide only (Ziauddin, et al., 1996). While this study does not rule out the possibility that ashwagandha could interfere with the activity of cyclophosphamide, the cytotoxic effects of cyclophosphamide on target tissues remained intact in the ashwagandha-treated mice. This suggests that the immunostimulatory actions of ashwagandha are the result of direct effects on the immune system.

Withaferin A, a compound found in ashwagandha, appears to have antineoplastic actions. An extract concentrated with withaferin A had a growth inhibitory effect on Chinese hamster V79 cancer cells. The withaferin A induced a G2/M block in vitro at higher doses (Devi, Akagi, Ostapenko, Tanaka, & Sugahara, 1996). The antitumor effect of *Withania somnifera* (ashwagandha) was also demonstrated against mouse tumor, Sarcoma 180 (Devi, Sharada, & Solomon, 1992). Another study assessed the antiproliferative effects of ashwagandha on laryngeal carcinoma (Mathur, et al., 2006). These findings suggest that the roots of *Withania somnifera* possess cell cycle disruption and antiangiogenic activity, which may be a critical mediator for its anticancer action.

Perhaps the most interesting indication for ashwagandha is to promote the tumor-kill effects of radiation therapy. *Withania somnifera* has been studied for its radiosensitizing properties. At least five studies in animals have confirmed a radiosensitizing effect of ashwagandha. Withaferin A, a steroidal lactone from *Withania somnifera* appeared to inhibit repair of radiation damage in tumor cells in a mouse model. While this in vivo data is compelling, the applicability to human patients remains unstudied and not definitively known. One issue that makes the translation from the preclinical to clinical scenario difficult is that the ashwagandha extracts used in many of the in vivo studies were intraperitoneal injections. It is unknown how oral dosing of ashwagandha in humans compares to intraperitoneal administration in rodents. In addition, it is unclear whether the radiosensitizing effect is localized to tumor cells only, or whether normal cells in the radiation field would also experience increased radiation effects. Nonetheless, the increased tumor response and prolonged survival time of rodents who received ashwagandha extracts along with radiation is encouraging and support the need for human trials.

State of the Evidence: Ashwagandha

Ashwagandha has potential as a multipronged antineoplastic agent. The immunostimulatory, anticarcinogenic, and radiosensitizing actions of this plant give it a unique place in the herbal armamentarium against cancer. While these actions have not been conclusively demonstrated in human trials, the preclinical evidence is encouraging.

Mycomedicinal Therapy in Oncology

Although in a kingdom of their own and not strictly encompassed by "botanical medicine" several species of higher fungi have been used traditionally as well as in modern times in the treatment of cancer. The most commonly used medicinal mushrooms are *Trametes versicolor* (Turkey Tail, formerly Coriolus versicolor), *Ganoderma lucidum* (Reishi), *Lentinus edodes* (Shiitake), *Grifola frondosa* (Maitake), and *Schizophyllum commune*. Mushrooms typically have not shown strong direct cytotoxic activity against tumor cells, but are rather used as immunomodulators. On the basis of what is known about the immunology of cancer, an effective immunomodulatory therapy could enhance innate immunity and tumor-specific adaptive immunity. Both of these immune response pathways are typically weakened due to tumor-induced immune suppression. Innate immune reactions that are typically suppressed in cancer states include NK cell tumoricidal activity, as well as maturation, recruitment and activation of antigen-presenting cells (APCs), such as macrophages and dendritic cells (DCs). Tumor-induced immune suppression appears to often also lead to down-regulation of type I inflammatory responses in APCs, which on encounter with tumor antigens, activate T cells that are needed for effective antitumor responses (Chung, Chen, Chan, Tam, & Lin, 2004). DC dysfunction has been shown to lead to immunosuppression in cancer states (Pinzon-Charry, et al., 2005), with a shift away from type I dendritic cell (DC1) and toward DC2 development (Rissoan, et al., 1999). This shift is hypothesized to promote regulatory T cell activation (Treg) and recruitment into tumor sites, and suppress T helper 1 (TH1)-dependent, cytotoxic T lymphocyte (CTL) responses. Thus, agents that could correct these immune imbalances and restore lymphocyte homeostasis, enhance APC-mediated delivery of adequate stimulation of antitumor effector cells, and inhibit Treg activity either systemically or locally would serve as excellent candidates in immune-based cancer therapy (Whiteside, 2006; Yamaguchi & Sakaguchi, 2006).

Because of their broad immune activity, medicinal mushrooms are a rich potential source of immunoceuticals. While other natural products from other plant species have known immunomodulatory activities (plant sterols, plant COX-2 inhibitors, thiol-containing allium vegetables), polysaccharides extracted from certain mushroom species have been the most thoroughly studied in preclinical and clinical studies.

TRAMETES VERSICOLOR (YUN ZHI, TURKEY TAIL MUSHROOM)

More than 270 recognized species of mushrooms are known to have specific immunotherapeutic properties (Ooi & Liu, 2000). Of these, 50 nontoxic mushroom species have yielded potential immunoceuticals in animal models, and of these, six species have been studied in human cancers (Kidd, 2000). An extract from one of these medicinal mushroom species, *Trametes versicolor*

(*Coriolus or Polyporus versicolor previously*), has been assessed in 31 Phase I, II, and III randomized clinical trials in over 9600 stomach, colorectal, esophageal, and breast cancer patients in Japan, Korea, and China.

  T. versicolor has a long history of medical use in Asia dating back hundreds of years in traditional Asian medicine. *T. versicolor* belongs to the more advanced Basidiomycetes class of fungi. It grows on tree trunks throughout the world in many diverse climates (Fig 6.2). In China it is called Yun Zhi or Cloud Fungus. According to Kidd (Kidd, 2000), the immunomodulatory activity of polysaccharide peptides in *T. versicolor* was discovered in 1965 in Japan by a chemical engineer who observed a case of cancer remission after ingesting Yun Zhi. Subsequent research revealed that there were two closely related proteoglycan constituents of *T. versicolor* with anticancer activity: polysaccharide-krestin (PSK, or Krestin and Polysaccharopeptide (PSP). PSK has been studied most extensively and is in wide clinical use as an adjunctive and adjuvant cancer therapy in Japan and China (Fisher & Yang, 2002; Kidd, 2000; Wasser, 2002). PSK was approved in 1977 as a cancer therapy by the Japanese National Health Registry and represents 25% of the total national costs of cancer care in Japan (Hobbs, 2004). The closely related PSP was first isolated in China in 1983. Adjunctive treatment with these *T. versicolor* polysaccharide-peptide fractions is a standard of oncologic care in mainstream modern Japanese and Chinese cancer management. However, while PSK and PSP have been extensively studied in Asia, there exists little data on the anticancer activity of the several distinct *T. versicolor* preparations now commercially available, despite their growing use in the United States.

  Most of the clinical research has focused on the effects of *T. versicolor* adjuvant therapy on disease-free survival and overall survival rates. In a randomized study of 158 esophageal cancer patients, survival of the group receiving

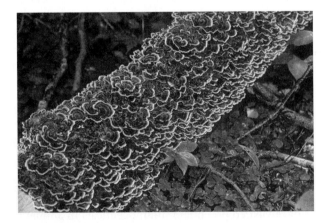

FIGURE 6.2. *Trametes versicolor.*

radiochemotherapy plus PSK (3,000 mg/day for 12 weeks) was significantly better than that of the group receiving radiochemotherapy alone (Ogoshi, et al., 1995). Since 2005, the results of five PSK trials in colorectal cancer have been published (Kanazawa, et al., 2005; Ohwada, et al., 2006; Takahashi, et al., 2005; Yoshino, et al., 2005), including one meta-analysis in 1094 colorectal cancer patients (Sakamoto, et al., 2006), all showing positive impact on clinical outcomes.

Current investigations of the mechanisms of action of *T. versicolor* have led to the hypothesis that β-1,3-D-glucans are the main immunologically active constituents present in the polysaccharide-peptide fractions PSK and PSP. Previously published studies assessing the effects of PSK on cytokine responses after oral administration in vivo have shown that PSK can enhance TNF-α, IFN-γ, IL-2, IL-8 and IL-12 protein concentrations. Data from epidemiological studies of immune deficiency in African-American women diagnosed with breast cancer, immune studies of the effect of chemotherapy drugs and radiotherapy on immune status, and the Asian literature on the clinical benefit of polysaccharide immune therapy together suggest that immune function may play a key role in primary and secondary prevention of breast cancer. High priority research areas for breast cancer immunotherapy include clinical trials of polysaccharide-peptide fractions (PSK and PSP) and *T. versicolor* biomass from which the polysaccharide fractions are extracted, in breast cancer patients. Two types of human trials are necessary to assess the potential for *T. versiocolor* in integrative cancer therapy. Clinical trials are required to assess the safety and effectiveness of *T. versiocolor* as a concurrent adjuvant therapy administered along with chemotherapy, radiotherapy, and Her2 neu monoclonal antibody therapy (Herceptin). In keeping with its potential role in secondary prevention as well as common use of *T. versiocolor* in Asian oncology, clinical trials of *T. versiocolor* immunotherapy after completion of standard cancer treatment are also needed. Breast cancer clinical trials currently rely on short-term surrogate markers of immune status toward the ultimate goal of improving breast cancer cure rates.

GANODERMA LUCIDUM (REISHI)

Ganoderma lucidum is another polysaccharide containing immunomodulatory polypore fungus. It has a long history of use in traditional Asian medicines. It is called *Lingzhi* in China and *Reishi* in Japan. Preclinical studies have established that the polysaccharide fractions of *G. lucidum* have diverse and potent immunomodulatory effects in vitro and in animal studies (Fig. 6.3).

Ganoderma is purported to have activity in breast and prostate cancer and has been shown to inhibit prostate and breast cancer cell migration. Sliva et al.

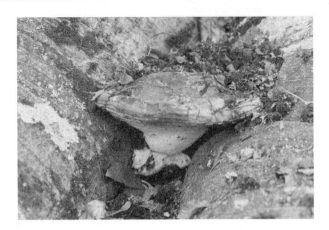

FIGURE 6.3. Ganoderma log.

(2003) compared commercially available *G. lucidum* spore and mycelial powder products and compared their ability to inhibit cancer cell migration and effect on NF-κB in vitro. Some products had strong activity against breast and prostate cancer cell lines and inhibited NF-κB, while others did not. Clinical evidence has been sparse until recently. Several clinical studies, mostly by research oncology groups in Asia and New Zealand, have been conducted on the effects of oral *G. lucidum* intake on immune parameters in advanced cancer patients. The studies have had mixed results that are difficult to interpret. Such inconsistencies may be due to the fact that the mycelia, fruiting body, and spores of the fungus may all have different biological properties; hence it is critical to know what part of the Ganoderma is being utilized.

Hot water extraction is believed by most traditional practitioners to yield the immunomodulatory polysaccharides from within medicinal mushrooms such as *G. lucidum* and *T. versicolor*. The effects of Ganopoly, a commercially available water-soluble polysaccharide product from *G. lucidum* at doses of 5.4 g/day, were studied in 36 advanced cancer patients (Gao, et al., 2005). The treatment had no significant effects on lymphocyte populations of CD3, CD4, CD8, CD56 or plasma concentrations of IL2, IL6, IFN-gamma, or NK cell activity. Doses of *G. lucidum* used in clinical trials range from 1500 mg/day to 5600 mg/day (1800 mg three times/day) (Tang, et al., 2005).

LENTINUS EDODES (SHIITAKE)

Lentinus edodes, called *shiitake* in Japanese and *xiang gu* or "fragrant mushroom in China, is the second most commonly cultivated edible mushroom

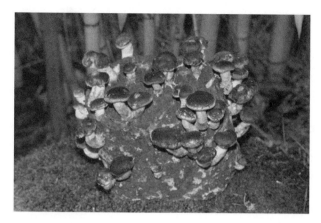

FIGURE 6.4. *Lentinus edodes.*

worldwide (Chang, 1996). The shiitake is a large, umbrella-shaped mushroom that is dark brown and is prized both for its culinary and medicinal properties (Fig 6.4). It has been renowned as a food and medicine for thousands of years and is a major ingredient of Chinese cuisine (Hobbs, 2000).

The shiitake mushroom contains components that have been shown to have many health and medicinal benefits. There are two preparations of *L. edodes* with well-studied pharmacological effects: *Lentinus edodes* mycelium (LEM), an extract from the powdered mycelia before the fruiting bodies develop and Lentinan, a highly purified, cell-wall constituent extracted from the fruiting bodies or mycelium (Hobbs, 2000). Lentinan was first isolated and studied in 1969 for its antitumor effects by Chihara and coworkers of the National Cancer Institute of Japan (Chihara, Hamuro, Maeda, Arai, & Fukuoka, 1970). Numerous animal studies demonstrate antitumor effect by activating different immune responses in the host (Aoki, 1981; Aoki, 1984; Dennert & Tucker, 1973; Herberman, 1981; Miyakoshi & Aoki, 1984; Miyakoshi, & Aoki, 1984; Mayell, 2001; Nanba, et al., 1987; Ng & Yap, 2002). Lentinan, a 1,3-β-glucan found in *L. edodes*, has been found to activate macrophages, T lymphocytes, and other immune effector cells that modulate the release of cytokines (Chang, 1996; Hamuro, 1985). Clinical trails have been done on Lentinan in Japan although none have been placebo-controlled and double-blinded (Zaidman, et al., 2005). In Japan, lentinan is often used to help support immune function in cancer patients during chemotherapy (Hobbs, 2000) and has been approved for clinical use there since the mid 1980's. It has been shown to increase overall survival of cancer patients, (Oka, et al., 1992; Yoshino, 1989), especially those with gastric and colorectal carcinoma (Furue, 1981; Hobbs, 2000; Taguchi, et al., 1985). A recent open label study (n = 62) by deVere White et al, however, showed that shiitake mushroom extract alone was ineffective in the treatment of clinical prostate cancer (deVere White, Hackman, Soares, Beckett, & Sun, 2002).

In human clinical studies shiitake extract has been given at an oral dose of 4 to 8 g/day. Other smaller studies used 9 g of dried mushrooms or 90 g of fresh mushrooms (Chang, 1996). Oral bioavailability of Lentinan is reportedly limited because of its molecular weight on the order of 400,000 to 1,000,000 daltons; therefore it is often administered intravenously. Lentinan seems to be safe when given to humans in the dosage range of 1 to 5 mg/day once or twice a week by IV injection (Hobbs, 2000).

GRIFOLA FRONDOSA

Maitake is the Japanese name for the edible fungus *Grifola frondosa*, which is characterized by a large fruiting body and overlapping caps. In the United States and Canada it is known as hen of the woods and sheep's head. It is a premier culinary mushroom with excellent taste and texture as well as a medicinal mushroom for health benefits. It is now being cultivated for food and use as a dietary supplement. It is estimated that commercial maitake production worldwide exceeds 40,000 tons (Mayell, 2001). In Japan, maitake has long been recognized as a tonic or adaptogen—a substance that balances bodily functions and enhances wellness, vitality, strength, and vigor (Fig 6.5) (Mayell, 2001).

Numerous animal studies have confirmed that maitake has prominent beneficial effects on immune function and cancer inhibition (Adachi,

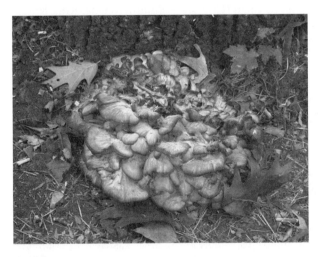

FIGURE 6.5. Grifola.

Nanba, & Kuroda, 1987; Mayell, 2001). Enhancement of the immune system by activation of macrophages, T cells, and NK cells has been demonstrated in tumor-bearing mice (Adachi, et al., 1987; Hishida, Nanba, & Kuroda, 1988; Kodama, Komuta, & Nanba, 2002; Kodama, Komuta, & Nanba, 2003; Mayell, 2001; Nanba, 1995; Nanba, 1997; Suzuki, Itani, et al., 1985; Suzuki, et al., 1989). In the early 1980s Japanese mycologist Hiroaki Nanba identified a D-fraction found in both the mycelia and the fruit body of the Maitake. The D-fraction is a standardized form of isolated β-glucan polysaccharide compounds (β-1,6 glucan and β-1,3 glucan) and a more purified extract, the MD-fraction, have shown particular promise as immunomodulating agents, and as an adjunct to cancer, specifically colon, lung, stomach, liver, prostate and brain (Mayell, 2001; Nanba, 1995; Nanba, 1997). Human studies are limited; however, nonrandomized clinical studies using D-fraction and whole maitake reduced the size of lung, liver, and breast tumors (Kodama, et al., 2002; Nanba, 1997). Maitake may also work in conjunction with chemotherapy to lessen its side effects, such as hair loss, pain, and nausea (Nanba, 1997).

Maitake is an edible mushroom that can be eaten as food or made into tea. A typical dosage of dried maitake in capsule or tablet form is 3 to 7 g daily. Most of the published studies to date have been animal studies; therefore, it is not known what doses may be safe or effective. Some references state that for disease prevention doses of 12 to 25 mg extract or .5 to 1 mg per kilogram daily should be taken in divided doses (Mayell, 2001). Because it has been used as a food in Japan for hundred of years, in amounts up to several hundred grams per day, it is thought to be safe (Kidd, 2000). Little is known about the safety of maitake in pregnancy and breastfeeding, and therefore its use as a supplement in these settings cannot be recommended.

SCHIZOPHYLLUM COMMUNE

Schizophyllum commune is called *Suehirotake* by the Japanese. The common name is "split gill or split-fold." *Schizophyllum commune* is one of the most common mushrooms in the world that grows on fallen trees in deciduous woodlands (Hobbs, 1995; Stamets, 2002). Schizophyllum is not generally available in North America or Europe for commercial trade. It is used primarily in Japan as an adjunctive antitumor polysaccharide with radiation therapy for cancer treatment and the commercial product (SPG, Sonifilan) is a pure β-glucan: β1–3, β1–6 D-glucan. *Schizophyllum commune* is similar to lentinan in composition and biological activity, and its mechanism of immunomoduation and antitumor action appears to be quite similar (Rowan, 2003).

Medicinal Mushrooms Summary

Mushroom polysaccharides are known to stimulate natural killer cells, T-cells, B-Cells and macrophage-dependent immune system responses (Wasser 2002). The immunomodulating action of mushroom polysaccharides is especially valuable as a means of prophylaxis, prevention, and co treatment with chemotherapy. The potential use of medicinal mushrooms for disease prevention and treatment is an expanding target for research and development. Given the rich background of medicinal mushroom for health benefits and the recent interest in research on mushroom extracts, it seems feasible that mushroom therapy may play an increased role in disease prevention and immunotherapy for adjunctive cancer therapy. Western-based clinical trials are needed to identify which mushroom extract is most effective against specific tumors in their ability to elicit cellular response and demonstrate safety.

Commercially Available Combination Herbal Therapies

Because botanical medicines have diverse mechanisms of action, including apoptotic, cytotoxic, autoantigenic, and immunomodulatory activities, both traditional and modern herbal cancer treatments involve multiple plants. Two commonly used commercially available combination botanical products are Essiac, and Zyflamend®. Zick et al. (2007) reported that women who used Essiac did not appear to have improved quality of life relative to non-users in a retrospective cohort study of 510 Canadian women (Zick, 2007) (See Chapter 26).

Zyflamend® has been studied in vitro, in animal experiments, and in Phase I clinical trial in men with prostate intraepithelial neoplasia. Zyflamend® is an encapsulated combination botanical medicine consisting of 10 standardized herbal extracts in olive oil (rosemary, tumeric, ginger, holy basil, green tea, Hu zhang, Chinese goldthread, barberry, oregano, and Baical skullcap). These herbs are among the richest sources of naturally occurring and chemically diverse cyclooxygenase-2 (COX-2) and 5-lipoxygenase (5-LO) inhibitor activity, both of which are upregulated in many tumors. Zyflamend® has undergone preclinical and clinical evaluation. Bennani-Baiti et al. (2006) at the Cleveland Clinic Brain Tumor Institute reported that Zyflamend® induced apoptosis in a human glioblastoma cell line and induced COX-2 and inhibited 5-LO expression while downregulating tubulin (Bennani-Bati, 2006). Newman et al. (2006) at MD Anderson Cancer Center reported that Zyflamend®

inhibited progression of oral carcinogenesis using the DMBA-induced hamster cheek pouch model (Newman, 2006).

Zyflamend® also has antiprostate cancer activity in in vitro and in vivo studies. Bemis et al. (2006) at Columbia University Medical Center treated human prostate cancer cells for 24 hours with 0.1 µL/mL Zyflamend® and observed a down-regulation of androgen receptors (Bemis, 2006). The interim results of a Phase I clinical trial of Zyflamend® in men with high-grade prostatic intra-epithelial neoplasia (PIN) were reported at the November 2006 meeting of the Society for Integrative Oncology. Of 29 African American high-risk PIN patients enrolled, 50% had a decrease in serum PSA values and one patient had a biopsy proven reversal of PIN (Pierorazio, 2006).

Botanical Interactions in Chemotherapy and Radiotherapy

Use of botanical therapy concurrent with chemo- and radiotherapy must be undertaken with caution. Many botanicals have hepatic effects that may have pharmacokinetic effects that alter plasma levels and half-lives of chemotherapeutic drugs. Some botanicals have antioxidant effects that could, in theory, affect the tumor cell killing ability of radiotherapy. Table 6.3 shows the predicted herb–chemotherapy drug interactions based on cytochrome P450 effects of a number of botanicals. Since many herbal medicines induce P450 enzymes, exogenous molecules, including chemotherapy drugs, are metabolized by the liver in a more efficient manner. This leads to reduced plasma levels of the drugs and thus lowers exposure of tumor cells to the chemotherapy. However, some botanicals have hepatic effects that would be predicted to increase the half-life of some chemotherapy agents. We can envision a future in integrative oncology in which selected botanicals will be administered concurrently with cyto-toxic drugs to improve efficacy. In the meantime, in the absence of detailed information on drug–herb interaction it is best to follow the motto, "When in doubt, leave it out." Chemotherapy represents a relatively small portion of the cancer patient's overall treatment plan. Co-administration of botanicals with chemotherapy drugs may risk reducing efficacy of chemotherapy, and thus, in the absence of data, it is best to suspend most herbal therapies during chemotherapy. There are notable exceptions, particularly those summarized in this chapter (see Table 6.4). Certain botanicals such as green tea, milk thistle, astragalus, and ashwaghanda are rarely contraindicated. Other botanicals such as curcumin, garlic, milk thistle, and ginseng are contraindicated with certain therapies, but well indicated with others. Some of most indicated herbal therapies are summarized in Table 6.4.

Table 6.3. Predicted Herbal-Chemotherapeutic Interactions
Mediated through Cytochrome Activities.

Botanicals	Chemotherapy Drugs	Cytochrome Enzymes	Expected Effect on Drug
Echinacea purpurea (coneflower)			
Ginkgo biloba (ginkgo)	Cyclophosphamide	2C8, 2C9, 2C19	Increased exposure
Harpagophytum procumbens (Devil's claw)	Ifosfamide	3A4	Decreased exposure
	Dacarbarzine	1A2	Increased exposure
	Paclitaxol	2C8, 3A4	Decreased exposure
Hypericum perforatum (St. John's wort)	Docetaxel	3A4	Decreased exposure
	Vinblastine	3A4	Decreased exposure
Mentha piperita (peppermint)	Vincristine	3A4	Decreased exposure
	Navelbine	3A4	Decreased exposure
Piper methysticum (kava-kava)	Etoposide	3A4	Decreased exposure
	Irinotecan	3A4, 3A5	Decreased exposure
Polygonum multiflorum (Fo-ti root)	Topotecan	3A4	Decreased exposure
	Tamoxifen	3A4, 1A2	Decreased exposure
	Armidex	3A4, 1A2, 2C8–9, 2C19	Decreased exposure
Tanacetum parthenium (feverfew)	Aromasin	3A4, 1A2, 2C8–9, 2C19	Decreased exposure
	Femara	3A4, 1A2, 2C8–9, 2C19	Decreased exposure
Trifolium pretense (red clover)	Iressa	3A4	Decreased exposure
Schisandra chinensis (wu wei)			
Valeriana officinalis (valerian)			

Zhou, et al., 2003; Gorski, et al., 2004; Iwata, et al., 2004; Jang, et al., 2004; Lefebvre, et al., 2004; Mannel, 2004; Sparreboom, et al., 2004; Unger & Frank, 2004.

Table 6.4. Selected Herbal Therapies for Co-administration
with Chemotherapy.

Chemotherapy Agent	Enhances Tumoricidal Actions	Reduces Toxicity
Cisplatin	Quercetin	Coriolus versicolor (and PS-K) Silybum marianum (silybin) Ginkgo biloba
Cyclophosphamide		Astragalus membranaceus, Withania somnifera, also Coriolus versicolor
Mitomycin-C	Panax ginseng	
Doxorubicin (Adriamycin) and Idarubicin	Green tea	Green tea
Tamoxifen	Green tea (EGCG) Panax quinquefolius	
Fluorouracils Interleukin-2	Curcumin Green tea Astragalus membranaceus Panax ginseng	—

Ichikawa, et al., 1998; Sadzuka, et al., 1998; Sugiyama & Sadzuka, 1998; Fukaya & Kanno, 1999; Masuda, et al., 2001; Sugiyama, et al., 2001; Hrelia, et al., 2004; Kim, et al., 2004; Koo, et al., 2004; Mei, et al., 2004; Du, et al., 2006.

Herbal Therapies Used to Mitigate Cancer Treatment Side Effects

A chapter on botanical oncology would not be complete without a mention of herbal therapies in common use by naturopathic physicians who specialize in the cancer care. Many of these treatments have not undergone clinical trial for either safety or efficacy. Nevertheless, most of the treatments have a long history of safe use. The integrative oncologist can feel comfortable using these treatments as therapeutic trials with patients with the following cancer treatment–related side effects.

RADIATION DERMATITIS

RayGel™ is a topical gel consisting of anthocyanins and glutathione. A small clinical study by Noel Peterson, ND showing prevention of radiotherapy-related skin burning was presented at the 2004 annual meeting of the American Association of Naturopathic Physicians (Miko Enomoto, et al., 2005). Aloe has not been shown to be effective. Aloe vera is widely prescribed and used for radiation burns but one controlled clinical trial reported that aloe vera gel did not significantly reduce radiation-induced skin side effects (Heggie, et al., 2002).

ANEMIA

Marrow Plus® is an encapsulated traditional Chinese herbal formulation for blood deficiency. This formula has been used in treating chemotherapy and zidovudine–related anemia.

LEUKOPENIA

Astragalus has been shown to be helpful. The strongest indication for astragalus in the context of oncology care is to help prevent the immunosuppression caused by chemotherapy agents. Additionally, there is some indication that astragalus may also potentiate the cytotoxic effects of certain chemotherapy agents. See previous section on Astragalus.

NAUSEA AND VOMITING

Ginger tea seems helpful for some patients. One placebo-controlled trial showed that ginger capsules were useful in lowering postoperative nausea and vomiting in 80 women undergoing gynecologic laparoscopic surgery (Pongrojpaw, & Chiamchanya, 2003). However, a single clinical trial showed that ginger capsules in 48 gynecologic cancer patients receiving cisplatin treatment was not more effective than metoclopramide (Manusirivithaya, Sripramote, et al., 2004).

HAND-FOOT SYNDROME

Chlorophyll and calendula cream has been helpful for some patients, usually in combination with Vitamin B$_6$ therapy.

INSOMNIA

Valerian has a long history of use as a sleep-promoting herb. Clinical trials are sparse and conflicting. Since valerian has been shown to have no effect on CYP3A4 or CYP2D6 activity in healthy humans (Donovan, DeVane, et al., 2004) it may be safe to use with cancer patients undergoing chemotherapy. However, most naturopathic physicians who specialize in cancer care will prescribe melatonin as a first-line sleep therapy because of cancer clinical trial evidence that concomitant oral melatonin in doses of 20 or 40 mg before bed improved chemotherapy outcomes.

APTHOUS ULCERS, STOMATITIS, AND MUCOSITIS

Slippery elm tea can reduce pain on eating and swallowing.

FATIGUE

Eleutherococcus senticosis (Siberian ginseng) is often prescribed by naturopathic physicians to treat radiotherapy-related fatigue.

DEPRESSION

St. John's wort is contraindicated with concurrent use of many chemotherapy drugs, but may be useful for both depression and menopausal hot flashes that are common sequela to completion of conventional cancer treatment.

MENOPAUSAL VASOMOTOR STABILITY

St. John's wort and hesperidin are both worth trying in cancer patients. Use caution during chemotherapy as hypericin can alter hepatic metabolism of several chemotherapy drugs.

Botanical Medicine as Secondary Prevention

Naturopathic physicians who specialize in oncology agree that herbal therapy plays a significant role in secondary prevention. Based on their safety and scientific evidence, most NDs include them in their core protocol for preventing cancer relapse in patients who have received primary conventional treatment (surgery, chemotherapy, radiation). The following botanicals are administered orally. Doses in common use are provided as well.

Garlic	3200 mcg allicin bid
Curcumin	3000–9000 mg/day
Camellia sinensis	500 mg bid
Quercetin	750 mg bid
Bromelain	750 mg bid
Silymarin officinalis	260 mg bid
Trametes versicolor	1500 mg tid

Conclusions, Future Directions, and Research Agenda

Plant medicines may fill gaps in current oncology treatment and offer useful immunomodulatory, antiinflammatory, apoptotic, and antiangiogenesis treatments.

Botanical oncology is an emerging field and research is desperately needed. Perhaps the most important question to answer is whether a botanical exists with chemopreventive, immunomodulatory, antiinflammatory, and antiangiogenic activity, effective in preventing recurrence of cancer following conventional treatment with surgery, radiation and chemotherapy? High priority studies include the following:

- Prospective outcomes study of naturopathic oncology clinics where science-based botanical medicine is being applied.
- Combination botanical oncology trials using active isolated molecular constituents from multiple plants that have anticancer activity utilizing multiple mechanisms.
- Combination natural product whole plant botanical oncology trials present methodological challenges that exceed those of conventional drug trials. These difficulties can be and must be overcome. An approach to standardization of both the chemical constituents and the biological activity of herbal products across trials must be adopted. In August 2007 NCCAM and NIH Office of Dietary Supplements sponsored a conference on botanical authentication held at Bastyr University. "White Paper" recommendations on chemical and biological methods for standardization will be published in 2008 to 2009.

- Single agent dose-escalating botanical trials in stage IV cancer patients.
- Phase I clinical trials of botanical medicines used by traditional shamans in South America, Central America, and Africa, including entheogenic plant medicines, to treat cancer.

ACKNOWLEDGMENT

Grateful acknowledgment to Bastyr library scientists Jane Saxton, MLS and Susan Banks, MLS.

We want to thank Paul Stamets and Tom Volk for providing the mushroom photos. Paul Stamets is a well-known mycologist, author and founder of Fungi Perfecti® a company specializing in gourmet and medicinal mushrooms-http://www.fungi.com. Tom Volk is Professor of Biology at the University of Wisconsin-La Crosse, WI, @ TomVolkFungi.net.

REFERENCES

Lamson, DW & Brignall MS. (1999). Antioxidants in cancer therapy: Their actions and interactions with oncologic therapies. *Alternative Medicine Review,* 4(5), 304–329.

Lamson, DW & Brignall MS. (2000a). Antioxidants and cancer therapy II: Quick reference guide. *Alternative Medicine Review,* 5(2), 152–163.

McCulloch M, See C, Shu XJ, Broffman M, Kramer A, Fan WY, et al. (2006). Astragalus-based Chinese herbs and platinum-based chemotherapy for advanced non-small-cell lung cancer: Meta-analysis of randomized trials. *Journal of Clinical Oncology,* 24(3), 419–430.

Nakachi K, Suemasu K, Suga K, Takeo T, Imai K, & Higashi Y. (1998). Influence of drinking green tea on breast cancer malignancy among Japanese patients. *Japanese Journal of Cancer Research,* 89(3), 254–261.

Sakamoto J, Morita S, Oba K, Matsui T, Kobayashi M, Nakazato H, et al. (2006). Efficacy of adjuvant immunochemotherapy with polysaccharide K for patients with curatively resected colorectal cancer: A meta-analysis of centrally randomized controlled clinical trials. *Cancer Immunology, Immunotherapy,* 55(4), 404–411.

Sharma RA, Euden SA, Platton SL, Cooke DN, Shafayat A, Hewitt HR, et al. (2004). Phase I clinical trial of oral curcumin: Biomarkers of systemic activity and compliance. *Clinical Cancer Research,* 10(20), 6847–6854.

Toi M, Hattori T, Akagi M, Inokuchi K, Orita K, Sugimachi K, et al. (1992). Randomized adjuvant trial to evaluate the addition of tamoxifen and PSK to chemotherapy in patients with primary breast cancer. 5-Year results from the Nishi-Nippon group of the adjuvant chemoendocrine therapy for breast cancer Organization. *Cancer,* 70(10), 2475–2483.

Tsang KW, Lam CL, Yan C, Mak JC, Ooi GC, Ho JC, et al. (2003). Coriolus versicolor polysaccharide peptide slows progression of advanced non-small cell lung cancer. *Respiratory Medicine,* 97(6), 618–624.

Wu AH, Yu MC, Tseng CC, Hankin J, & Pike MC. (2003). Green tea and risk of breast cancer in Asian Americans. *International Journal of Cancer. Journal International du Cancer,* 106(4), 574–579.

Zaidman BZ, Yassin M, Mahajna J, & Wasser SP. (2005). Medicinal mushroom modulators of molecular targets as cancer therapeutics. *Applied Microbiology and Biotechnology,* 67(4), 453–468.

(*A complete reference list for this chapter is available online at http://www.oup.com/us/ integrativemedicine*).

7

Cannabinoids and Cancer

DONALD I. ABRAMS AND MANUEL GUZMAN

KEY CONCEPTS

- Cannabis has been used in medicine for thousands of years before achieving its current status as an illicit substance.
- Cannabinoids, the active components of *Cannabis sativa*, mimic the effects of the endogenous cannabinoids (the so-called endocannabinoids), activating specific cannabinoid receptors, particularly cannabinoid receptor type 1 (CB1) found predominantly in the central nervous system and cannabinoid receptor type 2 (CB2) found in cells involved with immune function.
- Delta-9-tetrahydrocannabinol, the main psychoactive cannabinoid in the plant, has been available as a prescription medication approved for chemotherapy-induced nausea and vomiting and treatment of anorexia associated with the AIDS wasting syndrome.
- In addition to treatment of nausea and anorexia, cannabinoids may be of benefit in the treatment of cancer-related pain, possibly in a synergistic fashion with opioid analgesics.
- Cannabinoids have been shown to be of benefit in the treatment of HIV-related peripheral neuropathy, suggesting that they may be worthy of study in patients with chemotherapy-related neuropathic symptoms.
- Cannabinoids have a favorable drug safety profile, medical use predominantly limited by their psychoactive effects and their limited bioavailability.
- There is no conclusive evidence that chronic cannabis use leads to the development of any malignancies; some preclinical studies actually suggest a protective effect.
- Cannabinoids inhibit tumor growth in laboratory animal models by modulation of key cell-signaling pathways, inducing direct

growth arrest and tumor cell death, as well as by inhibiting tumor angiogenesis and metastasis.

- Cannabinoids appear to be selective antitumor compounds as they kill tumor cells without affecting their nontransformed counterparts.
- More basic and clinical research is needed to ascertain not only the role of cannabinoids in palliative cancer care, but also to delineate their role as potential anticancer agents with activity at a number of sites by way of multiple mechanisms of action.

■

Although long-recognized for its medicinal values and widely used by millions throughout the world, marijuana receives little attention in the standard literature because of its status as a controlled substance and classification in the United States as a Schedule I agent with a high potential for abuse and no known medical use. Data on the potential effectiveness of medicinal cannabis is difficult to find due to the limited numbers of clinical trials that have been conducted to date. As a botanical, cannabis shares those difficulties encountered in the study of plants that are grown in many climates and environments from diverse genetic strains and harvested under variable conditions. However, the potential benefits of medicinal cannabis have not been lost on a large number of people living with cancer, some of whom have been quite vocal in attributing their ability to complete their prescribed course of chemotherapy to the antiemetic effects of smoked cannabis. In the practice of integrative oncology, the provider is frequently faced with situations where being able to recommend medicinal cannabis seems like the right thing to do. A growing body of preclinical evidence suggests that cannabis may not only be effective for symptom management, but may have a direct antitumor effect as well. This chapter will be devoted to a review of the role of cannabinoids in cancer.

Cannabis as Medicine: A Brief History

Use of cannabis as medicine dates back at least 2000 years [1–4]. Widely employed on the Indian subcontinent, cannabis was introduced into Western medicine in the 1840s by W.B. O'Shaughnessy, a surgeon who learned of its medicinal benefits first hand while working in the British East India Company. Promoted for reported analgesic, sedative, anti-inflammatory, antispasmodic, and anticonvulsant properties, cannabis was said to be the treatment of choice for Queen Victoria's dysmennorhea. In the early 1900s, medicines that were indicated for each of cannabis' purported activities were introduced into the Western armamentarium making its use less widespread.

Physicians in the United States were the main opponents to the introduction of the Marihuana Tax Act by the Treasury Department in 1937. The legislation was masterminded by Harry Anslinger, director of the Federal Bureau of Narcotics from its inception in 1931 until 1962, who testified in Congress that "Marijuana is the most violence-causing drug in the history of mankind." The Act imposed a levy of $1 an ounce for medicinal use and $100 an ounce for recreational use, which in 1937 was a prohibitive cost. By using the Mexican name for the plant and associating it with nefarious South-of-the-Border activities, the proponents fooled many physicians. The Act was singly opposed by the American Medical Association who felt the objective evidence, that cannabis was harmful, was lacking and that its passage would impede further research into its medical utility. In 1942, cannabis was removed from the U.S. Pharmacopoeia.

Mayor Fiorello LaGuardia of New York commissioned an investigation into the reality of the potential risks and benefits of cannabis that reported in 1944 that the substance was not associated with any increased risk of criminal activity, addiction, or insanity as had been claimed. The LaGuardia Commission Report, as well as subsequent similar investigations that have been commissioned nearly every decade since, went largely ignored.

In 1970 with the initiation of the Controlled Substances Act, marijuana was classified as a Schedule I drug. Where both Schedule I and Schedule II substances have a high potential for abuse, Schedule I drugs are distinguished by having no accepted medical use. Other Schedule I substances include heroin, LSD, mescaline, methylqualone and, most recently, gammahydroxybutyrate (GHB). In 1973, President Nixon's investigation into the risks and benefits of marijuana, the Shafer Commission, concluded that it was a safe substance with no addictive potential and that it had medicinal benefits. Despite the fact that it was deemed to have no medical use, marijuana was distributed to patients by the US government on a case by case basis by way of a Compassionate Use Investigational New Drug (IND) program established in 1978.

In the late 1980s and early 1990s, many people living with human immunodeficiency virus-1 (HIV) developed a wasting syndrome as a preterminal event [5]. The wasting syndrome, characterized by anorexia, weight loss of greater than 10% body weight and frequent fever and diarrhea created hordes of cachectic individuals in search of any potential therapeutic intervention. Many turned to smoking marijuana [6–8]. Fearful that there might be a run on the Compassionate Use program, the Bush administration shut it down in 1992, the same year that dronabinol (delta-9-tetrahydrocannabinol, Marinol®) was approved for treatment of anorexia associated with the AIDS wasting syndrome.

Delta-9-tetrahydrocannbinol is one of the approximately 70 cannabinoids found in the cannabis plant and is felt to be the main psychoactive component. Overall, the plant contains about 400 compounds derived from its secondary metabolism, many of which may contribute to its medicinal effect. Synthetic delta-9-THC in sesame oil was first licensed and approved in 1986 for the treatment of chemotherapy-associated nausea and vomiting. Clinical trials done at that time determined that dronabinol was as effective, if not more so, as the available antiemetic agents [9]. The potent class of serotonin receptor antagonists that have subsequently revolutionized the ability to administer emetogenic chemotherapy had not yet come to market.

Dronabinol was investigated for its ability to stimulate weight gain in patients with the AIDS wasting syndrome in the late 1980s. Results from a number of trials suggested that although patients reported an improvement in appetite, no statistically significant weight gain was appreciated [10–11]. In one trial evaluating megesterol acetate and dronabinol alone and together, the cannabinoid seemed to negate some of the weight increase seen in those receiving only the hormone [12].

Cannabinoid Chemistry and Biologic Effects

Cannabinoids are a group of 21 carbon terpenophenolic compounds produced uniquely by *Cannabis sativa* and *Cannabis indica* species (Fig. 7.1) [13–14]. With the discovery of endogenous cannabinoids and to distinguish them from pharmaceutical compounds, the plant compounds may also be referred to as phytocannabinoids. Although delta-9-THC is the primary active ingredient in cannabis, there are a number of non-THC cannabinoids and non-cannabinoid compounds that also have biologic activity. Cannabinol, cannabidiol, cannabichromene, cannabigerol, tetrahydrocannabivirin and delta-8-THC are just some of the additional cannabinoids that have been identified. It is postulated that the secondary compounds may enhance the beneficial effects of delta-9-THC, for example, by modulating the THC-induced anxiety, anticholinergic, or immunosuppressive effects. In addition, cannabis associated terpenoids and flavonoids may increase cerebral blood flow, enhance cortical activity, kill respiratory pathogens, and provide anti-inflammatory activity.

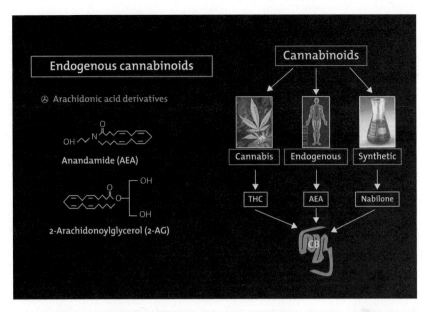

FIGURE 7.1. Cannabinoids. Cannabinoids are a group of 21 carbon terpenophenolic compounds. Delta-9-tetrahydrocannabinol is the most potent of the phytocannabinoids produced by the Cannabis species. The endogenous cannabinoids, anandamide (AEA) and 2-arachidonoylglycerol (2-AG), function as neurotransmitters. Synthetic cannabinoids have also been produced as phatrmaceutical agents.

The neurobiology of the cannabinoids has only been identified within the past 20 years, during which time an explosion of knowledge has occurred [15–18]. In the mid 1980s, researchers developed a potent cannabinoid agonist to be used in research investigations. In 1986 it was discovered that cannabinoids inhibited the accumulation of cyclic adenosine monophosphate (cAMP), suggesting the presence of a receptor-mediated mechanism. By attaching a radiolabel to the synthetic cannabinoid, the first cannabinoid receptor, CB1, was pharmacologically identified in the brain in 1988. The CB1 receptor is coupled to $G_{i/o}$ proteins. Its engagement inhibits adenylyl cyclase and voltage-gated calcium channels, and stimulates rectifying potassium conductances and mitogen-activated protein kinase activity. By 1990, investigators had cloned the CB1 receptor, identified its DNA sequence and mapped its location in the brain, with the largest concentration being in the basal ganglia, cerebellum, hippocampus, and cerebral cortex. In 1993 a second cannabinoid receptor, CB2, was identified outside the brain. Originally detected in macrophages and the marginal zone of the spleen, the highest concentration of CB2 receptors is located on the B lymphocytes and natural killer cells, suggesting a possible role in immunity.

The existence of cannabinoid receptors has subsequently been demonstrated in animal species all the way down to invertebrates. Are these receptors present in the body solely to complex with ingested phytocannabinoids? The answer came in 1992 with the identification of a brain constituent that binds to the cannabinoid receptor. Named *anandamide* from the Sanskrit word for bliss, the first endocannabinoid had been discovered. Subsequently 2-arachidonoylglycerol (2-AG) has also been confirmed as part of the body's endogenous cannabinoid system. These endocanabinoids function as neurotransmitters. As the ligands for the 7-transmembrane domain cannabinoid receptors, binding of the endocannabinoid leads to G-protein activation and the cascade of events transpires resulting in the opening of potassium channels, which decreases cell firing, and the closure of calcium channels, which decreases neurotransmitter release (Fig. 7.2).

The function of the endogenous cannabinoid system in the body is becoming more appreciated through advances in cannabinoid pharmacology. The

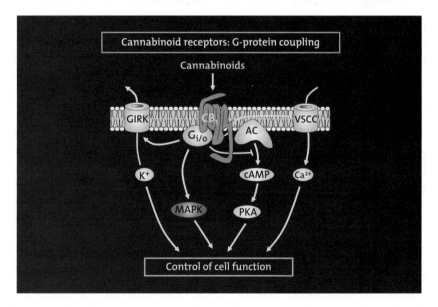

FIGURE 7.2. Signaling pathways coupled to the CB1 cannabinoid receptor. Cannabinoids exert their effects by binding to specific $G_{i/o}$ protein-coupled receptors. The CB1 cannabinoid receptor signals to a number of different cellular pathways. These include, for example, (i) inhibition of the adenylyl cyclase (AC)–cyclic AMP–protein kinase A (PKA) pathway; (ii) modulation of ion conductances, by inhibition of voltage-sensitive Ca^{2+} channels (VSCC) and activation of G protein-coupled inwardly-rectifying K^+ channels (GIRK); and (iii) activation of mitogen-activated protein kinase (MAPK) cascades. Other less established cannabinoid receptor effectors and the cross-talk among the different pathways have been omitted for simplification.

identification of the cannabinoid receptors has lead to a host of agonists and antagonists being synthesized. Utilizing these tools, investigators are discovering that the system is likely to be important in the modulation of pain and appetite, suckling in the newborn, and the complexities of memory (Michael Pollen in *The Botany of Desire* gives a particularly entertaining description of the natural function of endocannabinoids in memory) [19]. In addition to being utilized to learn more about the natural function of the endocannabinoid system, a number of these cannabinoid receptor agonists and antagonists are being developed as potential pharmaceutical therapies. In the meantime, dronabinol, nabilone (Cesamet®, a synthetic cannabinoid) and cannabis are the currently available cannabinoid therapies in the United States. Levonantradol (Nantrodolum®) is a synthetic cannabinoid administered intramuscularly, not used as much clinically since the oral agents became available. A whole cannabis extract (Sativex®) delivered as an oro-mucosal spray with varying combinations of THC and cannabidiol is available in Canada and undergoing late-phase testing in the United States and other countries.

Through the receptors described, cannabis delivered by way of inhalation or orally can produce a host of biologic effects. The Institute of Medicine report makes the following general conclusions about the biology of cannabis and cannabinoids [2].

- Cannabinoids likely have a natural role in pain modulation, control of movement, and memory.
- The natural role of cannabinoids in immune systems is likely multifaceted and remains unclear.
- The brain develops tolerance to cannabinoids.
- Animal research has demonstrated the potential for dependence, but this potential is observed under a narrower range of conditions than with benzodiazepines, opiates, cocaine, or nicotine.
- Withdrawal symptoms can be observed in animals but appear mild compared with those of withdrawal from opiates or benzodiazepines.

Pharmacology of Cannabis

When taken by mouth, there is a low (6%–20%) and variable oral bioavailability [13,20]. Peak plasma concentrations occur after 1 to 6 hours and remain elevated with a terminal half-life of 20 to 30 hours. When consumed orally, delta-9-THC is initially metabolized in the liver to 11-OH-THC, also a potent psychoactive metabolite. On the other hand, when smoked, the cannabinoids are rapidly absorbed into the bloodstream with a peak concentration in 2 to 10 minutes, which rapidly declines over the next 30 minutes. Smoking thus achieves a higher peak concentration with a shorter duration of effect. Less of the psychoactive 11-OH-THC metabolite is formed.

Cannabinoids can interact with the hepatic cytochrome P450 enzyme system [21–22]. Cannabidiol, for example, can inactivate CYP 3A4. After repeated doses, some of the cannabinoids may induce P450 isoforms. The effects are predominantly related to the CYP1A2, CYP2C, and CYP3A isoforms. The potential for a cannabinoid interaction with cytochrome P450 and, hence, possibly metabolism of chemotherapeutic agents has led to a small amount of data on the possibility of botanical–drug interactions. In one study, 24 cancer patients were treated with intravenous irinotecan (600 mg, n = 12) or docetaxel (180 mg, n = 12), followed 3 weeks later by the same drugs concomitant with medicinal cannabis taken as an herbal tea for 15 consecutive days, starting 12 days before the second treatment [23]. The carefully conducted pharmacokinetic analyses showed that cannabis administration did not significantly influence exposure to and clearance of irinotecan or docetaxel.

Cannabinoids and Cancer Symptom Management

ANTIEMETIC EFFECT

The nausea and vomiting related to cancer chemotherapy continues to be a significant clinical problem even in light of the newer agents that have been added to our armamentarium since the 1970s and 1980s when clinical trials of cannabinoids were first conducted [24]. In those days, phenothiazines and metoclopropramide were the main antiemetic agents used. Dronabinol, synthetic THC, and nabilone, a synthetic analog of THC, were both tested as novel oral agents in a number of controlled clinical trials. Nabilone was approved in Canada in 1982, but only recently became available in the United States. Dronabinol was approved as an antiemetic to be used in cancer chemotherapy in the United States in 1986.

Numerous meta-analyses confirm the utility of these THC-related agents in the treatment of chemotherapy-induced nausea and vomiting. Tramer et al. conducted a systematic review of 30 randomized comparisons of cannabis with placebo or antiemetics from which dichotomous data on efficacy and harm were available [25]. Oral nabilone, oral dronabinol, and intramuscular levonantradol were tested. No smoked cannabis trials were included. A total of 1366 patients were involved in the systematic review. Cannabinoids were found to be significantly more effective antiemetics than prochlorperazine, metoclopramide, chlorpromazine, thiethylperazine, haloperidol, domperidone, or alizapride. In this analysis, the number needed to treat (NNT) for complete control of nausea was six; the NNT for complete control of vomiting was eight. Cannabinoids were not more effective in patients receiving very low or very high emetogenic chemotherapy. In crossover trials, patients preferred cannabinoids for future chemotherapy cycles. Tramer identified some "potentially beneficial side effects" that occurred more often with cannabinoids including the "high," sedation or drowsiness, and euphoria. Less desirable side effects that occurred more frequently with cannabinoids included dizziness, dysphoria, or depression, hallucinations, paranoia, and hypotension.

A later analysis by Ben Amar reported that 15 controlled studies compared nabilone to placebo or available antiemetic drugs [26]. In 600 patients with a variety of malignant diagnoses, nabilone was found to be superior to prochlorperazine, domperidone and alizapride, with patients clearly favoring the nabilone for continuous use. Nabilone has also been shown to be moderately effective in managing the nausea and vomiting associated with radiation therapy and anesthesia after abdominal surgery [25,27,28]. In the same meta-analysis, Ben Amar reports that in 14 studies of dronabinol involving 681 patients, the cannabinoid antiemetic effect was equivalent or significantly greater than chlorpromazine and equivalent to metochlopramide, thiethylperazine and haloperidol. It is noted that the efficacy of the cannabinoids in these studies was sometimes outweighed by the adverse reactions and that none of the comparator antiemetics were of the serotonin receptor antagonist class that is the mainstay of treatment today.

There have been only three controlled trials evaluating the efficacy of smoked marijuana in chemotherapy-induced nausea and vomiting [26]. In two of the studies, the smoked cannabis was only made available after patients failed dronabinol. The third trial was a randomized, double-blind, placebo-controlled, cross-over trial involving 20 adults where both smoked marijuana and oral THC were evaluated. One-quarter of the patients reported a positive antiemetic response to the cannabinoid therapies. On direct questioning of the participants, 35% preferred the oral dronabinol, 20% preferred the smoked marijuana, and 45% did not express a preference. Four participants receiving dronabinol alone experienced distorted time perception or hallucinations, which were also reported by two with smoked marijuana and one with both substances. The University of California Center for Medicinal Cannabis Research also approved and funded a double-dummy design clinical trial to compare smoked cannabis, oral dronabinol, or placebo in patients with delayed nausea and vomiting, a condition for which the serotonin receptor antagonists are ineffective [29]. Unfortunately the trial was launched concurrently with the first release of aprepitant (Emend), the first commercially available drug from the new class of agents, the Substance P/neurokinin NK-1 receptor antagonists, which are approved for the treatment of delayed nausea [30]. The cannabis trial never accrued and the funding was withdrawn.

Both dronabinol and nabilone are FDA-approved for the treatment of nausea and vomiting associated with cancer chemotherapy in patients who have failed to respond adequately to conventional antiemetic therapy. Nabilone's extended duration of action allows for twice a day dosing of 1 or 2 mg commencing 1 to 3 hours before receiving chemotherapy. A dose of 1 or 2 mg the night before administration of chemotherapy might also be useful. It is recommended to commence dronabinol at an initial dose of 5 mg/m^2, also 1 to 3 hours before the administration of chemotherapy, then every 2 to 4 hours after chemotherapy, for a total of 4 to 6 doses/day. Should the 5 mg/m^2 dose prove to be ineffective, and in the absence of significant side effects, the dose may be escalated by 2.5 mg/m^2 increments to a maximum of 15 mg/m^2 per dose. Nabilone, with fewer metabolites and a lower dose range may be associated with fewer side effects. The need to dose 1 to 3 hours before chemotherapy is one factor that drives patients to prefer smoked cannabis where the delivery and effect peak within minutes. Patients also prefer the ability to more tightly titrate the dose of cannabinoids they receive when smoking compared to oral ingestion.

APPETITE STIMULATION

Anorexia, early satiety, weight loss, and cachexia are some of the most daunting symptom management challenges faced by the practicing oncologist. There are very few tools in the tool-box for addressing these concerns. Patients are not only disturbed by the disfigurement associated with wasting, but also by their inability to engage in the social interaction associated with breaking bread and partaking of a meal. For many the hormonal manipulation with megestrol acetate (synthetically derived progesterone) may be contraindicated or the side effects undesirable. Two small controlled trials demonstrated that oral THC stimulates appetite and may slow weight loss in patients with advanced malignancies [26]. In a larger randomized, double-blind, parallel group study of 469 adults with advanced cancer and weight loss, patients received either 2.5 mg of oral THC twice daily, 800 mg of oral megestrol daily or both. In the megestrol monotherapy group, appetite increased in 75% and weight in 11% compared to 49% and 3% respectively in the oral THC group. These differences were statistically significant. The combined therapy did not confer additional benefits. Of note, similar studies in patients with HIV-associated wasting syndrome also found that cannabinoids were more effective in improving appetite than in increasing weight. In our own study of the safety of smoked and oral cannabinoids in patients with HIV on protease inhibitor regimens, we did find an increase in weight in both cannabinoid groups compared to the placebo recipients; however, the study was not powered with weight gain as an endpoint [31,32].

Many animal studies have previously demonstrated that THC and other cannabinoids have a stimulatory effect on appetite and increase food intake. It is felt that the endogenous cannabinoid system may serve as a regulator of feeding behavior. For example, anandamide in mice leads to a potent enhancement of appetite [33]. It is felt that the CB1 receptors, present in the hypothalamus where food intake is controlled and in the mesolimbic reward system, may be involved in the motivational or reward aspects of eating. This has led to the development of the pharmaceutical CB1 antagonist rimonabant (Acomplia), now approved in Europe for the treatment of obesity on the basis of Phase III clinical trials where it was shown to induce a 4 to 5 kg mean weight loss with improved glycemic and lipid profiles [34]. This first of a new class of agents has not yet been approved in the United States because it was found to induce anxiety and depressive disorders that were deemed high risk.

Anecdotal as well as clinical trial evidence also supports the appetite-stimulating effect of smoking cannabis. In classic trials conducted in the 1970s in healthy controls, it was found that, especially when smoked in a social/communal setting, cannabis ingestion led to an increase in caloric intake, predominantly in the form of between meal snacks, mainly in the form of fatty and sweet foods. In cancer patients with anorexia as well as chemotherapy-induced nausea, it is worth noting that cannabis is the only antiemetic that also has orexigenic action. Although cannabis thus provides two potential benefits to the patient with cancer, the appetite stimulation does not always reverse cancer cachexia, which is a function of energy wasting in addition to decreased food intake.

ANALGESIA

Our understanding of the possible mechanisms of cannabinoid-induced analgesia has been greatly increased through study of the cannabinoid receptors, endocannabinoids and synthetic agonists and antagonists. The CB1 receptor is found in the central nervous system as well as in peripheral nerve terminals. Elevated levels of the CB1 receptor—like opioid receptors—are found in areas of the brain that modulate nociceptive processing [35]. In contrast, CB2 receptors are located in peripheral tissue and are present at very low expression levels in the CNS. Of the endogenous cannabinoids identified, anandamide has high affinity for CB1 receptors, whereas 2-AG has affinity for both CB1 and CB2 receptors. With the development of receptor-specific antagonists (SR141716 for CB1 and SR144528 for CB2), additional information has been obtained regarding the roles of the receptors and endogenous cannabinoids in modulation of pain [36,37]. Where the CB1 agonists exert analgesic activity in the CNS, both CB1 and CB2 agonists have peripheral analgesic actions [38,39].

Cannabinoids may also contribute to pain modulation through an anti-inflammatory mechanism—a CB2 effect with cannabinoids acting on mast cell receptors to attenuate the release of inflammatory agents such as histamine and serotonin and on keratinocytes to enhance the release of analgesic opioids [40–42]. Cannabinoids are effective in animal models of both acute and persistent pain. The central analgesic mechanism differs from the opioids in that it cannot be blocked by opioid antagonists. The potential for additive analgesic effects with opioids as well as the potential for cannabinoids to reduce nausea and increase appetite make a strong case for the evaluation of marijuana as adjunctive therapy for patients on morphine.

Medical literature cites evidence of the ability of cannabinoids to reduce naturally occurring pain, but few human studies have been performed. Early studies of cannabinoids on experimental pain in human volunteers produced inconsistent results. In some cases, the administration of cannabinoids failed to produce observable analgesic effects; in others, cannabinoids resulted in an increase of pain sensitivity (hyperalgesia). On review, Institute of Medicine researchers noted that these studies suffered from poor design and methodological problems and dubbed their findings inconclusive [2].

Encouraging clinical data on the effects of cannabinoids on chronic pain come from three studies of cancer pain. Cancer pain results from inflammation, mechanical invasion of bone, or other pain-sensitive structure, or nerve injury. It is severe, persistent, and often resistant to treatment with opioids. Noyes and colleagues conducted two studies on the effects of oral THC on cancer pain. Both studies used standard single-dose analgesic study methodology and met the criteria for well-controlled clinical trials of analgesic efficacy.

The first experiment measured both pain intensity and pain relief in a double-blind, placebo-controlled study of 10 subjects [43]. Observers compared the effects of placebo and 5, 10, 15 and 20 mg doses of delta-9-THC over a 6-hour period. Researchers reported that 15 and 20 mg doses produced significant analgesia, as well as antiemesis and appetite stimulation. Authors cautioned that some subjects reported unwanted side effects such as sedation and depersonalization at the 20 mg dose level. In a follow-up single-dose study of 36 subjects, Noyes et al. reported that 10 mg of THC produced analgesic effects over a 7-hour observation period comparable to 60 mg of codeine, and that 20 mg of THC induced effects equivalent to 120 mg of codeine [44]. Authors noted that respondents found higher doses of THC to be more sedative than codeine. However, in a separate publication, Noyes et al. reported that patients who had administered THC had improved mood, sense of well-being, and less anxiety [45]. A study by Staquet and colleagues on the effects of a THC nitrogen analogue on cancer pain yielded similar results [46]. Authors found the THC analogue equivalent to 50 mg of codeine and superior to both placebo and 50 mg of secobarbital in subjects with mild, moderate, and severe pain.

Cannabinoids have also been shown to be of potential benefit in an animal model of neuropathic pain [47]. Neuropathic pain is a troubling symptom in cancer patients, especially those treated with platinum-based chemotherapy or taxanes. A painful sensory peripheral neuropathy is also commonly encountered in patients with HIV infection either as a consequence of HIV itself or antiretroviral drugs used in treatment of the infection. We completed a randomized, controlled trial of smoked cannabis compared to placebo in 50 subjects with HIV-related peripheral neuropathy [48]. Smoked cannabis reduced daily pain by 34% compared to 17% with placebo ($P = 0.03$). Greater than 30% reduction in pain was reported by 52% in the cannabis group and by 24% in the placebo group ($P = 0.04$). The first cannabis cigarette reduced chronic pain by a median of 72% compared to 15% with placebo ($P < 0.001$). Cannabis also reduced experimentally-induced hyperalgesia to both brush and von Frey hair stimuli ($P \leq 0.05$) in a heat-capsaicin experimental pain model used to anchor the more subjective response of the chronic neuropathic pain. No serious adverse events were reported. Two recent placebo-controlled studies of cannabinioids for central neuropathic pain associated with multiple sclerosis produced results similar to the present study. In a crossover trial of synthetic delta-9-THC up to 10 mg/day, an NNT of 3.5 was reported [49]. A trial of a sublingual spray containing delta-9-THC alone or combined with cannabidiol showed a 41% pain reduction with active drug compared to a 22% reduction with placebo [50]. In this study, the cannabidiol-alone preparation was ineffective in pain relief. Improvement in sleep quality was also reported with the sublingual spray. To date, no clinical trials have examined the effectiveness of cannabinoid preparations in chemotherapy-induced neuropathic pain.

Synergism between opioids and cannabinoids has been postulated and subsequently demonstrated in a number of animal models [51–55]. The antinociceptive effects of morphine are predominantly mediated by mu receptors but may be enhanced by delta-9-THC activation of kappa and delta opioid receptors [55]. It has been further postulated that the cannabinoid:opioid interaction may occur at the level of their signal transduction mechanisms [56,57]. Receptors for both classes of drugs are coupled to similar intracellular signaling mechanisms that lead to a decrease in cAMP production by way of G_i protein activation [58–60]. There has also been some evidence that cannabinoids might increase the synthesis or release of endogenous opioids, or both. With this background, we are conducting a pharmacokinetic inter-action study to investigate the effect of concomitant cannabis on disposition kinetics of opioid analgesics. If cannabinoids and opioids are synergistic, it is possible that lower doses of opioids may be effective for longer periods of time with fewer side effects, clearly a benefit to the cancer patient with pain.

ANXIETY, DEPRESSION, AND SLEEP

In clinical trials of cannabis, euphoria is often scored as an adverse effect. Although not all patients experience mood elevation after exposure to can-nabis, it is a frequent outcome. Much depends on the "set and setting" and the individual's prior experience with cannabis. Some people develop dysphoria with or without paranoia upon exposure to cannabis; for them cannabis or its constituents may not be clinically useful. Sleepiness is another common side effect that can easily be recast as improved sleep quality as has been reported in trials of the sublingual spray cannabis-based medicine [61]. For the cancer patient suffering from anorexia, nausea, pain, depression, anxiety, and insom-nia, a single agent that can address all of these symptoms would be a valuable addition to the armamentarium.

Safety and Side Effects

Cannabinoids have an extremely favorable drug safety profile [13,14,24,62]. Unlike opioid receptors, cannabinoid receptors are not located in brainstem areas controlling respiration, so lethal overdoses due to respiratory suppression do not occur. The LD50 has been estimated to be 1500 pounds smoked in 15 minutes as extrapolated from animal studies where the median lethal dose was estimated to be several grams per kilogram of body weight [63].

The administration of cannabinoids to laboratory animals and humans does result in psychoactive effects. In humans, the central nervous system effects are both stimulating and depressing and are divided into four groups: affective (euphoria and easy laughter); sensory (temporal and spatial perception alterations and disorientation); somatic (drowsiness, dizziness, and motor incoordination); and cognitive (confusion, memory lapses, and difficulty concentrating).

As cannabinoid receptors are not just located in the central nervous sys-tem but are present in tissues throughout the body additional side effects of note include tachycardia and hypotension, conjunctival injection, bronchodilation, muscle relaxation and decreased gastrointestinal motility. Tolerance to the unwanted side effects of cannabis appears to develop rapidly in laboratory animals and humans. This is felt to occur because of a decrease in the number of total and functionally coupled cannabinoid receptors on the cell surface with a possible minor contribution from increased cannabinoid biotransformation and excretion with repeated exposure.

Although cannabinoids are considered by some to be addictive drugs, their addictive potential is considerably lower than other prescribed agents or substances of abuse. The brain develops tolerance to cannabinoids. Animal research demonstrates a potential for dependence, but this potential is observed under a narrower range of conditions than with benzodiazepines, opiates, cocaine, or nicotine. Withdrawal symptoms—irritability, insomnia with sleep EEG disturbance, restlessness, hot flashes, and rarely nausea and cramping—have been observed, but appear mild compared with the withdrawal from opiates or benzodiazepines and usually dissipate after a few days. Unlike other commonly used drugs, cannabinoids are stored in adipose tissue and excreted at a low rate (half-life 1–3 days), so even abrupt cessation of THC intake is not associated with rapid declines in plasma concentration that would precipitate withdrawal symptoms or drug craving.

The 1999 Institute of Medicine report addressed the frequent concern that marijuana is a "gateway drug" leading to use of other subsequent more potent and addictive substances of abuse [2]. The report recounts that marijuana is the most widely used illicit drug and, predictably, the first most people encounter. Not surprisingly, most users of other illicit drugs have used marijuana first. However, most drug users begin with alcohol and nicotine before marijuana; hence marijuana is not the most common and is rarely the first "gateway" drug. The report concludes that there is no conclusive evidence that the drug effects of marijuana are causally linked to the subsequent abuse of other illicit drugs and cautions that data on drug use progression cannot be assumed to apply to the use of drugs for medical purposes, which is certainly pertinent to the discussion of cannabis in cancer patients.

Cannabis and Cancer Risk

A study conducted by the National Toxicology Program of the US Department of Health and Human Services on mice and rats suggested that cannabinoids may have a protective effect against tumor development [64]. In this 2-year evaluation, rats and mice were given increasing doses of THC by gavage. A dose-related decrease in the incidence of both benign and malignant tumors was observed. Animals receiving THC dosing also survived longer than those receiving vehicle alone.

Mice and rats are not people and gavage is not equivalent to smoking a combusted botanical product. Many would find the combustion and inhalation of a therapeutic agent to be an undesirable and perhaps counter-intuitive way to deliver a drug. Most of the evidence available on the risk of cancer from marijuana smoking comes from epidemiologic studies, naturally, as prospective, randomized control trials are not possible. Over the years, reports of increased risks of lung cancer, oropharyngeal cancers, and prostate and cervical cancers have been most consistently reported. For each trial suggesting a possible increase in cancer incidence in chronic marijuana users, others have been published that appear to refute the association. A retrospective cohort study of 64,855 Kaiser Permanente health-care members seen between 1979 to 1985 and followed through 1993 yielded an interesting finding [65]. Men aged 15 to 49 were divided into four cohorts based on their use of tobacco and marijuana: never smoked either, smoked only cannabis, smoked only tobacco, smoked tobacco and cannabis. There were 5600 to 8200 men in each cell followed for an average of nearly nine years. In the men who never smoked, there were two cases of lung cancer diagnosed over the follow-up period. In the men who smoked tobacco, either alone or in addition to marijuana, the risk of lung cancer was increased 10-fold. In the over 50,000 person-years of follow-up of men who only smoked marijuana, there were no documented cases of lung cancer; less than in the never smokers!

A systematic review evaluating 19 studies that involved persons 18 years or older who smoked marijuana and examined premalignant or cancerous lung lesions concluded that observational studies failed to demonstrate significant associations between marijuana smoking and lung cancer after adjusting for tobacco use [66]. The authors site the selection bias, small sample size, limited generalizability, and overall young participant in stating that because of the biological plausibility of an association of marijuana smoking and lung cancer, physicians should still caution patients regarding potential risks until further rigorous studies permit definitive conclusions.

A population-based case–control study of the association between marijuana use and the risk of lung and upper aerodigestive tract cancers was performed in Los Angeles [67]. One thousand one hundred twelve incident cancer cases (611 of lung, 303 of oral, 108 of esophagus, 100 of pharynx, 90 of larynx) were matched to 1040 cancer-free controls on age, gender, and neighborhood. A standardized questionnaire used during face-to-face interview collected information on marijuana use expressed in joint-years, where 1 joint-year is the equivalent of smoking one marijuana cigarette per day for one year. The interviews also requested information on the use of other drugs including hashish, tobacco (all forms) and alcohol, sociodemographic factors, diet, occupational history, environmental factors including exposure to smoke, medical history, and family history of cancer. Data were presented as crude odds ratios and adjusted odds ratios using three models of covariate adjustment (with only Model 3 including tobacco use and pack/years). The results showed that although using marijuana for $\geq$30 joint-years was positively associated in the crude analysis with each cancer except pharyngeal, no positive associations were found when adjusting for several confounders including cigarette smoking. In fact, in the Model 3 analysis for lung cancer, the cohort who reported $>$0 to $<$1 joint-years of marijuana use had a 37% reduction in the risk of developing lung cancer compared to those who never smoked marijuana. Although this was the only cohort where the reduction in lung cancer risk reached statistical significance, in the model, all levels of marijuana use (including $\geq$60 joint-years) had adjusted odds ratios less than 1.0. The authors report adjusted ORs $<$1 for all cancers except oral cancer and found no consistent association of marijuana use with any malignant outcome. In what appears to be an overly aggressive attempt to delineate the possible limitations of their work, which could have led to such a consistent yet startling result, the authors mention that "it is possible that marijuana use does not increase cancer risk... Although the adjusted ORs $<$1 may be chance findings, they were observed for all non-reference exposure categories with all outcomes except oral cancer. Although purely speculative, it is possible that such inverse associations may reflect a protective effect of marijuana."

Cannabinoids as Anticancer Agents

There has been an increasing body of evidence over the past decade that cannabinoids may have a role in cancer therapy [62]. Evidence from cell culture systems as well as animal models have suggested that THC and other cannabinoids may inhibit the growth of some tumors by the modulation of signaling pathways that lead to growth arrest and cell death as well as by inhibition of angiogenesis and metastasis. The antiproliferative effects were originally reported in 1975 by Munson and colleagues, who demonstrated that delta-9-THC, delta-8-THC, and cannabinol inhibited Lewis lung adenocarcinoma cell growth in vitro as well as in mice. Curiously, there was no real follow-up of these findings for twenty years when the line of investigation was picked up by scientists in Spain and Italy who have remained at the forefront of this emerging field [62,68,69]. Since the late 1990s, several plant derived (THC and cannabidiol), synthetic (WIN-55,212-2 and HU-210) and endogenous cannabinoids (anandamide and 2-arachidonoylglycerol) have been shown to exert antiproliferative effects of a wide variety of tumor cells in culture systems. In addition to the original lung adenocarcinoma study, other tumor cells that have been shown to be sensitive to cannabinoid-induced growth inhibition include glioma, thyroid epithelioma, leukemia/lymphoma, neuroblastoma, and skin, uterus, breast, gastric, colorectal, pancreatic, and prostate carcinomas [70–81]. Perhaps even more compelling, cannabinoid administration to nude mice slows the growth of various tumor xenografts including lung and skin carcinomas, thyroid epitheliomas, melanomas, pancreatic carcinomas, lymphomas, and gliomas. The requirement of CB1 and/or CB2 receptors for the antitumor effect has been shown by various biochemical and pharmacological approaches already mentioned and the cumulative effects of CB signaling in the control of cell fate are expected to have important implications in the potential of cannabinoids for regulating tumor cell growth.

Cannabinoids may exert their antitumor effects by a number of different mechanisms including direct induction of transformed cell death, direct inhibition of transformed cell growth, and inhibition of tumor angiogenesis and metastasis [82,83]. A desirable property of antitumor compounds is their preferential targeting of malignant cells. Cannabinoids appear to kill tumor cells but do not affect their nontransformed counterparts and may even protect them from cell death (Fig. 7.3). This is best exemplified by glial cells. Cannabinoids have been shown to induce apoptosis of glioma cells in culture and induce regression of glioma cells in mice and rats. In contrast, cannabinoids protect normal glial cells of astroglial and oligodendroglial lineages from apoptosis mediated by the CB1 receptor.

Immunohistochemical and functional analyses in mouse models of gliomas and skin carcinomas have demonstrated that cannabinoid administration alters the vascular hyperplasia characteristic of actively growing tumors into a pattern characterized by small, differentiated, impermeable capillaries, thus thwarting angiogenesis. This is accompanied by a reduced expression of vascular endothelial growth factor (VEGF) and other proangiogenic cytokines, as well as of VEGF receptors. Activation of cannabinoid receptors in vascular endothelial cells inhibits cell migration and survival, also contributing to impaired tumor vascularization. Cannabinoid administration to tumor-bearing mice decreases the activity and expression of matrix metalloproteinase 2, a proteolyic enzyme that allows tissue breakdown and remodeling during angiogenesis and metastasis. This supports the inhibitory effect of cannabinoids in inhibiting tumor invasion in animal models (Fig. 7.4).

Further support comes from studies in human non–small cell lung cancer cell lines that overexpress epidermal growth factor receptor, in which THC inhibits epidermal growth factor-induced growth, chemotaxis, and chemoinvasion [84]. In an in vivo model using severe combined immunodeficient

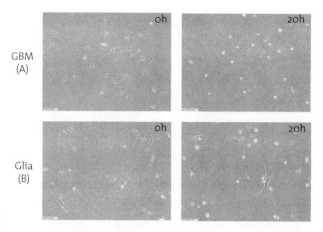

FIGURE 7.3. Delta-9-THC kills brain tumor cells at a concentration that is nontoxic to normal brain cells. Images obtained through a time-lapse microscope illustrate the selective induction of cell death in cultures of human glioblastoma multiforme (GBM) cells (A) compared to normal human glial cells (B). After 20 hours of treatment, death of nearly all of the GBM cells is evidenced by cells shrinking to inanimate white spheres. The normal cells exposed to the same concentration of delta-9-THC continue to migrate and divide. (Photo courtesy of McAllister and Yount.)

mice, subcutaneous tumors were generated by inoculating the animals with the same cell lines. Tumor growth in THC-treated animals was inhibited by 60% compared with vehicle-treated controls. The inhibition was significant both regarding the subcutaneous xenograft as well as the number and weight of lung metastases. Tumor specimens revealed antiproliferative and antiangiogenic effects of THC.

Most recently, another potential anticancer and particularly antimetastasis mechanism for cannabinoids has been identified. Id helix-loop-helix proteins control processes related to tumor progression [85]. Reducing Id-1 using antisense technology led to significant reductions in breast cancer cell proliferation and invasiveness in in vitro models and metastases in mice. Reducing Id-1 expression with antisense technology is not a possible intervention in humans with breast cancer at this time, however. Cannabidiol has been demonstrated to downregulate Id-1 expression in aggressive human breast cancer cells. The investigators suggest that cannabidiol represents the first nontoxic exogenous agent that can significantly decrease Id-1 expression in metastatic breast cancer cells leading to the downregulation of tumor aggressiveness.

Two additional potential mechanisms of anticancer activity warrant brief mention. Cannabinoids, both plant-derived and endogenous, are believed to have anti-inflammatory effects. Inflammation is being increasingly linked to the development of various malignancies. Perhaps one of the most obvious

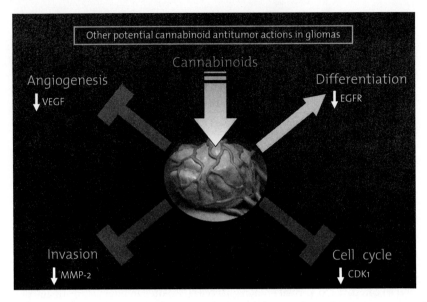

FIGURE 7.4. Other antitumor effects of cannabinoids. Besides inducing apoptosis of tumor cells, cannabinoid administration can decrease the growth of gliomas by other mechanisms, including at least: (i) reduction of tumor angiogenesis, by inhibition of the vascular endothelial growth factor (VEGF) pathway; (ii) inhibition of tumor cell invasion, by down-regulation of matrix metalloproteinase-2 (MMP-2) expression; (iii) induction of tumor cell differentiation, by down-regulation of epidermal growth factor (EGF) receptor expression; and perhaps (iv) arrest of the cell cycle, by down-regulation of cyclin-dependent kinase-1 (CDK1) expression. The relative contribution of these processes to the inhibition of tumor growth depends on various factors such as the type of tumor under study, the experimental model used and the intensity of cannabinoid signaling.

associations is the development of colorectal carcinoma in patients with inflammatory bowel disease. A mouse study has demonstrated that signaling of the endogenous cannabinoid system is likely to provide intrinsic protection against colonic inflammation. [86]. This finding has led to the development of a hypothesis that phytocannabinoids and endocannabinoids may be useful in the prevention and treatment of colorectal cancer [87].

Kaposi's sarcoma-associated herpesvirus/Human herpesvirus-8 (KSHV/HHV-8) and Epstein-Barr virus (EBV) are related and implicated in the cause of a number of malignant diseases including Kaposi's sarcoma and primary effusion lymphoma (KSHV) and Burkitt's lymphoma, primary central nervous system lymphoma, Hodgkin's disease, and nasopharyngeal carcinoma (EBV). A group of investigators has demonstrated that THC is a potent and selective antiviral agent against KSHV [88]. It is felt that THC may inhibit KSHV replication through the activation of cannabinoid receptors. The authors conclude that further studies on cannabinoids and herpesviruses are important as they may lead to development of drugs that inhibit reactivation of these oncogenic viruses. Counter to these findings, however, is the recent suggestion that delta-9-THC may actually enhance KSHV infection and replication and foster KSHV-mediated endothelial transformation [89]. These investigators caution that use of cannabinoids may thus place individuals at greater risk for the development and progression of Kaposi's sarcoma, although epidemiologic data have not supported these in vitro findings.

So with the body of evidence increasing, where are the clinical trials in humans with malignant disease? True, cannabinoids have psychoactive side effects, but these could be considered to be within the boundaries of tolerance for the toxicity profiles of cytotoxic chemotherapeutic and targeted small molecule therapies widely used in oncology. The Spanish Ministry of Health approved a pilot clinical trial carried out in collaboration between the Tenerife University Hospital and the Guzman laboratory in Madrid to investigate the effect of local administration of THC intracranially through an infusion catheter on the growth of recurrent glioblastoma multiforme [90]. In this groundbreaking pilot study, THC administration was shown to be safe and associated with decreased tumor cell proliferation in at least two of nine patients studied. Hopefully this pilot trial may open the door to further clinical investigations aimed at assessing the antitumor activity of cannabinoid therapies.

Alternative Delivery Systems

And what if clinical trials were to demonstrate that smoked marijuana may be of benefit to patients with a condition like, for example, recurrent glioblastma multiforme? It is not likely that even a meta-analysis of a number of similar studies in any condition would convince the necessary regulatory bodies that cannabis should be reinstated to the U.S. Pharmacopoeia and made widely available to patients who may benefit from its use. The Institute of Medicine Report in 1999 clearly stated that the accumulated data indicate a potential therapeutic value for cannabinoid drugs particularly in the areas of pain relief, control of nausea, and vomiting and appetite stimulation. They went on to suggest that the "goal of clinical trials of smoked marijuana would not be to develop it as a licensed drug, but as a first step towards the development of non-smoked, rapid-onset cannabinoid delivery systems" [2].

To this end, we conducted a trial in healthy marijuana smoker volunteers comparing the blood levels of cannabinoids achieved upon inhaling marijuana that has been vaporized in a device that heated the plant product to below the temperature of combustion and collected the volatilized gases with those obtained upon smoking a comparable dosed cigarette [91]. Eighteen healthy subjects were evaluated. One dose (1.7%, 3.4% ,or 6.8% tetrahydrocannabinol) and delivery system (smoked cannabis cigarette or vaporization system) was randomly assigned for each of the six inpatient study days. The peak plasma concentrations and 6-hour area under the plasma concentration-time curve of THC after inhalation of vaporized cannabis were similar to those of smoked cannabis.

Carbon monoxide levels were substantially reduced with vaporization suggesting less exposure to noxious substances. Neuropsychologic effects were equivalent and participants expressed a clear preference for vaporization as a delivery method.

No adverse events were observed. Vaporization of cannabis is a safe and effective mode of delivery of THC. Consequently, our ongoing evaluation of opioid:cannabinoid interactions is using the vaporizer as a smokeless delivery system.

Another nonsynthetic alternative to smoked or inhaled cannabis is the sublingual preparation of whole plant extract [50,61,92]. Sativex® was first approved as a prescription medication in Canada in 2005 for symptomatic relief of neuropathic pain in multiple sclerosis and subsequently as adjunctive therapy for patients with cancer pain on other analgesic medications. The cannabis-based medication is available in Spain, undergoing regulatory review by the European Union and is being evaluated in a Phase II/III clinical trial in patients with cancer-related pain in the United States.

Guidelines for Providers

The Institute of Medicine is aware that the development and acceptance of smokeless marijuana delivery systems "may take years; in the meantime there are patients with debilitating symptoms for whom smoked marijuana may provide relief." So what is a provider to do? Patients with cancer have a number of symptoms that may be responsive to cannabinoid therapies. As enumerated, these include nausea, vomiting, anorexia, pain, insomnia, anxiety, and depression. Many providers would frown upon the use of a relatively benign smoked psychotropic agent while freely writing prescriptions for pharmaceutical agents with significantly greater cost, potential for addiction or abuse, and more negative societal impact overall.

The Medical Board of California in their July 2004 Action Report provides a model for how states with medical marijuana legislation should advise physicians [93].

"The intent of the board at this time is to reassure physicians that if they use the same proper care in recommending medical marijuana to their patients as they would any other medication or treatment, their activity will be viewed by the Medical Board just as any other appropriate medical intervention.... If physicians use the same care in recommending medical marijuana to patients as they would recommending or approving any other medication or prescription drug treatment, they have nothing to fear from the Medical Board."

The Board recommends following the accepted standards that would be used in recommending any medication. A history and physical examination should be documented. The provider should ascertain that medical marijuana use is not masking an acute or treatable progressive condition. A treatment plan should be formulated. A patient need not have failed all standard interventions before marijuana can be recommended. The physician may have little guidelines in actually recommending a concrete dose for the patient to use [94]. As there are so many variables associated with effect, the physician and patient should develop an individual self-titration dosing paradigm that allows the patient to achieve the maximum benefit with tolerable side effects. Discussion of potential side effects and obtaining verbal informed consent are desirable. Periodic review of the treatment efficacy should be documented. Consultation should be obtained when necessary. Proper record keeping that supports the decision to recommend the use of medical marijuana is advised. Despite all these guidelines, the California Medical Board still reminds physicians that making a written recommendation "could trigger a federal action."

On a more positive note, in a unanimous vote, the Assembly of the American Psychiatric Association recently approved a strongly worded statement supporting legal protection for patients using medical marijuana with their doctor's recommendation [95]. The APA action paper reiterates that "the threat of arrest by federal agents, however, still exists. Seriously ill patients living in these states with medical marijuana recommendations from their doctors should not be subjected to the threat of punitive federal prosecution for merely attempting to alleviate the chronic pain, side effects, or symptoms associated with their conditions or resulting from their overall treatment regimens. ... [We] support protection for patients and physicians participating in state approved medical marijuana programs." Subsequently, the 124,000-member American College of Physicians issued a position paper supporting research into the therapeutic role of marijuana and urging protection for both physicians who participate in discussions regarding the use of medical cannabis and their patients who seek to use it [96].

Conclusion

It behooves the integrative oncologist to follow closely future studies of cannabinoids and cancer. It is likely that these agents will not only prove to be useful in symptom management and palliative care, but as antitumor agents as well.

REFERENCES

1. Joy JE, Watson SJ, & Benson JA (Eds.). (1999). *Marijuana and Medicine: Assessing the Science Base*. Washington, D.C: National Academy Press.
2. Grothenhermen F & Russo E. (Eds.) (2002). *Cannabis and Cannabinoids: Pharmacology, Toxicology, and Therapeutic Potential*. Binghamton, NY: The Haworth Press.
3. Tramer MR, Carroll D, Campbell FA, Reynolds DJ, Moore RA, McQuay HJ, et al. (2001). Cannabinoids for control of chemotherapy-induced nausea and vomiting: quantitative systematic review. *BMJ*, 323, 16–21.
4. Ben Amar M. (2006). Cannabinoids in medicine: A review of their therapeutic potential. *Journal of Ethnopharmacology*, 105, 1–25.
5. Walsh D, Nelson KA, & Mahmoud FA. (2003). Established and potential therapeutic applications of cannabinoids in oncology. *Support Care Cancer*, 11, 137–143.
6. Abrams DI, Jay C, Shade S, Vizoso H, Reda H, Press S, et al. (2007). Cannabis in painful HIV-associated sensory neuropathy: a randomized, placebo-controlled trial. *Neurology*, 68, 515–521.
7. Welch SP & Eads M. (1999). Synergistic interactions of endogenous opioids and cannabinoid systems. *Brain Research*, 848(1–2), 183–190.
8. Guzman M. (2003). Cannabinoids: potential anticancer agents. *Nature Reviews/ Cancer*, 3, 745–755.
9. Hashibe M, Morgenstern H, Cui Y, Tashkin DP, Zhang Z-F, Cozen W, et al. (2006). Marijuana use and the risk of lung and upper aerodigestive tract cancers: results of a population-based case-control study. *Cancer epidemiology, biomarkers & prevention*, 15, 1829–1834.
10. Bifulco M & DiMarzo V. (2002). Targeting the endocannabinoid system in cancer therapy: A call for further research. *Nature Medicine*, 8, 547–550.

(A complete reference list for this chapter is available online at http://www.oup.com/us/ integrativemedicine).

8

CAM: Chemo Interactions—What Is Known?

ALEX SPARREBOOM AND SHARYN D. BAKER

KEY CONCEPTS

- In the United States, 15 million adults combine herbal remedies with prescription medications; CAM use is more common among cancer patients than among individuals in the general population
- Many types of CAM, in particular herbs, have the potential to interact with prescription drugs, altering their pharmacokinetic characteristics and leading to clinically significant interactions.
- Many herbal preparations are known to either inhibit or induce the function of drug-metabolizing enzymes or drug transporters that are of putative relevance to the pharmacokinetic profile of anticancer drugs.
- Few clinical studies have been performed that specifically investigated the interaction potential of herbs with anticancer agents and those that have, have typically evaluated the herbs garlic, milk thistle, and St. John's wort and the anticancer agents docetaxel, imatinib, or irinotecan as model drugs.
- There appears to be little likelihood of significant pharmacokinetic interactions between most herbs and anticancer drugs; however, interactions between St. John's wort and most anticancer agents are likely to have clinical and toxicological implications.

The concept that chemotherapeutic agents are administered at a dose to the maximum a patient can tolerate, before the onset of unacceptable toxicity, is still in wide clinical use today. However, the therapeutic range for most cytotoxic anticancer agents is extremely narrow, and in most cases no information is available on the intrinsic sensitivity of a patient's tumor to a particular agent and the patient's tolerability of a given dose before therapy. Hence, the dosage of chemotherapeutic agents remains largely empirical and is typically only normalized to an individual's body surface area (Baker, et al., 2002).

There is often a marked variability in drug handling among individual patients resulting in variability in clearance, which, for many agents, contributes to variability in the pharmacodynamic profile—either toxic side effects or antitumor efficacy—of a given dose of a drug (Table 8.1). A combination of physiological variables, genetic characteristics, and environmental factors are known to alter the relationship between absolute drug dose and clearance

Table 8.1. Examples of Systemic Exposure as a Marker of Anticancer Drug Effects.

Drug	Side Effect	Drug	Response/Survival
Carboplatin	Thrombocytopenia	Carboplatin	Ovarian cancer
Cisplatin	Nephrotoxicity	Cisplatin	Head and neck cancer
Cyclophosphamide	Cardiotoxicity	Docetaxel	Nonsmall cell lung cancer
Docetaxel	Neutropenia	Etoposide	Nonsmall cell lung cancer
Doxorubicin	Neutropenia	5-Fluorouracil	Head and neck cancer
Epirubicin	Neutropenia	6-Mercaptopurine	Acute lymphoblastic leukemia
Erlotinib	Skin rash	Methotrexate	Acute lymphoblastic leukemia
5-Fluorouracil	Diarrhea, Mucositis	Teniposide	Lymphoma
Irinotecan	Diarrhea, Neutropenia		
Methotrexate	Mucositis		
Paclitaxel	Neutropenia		

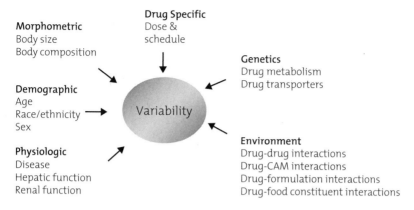

FIGURE 8.1. Potential sources of interindividual pharmacokinetic variability for anticancer drugs.

(Fig. 8.1). Accurate definition of the relationships between the pharmacokinetic variables of a drug and the drug's pharmacodynamic end points may allow the administration of the optimum dosage of that drug in any given patient such that it maximizes the likelihood of response and simultaneously minimizes the likelihood of severe toxicity.

In recent years, a wealth of evidence indicating that many types of CAM, in particular botanicals, may interact with prescription drugs, altering their pharmacokinetic characteristics and leading to clinically significant interactions has been generated. Over 100,000 deaths per year in the United States alone can be attributed to drug interactions, placing drug interactions between the fourth and sixth leading causes of death (Lazarou, Pomeranz, & Corey, 1998), and it has been suggested that the greater part of these might be linked to the use of herbs (Zhou, et al., 2003). Because (unintentional) changes in the systemic exposure to anticancer drugs may have catastrophic consequences for treatment outcome, there is an increasing need to understand possible adverse drug interactions in medical oncology (Sparreboom, Cox, Acharya, & Figg, 2004; Tascilar, de Jong, Verweij, & Mathijssen, 2006). This chapter reviews the existing data on known or suspected interactions between widely used, over-the-counter herbal medicines and conventional anticancer drugs, with further discussion of their clinical implications for the chemotherapeutic treatment of cancer.

Use of CAM by Cancer Patients

Interest in CAM usage has grown rapidly in the industrialized world. In particular, total sales for herbal dietary supplements in 2007 have shown continued growth for most channels of trade, indicating a steady increase since 2003 (Blumenthal, Cavaliere, & Rae, 2008). Some of the reasons for this increase relate to dissatisfaction with conventional allopathic therapies, a desire of patients to be involved more actively in their own health care, and because patients find these alternatives to be more congruent with their own philosophical orientations (Astin, 1998; Boon, et al., 2000). It has been estimated that up to a third of the entire population in the United States has turned to CAM use in the past 12 months, the majority of whom use herbal products on a routine basis (Jonas, 1998; Klepser, et al., 2000). An estimated 15 million adults combined herbal remedies with prescription medications, with more recent estimates putting this figure around 16% (Eisenberg, et al., 1998; Kaufman, Kelly, Rosenberg, Anderson, & Mitchell, 2002; Richardson, Sanders, Palmer, Greisinger, & Singletary, 2000). In view of the increasingly large number of people using botanicals combined with allopathic therapies, the risk for herb–drug interactions is a growing public health concern.

Interestingly, CAM use is more common among patients with cancer than among individuals in the general population (Ernst & Cassileth, 1998). By the late 1990s, surveys showed that CAM was widely used by cancer patients, with a prevalence ranging from 7% to 64% of patients sampled in 26 studies conducted worldwide (Tascilar, et al., 2006). Follow-up evaluations indicate that this use has steadily increased, with a current overall prevalence for CAM use of 37% to 83%, and for herbal preparations of 13% to 63%. Between 54% and 77% of patients receiving conventional therapy use CAM (Lippert, McClain, Boyd, & Theodorescu, 1999; Richardson, et al., 2000), and up to 72% do not inform their treating physician (Klepser, et al., 2000; Morris, Johnson, Homer, & Walts, 2000). It is also noteworthy that patients with breast cancer tend to use more CAM than individuals with other types of malignancy (Tesch, 2003), presumably because more women than men use CAM (Eisenberg, et al., 1998). Navo et al. recently reported on CAM use by women with breast cancer (Navo, et al., 2004), and found that 48% of the women used CAM, with 11% of participants using an herbal product. Twenty eight percent of these patients considered CAM supplements as a type of medication, and only about half informed their primary care givers that they were taking CAM in addition to chemotherapy. The most widely used botanicals used among cancer patients are shown in Table 8.2.

Oncologists should be aware of the potential for adverse interactions with herbs, question their patients on their use of these products, and urge patients to avoid or discontinue the use of herbs that could confound their cancer care.

Table 8.2. Top-Selling Herbal Supplements in the United States in 2007.[a]

Herb	Plant Name	Primary Clinical Indication(s)	Usage by Cancer Patients (%)[b]
Soy	Glycine max	Menopausal symptoms	unknown
Cranberry	Vaccinium macrocarpon	Urinary tract infection	<1.0
Garlic	*Allium sativum*	Hypercholesterolemia	4.2
Ginkgo	Ginkgo biloba	Dementia, intermittent claudication	9.6
Saw palmetto	Serenoa repens	Benign prostate hyperplasia	unknown
Echinacea	*Echinacea purpurea*[†]	Prevention of common cold	21.1
Black cohosh	Actaea racemosa	Menopausal symptoms	unknown
Milk thistle	Silybum marianum	Alcoholic cirrhosis and hepatitis	6.6
Ginseng	*Panax ginseng*	Physical and mental fatigue	3.0
St. John's wort	*Hypericum perforatum*	Mild depression	3.6
Green tea	*Camellia sinensis*	Anticarcinogen, hypercholesterolemia	1.8*
Evening primrose	*Oenothera biennis*	Premenstrual syndrome	19.9
Valerian	*Valeriana officinalis*	Insomnia, stress	3.0
Horny goat weed	*Epimedium* spp.	Impotence, asthma	unknown
Grape seed	*Vitis vinifera*	Allergic rhinitis	2.0

*Usage by up to 29.8% of patients enrolled onto Phase I clinical trials (Dy, et al., 2004)
[†]Other species include E. *angustifolia*, and E. *pallida*.

SOURCE: [a]Data obtained from Blumenthal, Cavaliere, & Rea, 2006; [b]Data obtained from Navo, et al., 2004; Werneke, Earl, Seydel, Horn, Crichton, & Fannon, 2004.

Potential Mechanisms for Pharmacokinetic Interactions

Combined use of botanicals with anticancer drugs may increase or reduce the effects of either component, possibly resulting in clinically important interactions. Obviously, synergistic therapeutic effects may complicate the dosing regimen of medications administered long-term, or lead to unfavorable toxicities. Herbal preparations may interact with conventional anticancer drugs at various anatomical or physiological sites, thereby changing the rate of elimination and/or the amount of drug absorbed. Although interactions are most likely to arise secondary to altered pharmacokinetics of the involved drugs (de Smet, 2002; Ioannides, 2002; Zhou et al., 2003), pharmacodynamic interactions (Izzo & Ernst, 2001; Miller, 1998), and/or intrinsic toxicity of several herbs have also been documented (Markman, 2002).

All aspects of pharmacokinetics might be affected when an herb is given in combination with anticancer drugs, including absorption (resulting in altered absorption rate or oral bioavailability), distribution (mostly caused by protein-binding displacement), metabolism, and excretion. Most known drug interactions are due to changes in metabolic routes. Conventionally, drug metabolism is broadly divided into phase I and phase II processes. Phase I processes include oxidation, reduction, hydrolysis, and hydration, resulting in the formation of functional groups (OH, SH, NH_2, or $COOH$) that impart the metabolite with increased polarity compared to the parent compound. Of the phase I processes, the cytochrome P450 (CYP) super family is responsible for the metabolism of a variety of xenobiotics. Human CYP isoforms that are involved in the biotransformation of xenobiotics include CYP1A1/2, CYP2B6, CYP2C8/9/19, CYP2D6, CYP2E1, CYP3A4/5, and CYP4A. Phase II processes include sulfation, methylation, acetylation, glutathione conjugation, fatty acid conjugation, and glucuronidation. The latter is catalyzed by uridine diphospho-glucuronosyltransferases (UGTs) and involves the transfer of the glucuronic acid residue from uridine diphosphoglucuronic acid to a hydroxy, either phenolic or alcoholic, or a carboxylic acid group on the compound. In humans, 16 different UGT isoforms have been classified into either 1A or 2B subfamilies. They metabolize a broad range of endogenous and exogenous substances with significant overlap in substrate specificity between isozymes.

Among the enzymes involved in either phase I or phase II metabolism, the CYP3A4 isoform has been most frequently implicated in interactions between allopathic medicine and herbal products. This is probably also true for anticancer drugs, as CYP3A4 is responsible for the oxidation of more than 35% of all currently prescribed oncology drugs (Lepper, et al., 2005). Elevated enzyme activity (induction), translated into a more rapid metabolic rate, may result in a decrease in plasma concentrations and to total loss of therapeutic effect. Conversely, suppression of enzyme activity (inhibition) may trigger a rise in plasma concentrations and lead to exaggerated toxicity commensurate with overdose.

Another principal mechanism that can explain interactions between botanicals and anticancer agents is the affinity for the so-called ATP binding-cassette (ABC) transporters expressed in the liver and kidney that are directed toward the lumen (Fig. 8.2). The three major classes of drug transporters, referred to as P-glycoprotein (ABCB1), multidrug resistance–associated protein-1 (MRP1; ABCC1), and its homologue MRP2 (cMOAT; ABCC2), and breast cancer–resistance protein (BCRP; ABCG2), may play a significant role in mediating transmembrane transport of anticancer drugs (Sparreboom, Danesi, Ando, Chan, & Figg, 2003). Many anticancer agents are also sensitive to transporters of the solute carrier family that are involved in both hepatocellular uptake and inward-directed transport from the blood into renal cells (Fig. 8.2). For anticancer drugs administered orally, extraction by extensive metabolism in the gut wall and/or the liver during first pass (i.e., before reaching the systemic circulation) is another potential mechanism involved in suspected interactions for various agents (Kruijtzer, Beijnen, & Schellens, 2002).

Chemical constituents in herbal products, similar to prescription drugs, are eliminated by various metabolic enzymes in the body and may be substrates for various transporters. The potential for involvement of drug metabolizing enzymes and transporters in the handling of herbal components leads to a predisposition of herb–drug interactions. It is of importance that potential drug–herb interactions be identified to prevent adverse outcomes in patients taking combinations of drugs and botanical supplements. Also, the identification of the mechanism involved in any such interaction will offer insight into the approaches to be taken to minimize their impact and to design appropriate studies in humans.

Known Herb–Anticancer Drug Interactions

Many botanicals are known to either inhibit or induce the function of drug-metabolizing enzymes or drug transporters that are of putative relevance to the pharmacokinetic profile of anticancer drugs (Table 8.3). However, only very few clinical studies, discussed in detail in the following paragraphs, have been

(A)

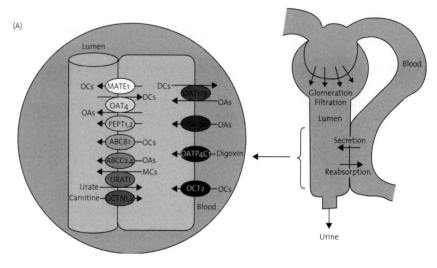

(B)

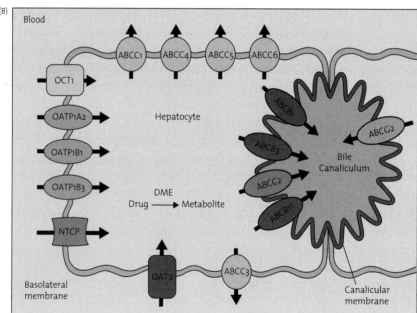

FIGURE 8.2. Common mechanisms for possible interactions between herbs and anticancer drugs in the kidney (A) and liver (B). OAs, organic anions; OCs, organic cations; DCs, dicarboxylates; MCs, monocarboxylates; DME, drug-metabolizing enzyme(s).

performed that specifically investigated the interaction potential of botanicals with anticancer agents. Although the information presented in Table 8.3 clearly documents the ability of various herbs to affect the pharmacokinetics of anticancer drugs, clinical studies will eventually be required to document the overall impact of such herbs on anticancer drug clearance. However, ethical concerns

Table 8.3. Effect of Commonly Used Botanicals on the Activity of Enzymes and Transporters in Humans.

Herb	Effect
Asian ginseng (*Panax ginseng*)	Weak inhibition of CYP2D6, CYP3A4; no influence on CYP1A2, CYP2E1
Baicalin (*Radix scutellariae*)	Induction of OATP1B1
Balloon vine (*Cardiospermum halicacabum*)	Potential inhibition of CYP1A2
Bitter orange (*Citrus aurantium*)	No influence on CYP1A2, CYP2D6, CYP2E1, or CYP3A4
Black cohosh (*Actaea racemosa*)	Weak inhibition of CYP2D6; no influence on CYP1A2, CYP2E1, CYP3A4, ABCB1
Black pepper (*Piper nigrum*)	Potential inhibition of CYP3A4, ABCB1
Bloodwort (*Sanguisorba officinalis*)	Potential induction of CYP1A2
Boldo-funigreek (*Peumus boldus*)	Potential inhibition of CYP2C9
Chinese skullcap (*Scutellaria baicalensis*)	Potential inhibition of CYP3A4, ABCB1
Cranberry (*Vaccinium macrocarpon*)	No influence on CYP2C9, CYP3A4, ABCB1
Dandelion (*Taraxacum mongolicum*)	Potential induction of CYP1A2
Danshen (*Salvia miltiorrhiza*)	Potential inhibition of CYP2C9; potential induction of CYP3A4
Devil's claw (*Harpagophytum procumbens*)	No conclusive data available
Dogbane (*Apocynum venetum*)	No influence on CYP3A4, ABCB1
Dong quai (*Angelica sinensis*)	Potential inhibition of CYP2C9
Echinacea (*Echinacea* spp.)	Potential induction of CYP3A4; no influence on CYP1A2, CYP2D6, CYP2E1, ABCB1
Fennel (*Foeniculum vulgare*)	Potential induction of CYP1A2
Feverfew (*Tanacetum parthenium*)	No conclusive data available
Fo-ti (*Polygonum multiflorum*)	No conclusive data available
Galic (*Allium sativum*)	Weak inhibition of CYP3A4, CYP2E1, ABCB1; weak induction of N-acetyl-transferase, no effect on CYP2C9

(*continued*)

Table 8.3. (Continued)

Herb	Effect
Gan cao (*Glycyrrhiza uralensis*)	Potential induction of CYP2C9, CYP3A4
Ginger (*Zingiber officinalis*)	No influence on CYP2C9
Ginkgo (*Ginkgo biloba*)	Strong induction of CYP2C19; weak inhibition of CYP3A4; no influence on CYP2C9
Goldernseal (*Hydrastis Canadensis*)	Strong inhibition of CYP2D6, CYP3A4
Grapefruit juice (*Citrus paradise*)	Strong inhibition of (intestinal) CYP3A4
Grape seed (*Vitis vinifera*)	Potential induction of (hepatic) CYP3A4
Green tea (*Camellia sinensis*)	No influence on CYP2D6, CYP3A4; potential induction of CYP1A2
Guar gum (*Cyamopsis tetragonoloba*)	No influence on ABCB1
Guggul tree (*Commiphora mukul*)	Potential induction of CYP3A4
Horny goat weed (*Epimedium* spp.)	No conclusive data available
I'm-Yunity (*Coriolus versicolor*)	No influence on CYP3A4
Japanese arrowroot (*Pueraria lobata*)	Potential inhibition of ABCC and OAT transporters
Kangen-Karyu	Potential inhibition of CYP2C9
Kava kava (*Piper methysticum*)	Strong inhibition of CYP2E1; no influence on CYP2D6, CYP3A4
Licorice (*Glycyrrhiza uralensis*)	Potential inhibition of CYP3A4
Milk thistle (*Silybum marianum*)	No influence on CYP1A2, CYP2D6, CYP2E1, CYP3A4, ABCB1
Peppermint oil (*Mentha piperita*)	Weak inhibition of CYP3A4
Pomelo juice (*Citrus grandis*)	Weak inhibition of CYP3A4 or ABCB1 (or both)
Red clover (*Trifolium pratense*)	No conclusive data available
Saw palmetto (*Serenoa repens*)	No influence on CYP1A2, CYP2D6, CYP2E1, CYP3A4

(continued)

Table 8.3. (Continued)

Herb	Effect
Shoseiryuto (*schisandra/ephedra/cinnamon*)	No influence on CYP3A4, CYP1A2, CYP2D6, XO, NAT2
Siberian ginseng (*Panax quinquefolius*)	No influence on CYP2D6, CYP3A4
Soy (*Glycine max*)	No influence on CYP3A4
St. John's wort (*Hypericum perforatum*)	Strong induction of CYP1A2, CYP2C8, CYP2C9, CYP2C19, CYP2E1, CYP3A4, ABCB1, no effect on CYP2D6
Tanner's Cassia (*Cassia auriculata*)	Potential inhibition of CYP1A2
Tian xian	Induction of CYP3A4 (activation of PXR)
Tortoise shell (*Quilinggao*)	Potential induction of CYP2C9
Turmeric (*Curcuma longa*)	No influence on CYP3A4, ABCB1
Valerian (*Valeriana officinalis*)	No influence CYP1A2, CYP2D6, CYP2E1, CYP3A4
Wheat bran (*Triticum aestivum*)	No influence on ABCB1; potential inhibition of CYP3A4
White peony (*Radix paeoniae alba*)	No influence on CYP3A4
Wolfberry (*Lycium barbarum*)	Potential inhibition of CYP2C9
Woohwangcheongsimwon	Potent inhibition of CYP2B6
Wu-Wei-Zi (*Schisandra chinensis*)	Potential induction of CYP2C9, CYP3A4
Wu-Chu-Yu (*Evodia rutaecarpa*)	Potential induction of CYP1A2

could make design of a clinical study involving exposure of cancer patients to the intentional combination of herbs with anticancer drugs difficult (Komoroski, Parise, Egorin, Strom, & Venkataramanan, 2005). Additionally, most chemo-therapeutic agents are potentially mutagenic, carcinogenic, or teratogenic and cannot be studied in a healthy volunteer population. Nonetheless, a few clinical investigations have been performed to evaluate the interaction potential between anticancer drugs and botanicals, and these studies have typically used docetaxel, imatinib, or irinotecan as model drugs. This is because of the potential to simultaneously study the effects of any herbal product on multiple enzymes and transporters involved in the absorption and disposition of these anticancer drugs (Fig. 8.3).

In vivo studies in humans have been carried out with various experimental designs. Typically subjects receive a single dose of a test drug or a cocktail of drugs that are markers for various enzymes on day one. This is followed by multiple daily dose treatment with the botanical and on the last day of treatment, administration of the test drug or the cocktail of drugs. A comparison

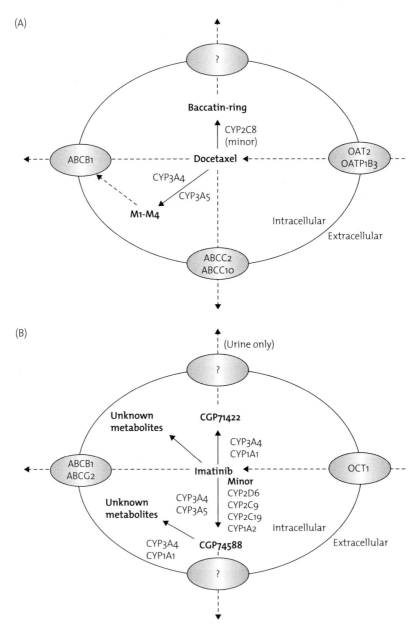

FIGURE 8.3. (Continued on next page)

(C)

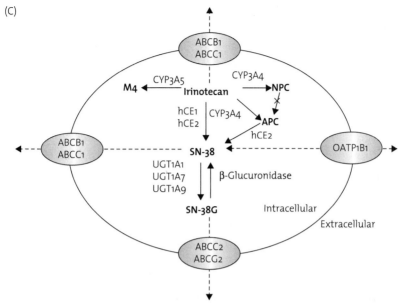

FIGURE 8.3. Hepatocellular enzymes and transporters involved in the pharmaco-kinetics of the model anticancer drugs docetaxel (A), imatinib (B), and irinotecan (C).

of the various pharmacokinetic parameters or phenotypic measures is used as a method to evaluate the effect of herbal products on the pharmacokinetics of test drug or activity of various drug metabolizing enzymes (Venkataramanan, Komoroski, & Strom, 2006). The evaluation of the interaction potential of anti-cancer drugs with botanicals has focused on some of the top-10 selling products that were most likely to result in altered pharmacokinetic profiles of the test drugs, namely garlic, milk thistle, and St. John's wort.

> The potential of botanicals to alter the pharmacokinetics of prescription drugs can rarely be accurately predicted from in vitro or animal studies. Such studies typically tend to overstate and overemphasize the herb–drug interac-tion *potential*.

GARLIC

Allicin, a sulfur compound and the active ingredient in garlic, is produced from alliin in the presence of the enzyme alliinase when fresh garlic is crushed or chewed (Lawson, Ransom, & Hughes, 1992). In vitro studies have shown that garlic constituents modulate the activity of various CYP isozymes. Extracts of fresh garlic, garlic oil, and freeze-dried garlic exhibit an inhibitory effect on CYP2C9, CYP2C19, CYP3A4, CYP3A5, and CYP3A7 metabolism, whereas no effect on CYP2D6 was observed (Chen, et al., 2003a; Foster, et al., 2001). Rats treated with diallyl sulfide, diallyl disulfide, allylmethyl sulfide, and allyl mercaptan had a suppression of CYP2E1 activity as a result of competitive inhibition (Brady et al., 1991; Guyonnet, et al., 2000; Haber, Siess, De Waziers, Beaune, & Suschetet, 1994). In addition, diallyl sulfone is known to be a suicide inhibitor of CYP2E1, forming a complex leading to autocatalytic destruction (Jin & Baillie, 1997). However, long-term administration (eg, more than 6 weeks) led to enhanced activity and increased expression of CYP1A, CYP2B (Dalvi, 1992; Haber et al., 1994; Sheen, Chen, Kung, Liu, & Lii, 1999), and CYP3A (Wu et al., 2002). Studies using in vitro and in vivo animal models have also indicated that various garlic constituents used at very high concentrations can induce the activity of CYP3A4 (Raucy, 2003) and conjugating enzymes such as glutathione S-transferases and quinone reductases (Guyonnet, Siess, De Waziers, Beaune, & Suschetet, 1999; Munday & Mundsay, 1999).

An almost 40% decrease in 6-hydroxychlorzoxazone/chlorzoxazone ratio reported in one study suggests that CYP2E1 activity is also inhibited in humans receiving garlic for a period of 4 weeks (Gurley, et al., 2002). Clinical studies using probe-drug cocktails have shown that garlic has no significant effect on the activity of CYP1A2 (caffeine), CYP2D6 (debrisoquine, dextromethorphan), and CYP3A4 (alprazolam, midazolam) (Gurley, et al., 2002; Markowitz, et al., 2003). Two previous trials indicated that garlic significantly decreases the systemic exposure to the HIV protease inhibitors saquinavir and ritonavir (Gallicano, Foster, & Choudhri, 2003; Piscitelli, Burstein, Welden, Gallicano, & Falloon, 2002a). These protease inhibitors are not only metabolized by CYP3A4 (Fitzsimmons & Collins, 1997), but are also substrates for ABCB1 (Kim, Dintaman, & Waddell, 1998). The data obtained using alprazolam and midazolam as probe substrates for CYP3A4 suggest that the pharmacokinetic alterations of saquinavir and ritonavir after garlic treatment are not due to induction of CYP3A4 but, more likely, to modulation of the activity of another (unknown) enzyme and/or a drug transporter, although an interaction at the level of ABCB1 is unlikely (Foster, et al., 2001).

A prospective pharmacokinetic study was performed on the basis of the considerations mentioned earlier, in which 10 patients acted as their own controls, during the first cycle of weekly docetaxel coadministered with a commonly used garlic supplement (Cox, et al., 2006). Docetaxel was administered as a 1-hour intravenous infusion once every week for three consecutive weeks (days 1, 8, and 15), with cycles repeated every 4 weeks, at a dose of 30 mg/m². Starting on day 5 and continuing through day 17, patients took 600 mg garlic tablets (containing 3,600 μg allicin per tablet) twice a day, orally. In this study, the mean clearance of docetaxel in the absence of garlic of 30.8 L/h/m² was reduced on days 8 and 15, with mean values of 23.7 L/h/m² and 20.0 L/h/m², respectively (P = 0.17). This suggests that garlic supplementation had no statistically significant effects on the pharmacokinetic profile of docetaxel when administered over the short term (4 days) or long term (12 days). Interestingly, the docetaxel area under the curve ratio on day 15 compared with day 1 was substantially increased in the three African Americans individuals, all expressing functional CYP3A5 (mean ratio, 3.74) as compared with the six individuals that did not express CYP3A5 (mean ratio, 1.02). Although this difference was not statistically significant (P = 0.38), this finding suggests that the ability to affect the pharmacokinetic profile of docetaxel is dependent on the presence of drug-metabolizing enzymes that exhibit clinically important and racially dependent polymorphisms. Overall, however, there appears to be little likelihood of significant interactions between garlic and anticancer drugs that are predominantly metabolized by CYP3A4.

MILK THISTLE

The principal constituent of milk thistle is silymarin, a mixture of flavonoids and phenyl-propanoids found in the fruit of the milk thistle plant, and consists mostly of silybin (about 50%–70%), but can also contain silychristin, silydianin, and other similar flavonoligans (Bilia, Bergonzi, Gallori, Mazzi, & Vincieri, 2002). Inhibition of certain hepatic enzymes secondary to silymarin ingestion has been reported (Letteron, et al., 1990), in addition to significant reductions in the glucuronidation of bilirubin and depletion of the UDP glucuronic acid pools (Chrungoo, et al., 1997). Furthermore, reports of reduced in vitro activity for CYP3A4 (up to 100% at 25 mM) (Beckmann-Knopp, et al., 2000; Venkataramanan, et al., 2000), CYP2D6, CYP2C9 (Beckmann-Knopp, et al., 2000), and UGT1A6/9 (Venkataramanan, et al., 2000) isozymes by milk thistle components have been published. However, at clinically achievable concentrations (about 0.6 μM at peak concentration) (Schandalik & Perucca, 1994; Weyhenmeyer, Mascher, & Birkmayer, 1992), silybin, dehydrosylibin, silydianin, and silycristin do not substantially inhibit the activity of CYP2D6, CYP2E1, and CYP3A4 in human liver microsomes (Zuber, et al., 2002). Similarly, the finding that silymarin at concentrations higher than 100 μM inhibits ABCB1 (Zhang & Morris, 2003) and ABCC1 (Nguyen, Zhang, & Morris, 2003) in some in vitro models is probably of unlikely clinical significance.

The effect of milk thistle, administered 3 times a day for a period of 2 or 3 weeks, on the pharmacokinetics of the HIV protease inhibitor indinavir was recently studied independently in three groups of volunteers (DiCenzo, et al., 2003; Mills, et al., 2005; Piscitelli et al., 2002b). In line with the in vitro findings, milk thistle did not significantly alter the overall exposure to indinavir, although the mean trough concentrations were 25% to 32% decreased in the two of the studies. Indinavir is a substrate for both CYP3A4 and ABCB1 that is highly susceptible to enzyme inhibition and induction (Barry, Gibbons, Back, & Mulcahy, 1997).

The potential interaction between milk thistle and irinotecan was recently studied in six cancer patients treated with the anticancer drug (dose, 125 mg/m^2) given as a 90-minute infusion once every week (van Erp, et al., 2005). Four days before the second dose, patients received 200 mg milk thistle, thrice a day, for 14 consecutive days. Short-term (4 days) or more prolonged intake of milk thistle (12 days) was found to have no significant effect on irinotecan clearance (mean, 31.2 vs 25.4 vs 25.6 L/h; $P = 0.16$). The area under the curve ratio of SN-38 (the active metabolite) and irinotecan was slightly decreased by milk thistle (2.58% vs 2.23% vs 2.17%; $P = 0.047$), whereas the relative extent of glucuronidation of SN-38 was similar (10.8 vs 13.5 vs 13.1; $P = 0.64$). Likewise, the area under the curve ratio of the inactive metabolite APC and irinotecan was unaffected by milk thistle (0.332 ves 0.285 vs 0.337; $P = 0.53$). The underlying reasons for the inconsistency between the various in vitro and in vivo observations related to the effect of milk thistle on enzyme and transporter function with the outcome of the irinotecan study are unknown. It is possible that the lack of effects in vivo is related to poor absorption in conjunction with large interindividual variability of the various milk thistle constituents. Indeed, the oral absorption of silybin has previously been reported to be low due to the poor solubility. In the patients treated with irinotecan, the highest concentration of silybin measured at steady state in plasma was ~0.26 μmol/L. Prior in vitro studies showed that silybin concentrations of >1.4 μmol/L are required for inhibition of UTG1A1, whereas only concentrations of >32 μmol/L are associated with inactivation of CYP3A4 function (Venkataramanan, et al., 2000). Therefore, the plasma concentrations of silybin at the manufacturer-recommended doses of milk thistle as applied in this study may be too low to affect the various disposition pathways of irinotecan. Overall, this suggests that milk thistle is unlikely to alter the pharmacokinetics of anticancer drugs that are predominantly eliminated by CYP3A and/or UGT1A.

ST. JOHN'S WORT

St. John's wort is composed of a very complex mixture of over two dozen compounds, including catechin-type tannins and condensed-type proanthocyanidins; flavonoids (mostly hyperoside, rutin, quercetin, and kaempferol); biflavonoids (eg, biapigenin); phloroglutinol derivatives like hyperforin, phenolic acids, volatile oils and naphtodianthrones, including hypericin and pseudohypericin (Barnes, Anderson, & Phillipson, 2001).

Various in vitro studies have shown that St. John's wort is a potent inducer of CYP1A2 (Karyekar, Eddington, & Dowling, 2002), CYP2B6 (Goodwin, Moore, Stoltz, McKee, & Kliewer, 2001), CYP2C9, CYP2C19 (Zou, Harkey, & Henderson, 2002), and CYP3A4 (Moore et al., 2000; Wentworth, Agostini, Love, Schwabe, & Chatterjee, 2000), but not of CYP2D6 (Zhou, et al., 2003), CYP3A5, CYP3A7, and CYP3A43 (Krusekopf, Roots, & Kleeberg, 2003). The inducing effects on CYP2B6 (Goodwin, et al., 2001), CYP2C19 (Chen, Ferguson, Negishi, & Goldstein, 2003b), and CYP3A4 (Bertilsson, et al., 1998; Lehmann, et al., 1998; Watkins, et al., 2003) have been linked to hyperforin-induced ligand activation of a steroid- and xenobiotic-regulated transcription factor known as the pregnane X receptor (also known as PXR or NR1I2) (Fig. 8.4). Using cDNA-expressed models, St. John's wort extracts have also been reported to inhibit the activity of several enzymes including CYP1A2, CYP2C9, CYP2C19, CYP2D6, and CYP3A4 through both competitive and noncompetitive actions

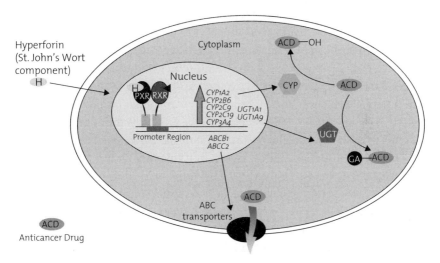

FIGURE 8.4. Induction of cytochrome P450 (CYP) isozymes, UDP glucuronosyltransferase (UGT) isozymes, and ATP binding cassette (ABC) transporter proteins by the St. John's wort constituent, hyperforin, through activation of the human pregnane X receptor (PXR; also known as Nr1i2). PXR binds to DNA via a pregnane response element as a heterodimer with the 9-cis retinoic acid receptor (RXR), and transduces phase I metabolism (e.g., hydroxylation), Phase II metabolism (e.g., glucuronic acid [GA] conjugation), and active, outward-directed transport of many commonly used anticancer drugs (ACD).

(Budzinski, Foster, Vandenhoek, & Arnason, 2000; Foster, et al., 2003; Obach, 2000).

Animal studies using probe drugs have provided compelling evidence that St. John's wort is also a potent modulator of CYP3A activity in vivo both in mice (Bray, Perry, Menkes, & Rosengren, 2002b; Cantoni, Rozio, Mangolini, Hauri, & Caccia, 2003) and rats(Durr et al., 2000). However, short-term treatment of St. John's wort, hypericin, or hyperforin failed to induce CYP isoforms (Bray, Brennan, Perry, Menkes, & Rosengren, 2002a; Noldner & Chatterjee, 2001). Human studies indicated that long-term (i.e. more than 2 weeks) administration of St. John's wort significantly induced intestinal and hepatic CYP3A4 (Dresser, Schwarz, Wilkinson, & Kim, 2003; Durr, et al., 2000; Gurley, et al., 2002; Kerb, Bauser, Brockmoller, & Roots, 1997; Roby, Anderson, Kantor, Dryer, & Burstein, 2000; Wang, et al., 2001), but did not alter CYP2C9 (Wang, et al., 2001), CYP1A2 (Gurley, et al., 2002; Wang, et al., 2001), or CYP2D6 (Gurley, et al., 2002; Markowitz, et al., 2000; Roby, Dryer, & Burstein, 2001; Wang, et al., 2001). As predicted from the animal experiments, induction of CYP3A4 by St. John's wort is subject to the dosing regimen, and schedules involving administration of the herb for less than 8 days are unlikely to activate PXR (Ereshefsky, Gewertz, Francis Lam, Vega, & Ereshefsky, 1999; Markowitz, et al., 2000). The cited studies have also indicated that St. John's wort contains both inhibitory and activating constituents for the CYP system, causing temporally distinguishable inhibition and induction depending on the dose, duration of administration, and the formulation and source of the herb.

LS-80 intestinal carcinoma cell exposed to St. John's wort or hypericin have shown strong induction of ABCB1 in a dose-dependent fashion (Perloff, Von Moltke, Stormer, Shader, & Greenblatt, 2001). Similarly, the administration of St. John's wort significantly increases the intestinal expression of ABCB1 in rats and humans (Durr, et al., 2000), as well as its expression in peripheral blood lymphocytes (Hennessy, et al., 2002). Given the broad substrate specificity of this protein, these findings have been used to support the importance of ABCB1 in addition to CYP3A4 as a mechanism to reduce oral absorption of substrate drugs given combined with St. John's wort.

The mechanism for most of the interactions observed in subsequent clinical trials remains unclear, although for some agents induction of CYP3A4 (e.g., indinavir, midazolam, simvastatin), ABCB1 (e.g., digoxin, fexofenadine), or both (e.g., cyclosporin, tacrolimus) may explain their increased clearance. Nonetheless, although common molecular mechanisms may be involved, the quantitative aspects of CYP3A4 and ABCB1 induction are complex and depend on the particular drug and the relative contribution of both proteins to its absorption and disposition (Dresser, et al., 2003). Another factor adding to the complexity is the recent finding that St. John's wort produced significantly greater increases in CYP3A4 expression in females compared to males, which appeared to be unrelated to body mass index (Gurley et al., 2002).

Although no differences have been noted in the extent of inducibility by St. John's wort among six different ethnic groups (Xie et al., 2005), the effects of this herb remain unpredictable, especially when based on in vitro or animal studies. For example, St. John's wort did not alter the pharmacokinetics of the CYP3A4 substrate carbamazepine (Burstein et al., 2000), presumably because repeated intake of the drug already maximizes enzyme induction. More recently, it was shown that various transcription factors, including the pregnane X receptor, regulate constitutive expression of mouse Ugt1a1 and Ugt1a9 (Mackenzie et al., 2003), and human UGT isoforms (Xie et al., 2003). However, in a clinical study, St. John's wort had no effect on the extent of glucuronidation of SN-38, the active metabolite of the anticancer drug irinotecan (Mathijssen, Verweij, de Bruijn, Loos, & Sparreboom, 2002), which is a known substrate for UGT1A1 and UGT1A9 (Hanioka, et al., 2001). Regardless, the modulation of CYP3A4 activity and subsequently reduced exposure to SN-38 observed in the study with St. John's wort administered to cancer patients receiving irinotecan is particularly worrying bearing in mind that the degree of drug-induced myelo-suppression, and likely also the antitumor activity, was substantially reduced in the presence of the botanical (Mathijssen, et al., 2002). Animal studies have further suggested that St. John's wort may modulate irinotecan-induced toxicity by mechanisms that are unrelated to altered drug clearance (Hu, et al., 2005; Hu, et al., 2006). On the basis of in vitro data obtained in human hepatocyte cultures, increased docetaxel metabolism can also be expected in patients using St. John's wort chronically (Komoroski, et al., 2005). Because of the extensive reduction in the plasma levels of SN-38, patients should be advised to refrain from taking St. John's wort to prevent undertreatment.

The same advice could be given to patients that are going to be treated with imatinib. In two clinical trials, healthy subjects taking imatinib combined with St. John's wort showed on average a 30% to 32% lower mean area under the curve (Frye, Fitzgerald, Lagattuta, Hruska, & Egorin, 2004; Smith, et al., 2004). It should be noted that the main metabolite formed after metabolism of imatinib, an N-desmethylated piperazine derivative, has been shown to have antitumor activity comparable with that of imatinib. Since St. John's wort had no substantial influence on the systemic exposure to this metabolite, the clinical implications of the reduced plasma levels of imatinib after St. John's wort intake is therefore unclear and requires further investigation (Meijerman, Beijnen, & Schellens, 2006). Overall, however, the reported data suggest that interactions between St. John's wort and most anticancer agents are likely to have clinical and toxicological implications (Table 8.4), and that rigorous testing for possible interactions is urgently needed.

Table 8.4. Suspected Interaction of St. John's Wort with Anticancer Drugs

Anticancer Drug	Main Proteins Involved in Drug Absorption and/or Elimination	Expected Effect of Chronic St. John's Wort Coadministration
6-Mercaptopurine	Thiopurine methyltransferase, ABCC4	None
6-Thioguanine	N/a	None
Anastrazole	CYP2C9, CYP3A4	Decreased exposure
Arsenic trioxide	Non CYP methylation	None
Asparaginase	N/a	None
Bleomycin	N/a	None
Busulfan	CYP3A4	Decreased exposure
Capecitabine	carboxylesterases, cytidine deaminase	None
Carboplatin	N/a	None
Chlorambucil	ABCC2	Decreased exposure
Cisplatin	OCT2, ABCC2	Decreased exposure
Cyclophosphamide	CYB2B6, CYP2C9, CYP3A4	Decreased exposure
Cytarabine	Cytidine deaminase	None
Dacarbazine	CYP2E1	Decreased exposure
Docetaxel	CYP3A4, CYP3A5, ABCB1	Decreased exposure
Doxorubicin	CYP3A4, CYP2D6, ABCB1	Decreased exposure
Epirubicin	CYP3A4	Decreased exposure
Erlotinib	CYP3A4, CYP1A2	Decreased exposure
Estramustine	N/a	None
Etoposide	CYP3A4, ABCB1, ABCC1, ABCC2	Decreased exposure
Exemestane	CYP3A4	Decreased exposure
Fluorouracil	Dihydropyrimidine dehydrogenase	None
Gefitinib	CYP3A4, ABCG2	Decreased exposure

(*continued*)

Table 8.4. (Continued)

Anticancer Drug	Main Proteins Involved in Drug Absorption and/or Elimination	Expected Effect of Chronic St. John's Wort Coadministration
Gemcitabine	Deaminases	None
Hydroxyurea	N/a	None
Ifosfamide	CYP2B6, CYP3A4	Decreased exposure
Imatinib	CYP2C9, CYP2C19, CYP3A4, ABCB1, ABCG2	Decreased exposure
Irinotecan	CYP3A4, CES2, UGT1A1, ABCC2, ABCG2	Decreased exposure
Ixabipelone	CYP3A4	Decreased exposure
Letrozole	CYP2A6, CYP3A4	Decreased exposure
Melphalan	N/a	None
Mesna	N/a	None
Methotrexate	ABCC1, ABCC2, ABCG2	Decreased exposure
Mitomycin C	N/a	None
Mitoxantrone	ABCB1, ABCG2	Decreased exposure
Oxaliplatin	OCT2	None
Paclitaxel	CYP3A4, CYP2C8, ABCB1	Decreased exposure
Tamoxifen	CYP2B6, CYP3A4, CYP1A2, CYP2E1	Decreased exposure
Temozolomide	N/a	None
Teniposide	CYP3A4, ABCB1	Decreased exposure
Thiotepa	N/a	None
Topotecan	CYP3A4, ABCB1, ABCG2	Decreased exposure
Tretinoin	CYP2C8, CYP2C9, CYP3A4	Decreased exposure
Vinblastine	CYP3A4, ABCB1	Decreased exposure
Vincristine	CYP3A4, CYP3A5, ABCB1	Decreased exposure
Vinorelbine	CYP3A4	Decreased exposure

N/a, information not available.

St. John's wort is currently the only top-selling botanical for which sufficient clinical data is available that warrants labeling a contraindication for its concurrent or concomitant use with prescription anticancer drugs.

Conclusions and Future Research

In recent years, a wealth of evidence has been generated from in vitro and in vivo studies showing that many herbal preparations interact extensively with drug-metabolizing enzymes and drug transporters. Moreover, a number of clinically important pharmacokinetic interactions have now been recognized, although causal relationships have not always been established. Most of the observed interactions point to the botanicals affecting several isoforms of the CYP family, either through inhibition or induction. These enzymes have a crucial role in the elimination of various anticancer drugs, and concurrent use of at least some herbs with chemotherapy is destined to have serious clinical and toxicological implications (Table 8.5). Therefore, rigorous testing for possible

Table 8.5. Specific Botanicals to Discourage and Avoid
during Chemotherapy.

Herb	Concurrent Chemotherapy/Condition (Suspected Effect)
Echinacea	Caution with camptothecins, cyclophosphamide, TK inhibitors, epipodophyllotoxins, taxanes, and Vinca alkaloids (CYP3A4 induction)
Ephedra	Avoid with all cardiovascular chemotherapy (synergistic increase in blood pressure)
Ginkgo	Caution with camptothecins, cyclophosphamide, TK inhibitors, epipodophyllotoxins, taxanes, and Vinca alkaloids (CYP3A4 and CYP2C19 inhibition); discourage with alkylating agents, antitumor antibiotics, and platinum analogues (free-radical scavenging)
Ginseng	Discourage in patients with estrogen-receptor positive breast cancer and endometrial cancer (stimulation of tumor growth)
Green tea	Discourage with erlotinib (CYP1A2 induction)

(*continued*)

Table 8.5. (Continued)

Herb	Concurrent Chemotherapy/Condition (Suspected Effect)
Japanese arrowroot	Avoid with methotrexate (ABCC and OAT transporter inhibition)
Soy	Avoid with tamoxifen (antagonism of tumor growth inhibition), and treatment of patients with estrogen-receptor positive breast cancer and endometrial cancer (stimulation of tumor growth)
St. John's wort	Avoid with all concurrent chemotherapy (CYP2B6, CYP2C9, CYP2C19, CYP2E1, CYP3A4, and ABCB1 induction)
Valerian	Caution with tamoxifen (CYP2C9 inhibition), cyclophosphamide, and teniposide (CYP2C19 inhibition)
Kava-kava	Avoid in all patients with preexisting liver disease, with evidence of hepatic injury (herb-induced hepatotoxicity), and/or in combination with hepatotoxic chemotherapy; caution with camptothecins, cyclophosphamide, TK inhibitors, epipodophyllotoxins, taxanes, and Vinca alkaloids (CYP3A4 induction)
Grape seed	Caution with camptothecins, cyclophosphamide, TK inhibitors, epipodophyllotoxins, taxanes, and Vinca alkaloids (CYP3A4 induction), and with alkylating agents, antitumor antibiotics, and platinum analogues (free-radical scavenging)

TK, tyrosine-kinase.

pharmacokinetic interactions of anticancer drugs with widely used herbs is urgently required. An additional consideration for cancer chemotherapy is that herb-mediated induction of various enzymes and transporters may also take place in tumor cells, and subsequently result in resistance to anthracyclines, epipodophyllotoxins, taxanes, and Vinca alkaloids (Broxterman, Lankelma, & Hoekman, 2003). Likewise, catalytic inhibition of topoisomerase IIα in tumor cells by some botanicals (Peebles, Baker, Kurz, Schneider, & Kroll, 2001) might diminish therapeutic responses to anthracyclines, dactinomycin, and etoposide (Mansky & Straus, 2002). Because of the high worldwide prevalence of herbal medicine use, physicians should include herb usage in their routine drug histories to have an opportunity to outline to individual patients which potential hazards should be taken into consideration (de Smet, 2002; Weiger, et al., 2002).

REFERENCES

de Smet PAGM. (2002). Herbal Remedies. The New England Journal of Medicine, 347, 2046–2056.

Dresser GK, Schwarz UI, Wilkinson GR, & Kim RB. (2003). Coordinate induction of both cytochrome P4503A and MDR1 by St John's wort in healthy subjects. Clinical Pharmacology and Therapeutics, 73, 41–50.

Eisenberg DM, Davis RB, Ettner SL, Appel S, Wilkey S, & van Rompay M. (1998). Trends in alternative medicine use in the United States, 1990–1997: results of a follow-up national survey. JAMA, 280, 1569–1575.

Frye RF, Fitzgerald SM, Lagattuta TF, Hruska MW, & Egorin MJ. (2004), Effect of St John's wort on imatinib mesylate pharmacokinetics. Clinical Pharmacology and Therapeutics, 76, 323–329.

Izzo AA & Ernst E. Interactions between herbal medicines and prescribed drugs: a systematic review. Drugs, (2001) 61, 2163–2175.

Mathijssen RH, Verweij J, de Bruijn P, Loos WJ, & Sparreboom A. (2002). Effects of St. John's wort on irinotecan metabolism. Journal of the National Cancer Institute, 94, 1247–1249.

Meijerman I, Beijnen JH, & Schellens JH. (2006). Herb-drug interactions in oncology: Focus on mechanisms of induction. Oncologist, 11, 742–752.

Sparreboom A, Cox MC, Acharya MR, & Figg WD. (2004). Herbal remedies in the United States: potential adverse interactions with anticancer agents. Journal of Clinical Oncology, 22, 2489–2503.

van Erp NP, Baker SD, Zhao M, Rudek MA, Guchelaar HJ, Nortier JW, et al. (2005). Effect of milk thistle (Silybum marianum) on the pharmacokinetics of irinotecan. Clinical Cancer Research, 11, 7800–7806.

Zhou S, Gao Y, Jiang W, Huang M, Xu A, & Paxton JW. (2003). Interactions of herbs with cytochrome P450. Drug Metabolism Reviews, 35, 35–98.

(A complete reference list for this chapter is available online at http://www.oup.com/us/ integrativemedicine).

9

The Antioxidant Debate

ELENA LADAS AND KARA M. KELLY

KEY CONCEPTS

- Patients with cancer are taking antioxidant supplements in combination with conventional chemotherapy and radiotherapy to enhance the anticancer activity and to reduce the side effects of conventional treatment.
- Many oncologists are concerned that the protective mechanisms of antioxidants may not distinguish between normal and malignant cells, so that supplements may interfere with the anticancer activity of the conventional therapies.
- Not all antioxidant supplements are equivalent; antioxidants counteract free radical activity through multiple mechanisms of action.
- Not all chemotherapy agents rely on oxidative stress for anticancer activity, so risk of interaction with antioxidant supplements is also dependent on the type of conventional chemotherapy.
- Several studies have shown that plasma concentrations of antioxidants are depleted in individuals undergoing treatment for cancer; some studies suggest that this decrease may be associated with therapy-related toxicities.
- Few randomized controlled trials have investigated the efficacy of antioxidants as a *treatment* for cancer, most of the trials published have been case series or nonrandomized trials.
- Most of the clinical trials published have described the use of antioxidants as supportive care agents; the results of these trials have been mixed.
- Based on the findings from a large randomized controlled trial, the combined use of β-carotene and vitamin E supplements in conjunction with radiation therapy is contraindicated and should be avoided until further research is available.

- As few randomized controlled trials have addressed the use of antioxidant supplements during chemotherapy, health care providers should be cautious about recommending antioxidant supplements during chemotherapy until further research is available to guide clinical practice.

■

The use of antioxidant supplements by patients during conventional cancer treatment is among one of the most controversial areas in oncology. Past estimates of antioxidant use by patients with cancer have varied considerably, with rates ranging from 13%–87% depending on the survey, the type of cancer studied, and a variety of other individual and demographic factors (Block, et al., 2007; Branda, Naud, Brooks, Chen, & Muss, 2004; Burstein, Gelber, Guadagnoli, & Weeks, 1999; Clemens, Waladkhani, Bublitz, Ehninger, & Gey, 1997; Kelly, et al., 2000; Legha, et al., 1982; Lesperance, et al., 2002). In one large study, the Women's Health Eating Initiative, 58% of women with breast cancer reported taking multivitamin supplements, 46% used Vitamin E, 42% took vitamin C and 10% supplemented with an antioxidant mixture (Rock, Newman, Neuhouser, Major, & Barnett, 2004). However, data is still lacking on the use of antioxidant supplements among patients with other types of cancer, and the doses used in conjunction with conventional therapies.

Antioxidants are substances that counteract free radicals and prevent them from causing tissue and organ damage (Ratnam, Ankola, Bhardwaj, Sahana, & Kumar, 2006). Evidence supporting the potential role of antioxidants in preventing and treating disease include preclinical studies, which have correlated oxidative stress and an antioxidant-depleted diet with the development of diseases including cancer (Salganik, et al., 2000). Some epidemiologic studies have observed an association between an increased intake of dietary antioxidants and a decreased risk of developing lung (Mannisto, et al., 2004; Yong, et al., 1997), esophageal (Mark, et al., 2000), and gastrointestinal (Bjelakovic, Nikolova, Simonetti, & Gluud, 2004; Jenab, et al., 2006a; Jenab, et al., 2006b) cancer. Antioxidants are most commonly taken in conjunction with conventional cancer treatment rather than as its replacement. At the current time, the precise role of antioxidant supplementation in the patient with established cancer remains to be determined.

Table 9.1. Oxidative Stress and Chemotherapy.

	Class	Examples
High	Anthracyclines	Doxorubicin, daunorubicin
	Alkylating agents	Cyclophosphamide, ifosfamide, procarbazine, dacarbazine, melphalan
	Platinum-containing complexes	Cisplatin, carboplatin
	Topoisomerase 1 inhibitors	Irinotecan
	Topoisomerase 2 inhibitors	Etoposide
Low	Purine/pyrimidine analogues	6-Mercaptopurine, 6-thioguanine
	Antimetabolites	Methotrexate, L-asparaginase
	Monoclonal antibodies	Rituximab
	Vinca alkaloids	Vincristine, vinblastine
	Taxanes	Paclitaxel
	Corticosteroids	Prednisone, dexamethasone
Insufficient data	Antiangiogenic agents	Bevacizumab
	Tyrosine kinase inhibitors	Imatinib

Chemotherapy agents vary in their risk for interaction with antioxidant supplements. Table 9.1 lists chemotherapy agents by association with the generation of oxidative stress, with "high oxidative stress" agents being at potentially increased risk for interaction with antioxidant supplements.

Much of the controversy surrounding antioxidants and cancer therapy has arisen because certain classes of chemotherapy agents exert some of their anticancer effects by generating reactive oxygen species, or free radicals (Moss, 2006). Some of these agents include the anthracyclines (e.g., doxorubicin), platinum-containing complexes (e.g., cisplatin, carboplatin), and alkylating agents (e.g., cyclophosphamide, ifosfamide), as well as radiation therapy. The theoretical concern is that antioxidants might somehow interfere with or counteract the activities of these anticancer agents. However, many chemotherapy agents have multiple mechanisms of action and do not necessarily rely on the generation of free radicals (Table 9.1).

Free radical–mediated damage to normal tissues often manifests as side effects of chemotherapy, such as anthracycline-associated cardiomyopathy, or hearing loss or kidney failure caused by platinum-based agents. Antioxidant supplementation may facilitate anticancer treatment by protecting normal tissues and allowing for higher doses of chemotherapy to be administered.

Additionally, at certain concentrations, they might also be able to directly affect cancer cells through prooxidant effects.

Many proponents for combining antioxidant supplements with conventional cancer therapy justify this approach because observational studies have identified the depletion of antioxidant levels during treatment with radiation and chemotherapy, particularly with the use of conditioning regimens before stem cell transplantation (Durken, et al., 2000; Kennedy, Ladas, Rheingold, Blumberg, & Kelly, 2004a; Kennedy, et al., 2004b).

The use of accepted pharmaceutical protective agents that work through antioxidant mechanisms further supports the use of antioxidant supplements during chemotherapy. Mesna, for example, minimizes the risk of hemorrhagic cystitis by forming nontoxic compounds in the bladder with acrolein, 4-hydroxy-metabolites, and other urotoxic metabolites of oxazaphosphorines related to ifosfamide and cyclophosphamide metabolism. The thiol metabolite of amifostine is readily taken up by cells where it binds to and detoxifies reactive metabolites of platinum and alkylating agents as well as scavenges free radicals. Tumor cells are generally not protected because amifostine and metabolites are present in normal cells at 100-fold greater concentrations than in tumor cells (Creagan, et al., 1979; Culy & Spencer, 2001, 2002; McEvoy, 2002; Moertel, et al., 1985). The use of these cytoprotective agents is based on the results of preclinical studies and evidence accumulated from clinical trials to date, which is still lacking for most antioxidant supplements.

A limited number of clinical trials have investigated antioxidant supplementation for the treatment of specific cancers, or for the reduction in or prevention of common adverse effects associated with anticancer therapy (Bairati, et al., 2005; Drisko, Chapman, & Hunter, 2003a; Drisko, Chapman, & Hunter, 2003b; Hoenjet, et al., 2005; Ladas, et al., 2004; Pathak, et al., 2005). Several systematic reviews have evaluated the health advantages of using antioxidant supplements concomitantly with chemotherapy (Block, et al., 2007; Ladas, et al., 2004; Simone, Simone, Simone, & Simone, 2007a, 2007b). Most clinical trials have been limited by inadequate sample sizes, heterogeneous patient populations, variation in the routes of antioxidant administration, or study designs that lacked appropriate blinding to randomization (Ladas, et al., 2004). Although the data on antioxidant use during chemotherapy has not been associated with an attenuation of the effects of the particular anticancer treatment on tumor control, the studies have not yet thoroughly investigated this issue to allow for the routine recommendation of antioxidant supplementation. This chapter provides an overview of the issues surrounding this very controversial topic, with a summary of the key clinical trial evidence that has been reported to date.

Classes of Antioxidants

Antioxidant is a broad term that refers to a myriad of different compounds. Because of the disparity in the biological actions and targets of antioxidants, there is no simple paradigm for advising patients of their safe use during conventional chemotherapy and radiotherapy. Antioxidants function through a variety of mechanisms and each may belong to more than one functional category (Papas, 1999).

There are **two general categories** of antioxidants:

- Enzymatic antioxidants such as catalase, superoxide dismutase, and glutathione peroxidase
- Nonenzymatic antioxidants, such as vitamin C, vitamin E, coenzyme Q10, melatonin, and pycnogenol

Within these two broad categories, there are **four functional subclasses**:

- Preventative agents that suppress the formation of free radicals
- Radical scavenging agents that inhibit chain initiation and/or propagation
- Repair and de novo enzymes that repair and reconstitute cell membranes
- Adaptation agents that generate appropriate antioxidant enzymes and transfer them to the site of action

The wide spectrum of activity of antioxidant compounds further complicates the counsel for patients on the safety of taking antioxidants in combination with conventional cancer therapy.

Most nonenzymatic antioxidant compounds or their precursors are obtained orally, either through foods or dietary supplements. Although dietary intake of antioxidant-rich foods has been shown to elevate human plasma antioxidant levels, it is unlikely that intake from the typical 2500-calorie American adult diet could effectively achieve the steady state levels required to interact with the chemotherapy concentrations used in anticancer treatments. Although one study in children being treated for acute lymphoblastic leukemia found that an increased dietary intake of antioxidant nutrients was associated with reductions in chemotherapy-associated side effects (Kennedy, et al., 2004b), this observation has not been confirmed in larger studies. It is conceivable that the regular use of antioxidant supplements could achieve steady state levels that might interact with chemotherapy or radiation therapy. Nonetheless, the dose, duration, and particular type of antioxidant that might be able to create an interactive effect have not yet been established.

The bioavailability of antioxidant compounds varies according to their source, route of administration, and form (Ratnam, et al., 2006). Lycopene, for example, is more readily absorbed in cooked rather than raw form, and intravenous administration of vitamin C has a biological activity that differs from its oral form (Padayatty, et al., 2004; Ratnam, et al., 2006).

Studies evaluating antioxidant supplementation during chemotherapy are further complicated by the individual variation in the genes that code for antioxidant enzymes as well as variation in the enzymes involved in the metabolism of chemotherapeutic agents, thus potentially impacting the effectiveness of the antioxidant. Individuals with limited or no activity in specific antioxidant genes, such as glutathione-S-transferase, may have decreased ability to exert antiradical activity which may impact the incidence of toxicity and influence treatment outcomes (Ambrosone, et al., 2005; Davies, et al., 2001). The overall antioxidant status of the patient will further impact their effectiveness. Children with acute lymphoblastic leukemia with a higher antioxidant status, measured by the oxygen radical absorbance assay, have been shown to experience fewer side effects associated with cancer therapy (Kennedy, et al., 2004b). The safety of antioxidant supplementation during chemotherapy and radiation therapy is likely to depend on the specificity of the antioxidant and the chemotherapy agent. The opinion that all antioxidants are contraindicated within the context of anticancer treatment is narrow and oversimplified.

Antioxidants for the Treatment of Cancer

Although there is extensive preclinical data supporting a possible role for antioxidant supplements as anticancer agents, the evidence from clinical trials remains quite limited. In a systematic review of studies that evaluated the effects of antioxidants during chemotherapy, six studies investigated the effects of antioxidant supplementation on recurrence rates and survival (Ladas, et al., 2004). Two studies reported survival benefits with antioxidant supplementation (Jaakkola, et al., 1992; Lockwood, Moesgaard, Hanioka, & Folkers, 1994), while one study found antioxidant supplementation was associated with short-, but not long-term survival advantage (Lamm, et al., 1994). In three studies, no overall survival benefit was observed with antioxidant supplementation (Clemens, et al., 1997; Legha, et al., 1982; Mills, 1988). Several clinical studies that have evaluated antioxidants as either primary or adjunctive cancer treatment are presented in the following paragraphs.

Single Antioxidant Supplements

Vitamin C, a strong reducing agent, functions as a metal chelator and cellular protector. Vitamin C was postulated to have an important role in the treatment of cancer, based upon the observations that vitamin C is involved in host resistance to cancer and that patients with cancer are often found to be depleted of vitamin C. Supplementation with vitamin C was suggested for its potential role to increase host resistance to cancer by stimulating immune function, increasing resistance to intercellular ground substance hydrolysis by hyalurinidase elaborated by tumor cells, stabilizing the production of hormones, and by protecting the pituitary–adrenal axis from the effects of stress (Cameron, Pauling, & Leibovitz, 1979; Wittes, 1985). Case studies of terminal-stage cancer patients treated with a combination of high-dose oral and intravenous vitamin C who demonstrated prolonged survival were reported (Cameron & Pauling, 1976; Cameron & Pauling, 1978; Cameron, et al., 1979; Cameron, 1991). Two subsequent double-blind randomized placebo-controlled trials showed no survival advantage with high-dose oral vitamin C supplementation as a treatment for cancer (Creagan, et al., 1979; Moertel, et al., 1985). More recent work has shown that vitamin C is cytotoxic to tumor cell lines at concentrations that can be achieved in plasma only by intravenous administration (Koh, et al., 1998). Intravenous vitamin C is also associated with better tissue distribution and saturation (Padayatty, et al., 2004). Whether similar effects would occur in vivo has not been addressed. Recent case studies have reported a beneficial effect of intravenous administration of vitamin C on tumor control (Padayatty, et al., 2006). Clinical studies with intravenous vitamin C are currently in progress.

Vitamin C has also been investigated as an adjunctive agent to conventional chemotherapy. The combination of melphalan, arsenic trioxide, and intravenous vitamin C was shown to be feasible and associated with considerable objective responses in a phase II study in relapsed or refractory multiple myeloma (Berenson, et al., 2006).

Melatonin is an endogenous hormone that is synthesized and secreted by the pineal gland from the amino acid tryptophan. Melatonin protects against oxidative stress through its ability to upregulate antioxidant enzymes such as superoxide dismutases, peroxidases, and enzymes of glutathione supply; to downregulate prooxidant enzymes such as nitric oxide synthases and lipoxygenases; and also to govern some of the actions of quinone reductase 2 (Hardeland, 2005). In addition to its antioxidant effects, melatonin stimulates apoptosis, reduces tumor growth factors, decreases endothelial growth factor, and exerts anti-inflammatory properties (Lissoni, 2002). At physiologically attainable concentrations, melatonin inhibits cancer cell division and with administration of higher oral doses (20–40 mg/day), melatonin is cytotoxic (Mahmoud, Sarhill, & Mazurczak, 2005).

A systematic review has suggested that melatonin supplementation may improve survival in a number of solid tumors (Mills, 2005). Although the effects of melatonin on prolonging survival are intriguing, the studies demonstrating cancer survival were all conducted by the same research group and thus should be confirmed in larger phase III trials.

Melatonin has also been studied as an adjunctive agent to chemotherapy. The addition of melatonin to interferon therapy in the treatment of 22 patients with progressive metastatic renal cell carcinoma was associated with remission in seven patients (three complete) and achievement of stable disease in nine others (Neri, et al., 1994). In conjunction with cisplatin and etoposide, melatonin has also been studied as a treatment for nonsmall cell lung cancer (Lissoni, Chilelli, Villa, Cerizza, & Tancini, 2003). The addition of melatonin to irinotecan in 30 patients with metastatic colorectal cancer who were progressing on 5-fluorouracil therapy was well-tolerated and was associated with partial responses to treatment and the ability to decrease irinotecan dose by 50% without attenuating its efficacy (Cerea, et al., 2003).

Mixtures of Antioxidant Supplements

The administration of antioxidant mixtures has been investigated in the treatment of several different cancer types, with largely insignificant results.

- A randomized trial of chemotherapy alone or chemotherapy with antioxidants [vitamin C 6100 mg/day; DL-α-tocopherol 1050 mg/day; and β-carotene 60 mg/day] for treatment of 136 patients with stage IIIb and stage IV non–small cell lung cancer observed no difference in tumor response rate or chemotherapy associated toxicities (Pathak, et al., 2005).
- A case–control study investigating megadoses of vitamins in 90 women with unilateral nonmetastatic breast cancer noted no improvement in disease-free survival in the supplemented group; in fact, the supplemented group had lower survival overall, albeit nonsignificantly (Lesperance, et al., 2002).
- In men with androgen-insensitive prostate cancer, combination antioxidant treatment (750 mg of vitamin C, 200 mg selenium, 350 mg vitamin E, and 200 mg of coenzyme Q10) was not associated with significant effects on PSA levels (Hoenjet, et al., 2005).

- However, building on reports of prolonged remission in two women with advanced epithelial ovarian cancer supplementation with vitamin C (3000–9000 mg/day), vitamin E (1200 IU/day), β-carotene (25 mg/day), and vitamin A (5000–10,000 IU/day) (Drisko, et al,. 2003b), a randomized, controlled trial is currently underway (Drisko, et al., 2003a).

Antioxidants for Supportive Care

Several trials have investigated the efficacy of antioxidants as supportive care agents in individuals receiving conventional anticancer therapy. While many trials investigating the role of antioxidants as supportive care agents have been published, very few have been double-blind randomized trials (Tables 9.2 and 9.3). Summarized here are the results from select studies of antioxidants for cancer-related toxicities, categorized by symptoms.

CANCER RELATED CACHEXIA

Cancer-related wasting, or cachexia, is characterized by early satiety, weight loss, anemia, and asthenia (Langer, Hoffman, & Ottery, 2001). A variety of tumor-related factors and increased catabolism often incite cachexia, and its progression is associated with the depletion of intracellular glutathione (GSH) as well as increases in markers of oxidative stress. Supplementation with a GSH-repleting agent has been shown to be effective in treating cachexia associated with human immunodeficiency virus infection (Pacheo, Goldhart, Guilford, Kwyer, & Kongshavn, 1997). A small pilot study in children with cancer at high risk for developing cachexia investigated the effects of an undenatured whey-protein derivative that provides a form of GSH precursor that can be efficiently utilized by cells. Improvements in clinical status including weight gain and increased levels of reduced glutathione were observed (Melnick, et al., 2005).

Supplementation with a mixture of antioxidants may also prevent or ameliorate cancer cachexia. A phase II open label study that investigated the efficacy and safety of a multiagent protocol that included the antioxidants α-lipoic acid (300 mg), vitamin E (400 mg), and vitamin C (500 mg) in 44 adult patients with various malignancies was associated with significant increases in appetite, body weight, and lean body mass (Mantovani, et al., 2006).

Table 9.2. Studies of Antioxidant Supplements for Supportive Care during Cancer Therapy in Adults.

Author, Year	Antioxidant (Dose)	Indication	Type of Cancer	Outcome
Mantovani, et al., 2006	α-Lipoic acid (300 mg) Vitamin E (400 mg) Vitamin C (500 mg)	Cachexia	Advanced cancer	↑ lean body mass, appetite, and body weight ↓ proinflammatory cytokines and tumor necrosis factor ↑ quality of life ↓ fatigue
Iarussi, et al., 1994	Coenzyme Q10 (200 mg)	Cardiotoxicity	Acute lymphoblastic leukemia Non−Hodgkin lymphoma	↓ % left ventricular fractional shortening ($P < 0.05$; placebo; $P < 0.002$ intervention group) ↓ septum wall thickening (control only, $P < 0.01$)
Okuma, et al., 1984	Coenzyme Q10 (90 mg)	Cardiotoxicity	Various malignancies	Prolongation of QTc observed in controls compared to intervention group ($P < 0.05$)
Takimoto, et al., 1982	Coenzyme Q10 (90 mg)	Cardiotoxicity	Various malignancies	↑ in cardiothoracic ratio in controls compared to intervention ($P < 0.01$) No significant differences in pulse rates or QRS voltage
Lenzhofer, et al., 1983	α-Tocopherol (200 mg)	Cardiotoxicity	Metastatic breast cancer	After 6 hrs of doxorubicin, ↑ in PEPI:LVETI ratio in controls ($P < 0.001$) Doxorubicin distributed and eliminated faster in subjects ($P < 0.05$) In controls, correlation between change in PEPI:LVETI ratio and doxorubicin concentration ($P < 0.001$)

Study	Supplement	Toxicity	Cancer type	Findings
Legha, et al., 1982	α-Tocopherol (2 gm/m^2)	Cardiotoxicity	Metastatic breast cancer	No significant findings
Wagdi, et al., 1996	Vitamin C (1gm), Vitamin E (600 mg)	Cardiotoxicity	Various malignancies	No significant findings
Weitzman, et al., 1980	DL-α-tocopherol (1800 IU)	Cardiotoxicity	Various malignancies	No significant findings
Argyriou, et al., 2005	α-Tocopherol (600 mg)	Neurotoxicity	Nonmyeloid malignancies	↓ incidence of neurotoxicity ($P = 0.019$) ↓ risk of developing neuropathy (RR = 0.34; CI = 0.14–0.84)
Argyriou, et al., 2006	DL-α-tocopheryl acetate (600 mg)	Neurotoxicity	Solid malignancies	↓ incidence of neurotoxicity ($P = 0.03$) ↓ risk of developing neuropathy (RR = 0.3; CI = 0.1–0.9)
Weijl, et al., 2004	Vitamin C (1000 mg), DL-α-tocopherol acetate (400 mg), and selenium (100 μg)	Cisplatin-induced ototoxicity and nephrotoxicity	Various malignancies	No significant findings
Sieja, 2000	Selenium (50 μg), vitamin C (200 mg), vitamin E (36 mg), and β-carotene (15 mg)	Chemotherapy-related toxicities	Ovarian cancer	↑ neutrophil count and % after 12 weeks in treatment group vs. controls ($P <0.05$) ↓ in severity of sideeffects in treatment group vs. controls after 12 wks ($P <0.05$)

(continued)

Table 9.2. (Continued)

Author, Year	Antioxidant (Dose)	Indication	Type of Cancer	Outcome
Hu, et al., 1997	Selenium (4000 µg)	Cisplatin-induced toxicities	Various malignancies	Leukocytes ↑ during treatment on Days 7 ($P < 0.05$), 10 ($P < 0.05$), and 14 ($P < 0.05$) ↓ need of blood transfusions and use of Granulocyte Colony Stimulating Factor due to leucopenia during treatment ($P < 0.05$, $P < 0.05$)
Blanke, et al., 2001	D-α-tocopherol (3200 IU)	Chemotherapy-related toxicity Survival	Advanced cancer	No patient had complete or partial response No effect on chemotherapy-related toxicity
Branda, et al., 2004	Multivitamins (various doses; various vitamins)	Chemotherapy-related toxicities	Breast cancer	↓ neutrophils in patients taking supplements vs. no supplements ($P = 0.01$) ↓ neutrophils in patients taking multivitamins (p = 0.01) or vitamin E ($P = 0.03$)
Babu, et al., 2000	Vitamin C (500 mg) Vitamin E (400 mg)	Tamoxifen-induced hypertriglyceridemia	Breast cancer	↓ cholesterol ($P < 0.001$), ↓ triglycerides ($P < 0.001$) ↑ high-density lipoprotein ($P < 0.01$)
Hille, et al., 2005	Vitamin E and pentoxifylline	Radiation-induced proctitis/enteritis	Various malignancies	15 of 21 patients (71%) experienced a relief of their symptoms, with seven patients achieving a reduction from grade I/II to grade 0 toxicity and eight going from grade II to grade I toxicity No significance reported

Study	Intervention	Outcome	Cancer type	Results
Brooker, et al., 2006	Grape seed proanthocyanidin extract (300 mg)	Radiation-induced tissue induration	Breast cancer	No significant results
Wadleigh, et al., 1992	β-Carotene (250 mg) or topical vitamin E oil (400 mg)	Radiation-induced mucositis	Various malignancies	Resolution of mucositis was shorter in subjects vs. controls ($P = 0.025$)
Mills, 1998	β-Carotene (250 mg)	Mucositis	Various malignancies	Subjects had ↓ in severe mucositis (Grade III or IV) ($P < 0.025$) No significant differences in rates of remission in subjects vs. controls
Ferreira, et al., 2004	Vitamin E (400 mg)	Mucositis Survival	Head and neck cancer	↓ of mucositis in cases vs. controls ($P = 0.038$) ↓ pain in cases vs. controls ($P = 0.0001$) No significant difference in survival
Bairati, et al., 2005	DL-α-tocopherol (400 IU/day) and β-carotene (30 mg/day)	Radiation-induced toxicities; Survival	Head and neck cancer	↑ radiation-induced side effects (odds ratio 0.72; CI 0.52–1.02) ↑ mortality in intervention group vs. placebo (hazard ratio: 1.38, 95% confidence interval 1.03–1.85)
Misirlioglu, et al., 2006	600 mg α-tocopherol	Survival	Stage IIIB non–small cell lung cancer	↑ survival in cases vs. controls ($P = 0.0175$)

Table 9.3. Studies of Antioxidant Supplements for Supportive Care during Cancer Therapy in Children.

Author, Year	Antioxidant (Dose)	Indication	Type of Cancer	Outcome
Melnick, et al., 2005	Immunocal	Cachexia	Children with solid tumors	↑ weight gain ↓ toxicity (mucositis, nausea/vomiting)
Letur-Könirsch, et al., 2002	α-Tocopherol (1000 IU) with pentoxifylline	Fibroatrophic uterine lesions	Survivors of childhood cancer	Improvements in endometrial thickness, uterine volume, and uterine artery blood flow No significance reported

CARDIOTOXICITY

Cardiomyopathy with ventricular failure is a significant cause of long-term morbidity in patients treated with anthracycline chemotherapeutic agents. Coenzyme Q10 (CoQ10), also known as ubiquinone, is an endogenous compound that functions as an antioxidant, promotes membrane stabilization, and acts as a cofactor in many metabolic pathways, including the production of adenosine triphosphate in oxidative respiration. The most researched antioxidant supplement for the prevention of anthracycline-induced cardiotoxicity, CoQ10, may have a cardioprotectant effect by replenishing or scavenging free radicals in cardiac myocytes (Greenberg & Frishman, 1990). Plasma CoQ10 levels have been observed to be low in patients with melanoma, breast, and lung cancer (Folkers, Osterborg, Nylander, Morita, & Mellstedt, 1997; Rusciani, et al., 2006; Shinkai, et al., 1984). A systematic review of clinical trials investigating the efficacy of CoQ10 reported some benefits; however, many of the trials were hampered by small sample sizes, inclusion of patients with a mixture of cancer diagnoses, and poor study design or methodology (Roffe, Schmidt, & Ernst, 2004).

Four separate clinical studies have evaluated vitamin E supplementation for cardioprotection. Although one study reported improvements in cardiac function with nifedipine and vitamin E supplementation (α-tocopherol 200 mg by intramuscular route) (Lenzhofer, Ganzinger, Rameis, & Moser, 1983) given to women with metastatic breast cancer, cardioprotective effects of vitamin E were not confirmed in three other studies (Legha, et al., 1982; Wagdi, Fluri, Aeschbacher, Fikrle, & Meier, 1996; Weitzman, Lorell, Carey, Kaufman, & Stossel, 1980).

NEUROTOXICITY

Neurotoxicity is a frequent chemotherapy dose-limiting toxicity in patients treated with vinca alkaloids (vincristine, vinblastine) or platinum complexes, particularly cisplatin. Decreased vitamin E levels have been observed in patients who have received treatment with cisplatin (Weijl, et al., 1998) and vitamin E deficiency has clinical similarity to cisplatin-induced neuropathy (Leonetti, et al., 2003). Animal studies in male CD-1 nude mice reported that vitamin E decreased cisplatin-induced neuropathy by neutralizing oxidative stress that occurs at the dorsal root ganglia, the target of cisplatin neurotoxicity, as measured by histologic analysis (Leonetti, et al., 2003). In a small pilot study, neurotoxicity developed in only 4 of 16 patients supplemented with vitamin E along with cisplatin, paclitaxel, or their combination regimens, versus 11 of 15 patients receiving chemotherapy alone ($P = 0.019$, overall RR= 0.34) (Argyriou, et al., 2005). In a randomized controlled trial, vitamin E supplementation was associated with a reduction in the incidence of paclitaxel-induced neuropathy (Argyriou, et al., 2006).

OTOTOXICITY

Otoxicity, a dose-limiting toxicity of cisplatin therapy, can develop with oxidative stress-induced injury in the organ of Corti. (Ravi, Somani, & Rybak, 1995) Although reductions in plasma antioxidant status in patients receiving cisplatin-based chemotherapy have been observed (Weijl, et al., 1998), only one clinical trial has been completed to investigate the effects of antioxidant supplementation in preventing hearing loss. In a study of 48 patients treated with cisplatin-based therapy and a mixture of antioxidants (1000 mg vitamin C, 400 mg DL-α-tocopherol acetate, and 100 µg selenium), no significant differences in the incidence of ototoxicity, nephrotoxicity, or bone marrow toxicity were observed, despite the observation of elevated levels of plasma antioxidants in the intervention group (Weijl, et al. 2004). A significant correlation, unrelated to the treatment group, was observed between higher reduced–oxidized vitamin C ratios and lower malondialdehyde levels—markers of oxidative stress—and the incidence of otoxicity and nephrotoxicity. This study was complicated by the poor compliance to the treatment assignment, as 64% and 46% of subjects, respectively, did not adhere to antioxidant protocol in the intervention and placebo arms.

GENERAL CHEMOTHERAPY-RELATED TOXICITIES

Reductions in plasma levels of antioxidants in patients undergoing treatment for cancer or receiving conditioning regimens in preparation for stem cell transplants have been observed (Ladas, et al., 2004), leading researchers to investigate the effect of different mixtures of antioxidants on frequently encountered chemotherapy-related toxicities, such as anemia and myelosuppression. In a study of women being treated for ovarian cancer, supplementation with selenium (50 μg), vitamin C (200 mg), vitamin E (36 mg), and β-carotene (15 mg) was associated with increases in neutrophil counts and decreased incidence of chemotherapy-associated side effects (Sieja, 2000). While one study reported improvements in blood indices in patients supplemented with 4000 μg of selenium, (Hu, et al., 1997) another noted no difference in the incidence of general toxicities in a group of patients who took supplements containing D-α-tocopherol (3200 IU) (Blanke, et al., 2001). Significant improvements in neutrophil recovery was observed among 35 women with breast cancer who took either a multivitamin or vitamin E, although decreased neutrophil recovery was observed in the women in this study taking folic acid (Branda, et al., 2004). Additionally, supplementing with vitamin C (500 mg) and vitamin E (400 mg) in an attempt to prevent tamoxifen-induced hypertriglyceridemia was associated with improvements in plasma lipid and lipoprotein levels in postmenopausal women with resectable breast cancer (Babu, et al., 2000).

RADIATION-INDUCED SIDE EFFECTS

Because one of the major ways that radiation therapy exerts its anticancer effect is by generating free radicals, there has been much controversy and uncertainty surrounding the use of antioxidants during radiation treatment. To date, several research studies have investigated the effect of different antioxidant mixtures on the risk of developing acute and long-term radiation-associated side effects and their ability to influence survival.

A few small trials have investigated the effect of antioxidants for the prevention of proctitis or enteritis, tissue induration, and mucositis associated with radiation therapy.

- Twenty-one patients with grade I–II radiation-induced proctitis/enteritis were treated with a combination of vitamin E and pentoxifylline, a radiosensitizing agent (Hille, et al., 2005). In the pentoxifylline/

vitamin E treatment group, 15 of 21 patients (71%) experienced a reduction of symptoms, with 7 patients achieving a reduction from grade I/II to grade 0 toxicity and 8 achieving a reduction from grade II to grade I toxicity.

- Grape seed proanthocyanidin extract was administered for 6 months to 66 women for the prevention of tissue induration following radiation to the breast (Brooker, et al., 2006). No significant differences were observed at 6 and 12 months following completion of radiation.
- Other studies have observed that the topical application of β-carotene (250 mg) or topical vitamin E oil (400 mg) for the prevention of mucositis is associated with reductions in the severity or duration of mucositis (Mills, 1988; Wadleigh, et al., 1992).
- A small case series investigating the effect of antioxidants among survivors of childhood cancer reported that six women who had received pelvic radiation as children had reductions in fibroatrophic uterine lesions following the administration of vitamin E with pentoxifylline.

A survival benefit was reported with pentoxifylline and vitamin E supplementation in a randomized nonplacebo controlled trial among 66 patients receiving radiotherapy for stage IIIB non–small cell lung cancer (Misirlioglu, Erkal, Elgin, Ugur, & Altundag, 2006). In the group receiving the supplements, 2-year overall survival and progression-free survival were 30% and 23%, respectively, versus 18% and 14%, respectively for the control group ($P = 0.0175$; $P = 0.0223$, respectively).

In a double-blind randomized controlled trial among 54 patients with head and neck cancer, an orally administered vitamin E rinse during radiotherapy was associated with a 36% risk reduction in symptomatic mucositis. (Ferreira, et al., 2004) However, 2-year overall survival was reduced in the supplementation group (vitamin E group: 32.2%; placebo group 62.9%), although this difference was not statistically significant.

A single large, well-designed trial investigated the efficacy of antioxidant supplementation for prevention of radiotherapy associated mucositis and reduction of second primary cancers in 540 head and neck cancer patients during radiation therapy (Bairati, et al., 2005). Patients took the antioxidant supplements, DL-α-tocopherol (400 IU/day) and β-carotene (30 mg/day), both during and for 3 years following the completion of radiation therapy. β-Carotene supplementation was discontinued early due to ethical concerns following the observations of significantly increased risks of lung cancer in patients supplemented with antioxidants that included β-carotene in large cancer chemoprevention trials (The Alpha-Tocopherol, Beta-carotene Cancer Prevention Study Group, 1994; Omenn, et al., 1996). In this study, patients in the intervention arm experienced less severe acute side effects from radiation therapy. The rate of local recurrence was higher among patients randomized to antioxidant supplementation, although the increased risk was seen in patients receiving the combination of DL-α-tocopheral and β-carotene, rather than those patients assigned to DL-α-tocopheral alone. With longer follow-up, overall survival was significantly compromised in the antioxidant supplemented group. Further analyses demonstrated that all-cause mortality was significantly increased in the supplement arm (hazard ratio: 1.38, 95% confidence interval 1.03–1.85), and cause-specific mortality rates tended to be higher in the supplement arm than in the placebo arm (Bairati, et al., 2006). Other investigators have countered that differences in doses, sources (synthetic vs. natural antioxidants), and dose schedules may have accounted for the adverse effects of antioxidant supplementation on long-term prognosis in this trial (Prasad & Cole, 2006).

Conclusion

Clinical studies of antioxidant supplementation and changes in oxidative status, disease risk, or disease outcome have been performed among healthy individuals, populations at risk for cancer, and patients undergoing cancer treatment. However, when the evidence is evaluated as a whole, the published clinical trials have not incorporated consistent sample populations, utilized standardized treatment regimens, or reported consistent outcomes. These inconsistencies preclude definitive conclusions in regard to the safety and efficacy of antioxidant supplementation for chemotherapy- or radiation therapy-related toxicities or survival from cancer. Until crucial additional clinical trials are completed, algorithms for evaluating possible interactions of supplements and conventional cancer therapies, as well as systematic approaches to review the published literature may serve as guides (Seely, Stempak, & Baruchel, 2007; Weiger, et al., 2002). Broad rejection or recommendation for the concurrent use of antioxidants with chemotherapy or radiation therapy is not justified at the present time.

Recommendations for clinical practice at the current time include the following:

- Since the clinical research on antioxidant supplementation has not yet adequately demonstrated that the benefits of supplementation clearly outweigh the risks, the possibility of harm must be strongly considered.
- Patients should therefore be advised to avoid dietary antioxidant supplements above the basic nutritional requirements during radiation therapy.

- Patients should exert caution in supplementing with antioxidants while receiving treatment with chemotherapy agents (Table 9.1) until their combined use is found to be safe and does not compromise the efficacy of chemotherapy agents.

There are theoretical reasons to support that the role for some antioxidants in either the enhancement of the effects of some chemotherapy or radiation regimens or the reduction of treatment-related toxicities, without interfering with anticancer activity. Future trials evaluating the safety and efficacy of antioxidants must consider the diagnosis, the specific type of conventional treatment, and the type and form of antioxidant to be used.

Suggestions for future antioxidant research include the following:

- Preliminary evidence supports a beneficial role for melatonin during cancer treatment; large randomized phase III trials cohorts should be performed to confirm.
- Despite the widespread prevalence of cachexia in patients with cancer, no consistent approaches have been developed. Future research should investigate potential antioxidant treatments and identify the appropriate mixtures, dosing, duration, and timing of supplementation.
- Findings from a meta-analysis support the efficacy of coenzyme Q10 for its cardioprotectant effects; this finding needs to be investigated in a large, phase III randomized trial with appropriate markers of acute and long-term cardiotoxicity.
- Antioxidants may adversely affect outcome in patients with head and neck cancer receiving radiation therapy. Additional trials are needed to ascertain the safety of antioxidant supplementation in patients with other types of malignancies undergoing radiation treatment.
- Antioxidant status may impact risk for developing chemotherapy-related toxicities, particularly in patients treated with antioxidant-depleting regimens. Further research is needed to evaluate the role of antioxidant supplementation for supportive care, which may allow administration of the recommended doses of conventional therapies and minimization of therapy delays and dose reductions. However, before broad recommendations can be made for antioxidant supplementation for the prevention or treatment of general chemotherapy-related toxicities, more research is needed to determine the biological mechanisms, appropriate antioxidant mixtures and dosing for each clinical setting.
- The majority of published clinical trials have been performed in adults with cancer. Investigations of antioxidant supplementation in children and adolescents with cancer are also needed.

REFERENCES

Bairati I, Meyer F, Jobin E, Gelinas M, Fortin A, Nabid A, et al. (2006). Antioxidant vitamins supplementation and mortality: A randomized trial in head and neck cancer patients. *International Journal of Cancer,* 119, 2221–2224.

Block KI, Koch AC, Mead MN, Tothy PK, Newman RA, & Gyllenhaal C. (2007). Impact of antioxidant supplementation on chemotherapeutic efficacy: A systematic review of the evidence from randomized controlled trials. *Cancer Treat Reviews,* 33(5), 407–418.

Cameron E, Pauling L, & Leibovitz B. (1979). Ascorbic acid and cancer: review. *Cancer Research,* 39, 663–681.

Ladas EJ, Jacobson JS, Kennedy DD, Teel K, Fleischauer A, & Kelly KM. (2004). Antioxidants and cancer therapy: A systematic review. *Journal of Clinical Oncology,* 22, 517–528.

Moertel CG, Fleming TR, Creagan ET, Rubin J, O'Connell MJ, & Ames MM. (1985). High-dose vitamin C versus placebo in the treatment of patients with advanced cancer who have had no prior chemotherapy. A randomized double-blind comparison. *The New England Journal of Medicine,* 312, 137–141.

Moss RW. (2006). Should patients undergoing chemotherapy and radiotherapy be prescribed antioxidants? *Integrative Cancer Therapies,* 5, 63–82.

Prasad KN & Cole WC. (2006). Antioxidants in cancer therapy. *Journal of Clinical Oncology,* 20;24, e8–e9.

Ratnam DV, Ankola DD, Bhardwaj V, Sahana DK, & Kumar MN. (2006). Role of antioxidants in prophylaxis and therapy: A pharmaceutical perspective. *Journal of Controlled Release,* 20;113, 189–207.

Rock CL, Newman VA, Neuhouser ML, Major J, & Barnett MJ. (2004). Antioxidant supplement use in cancer survivors and the general population. *The Journal of Nutrition,* 134, 3194S–3195S.

Seely D, Stempak D, & Baruchel S. (2007). A Strategy for Controlling Potential Interactions Between Natural Health Products and Chemotherapy: A Review in Pediatric Oncology. *Journal of Pediatric Hematology and Oncology,* 29, 32–47.

(A complete reference list for this chapter is available online at http://www.oup.com/us/ integrativemedicine).

10

Physical Activity and Cancer

CLARE STEVINSON AND KERRY S. COURNEYA

KEY CONCEPTS

- Research has established that physical activity plays an important role in the prevention and management of many chronic medical conditions.
- Physical activity helps to protect against colon and breast cancer, and possibly endometrial, lung, and prostate cancer.
- Physical activity is essential for maintaining a healthy body weight, which is important since obesity is a major risk factor for many cancers.
- Some preliminary data suggest that postdiagnosis physical activity may be associated with increased survival in colon and breast cancer.
- Physical activity can improve general health and strength, contributing to enhanced functional status and ability to cope with disease- and treatment-related symptoms and side effects.
- Current evidence suggests that by adhering to a graded exercise program, cancer survivors can maintain or increase their level of conditioning function and thereby avoid becoming trapped in a perpetuating cycle of deteriorating physical function and increasing fatigue.
- Physical activity can also enhance quality of life, and help to prevent other chronic conditions (e.g., diabetes or cardiovascular disease) for which cancer survivors are at increased risk.
- The risk/benefit profile of physical activity is favorable, assuming that key safety issues are considered for each individual before initiating an exercise program.

A growing body of research has established an important role for physical activity in the prevention and management of various chronic medical conditions, including coronary heart disease (Taylor, et al., 2004), stroke (Gordon, et al., 2004), hypertension (Pescatello, et al., 2004), noninsulin dependent diabetes (Albright, et al., 2000), obesity (Jakicic, et al., 2001), musculoskeletal disorders (Vuori, 2001), and mental health problems (Callaghan, 2004). Evidence of the effects of physical activity in protecting against cancer has been accumulating over the last five decades. More recently, attention has also turned to the potential benefits of exercise for individuals already diagnosed with cancer.

In 2001, Courneya and Friedenreich published the PEACE (Physical Exercise Across the Cancer Experience) framework (Fig. 10.1), identifying key periods during which exercise has potential benefit (Courneya & Friedenreich 2001). These include the primary prevention of cancer, preparing for cancer treatments, coping with side effects during treatment, rehabilitation after treatment, long-term health promotion for those with good outcomes, and palliative care for those unlikely to be cured. The majority of research so far has focused on three broad questions: (1) Can physical activity help prevent cancer? (2) Can physical activity contribute to increased survival in those diagnosed with cancer? (3) Can physical activity improve quality of life outcomes in

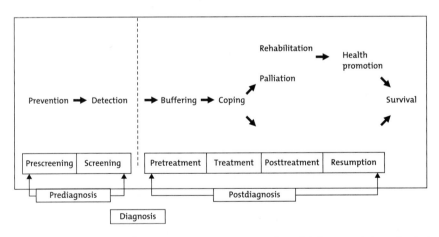

FIGURE 10.1. Framework PEACE: An organizational model for examining physical exercise across the cancer experience. Reprinted with permission from Courneya KS & Friedenreich CM. (2001). Framework PEACE: An organizational model for examining physical exercise across the cancer experience. *Annals of Behavioral Medicine*, 23(4), 263–272. Copyright 2001, Lawrence Erlbaum Associates, INC.

patients during and after cancer therapy? This chapter summarizes the evidence available so far in these areas and provides guidelines for appropriate levels of physical activity for cancer prevention and rehabilitation.

Cancer Prevention

The evidence for a preventative role of physical activity against cancer has been accumulating since a seminal study of railway workers in 1962 that demonstrated a 30% reduced risk in cancer mortality among section men, compared with clerks (Taylor, et al., 1962). A comprehensive review published by the American Institute for Cancer Research in 2005 (AICR, 2005) concluded that the totality of evidence from more than 180 epidemiological studies confirms a protective effect. Furthermore, it reported no consistent evidence of an increased risk of any cancer in association with physical activity. In terms of specific cancers, the protective effect was classified as "convincing" for colon and breast cancer. The results of a meta-analysis of 47 studies indicate a risk reduction for colon cancer of approximately 20% but no effect on rectal cancer (Samad, Taylor, Marshall, & Chapman, 2005). The AICR concluded that the evidence for a protective role of physical activity was "probable" for endometrial cancer and "possible" for prostate and lung cancer. Further evidence of a preventive effect for lung cancer is provided by a meta-analysis of nine studies indicating a reduced risk with higher levels of leisure-time physical activity (Tardon, et al., 2005). However, a recently updated meta-analysis of 41 prostate cancer studies found the evidence still weak and inconsistent (Lee, 2006). Although reduced risk in association with physical activity has been observed for other cancers (e.g., testicular, ovarian, kidney, pancreatic), the AICR report considered the evidence to be "insufficient" because of the small number of studies.

MECHANISMS

The reasons for the apparent cancer-protective effects of physical activity have not yet been determined. It is conceivable that independent factors that influence both ability to exercise, and susceptibility to cancer, might explain the relationship, such as preexisting disease or healthy lifestyle. However, there are also various plausible biological explanations, and research efforts are focused on understanding the role of these potential mechanisms (Rundle, 2005). Table 10.1 summarizes the possible mechanisms operating at either a systemic level to reduce overall cancer risk or a site-specific level to help prevent particular cancers. The role of physical activity in maintaining a healthy body weight is

Table 10.1. Potential Biological Mechanisms for Protective Effect
of Physical Activity against Cancer.

Systemic Effects

Regulation of energy balance and fat distribution

Modification of metabolic hormones (e.g. insulin, glucose) and growth
factors (e.g. insulin-like growth factors)

Improvement of the antitumor immune defence system

Improvement of antioxidant defence and DNA repair activity

Site-specific effects

Colon: reduction in gastrointestinal transit time may reduce exposure
to carcinogens; changes to levels of insulin, prostaglandin and bile acids
may inhibit colonic cell proliferation.

Lung: improvement of pulmonary ventilation and perfusion may
minimize the interaction time of carcinogens in the airways

Breast, ovary, endometrium: reduction in estrogen exposure; increase
in sex hormone-binding globulin
Prostate: modulation of testosterone levels

considered particularly important since obesity is a major risk factor for many
cancers. However, results of studies that have controlled for energy intake or
body size indicate that activity influences cancer risk independently of weight
control. It is considered most likely that multiple mechanisms are responsible for
the anticarcinogenic properties of physical activity (Westerlind, 2003).

> The American Institute for Cancer Research reports that obesity increases the
> risk for breast, colon, endometrial, esophageal, kidney, and prostate cancers
> by 25 to 33 percent.

Cancer Survival

Given the important role identified for physical activity in the primary prevention of cancer, it is conceivable that the mechanisms thought to be responsible
for this, may also play a part in secondary prevention. However, there is, so
far, only preliminary evidence to indicate that exercise may directly influence
disease progression or survival (Courneya, et al., 2004).

Results from animal studies are ambiguous in this respect. Although several studies demonstrate that exercise protects against tumor metastasis in rodents (Hoffman, 1994), findings are strongly influenced by the specific tumor and animal models used (Hoffman, 2003). Furthermore, the high volume of the exercise protocols used in many of these studies does not represent a realistic level of physical activity for human cancer patients, hence the generalizability of the findings is severely limited.

A small number of clinical trials with cancer patients have examined the effect of exercise interventions on intermediate biological markers that are thought to lie on the causal pathway between physical activity and cancer recurrence or mortality. There is some evidence of increases in natural killer cell cytotoxic activity and other immune function parameters following exercise programs, beyond that expected through normal recovery (Fairey, Courneya, Field, & Mackey, 2002; Fairey, et al., 2005). Changes in sex steroid hormones such as estrodial, estrone, and testosterone were not observed in studies of breast and prostate cancer patients (McTiernan, et al., 1998; Segal, et al., 2003), which may reflect the effects of hormonal treatments received by these patients. In two trials examining the effects on metabolic hormones, fasting glucose, insulin, and insulin resistance were not influenced by aerobic (Fairey, et al., 2003) and resistance (Schmitz, Ahmed, Hannan, & Yee, 2005) exercise programs in breast cancer survivors. Although, few studies exist so far, this is an area generating considerable interest, leading to a growth in transitional research that attempts to validate biomarkers, and understand the effects of exercise on these intermediate outcomes, in order to determine the clinical implications for patients in terms of disease progression and survival.

The most encouraging data suggesting that physical activity may improve cancer survival, come from epidemiological investigations. In one of the first studies to directly address this question, 2987 women who were diagnosed with breast cancer while participating in the Nurses Health Study, were monitored for up to 18 years, with physical activity assessed every 2 years (Holmes, et al., 2005). After adjusting for various demographic and medical variables, women who reported 9 to 15 metabolic equivalent task (MET)-hours of physical activity per week (equivalent to 3–5 hours of brisk walking), had a 50% decreased risk of cancer-specific mortality, compared with women who reported less than 3 MET-hours per week (e.g., 1 hour of walking). Similar risk reductions were observed for breast cancer recurrence and all-cause mortality.

Another analysis from the Nurses Health Study involved 573 women diagnosed with colorectal cancer (Meyerhardt, et al., 2006). Disease-specific mortality and all-cause mortality were reduced by approximately 50% in women performing at least 18 MET-hours per week of physical activity, compared with those reporting less than 3 MET-hours per week. The analyses indicated that it was postdiagnosis physical activity that was related to survival, and not activity performed before disease onset.

In a further study, 816 patients with stage III colon cancer who were part of a clinical trial of adjuvant chemotherapy completed physical activity measures during treatment and 6 months afterward (Meyerhardt, et al., 2006). Increases in recurrence-free survival, disease-free survival, and overall survival were observed in association with increasing volumes of physical activity. After controlling for various demographic and medical variables, those performing at least 18 MET-hours of exercise per week had a 49% reduction in risk of recurrence or death compared with those performing less than 3 MET-hours per week, over a 3-year period following treatment.

The implication from these studies that a lifestyle factor such as physical activity can have prognostic value is of obvious interest and importance. Results from further studies investigating the impact of physical activity performed after diagnosis on disease progression and survival are keenly awaited.

Cancer Rehabilitation

Regardless of whether or not physical activity will ultimately prove to have specific effects on disease or survival outcomes, there is, nonetheless, increasing acceptance of the importance of cancer patients being physically active in order to maximize their functional status and cope with disease- and treatment-related symptoms.

Cancer treatments such as surgery, chemotherapy, and radiation, typically involve damage to healthy tissue as well as the destruction of malignant cells. Patients may experience a range of possible side effects (e.g. pain, nausea, fatigue, alopecia, neutropenia, peripheral neuropathy), and psychological sequelae (e.g. anxiety, depression). Furthermore, overall physical function is generally diminished due to losses of aerobic capacity, muscle tissue, and range of motion. Therefore, great importance is placed on preserving physical and psychosocial functioning as far as possible during treatment and restoring it afterward.

The results of a recent survey illustrate the reduction in physical function experienced by cancer patients. The physical performance limitations of 279 short-term ($<$5 years) and 434 long-term ($\geq$5 years) cancer survivors were compared with 9370 individuals with no cancer history (Ness, Wall, Oakes, Robison, & Gurney, 2006). The results indicated that over half of the cancer survivors (54% of short-term and 53% of long-term survivors) had performance limitations, compared with 21% of the individuals with no cancer history.

The most commonly reported difficulties were crouching/kneeling, standing for 2 hours, lifting/carrying 10 pounds, and walking quarter of a mile. Given the importance of such actions to performing activities of daily living (e.g., dressing, housework, childcare, shopping, gardening), there is a clear need for rehabilitation interventions focusing on building physical endurance and strength. Furthermore, this study demonstrates that these needs are not restricted only to patients who have recently completed treatment but also apply to longer-term survivors.

EVIDENCE BASE

Since the pioneering work of Maryl Winningham of Ohio State University College of Nursing during the 1980s (Winningham, 1983; Winningham, MacVicar, & Burke, 1986) the number of exercise intervention studies with cancer patients has grown exponentially. There are now at least 20 review articles published that attempt to summarize the results and implications of individual studies. Table 10.2 lists the conclusions of systematic reviews published since 2004 that have evaluated the evidence from intervention trials (Oldervoll, Kaasa, Hjermstad, Lund, & Loge, 2004; Stevinson, Lawlor, & Fox, 2004; Douglas, 2005; Galväo & Newton, 2005; Knols, Aaronson, Uebelhart, Fransen, & Aufdemkampe, 2005; Schmitz, et al., 2005; Conn, Hafdahl, Porock, McDaniel, & Nielsen, 2006; McNeely, et al., 2006a).

Conclusions from reviews have been consistently positive regarding the potential benefits of physical activity during cancer therapy and after treatment completion. Nonetheless, all include caveats regarding the inconsistencies among results and the heterogeneity and methodological limitations of trials. Encouragingly, methodological rigor has improved in more recent trials, demonstrating more modest outcomes, but increasing the validity of the reported findings.

PHYSICAL FUNCTION

The most consistent and positive effects demonstrated in randomized clinical trials relate to physical function outcomes. Results of meta-analyses show moderate improvements in cardiorespiratory fitness among cancer survivors engaging in aerobic exercise programs during, and after, cancer treatment (Stevinson, et al., 2004; Schmitz, et al., 2005; Conn, et al., 2006; McNeely, et al., 2006a). The benefits of preserving fitness during treatment, and gradually increasing it

Table 10.2. Recent Systematic Reviews of Exercise Interventions
for Cancer Survivors.

Authors	Review	Conclusions
McNeeley, et al., 2006	Systematic review of 14 randomized breast cancer trials with meta-analysis	Exercise is an effective intervention to improve quality of life, cardiorespiratory fitness, physical functioning, and fatigue
Conn, et al., 2006	Systematic review of 30 intervention studies with meta-analysis	Exercise interventions resulted in small positive effects on health and well-being outcomes
Schmitz, et al., 2005	Systematic review of 32 controlled trials with meta-analysis	Physical activity improves cardiorespiratory fitness during and after cancer treatment, symptoms and physiological effects during treatment, and vigor post treatment
Knols, et al., 2005	Systematic review of 34 controlled trials	Cancer patients may benefit from physical exercise both during and after treatment
Douglas, 2005	Systematic review of 21 intervention studies	There is a growing body of evidence to justify the inclusion of exercise programmes in the rehabilitation of cancer patients returning to health after treatment
Galväo & Newton, 2005	Systematic review of 26 intervention studies	Preliminary positive physiological and psychological benefits from exercise when undertaken during or after traditional cancer treatment
Stevinson, et al., 2004	Systematic review of 33 controlled trials with meta-analysis	Exercise interventions for cancer patients can lead to moderate increases in physical function and are not associated with increased symptoms of fatigue
Oldervoll, et al., 2004	Systematic review of 12 randomized controlled trials	Cancer patients benefit from maintaining physical activity balanced with efficient rest periods

again afterward, are considerable in terms of being able to perform daily activities and continue with leisure pursuits.

Similarly, encouraging functional outcomes have been demonstrated in trials that have focused on resistance exercise training. Reductions in shoulder pain and disability were reported in head and neck cancer survivors who had undergone spinal accessory neuropraxia/neurectomy (McNeely, et al., 2004), and increases in muscular fitness (Segal, et al., 2003) and muscle mass (Marcora, Oliver, Callow, Lemmy, & Stuart, 2005) were demonstrated for prostate cancer patients receiving androgen deprivation therapy. Increased muscle mass was also reported in breast cancer survivors following a 6-month weight training program (Schmitz, et al., 2005). If resistance exercise helps prevent or reverse the loss of muscle tissue that can result from inactivity, inadequate nutrition, or cachectic processes, it would make a significant contribution to maintaining functional ability.

TREATMENT SIDE EFFECTS

There is some preliminary evidence from meta-analysis that exercise can help in the management of treatment-related symptoms or side effects (Schmitz, et al., 2005). One trial involving inpatients receiving high-dose chemotherapy following peripheral blood stem cell transplantations demonstrated a range of positive outcomes for those exercising daily on a supine cycle ergometer, compared with control participants (Dimeo, Fetscher, Lange, Mertelsmann, & Keul, 1997). These outcomes included lower pain severity and less use of analgesics, lower severity of diarrhea, shorter duration of thrombopenia and neutropenia, and shorter hospitalization.

Cancer-related fatigue has been identified as one of the most common and distressing symptoms reported by patients and also as one of the most difficult to treat (Curt, 2001). An overemphasis on rest carries the risk of increased fatigue, due to individuals becoming caught in a vicious cycle of inactivity leading to further deconditioning, hence greater fatigue upon even minimal exertion. Results of meta-analyses provide encouraging evidence that fatigue is not increased by exercise (Stevinson, et al., 2004; Schmitz, et al., 2005) and may actually be reduced (Conn, et al., 2006; McNeely, et al., 2006a). This is an important finding with respect to the understandable concerns of patients and caregivers that exercise may cause or exacerbate existing fatigue. Instead, current evidence suggests that by adhering to a graded exercise program, cancer survivors can maintain or increase their level of conditioning and function, thereby avoiding becoming trapped in a perpetuating cycle of deteriorating physical function and increasing fatigue. Only one trial has demonstrated greater reductions in fatigue among the control group than the exercisers (Thorsen, et al., 2005). These participants were cancer patients recruited straight after completion of chemotherapy, and the authors suggested that a period of spontaneous recovery before commencing exercise may be optimal for fatigue reduction.

Exercise has been suggested as useful method of reversing unwanted weight gain in cancer survivors (Schwartz, 2000). Although a few studies have reported improved body composition (i.e. improved lean/fat tissue ratio) (e.g. Courneya, et al., 2003; Schmitz, et al., 2005; Winningham, MacVicar, Bondoc, Anderson, & Minton, 1989), there is no evidence of significant changes in total body weight (Schmitz, et al., 2005; McNeely, et al., 2006a). It may be that most clinical trials of exercise have been of insufficient duration to influence body weight, and that this outcome is better addressed in longer-term health promotion protocols. A recent systematic review of 14 trials in breast cancer survivors concluded that the evidence for improved body composition was sketchy, but encouraging (Ingram, Courneya, & Kingston, 2006).

> Specific exercises are often prescribed for side effects related to specific cancer types. For instance, pelvic exercises (commonly known as Kegels) can help restore continence following treatment for prostate cancer.

QUALITY OF LIFE

Many trials have assessed the effect of exercise interventions on dimensions of quality of life. Meta-analysis results indicate small advantages in overall quality of life for cancer survivors who exercise, over those in control groups, with the strongest effects demonstrated for those who are post treatment (Schmitz, et al., 2005; Conn, et al., 2006; McNeely, et al., 2006). Several of the more recent and rigorous trials have demonstrated significant quality of life benefits. These studies have included breast cancer survivors post treatment following resistance training (Ohira, Schmitz, Ahmed, & Yee, 2006) and aerobic exercise (Courneya, et al., 2003) interventions, and men with prostate cancer undergoing androgen deprivation therapy and resistance training (Segal, et al., 2003). A heterogeneous sample of cancer survivors who followed a walking intervention in combination with group psychotherapy improved functional aspects of quality of life more than those receiving only group psychotherapy (Courneya, et al., 2003).

Physical Activity Guidelines

CANCER PREVENTION

Many public health organizations provide general recommendations for physical activity in the context of reducing risk of cancer. Table 10.3 summarizes the recommendations of some major international and national cancer

Table 10.3. Physical Activity Recommendations for Cancer Prevention from Public Health Organizations.

Organization	Recommendation
International Agency for Research on Cancer (2002)	Continuous physical activity on most days of the week. More vigorous activity, such as fast walking, several times per week may give some additional benefits regarding cancer prevention
World Cancer Research Fund / American Institute for Cancer Research (1997)	If occupational activity is low or moderate, take an hour of brisk walk or similar exercise daily, and also exercise vigorously for a total of at least 1 hour in a week
American Cancer Society (Kushi, et al., 2006)	Engage in at least 30 minutes of moderate to vigorous physical activity, above usual activities, on 5 or more days of the week; 45 to 60 minutes of intentional physical activity are preferable
Canadian Cancer Society (2003)	60 minutes of light physical activity daily, or 30 to 60 minutes of moderate physical activity 4 days/week, or 20 to 30 minutes of vigorous physical activity at least 3 days/week
The Cancer Council Australia (2005)	30 minutes/day of moderate intensity activity is recommended for general good health. 60 minutes/day of moderate intensity or 30 minutes/day vigorous activity is more likely to reduce cancer risk
Cancer Research UK (2006)	30 minutes of moderate exercise 5 days a week can reduce your cancer risk. 30 minutes a day is a minimum recommended level. Studies have shown that you can reduce your breast and bowel cancer risk even more by exercising: more frequently, more intensely, for longer periods of time, and throughout your lifetime
Europe against Cancer (2003)	Undertake some brisk physical activity every day. More vigorous activity several times per week may give some additional benefits regarding cancer prevention

organizations. Most advise a minimum of 30 to 60 minutes of moderate to vigorous intensity activity 5 to 7 days per week. These recommendations are in line with general health promotion guidelines regarding physical activity (US Department of Health and Human Services, 1996; Australian Government Department of Health and Ageing, 1999; UK Department of Health, 2004).

The American Cancer Society recently modified their recommendations to advise a minimum of 30 minutes of moderate to vigorous physical activity, above usual activities, on five or more days of the week, with 45 to 60 minutes of intentional physical activity being preferable (Kushi, et al., 2006). It is likely that public health guidelines will need revision in the future as more precise evidence emerges regarding the optimal frequency, duration, and intensity of physical activity required for risk reduction.

> The American Cancer Society makes a general recommendation for adults of at least 30 minutes of moderate physical activity 5 days a week. Further evidence suggests that vigorous physical activity 5 days a week may reduce the risk of breast and colon cancer.

CANCER REHABILITATION

Humpel & Iverson systematically reviewed published guidelines/recommendations regarding exercise for cancer survivors from journal articles, books, and cancer-related websites (Humpel & Iverson 2005). Recommendations for aerobic exercise typically covered a broad range of three to five times weekly for 10 to 60 minutes at a low to moderate intensity. Recommendations for resistance training were within the range of 1 to 3 times weekly with 1 to 3 sets of 8 to 15 repetitions at low resistance. The need to individualize the prescription according to medical treatments, comorbidities, and fitness levels was emphasized in most cases. Although recommendations were generally consistent across the different sources, supportive scientific evidence was not routinely cited and the reviewers concluded that none met criteria for evidence-based guidelines.

In a recent review of the potential therapeutic role of exercise training in the cancer setting, McNeely and colleagues proposed recommendations for integrating exercise programming into clinical practice (McNeely, Peddle, Parliament, & Courneya, 2006b). They suggested formal exercise training as part of a supervised outpatient rehabilitation program immediately following treatment completion. The exercise prescription may involve aerobic training for cardiorespiratory fitness, resistance training for muscular strength and endurance, and flexibility exercises for increasing range of motion and muscle length. An initial program of at least 8 weeks was recommended, with the exercise prescription cautiously progressed over time and allowing for modifications where appropriate. A summary of these guidelines is presented in Figure 10.2.

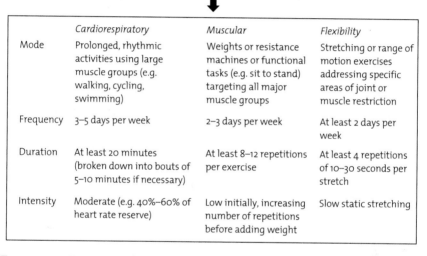

Screening

- Medical history, physical examination, laboratory tests (e.g. complete blood count, lipid profile, pulmonary function), and physician clearance
- Exercise tolerance tests (e.g. maximal or submaximal oxygen uptake; 1-repetition maximum or standard load test)

Prescription

- Individualize prescription based on all available clinical data and exercise tolerance tests
- Consider goals and preferences of patient and identify potential barriers
- Include warm-up and cool-down phases
- Progressively increase total exercise to allow for physiological adaptation
- Reevaluate prescription regularly and modify where appropriate

	Cardiorespiratory	*Muscular*	*Flexibility*
Mode	Prolonged, rhythmic activities using large muscle groups (e.g. walking, cycling, swimming)	Weights or resistance machines or functional tasks (e.g. sit to stand) targeting all major muscle groups	Stretching or range of motion exercises addressing specific areas of joint or muscle restriction
Frequency	3–5 days per week	2–3 days per week	At least 2 days per week
Duration	At least 20 minutes (broken down into bouts of 5–10 minutes if necessary)	At least 8–12 repetitions per exercise	At least 4 repetitions of 10–30 seconds per stretch
Intensity	Moderate (e.g. 40%–60% of heart rate reserve)	Low initially, increasing number of repetitions before adding weight	Slow static stretching

FIGURE 10.2. Recommendations for supervised exercise rehabilitation programming for cancer patients (McNeely, et al., 2006a).

RISKS OF EXERCISE

Clearly, for exercise to be considered a valuable intervention that can be routinely recommended to cancer survivors it must have a positive risk/benefit ratio. The risks associated with exercise at levels required for health promotion are low in the general population. For cancer patients, concerns relate to the possibility of exercise leading to immunosuppression, falls, bone fractures, complications of cardiotoxic treatments, exacerbation of pain and other symptoms, and interference with treatment completion or efficacy. McNeely et al. (2006b) have identified key safety considerations for prescribing exercise to cancer patients, and have provided a list of contraindications and precautions to exercise testing and training (Table 10.4).

Table 10.4. Contraindications and Precautions to Exercise Testing and Training.

	Contraindications to Exercise Testing and Training	*Precautions Requiring Modification and/or Physician Approval*
Factors related to cancer treatment	No exercise on days of intravenous chemotherapy or within 24 hours of treatment No exercise prior to blood draw Severe tissue reaction to radiation therapy	Caution if on treatments that affect lungs and/ or heart: recommend medically supervised exercise testing and training Mouth sores/ulcerations: avoid mouthpieces for maximal testing; use face masks
Hematologic	Platelets <50,000/mm^3 White blood cells <3,000/mm^3 Hemoglobin <10 g/dl	Platelets >50,000 to 150,000/mm^3: avoid tests that increase risk of bleeding White blood cells >3000 to 4000/mm^3: ensure proper sterilization of equipment Hemoglobin >10 g/dL to 11.5/13.5 g/dL: caution with maximal tests
Musculoskeletal	Bone, back, or neck pain of recent origin Unusual muscular weakness Severe cachexia Unusual/extreme fatigue Poor function status: avoid exercise testing if Karnofsky Performance Status score ≤60%	Any pain or cramping: investigate Osteopenia: avoid high impact exercise if risk of fracture Steroid-induced myopathy: Cachexia: multidisciplinary approach to exercise Mild to moderate fatigue: closely monitor response to exercise

(*continued*)

Table 10.4. (Continued)

	Contraindications to Exercise Testing and Training	Precautions Requiring Modification and/or Physician Approval
Systemic	Acute infections Febrile illness: fever >100°F (38°C) General malaise	Recent systemic illness or infection: avoid exercise until asymptomatic for >48 hours
Gastrointestinal	Severe nausea Vomiting or diarrhea within 24 to 36 hours Dehydration Poor nutrition: inadequate fluid and/or intake	Compromised fluid and/or food intake: recommend multidisciplinary approach/consultation with nutritionist
Cardiovascular	Chest pain Resting pulse >100beats/min or <50 beats/min Resting blood pressure >145 mm Hg systolic and 95 mm Hg diastolic Resting blood pressure < 85 mm Hg systolic Irregular pulse Swelling of ankles	Caution if at risk of cardiac disease: recommend medically supervised exercise testing and training If on blood pressure medication that controls heart rate, target heart rate may not be attainable; avoid overexertion Lymphedema: wear compression garment on limb when exercising
Pulmonary	Severe dyspnea Cough, wheezing Chest pain increased by deep breath	Mild-to-moderate dyspnea: avoid maximal tests
Neurological	Significant decline in cognitive status Dizziness/lightheadedness Disorientation Blurred vision Ataxia	Mild cognitive changes: ensure that patient is able to understand and follow instructions Poor balance/peripheral sensory neuropathy: use well-supported positions for exercise

Source: Reprinted with permission from McNeely, Peddle, Parliament, & Courneya. Cancer rehabilitation: recommendations for integrating exercise programming in the clinical practice setting. Current Cancer Therapy Reviews (2006). Copyright 2006, Bentham Science Publishers Ltd.

Systematic reviews of trials with cancer survivors have reported few adverse events associated with exercise (Stevinson, et al., 2004; Schmitz, et al., 2005; McNeely, et al., 2006a). However, it should be noted that clinical trials have rigorous screening criteria and generally exclude participants for whom exercise may pose a potential risk (e.g. those with uncontrolled cardiovascular or pulmonary disease, existing musculoskeletal disorders, or cancer-related conditions such as cachexia, anemia, neutropenia, thrombocytopenia, or metastatic bone disease). Studies that have addressed the role of exercise in causing or worsening lymphedema in breast cancer survivors who have undergone axillary node dissection have found no increased risk with upper body physical training (Ahmed, Thomas, Yee, & Schmitz, 2006; Harris & Niesen-Vertommen, 2000; McKenzie & Kalda, 2003).

In assessing the risk/benefit ratio of exercise, it is important to consider the potential harm to cancer survivors of remaining inactive alongside the possible hazards of exercise. Physical inactivity leads to deconditioning, bone loss, and muscle atrophy, decreases in glucose metabolism, insulin sensitivity, digestive function and immunosurveillence, and increases in cardiovascular risk factors (e.g., lipid levels, blood pressure). Maintaining regular activity is essential therefore for reducing the risk of developing other chronic conditions (e.g., diabetes, cardiovascular disease, osteoporosis), and particularly so for cancer survivors who may be at increased risk of further disease (Brown, Brauner, & Minnotte, 1993; Mahon, 1998; Penedo, Schneiderman, Dahn, & Gonzalez, 2004).

Summary

In terms of prevention, there is compelling evidence that regular physical activity reduces the risk of colon and breast cancer. However, the optimal type and volume has not yet been determined. Similarly, there is currently insufficient evidence to establish if physical activity protects against other cancers. Regarding survival, there is some intriguing data suggesting that physical activity performed after diagnosis is associated with lower cancer mortality, but more studies of this type are needed before conclusions can be drawn. The evidence base on rehabilitation is expanding and currently indicates positive effects on outcomes relating to physical functioning and quality of life, both during cancer therapy, and after treatment completion. Research is ongoing in all these areas in the attempt to understand and maximize the benefits of physical activity in relation to cancer.

ACKNOWLEDGMENTS

Clare Stevinson is supported by a Postdoctoral Fellowship from the Faculty of Physical Education and Recreation, University of Alberta. Kerry S. Courneya is supported by the Canada Research Chairs Program and a Research Team Grant from the National Cancer Institute of Canada with funds from the Canadian Cancer Society and the Sociobehavioral Cancer Research Network.

REFERENCES

Courneya KS & Friedenreich CM. (2001). Framework PEACE: An organizational model for examining physical exercise across the cancer experience. *Annals of Behavioral Medicine,* 23, 263–272.

Holmes M, Chen WY, Feskanich D, Kroenke CH, & Colditz GA. (2005). Physical activity and survival after breast cancer diagnosis. *Journal of the American Medical Association,* 293, 2479–2486.

Humpel N & Iverson DC. (2005). Review and critique of the quality of exercise recommendations for cancer patients and survivors. *Supportive Care in Cancer,* 13, 493–502.

International Agency for Research on Cancer. (2002). *Weight control and physical activity, IARC handbook of cancer prevention* (Vol 6). Lyon, France, IARC Press.

Kushi LH, Byers T, Doyle C, Bandera EV, McCullough M, Gansler T, et al. (2006). American cancer society guidelines on nutrition and physical activity for cancer prevention: Reducing the risk of cancer with healthy food choices and physical activity. *CA A Cancer Journal for Clinicians,* 56, 254–281.

McNeely ML, Peddle C, Parliament M, & Courneya KS. (2006b). Cancer rehabilitation: Recommendations for integrating exercise programming in the clinical practice setting. *Current Cancer Therapy Reviews,* 2, 351–360.

Ness KK, Wall MM, Oakes M, Robison LL, & Gurney JG. (2006). Physical performance limitations and participation restrictions among cancer survivors: A population-based study. *Annals of Epidemiology,* 16, 197–205.

Rundle A. (2005). Molecular Epidemiology of Physical Activity and Cancer. *Cancer Epidemiology, Biomarkers & Prevention,* 14, 227–236.

Schmitz KH, Holtzman J, Courneya KS, Mâsse LC, Duval S, & Kane R. (2005). Controlled physical activity trials in cancer survivors: A systematic review and meta-analysis. *Cancer Epidemiology, Biomarkers & Prevention,* 14, 1588–1595.

Westerlind KC. (2003). Physical activity and cancer prevention—mechanisms. *Medicine and Science in Sports and Exercise,* 35, 1834–1840.

(A complete reference list for this chapter is available online at http://www.oup.com/us/ integrativemedicine).

11

Massage Therapy

LISA W. CORBIN

KEY CONCEPTS

- Patients with cancer often suffer physical symptoms and psychological stress. Massage therapy, widely used by healthy people for relaxation, may have other specific benefits for patients in all stages of cancer treatment.
- The use of massage therapy, with specific precautions in certain situations, is safe for patients with cancer.
- There are few large, well-designed trials of massage therapy for patients with cancer; existing research suggests the most benefits for lymphedema and anxiety.
- Though there is even less substantial research to support other claims, massage is often suggested for improved postoperative wound healing, sleep, pain, fatigue, constipation, and improved immune function
- Physicians caring for patients with cancer should ask all patients about the use of massage, consider recommending massage for anxiety and distress, and help guide the patient to a qualified massage therapist.

■

Massage therapy, a complementary therapy known primarily for its use in relaxation, may also benefit patients with cancer in other ways. However, the use of massage techniques in patients with cancer requires special considerations. While safe and efficacious for some patients, it may be harmful or ineffective in other situations. Risks can be minimized and benefits maximized when the clinician feels comfortable discussing massage with his or her patients. This chapter reviews and summarizes the literature on massage and cancer to provide the clinician with reliable information regarding the safe, appropriate use of massage therapy for patients with cancer, and thus to help facilitate discussions with patients.

Defined by the National Center for Complementary and Alternative Medicine (NCCAM), "massage therapy" is classified within the category of "manipulative and body-based therapies" as an "assortment of techniques involving manipulation of the soft tissues of the body through pressure and movement" (http://nccam.nih.gov/). There are many different styles of massage therapy (such as Swedish, Rolfing, Deep Tissue, and Neuromuscular). A detailed comparison of techniques is not relevant to this text; instead, the clinician should work with a massage therapist skilled in treating patients with cancer and who can employ the techniques appropriate for the situation.

Almost all cultures have developed massage therapy as it seems instinctual to rub and press an area of muscular pain. References date back at least as far as 1600 BC. Hippocrates mentioned massage (around 400 BC), and massage was used and referenced as a medical therapy until the focus of medical care shifted to the biological sciences in the early 20th century. In the 1970s, massage in the United States found renewed interest, especially for athletes. Over the past 25 years, the therapeutic uses of massage have broadened, and research has sought to investigate its physical, physiological, and psychological effects.

Proposed theories abound to explain the mechanism of action of massage therapy. Few of these theories are well-tested, however, and there is little to no correlation of bench research (such as the observation of an acute increase in natural killer cell number and activity following massage (Hernandez-Reif, 2005; Zeitlin, Keller, Shiflett, Schleifer, & Bartlett, 2000)) to clinical outcomes (such as improved disease-free survival for patients with cancer). Theories on mechanisms of action are summarized in Box 11.1 (Field, et al., 1998; Moyer, 2004). The lack of a thorough understanding of mechanism of action or clinical correlation should not necessarily dissuade the physician from recommending massage therapy, however, as these theories lend plausibility to the anecdotal reports and small studies supporting efficacy discussed in a subsequent section. Ideally, the physician will have a candid discussion with his or her patient about the potential benefits and safety issues framed in the context of studies which support benefit.

Patients with cancer may suffer physical symptoms and psychological stress. Physical symptoms such as pain or early satiety may be due to the location of the tumor; other symptoms, such as constipation or nausea, can result from the medications used to treat these symptoms. Patients who have undergone cancer treatment may have symptoms related to the treatment, such as postsurgical

Box 11.1. Theories of Mechanism of Action of Massage Therapy

Theory	Explanation
Gate control theory of pain reduction	Massage therapy creates a physical stimulus; the brain has difficulty processing and perceiving competing stimuli, thus, other physical stimuli, such as pain, are less recognized
Increasing parasympathetic activity	Massage therapy may shift the autonomic nervous system from the sympathetic ("fight or flight") to parasympathetic (relaxation), with a subsequent reduction of stress hormones (such as cortisol), increased immune response, increased alertness, and general feelings of well-being
Increasing serotonin and endorphins	Some studies have linked massage therapy with increases in these "feel-good" neurotransmitters
Improved blood flow	Massage has been theorized to improve blood flow, thus helping to clear waste products (such as lactic acid, thus reducing muscle pain) or to promote wound healing
Improved lymphatic circulation	Massage therapy may improve lymphatic circulation and is used to reduce lymphedema
Interpersonal attention	Some theorize that the effects of massage therapy are due to the attention given to the patient by the therapist and less to the actual physical treatment

pain or lymphedema. The burden of psychological stress, anxiety, and depression in cancer patients cannot be overemphasized. Depression has been estimated to be four times as common in cancer patients as compared with that in the general population. Anxiety may lead to patients overestimating the risks associated with treatments or worsen their perception of their physical symptoms. Because of undertreated psychological symptoms, patients with cancer may not follow through with treatment recommendations or may report a higher severity of physical symptoms.

Massage therapy has been increasingly employed and investigated as a therapeutic intervention to reduce symptoms in cancer patients. Studies are typically small or poorly designed, however, making it difficult to draw firm conclusions (see section on benefits).

Indeed, studies have shown that patients with cancer are increasingly drawn to massage therapy in an attempt to alleviate symptoms (Ashikaga, Bosompra, O'Brien, & Nelson 2002; Coss, McGrath, & Caggiano, 1998; Lengacher, 2002). In a study published in 2000, 26% of 453 adult patients surveyed at MD Anderson Cancer Center acknowledged using massage therapy (Richardson, Sanders, Palmer, Greisinger, & Singletary, 2000); in 2001, 20% of 100 patients seeking care at a private cancer center reported having received massage therapy (Bernstein & Grasso, 2001); although in a prospective study of 50 patients receiving radiation for prostate cancer only 7% of patients reported receiving massage therapy (Kao & Devine, 2000). 60% of 169 hospices responding to a survey published in 2004 reported that they offered complementary medicine services at their hospices, with massage therapy the most commonly offered service (available at 83% of the hospices offering CAM therapies) (Demmer, 2004). Despite the popularity and availability of massage therapy for patients with cancer, some patients and their family members remain unaware of the potential uses of massage as a therapy for symptom control.

> Over 20% of patients with cancer report using massage therapy as an adjunct to conventional care. Massage is the most commonly available CAM therapy in US hospices.

Clinicians are aware that patients use complementary therapies, including massage therapy, but often do not discuss it with patients (Bourgeault, 1996). It has been widely postulated that open discussion between physicians and patients about CAM may result in an enhanced physician/patient relationship and encourage enhanced compliance with recommended treatments.

Safety of Massage Therapy

Overall, therapeutic massage is widely considered to be safe, though adverse events have been reported. Healthy patients may experience an allergic reaction to the lubricants used, bruising, swelling of massaged muscles, or a temporary increase in muscular pain; absolute risk of these events is unknown. Pregnant women should avoid prolonged positioning on their back. Case reports have reported or theorized serious adverse events, including fractures

Table 11.1. Circumstances with Potential for Massage-Related Adverse Events.

Situation	Potential Harm	Modification Necessary
Coagulation disorder (low platelet count, warfarin, heparin, or aspirin therapy)	Bleeding (ranging from minor bruising to internal hemorrhaging)	Lighter pressure and avoidance of deep tissue massage
Metastatic cancer in bones	Fracture	Knowledge of location of metastases and lighter pressure over those areas
Open wounds; radiation dermatitis	Increased pain, infection	Avoid massage directly over open or healing wounds or dermatitis

and dislocations; internal hemorrhage, and hepatic hematoma (Trotter, 1999); dislodging of deep venous thrombosis and resultant embolism of the renal artery (Mikhail, Reidy, Taylor, & Scoble, 1997); and displacement of a ureteral stent (Kerr, 1997). A recently published review of cases reported in the literature and randomized controlled trials of massage therapy found that few reported adverse events (Ernst, 2003). Cancer patients may be at higher risk for these problems, requiring modification of technique to avoid them. Table 11.1 shows specific situations often encountered with cancer patients, the potential harm of massage in these situations, and suggestions on ways to decrease risk. There has been no evidence that massage therapy can spread cancer, although direct pressure over a tumor is usually discouraged.

There is no evidence that therapeutic massage can spread cancer.

Certainly, massage should never be advocated as a *substitute* for potentially curative oncological care. Health care providers should also realize that while massage therapy can be safe for their patients with cancer, massage therapists may also be suggesting certain herbs or other complementary medicine therapies to their patients that may put the patient at risk.

Benefits of Massage Therapy

Few studies have adequate numbers of patients to investigate efficacy of massage therapy for symptoms in cancer patients. A meta-analysis (see following text) found only eight randomized clinical trials, with a total of only 357 patients. Investigators have found large trials difficult to design and carry out; one report described unforeseen challenges including late-stage cancer patients being too ill to participate and health care providers withholding referrals to the study because of a bias against having their patients possibly randomized to the non-massage therapy control group (Westcombe, 2003).

A meta-analysis by the Cochrane collaborative group reviewed randomized controlled trials published prior to May 2002 that investigated the use of massage to reduce symptoms in patients with cancer. Their search strategy yielded eight randomized controlled trials with a total of 357 patients. The authors noted that a reduction in anxiety (19% to 32% in four studies; 207 patients) was most commonly seen. Only three studies with a total of 117 patients measured pain; a decrease was noted in just one study. Criticisms of these studies included the small number of subjects enrolled and the use only of standardized massages that did not allow the therapist to direct the massage based on the patient's specific situation. Similarly, only two studies (71 patients) demonstrated a reduction in nausea. Individual studies showed improvement in other common symptoms, such as sleep (Fellowes, Barnes, & Wilkinson, 2004).

A few randomized controlled trials have been published since the meta-analysis. In the United Kingdom, Soden et al. randomized 42 hospice patients with cancer to receive massage, massage plus aromatherapy, or no intervention over a 4-week period. They did not find any significant benefits for pain, anxiety, or quality of life, although statistically significant improvements in sleep were seen in both massage groups, and a reduction in depression was noted in the massage-only group. Patients with higher initial levels of psychological distress had more response to the massage interventions (Soden, Vincent, Craske, Lucas, & Ashley, 2004).

The largest study on massage for symptom reduction in cancer patients to date was published by Post-White et al. in 2003. This group randomized 230 cancer outpatients to receive a standardized massage, healing touch (an intervention whereby the practitioner is believed to modify a patient's energy fields by motion of his or her hands near or gently on the patient), or the presence of a staff member in the room in a crossover design. Each intervention was given weekly for 45 minutes for 4 weeks. Physiological effects such as decreased heart rate and respirations were seen in all three groups; massage therapy lowered pain (with a reduction in the use of nonsteroidal anti-inflammatory medications also noted) and anxiety, and therapeutic touch also lowered anxiety (Post-White, et al., 2003).

A nonrandomized study of a simple 10-minute foot massage by nurses showed immediate benefits for pain, nausea, and anxiety in 87 hospitalized patients with cancer. Though conclusions cannot be drawn without a control group, further study is warranted as this intervention would be relatively simple and easy to deliver (Grealish, Lomasney, & Whiteman, 2000).

A large, retrospective, observational study of pre- and postmassage symptom scores of 1290 in- and outpatients seen over a 3-year period at Memorial Sloan Kettering Cancer Center (3609 massages delivered) showed an average 50% reduction in symptoms (ranging from 21% improvement for nausea to 52% for anxiety) following massage. Follow-up surveys at 48 hours showed persistence of the benefit. Patients rated symptoms including pain, fatigue, anxiety, nausea, and depression on a 0 to 10 scale. For whatever symptom rated the highest on premassage assessment, improvement was 54%. Results were felt to be clinically significant and, although the study did not have a randomized design, it certainly supports the idea of massage's utility in symptom control for patients with cancer (Cassileth & Vickers, 2004).

Massage also has been proposed to reduce stress and increase relaxation for caregivers of patients with cancer. One study investigated these symptoms in 42 spouses of patients with cancer randomly assigned to a trial group receiving a single 20-minute therapeutic back massage or to a control group. Mood assessed preintervention, immediately postintervention, and 20 minutes postintervention showed improvement postintervention in the massage group (Goodfellow, 2003). A separate trial assigned 36 caregivers of patients undergoing autologous hematopoetic stem cell transplant to receive two 30-minute massage sessions (13 participants), two 30-minute healing touch sessions (10 participants), or one 10-minute nurse visit (13 patients). Anxiety and depression as well as fatigue were significantly reduced in the massage group (Rexilius, Mundt, Eckson Megel, & Agrawal, 2002).

Massage therapy may also reduce stress and anxiety for caregivers of oncology patients.

A specific massage technique, "manual lymphatic drainage" (MLD), has been employed to decrease breast cancer related lymphedema and is commonly used in combination with support/compression garments, skin care, and exercise. Despite widespread use, MLD has not been rigorously studied. An exhaustive Cochrane collaboration search identified just two randomized studies, noted here (Preston, Seers, & Mortimer, 2008). A randomized crossover design study specifically examined this technique in 31 women with breast cancer-related lymphedema and showed significantly reduced limb volume as well as symptoms such as pain and heaviness. Quality of life was positively affected, and sleep improved (Williams, Vadgama, Franks, & Mortimer, 2002). However, in a study of 42 women with mastectomy-related lymphedema comparing

MLD along with compression garments versus compression garments alone, the addition of MLD did not offer additional improvement in lymphedema (Andersen, Hojris, Erlandsen, & Anderson, 2000).

Abdominal massage has been advocated to reduce constipation; a review of trials of massage for chronic constipation in 1999 concluded that the numbers of patients studied was too small to make definitive statements on efficacy (Ernst, 1999). Massage has been promoted to improve immune function, but actual studies are small and inconclusive (Field, 2001). Massage therapy is also commonly advocated to cancer patients to help promote postoperative wound healing and reduce scar tissue formation, and to help release metabolic waste by improving circulation. A Medline search failed to locate any published trials demonstrating the efficacy of massage therapy for these indications. Future well-designed trials may wish to look at massage therapy for these indications.

Research on the benefits of massage therapy is ongoing. For the clinician who is interested in information on current clinical trials involving massage and cancer can be found by searching the NIH CRISP database (http://clinicaltrials.gov). As of August 2008, there were 11 open and recruiting studies listed on this site investigating the effects of massage therapy on patients with cancer. Six of the 11 have pain and other physical and functional symptoms as the primary outcomes; three are looking at MLD for breast cancer related lymphedema. Two of the larger trials are discussed in the subsequent paragraphs.

One recently completed NIH-funded multi-site randomized controlled trial enrolled 380 patients with advanced cancer (90% of whom were in hospice care) and pain (at least 4 on a 0–10 point pain scale) to either 6 30 minute massage therapy visits or 6 30 minute visits of non–moving touch (administered by a volunteer instructed to place his/her hands in predefined locations on the patient's body for a total of 30 minutes) over a 2-week period. Participants received an average of 4.1 visits. The non–moving touch control was chosen to control for the benefits of attention and simple touch. Pain was reduced over the course of the study to a similar extent in both groups; however, massage therapy showed a greater benefit in short-term pain control. Massage therapy was safe in this population, though patients with known coagulopathies or unstable spines were excluded. (Kutner JS, Smith MC, Corbin L, Hemphill L, Benton K, et al., 2008. In press)

The NIH is also funding a study of massage therapy to reduce fatigue in patients with certain cancer types; this study (currently in analysis phase) randomized patients to massage, sham bodywork, or usual care and was based at the University of California San Francisco. Final results are not yet available.

In summary, trials of massage therapy in cancer patients give the strongest evidence for its ability to decrease anxiety and distress. Massage may likely decrease pain but the number of patients studied is small; the efficacy of massage on other symptoms associated with cancer as well as on the number of medications used for symptom control also warrants more study. If massage therapy is indeed beneficial in cancer patients, perhaps more care centers for patients with cancer will make massage therapy available.

Discussing the Use of Massage Therapy with Cancer Patients

Cancer patients often use complementary medical therapies, including massage therapy, in conjunction with conventional treatment. Although massage is generally safe, cancer patients, particularly those undergoing active treatment, are at higher risk for complications. The clinician should note the presence of comorbid conditions which may put the patient at higher risk for complications, such as anticoagulant use, heart failure, deep venous thrombosis, cellulitis, the presence of catheters, pregnancy, or bone metastases. If the patient has any of these comorbidities, he or she should be advised to work with a therapist experienced in medical massage or cancer massage who will feel comfortable making the appropriate modifications in technique necessary to decrease risk. Secondarily, patients should be encouraged to consider the use of massage therapy for adjunctive management of pain and anxiety. If a patient is interested in using massage therapy, the physician should help them find a qualified therapist (see Box 11.2 for further details).

Philosophy and education of therapists is variable, with some massage therapists under the mistaken belief that cancer is a contraindication for massage and others perhaps discouraging patients from receiving potentially curative conventional care or promoting potentially harmful therapies. Thus, finding a massage therapist experienced and comfortable with both cancer patients and the conventional care commonly used is paramount.

Clinicians can help patients find a qualified massage therapist. Given that many cancer centers, hospitals, and hospices now have Integrative Medicine programs offering massage therapy, clinicians can ideally refer patients to seek treatment in these settings. If no such programs are available, the clinician should encourage the patient to interview potential therapists or should do so himself or herself to establish an ongoing consultant relationship for future referrals.

When interviewing a potential massage therapist, ask about education and experience including licensing and certification. Consider only massage therapists who have a minimum of 500 hours of training. Massage therapy schools voluntarily meeting criteria set by the Commission on Massage Therapy Accreditation have achieved and maintained a level of quality, performance, and integrity that meets meaningful standards. A directory of accredited programs is available on the Commission's web site (http://www.comta.org/

Box 11.2. Finding a Qualified Massage Therapist

Standard	Minimum qualifications	Preferred Qualifications (in Addition to the Minimum)
Education	500 hours Accredited school Experience working with cancer patients	Advanced training in oncology massage
Licensure and certification	Licensed, if required by state (LMT or LMP) Certified, if no licensure required (CMT)	Certified by NCTMB
Philosophy	View selves as extension of patient's health care team, not as a stand-alone therapy Will communicate with other health-care providers Aware that massage is not contraindicated in patients with cancer but that special considerations may be necessary	

Home.htm). Specialized programs for advanced training in massage care of the patient with cancer are also available; additional education and experience in working with cancer patients is a must. Specialized programs are not standardized, however. Overall, studies of massage in other conditions have suggested that the greatest benefits are seen with the most experienced massage therapists (Furlan, Brosseau, Imamura, & Irin, 2002).

Not all states regulate massage therapists. A current list is available from the American Massage Therapy Association (http://www.amtamassage.org/about/lawstate.html). If a therapist is licensed, the initials "LMT" (Licensed Massage Therapist) or "LMP" (Licensed Massage Practitioner) are used after the therapist's name. In other nonlicensing states, a therapist should have "CMT" (Certified Massage Therapist) as a minimum qualification. Beyond this, the initials NCTMB indicate that the therapist has voluntarily taken and passed an exam given by the National Certification Board of Therapeutic Massage and Bodywork.

The right massage therapist will be knowledgeable about risks and benefits of massage in a cancer population and should be comfortable communicating with the referring physician on an ongoing basis. They should see themselves as an extension of the patient's healthcare team, not as a replacement. Some massage therapists may have experience with other complementary therapies and should agree to encourage the patient to discuss any suggestions on other therapies with their clinician.

The cost of massage therapy visits is relatively trivial when compared with the cost of some medications and other conventional treatments for symptom control, but may be prohibitive for some patients nonetheless as it is often not covered by insurance. There may be funds available for patients through charitable organizations, and this option should be explored. The cost of massage therapy will typically qualify for reimbursement through medical flexible spending accounts and usually will count toward medical expenses that can be itemized on federal taxes. Patients should be encouraged to verify this with their employer and/or tax accountant or attorney. A relatively new and intriguing area of research in massage therapy is exploring the idea of teaching caregivers to massage patients undergoing cancer treatment. If this approach can be shown to be feasible and effective in terms of reduced symptoms in cancer patients, it will present a much more cost-effective and convenient approach.

Summary and Conclusions

Over 20% of patients with cancer use massage therapy, with most patients using massage and other complementary therapies along with conventional treatments. Though physicians increasingly recognize that patients use complementary therapies, many are reluctant to bring the subject up with their patients. Discussion of CAM with patients may enhance the doctor–patient relationship, improve compliance with conventional treatments, and allow the physician to promote nonpharmacological approaches to symptom management. A nice general review of discussion complementary and alternative medical therapies with cancer patients was published in 2002 (Weiger, et al., 2002).

Given what is known from research studies, massage should be promoted to cancer patients as a therapy to help reduce stress and anxiety. Though the ability of massage therapy to reduce symptoms other than anxiety has not yet been conclusively demonstrated, the low likelihood of harm and studies leaning towards proving benefit for pain and other symptoms makes massage therapy an attractive adjunct to conventional care. Massage should not be used as a substitute for conventional cancer care, and clinicians should recognize and discuss that massage practitioners may promote other potentially harmful unconventional therapies. Massage therapy should be accepted and condoned as a potentially beneficial intervention for symptomatic relief in patients with cancer, and can be safely incorporated into conventional care of cancer patients.

GENERAL REFERENCES

National Cancer Institute (www.cancer.gov/cancerinfo/treatment/cam) the massage research database maintained by the American Massage Therapy Association (http://www.amtafoundation.org/researchdb.html), the database maintained by the Touch Research Institutes (http://www.miami.edu/touch-research/).
(http://nccam.nih.gov/)

REFERENCES

Ernst E. (2003). Safety of massage therapy. *Rheumatism*, 42, 1101–1106.

Fellowes D, Barnes K, & Wilkinson S. (2004). Aromatherapy and massage for symptom relief in patients with cancer. *Cochrane Database of Systematic Reviews*, (2), CD002287.

Kutner JS, Smith MC, Corbin L, Hemphill L, Benton K, Mellis K et al. (2008). Massage Therapy vs. Simple Touch to Improve Pain and Mood in Patients with Advanced Cancer: A Randomized Trial. Accepted for publication 2008, Ann Int Med.

Weiger WA, Smith M, Boon H, Richardson MA, Kaptchuck TJ, & Eisenberg DM. (2002). Advising patients who seek complementary and alternative medical therapies for cancer. *Annals of Internal Medicine*, 137, 889–903.

(*A complete reference list for this chapter is available online at http://www.oup.com/us/integrativemedicine*).

12

Mind-Body Medicine in Integrative Cancer Care

MARTIN L. ROSSMAN AND DEAN SHROCK

KEY CONCEPTS

- A serious cancer diagnosis carries unique psychological challenges. A compassionate physician with an integrative perspective can be a key ally.
- The ubiquity of the placebo effect suggests that every communication between a doctor and patient is a mind-body interaction that can have effects as potent as a scalpel or cytotoxic agent. Professionals need to be aware of the power of their communications and use them skillfully.
- There are a wide range of mind-body approaches that allow professionals to help cancer patients, and allow patients to help themselves. They can be delivered as self-care tools, in groups, or in individual sessions.
- The issue of whether mind-body approaches can influence survival is unresolved, but the evidence that mind-body approaches improve quality of life is consistent, abundant, and unequivocal.
- Mind-body therapies can reduce anxiety and depression, temper adverse effects of cancer treatments, relieve pain, stimulate immune responses, and help people deal with a wide range of cancer-related stress including relationships, decision making, planning for the future, dealing with loss, and if necessary, coming to terms with end-of-life issues.
- Mind-body approaches have minimal risk, significant benefits, and low cost and should be standard of care with every cancer patient.

A cancer diagnosis is one of the most common traumatic events faced in developed cultures. A serious cancer diagnosis carries with it a unique set of challenges for patients, their family, and health-care professionals. Patients newly diagnosed with cancer, and their support people, are frequently in shock, fearful, and emotionally regressed. During this difficult emotional time they are called on to make difficult treatment decisions, to evaluate complex information and opinions that often are in conflict, and all in an atmosphere of urgency. They can feel pressured to sort through an overwhelming amount of information, and may feel torn between conventional, complementary, and alternative treatment advice. Finally, cancer patients often are asked to choose treatments that can have difficult, disfiguring, and sometimes life-threatening effects of their own, which makes them difficult to choose, even when they offer potential benefits.

For all these reasons, a physician with an integrative perspective can be a critical ally in helping patients choose the optimal approach to their management and treatment.

The Mind-Body Effects of Physician-Patient Communications

The National Institutes of Health (NIH) define mind-body therapies as interventions designed to facilitate the mind's capacity to affect bodily function and symptoms. In actuality, all therapeutic encounters have a mind-body aspect. Usually called the placebo effect, it is the most ubiquitous phenomenon in all of medicine. It is an effect that results from the patients' hopes, beliefs, and expectations, and it can be potentiated or depotentiated by both the physicians' beliefs and the way that physicians communicate. The fact that the expectations of both the patients' and physicians' expectations impact treatment effects is the reason that we go to the immense trouble and expense to do double-blinded studies. While researchers want to eliminate the placebo effect, patients and clinicians want to maximize its benefit, and use it to therapeutic advantage.

The ubiquity of the placebo effect suggests that every communication between a doctor and patient can have consequences as potent as a scalpel or cytotoxic agent. As Norman Cousins said, "Communications from doctor to patient can set the stage for a heroic response or a collapse into despair." Telling patients that they have cancer is not easy, but there are ways of communicating this news that tells the truth but leaves room for hope. Carl Simonton, MD, a radiation oncologist who pioneered in the mind-body treatment of cancer patients, uses the phrase, "This is a serious illness, and you may be able to do something about it."

Following this communication model can help prevent creating what can amount to an iatrogenic post-traumatic stress disorder. We have seen too many patients who say "I will never forget the look on my doctor's face when he told me I have cancer." Patients often have great trouble overcoming such memories and its discouraging effects in spite of intensive counseling. If we could instill confidence and calmness as easily and powerfully as we can instill terror, we would be great physicians indeed. The best opportunity we have is when we first deliver the diagnosis, and we need to be mindful of what and how we are communicating.

Major Mind-Body Approaches Used in Cancer Care

There are a wide range of mind-body approaches that allow professionals to help cancer patients, and allow patients to help themselves. The most researched and frequently used are: relaxation training, guided and Interactive Guided Imagery, meditation, hypnosis, biofeedback, and forms of group social support.

Almost all mind-body techniques involve a combination of relaxation and imagery, which is why we think it is crucial for practitioners to familiarize themselves with these modalities. The most common form of imagery is worry, and cancer patients often spend far too much time focusing involuntarily on their fears and concerns, which is not only frightening but also exhausting and self-reinforcing. Teaching them more productive uses of their thoughts and imagination is an essential part of their care and treatment, and offers multiple benefits detailed later in this chapter.

> We think it is important for people to be introduced to mind-body approaches as early as possible after their diagnosis: 1) it gives them a positive focus and a sense of participation; 2) it distracts from worrying and catastrophizing; 3) it gives them the message that you think there is reason to hope; and 4) they can learn and practice these skills before their concentration abilities are affected by chemotherapy or radiation.

1. *Relaxation techniques* utilizing abdominal breathing, muscle relaxation, autogenic suggestions, and simple imagery are the most widely used, easily learned, and generally useful mind-body techniques. Because stress is such

a common experience in cancer, reducing it through regular relaxation practice allows a patient to interrupt obsessive worry, regain some sense of control, and create periods of respite from the ongoing challenges of cancer and its treatment.

2. *Guided imagery* is the mental picturing, or sensing, thinking, and feeling of a desired outcome or focus of inquiry. It includes a range of techniques from simple visualization and direct imagery-based suggestion to metaphor and story-telling. Guided imagery is used to help teach psycho-physiologic relaxation, to relieve symptoms, to stimulate healing responses in the body, to access inner resources, and to help people tolerate procedures and treatments more easily.

3. *Social support and psychoeducational groups* consistently demonstrate improved quality of life for cancer patients, and they may contribute to better survival. Feeling listened to, cared for, supported, and learning how to live fully despite a cancer diagnosis are essential components of cancer care. Not everyone benefits from support groups, but almost everyone benefits from support, whether from professionals, family, friends, their spiritual community, or counseling.

4. *Meditation* involves concentrating the mind on either a neutral or meaningful focus: a word, image, external object, one's breath, or whatever is occurring at the time. Meditation distracts the mind from worrisome imagery, tends to create a physiologically relaxed state, and helps develop peace of mind. There are many forms of meditation; some are connected to particular religious belief systems, and others are non-secular and compatible with any belief system.

5. *Biofeedback* uses sensitive physiological monitors to display the reactions the body is having in response to thoughts and feelings. By being able to see, hear, or otherwise experience changes the body makes in response to mental contents, it is possible to gain control over physical functions normally out of conscious control. When people see how quickly and effectively the body responds to thoughts, it gives them confidence to use their mind to affect their bodies.

6. *Hypnosis* is a term used to describe a state of relaxed focused attention in which response to suggestions is enhanced. While words are used to create suggestions, the most effective suggestions involve mental imagery. In actual practice, guided imagery and hypnosis often are often indistinguishable, although people's beliefs associated with each term can affect their responses.

7. *Interactive Guided Imagery*ˢᵐ (IGI) is a specific way of using imagery that is particularly effective in helping patients use their inner resources most effectively. Patients are guided to work with their own personal imagery and insights

about their illness and healing, to clarify any issues that may be involved, and to learn to use the mind to support their own healing. IGI principles can be used in self-care approaches but often are best facilitated by a trained health professional, especially where highly emotional issues are involved, as they often are with cancer.

All of these therapies have the potential to affect the psychological and treatment issues that arise in the diagnosis, treatment, and care of cancer patients and their families. Mind-body therapies can make a substantial impact by helping patients and families reduce anxiety and depression, manage their emotions, help in their decision making, reduce adverse effects of cancer treatments and procedures, manage pain, stimulate an immune response, deal with loss, plan for the future, support the will to live, and, if necessary, come to terms with end-of-life issues.

Evidence Supporting Mind-Body Approaches with Cancer

Here we will review research that supports the use of mind-body approaches to address five important aspects of working with cancer patients: (1) the psychological and emotional issues of being diagnosed with cancer; (2) coping with and reducing adverse effects of cancer treatments; (3) stimulating immunity, blood flow, and other healing responses; (4) reducing or relieving cancer-related pain; and (5) influencing the progression or outcome of the diagnosis.

EARLY PSYCHOLOGICAL AND EMOTIONAL ISSUES OF BEING DIAGNOSED WITH CANCER

Almost everyone responds to the diagnosis of cancer with a period of shock, numbness, and disbelief. Approximately 40% to 60% of cancer patients are significantly fearful and distressed following their diagnosis (Graves, et al., 2006; Hegel, et al., 2006), and these emotions can affect their ability to follow through with treatment plans. Depression is common, but often under-recognized by oncologists and nurses (Passik, et al., 1998).

There is so much evidence that mind-body interventions reduce or relieve anxiety and depression in cancer patients that we will quote only selected reviews and papers for the reader who wants to investigate this in more depth. Reviews of the literature and meta-analyses (Barsevick, Sweeney, Haney, & Chung, et al., 2002; Greer, 2002) consistently conclude that psychosocial interventions, including relaxation, guided imagery, cognitive behavioral, psychoeducational, and supportive–expressive group therapies, reduce anxiety and depression, and improve mood and quality of life in cancer patients. More recent studies (Cameron, Booth, Schlatter, Ziginskas, & Harman et al., 2006; Burgess, et al., 2005) recommend group emotional and social support to help patients manage their anxiety and depression in the first year following diagnosis.

COPING WITH AND REDUCING ADVERSE EFFECTS OF CANCER TREATMENTS

While medical treatments including surgery, chemotherapy, and radiation can be powerful weapons in fighting cancer, side effects including fatigue, pain, and nausea can be debilitating and even cause patients to forego or discontinue treatment. Randomized studies demonstrate that mind-body therapies can reduce or eliminate emotional and physical side effects of surgical, radiation, and chemotherapy treatments.

Relaxation with guided imagery, self-hypnosis, and giving patients reassuring information before surgery have been shown to be highly effective in reducing anxiety before, during, and after surgery (Ashton, et al., 2000; Bugbee, et al., 2005; Faymonville, et al., 1995; Huth, Broome, & Good, et al., 2004; Lang, Joyce, Spiegel, Hamilton, & Lee, 1996; Laurion, & Fetzer, 2003; Ludwick-Rosenthal & Newfeld, 1993), including pediatric patients (Calipel, Lucas-Polomeni, Wodey, & Ecoffey, 2005).

The same mind-body techniques can shorten surgical procedures (Lang, et al., 2000; Tusek, Church, Strong, Grass, & Fazio, 1997) and significantly reduce pain and the need for pain medication post-operatively (Antall & Kresevec, 2004; Ashton, et al., 2000; Disbrow, Bennett, & Owings, 1993; Faymonville, et al., 1995; Huth, et al., 2004; Lang, et al., 2000; Manyande, et al., 1995; Pellino, et al., 2005; Rensi, Peticca, & Pescatori, 2000; Syrjala, Donaldson, Davis, Kippes, & Carr, 1995; Tusek, et al., 1997; Weinstein & Au, 1991). Guided imagery and suggestion reduces the time it takes for patients' bowels to return to normal functioning (Disbrow, et al., 1993; Tusek, et al., 1997), and shortens hospital stays (Cowan, Buffington, Cowan, & Hathaway, 2001; Disbrow, et al., 1993; Meurisse, et al., 1996; Rapkin, Straubing, & Holroyd, 1991; Tusek, et al., 1997). There is also evidence that these techniques can reduce blood loss (Enqvist, von Konow, & Bystedt, 1995; Lucas, 1975; Meurisse, et al., 1996) and speed wound healing (Holden-Lund, 1988; Jones, 1977). In a prospective, randomized, controlled trial Burgio et al. (2006) studied 125 prostate cancer patients after radical prostatectomy, and found that preoperative biofeedback hastened the recovery of urine control and decreased the severity of incontinence.

Several sources, including Blue Shield of California and Cedars Sinai Medical Center (Los Angeles), have reported that 88% of patients who used guided imagery tapes to prepare for surgery were very satisfied with them. It also reduced their average bill by nearly $800 (Fontana, 2000; Holden-Lund, 1988).

As many as 25% of cancer patients have nausea and vomiting in anticipation of chemotherapy, an effect clearly mediated by expectations. Morrow and Morrell (1982) showed that systematic desensitization, (a behavioral treatment using relaxation and guided imagery), had a significant anti-emetic effect in these patients.

Vasterling et al. (1993) reported that both cognitive distraction and relaxation training reduced nausea and blood pressure in patients on chemotherapy. Burish and Jenkins (1992) found that biofeedback combined with relaxation training decreased nausea and anxiety during chemotherapy, and physiological arousal after chemotherapy. Given et al. (2004) reported that a cognitive-behavioral intervention (which included self-care management, problem solving, communication, and counseling and support) for 237 patients undergoing chemotherapy resulted in significantly lower levels of symptom severity for all symptoms measured. Molassiotis et al. (2002) concluded that progressive muscle relaxation training and guided imagery considerably decreased the duration of nausea, vomiting, and overall mood disturbance in a study of 71 chemotherapy-naïve breast cancer patients. Eller (1999) found 46 studies that suggested the effectiveness of guided imagery in the management of stress, anxiety, and depression, and for the reduction of blood pressure, pain and other side effects of chemotherapy. A clinical trial with 110 patients demonstrated that preparatory information, cognitive restructuring, relaxation and guided imagery significantly reduced nausea and fatigue 7 days after autologous bone marrow and/or peripheral blood stem cell transplantation when the side effects of treatment are usually most severe (Gaston-Johansson, et al., 2000). Yoo et al. (2005) assessed the effectiveness of progressive muscle relaxation training and guided imagery in a randomized study of 60 patients with breast cancer. The treatment group had a better quality of life with significantly less anxiety, depression, and hostility than the control group. They also had less anticipatory and post chemotherapy nausea and vomiting. Mundy et al. (2003) reviewed 67 studies of behavioral interventions for cancer treatment, and reported that they effectively control anticipatory nausea and vomiting from chemotherapy, can decrease levels of anxiety and distress associated with cancer diagnosis and treatments, and can help control cancer-related pain. Methods involving relaxation and guided imagery have the greatest research support.

Self-help interventions can reduce depression, fatigue, and nausea associated with radiation therapy for cancer (Badger, et al., 2001). In a randomized comparison study, women undergoing radiation therapy for breast cancer who learned muscular relaxation or relaxation and guided imagery from audiotapes had relief from depression, with the group utilizing imagery improving more than the relaxation group. The control group, where women were encouraged to talk about their feelings, had worsened depression during the same time (Bridge, et al., 1988). Audiotapes were also found to be effective in improving self-care and increasing comfort in breast cancer patients undergoing radiation therapy (Hagopian, 1996; Kolcaba & Fox, 1999).

Few approaches in medicine have the risk/benefit ratio and cost-effectiveness of mind-body approaches. For reducing adverse effects of treatment, most people can learn to use relaxation, imagery, and auto-suggestion from inexpensive CDs that allow unlimited home practice. If these results could be obtained from a medication, they would be routinely prescribed for every surgery and chemotherapy patient.

STIMULATING IMMUNITY AND OTHER HEALING RESPONSES

In 1981 Ader and Cohen discovered that the immune system could be classically conditioned, which demonstrated the link between the central nervous and immune systems. Ader (1981) coined the term "psychoneuroimmunology" (PNI) to describe the field that examines the basis and phenomena of this relationship.

From PNI research we now know that there is direct innervation to the thymus gland and lymph nodes, and that lymphocytes not only have receptor sites to all known neurotransmitters, they also produce neurotransmitters that can cause neurological and emotional symptoms. Thus, a biochemical mechanism has been established to explain how depression, anxiety, and related negative or positive emotional states could affect immunity.

Bakke et al. (2002) concluded that hypnosis and guided imagery could enhance both psychological well-being and immune function in patients treated for stage I or II breast cancer. Fawzy et al. (1993b) evaluated the immediate and long-term effects on immune function of a 6-week psycho-educational group with 61 patients with malignant melanoma. They reported reduction in levels of psychological distress, greater use of active coping methods, and significant increases in the percent of large granular lymphocytes and natural killer cells. Gruber and Hall et al. (1993) found that when patients with breast cancer used guided imagery to increase an immune response, they significantly increased numbers and aggressiveness of natural killer cells, an effect which increased with time. In a review of 24 studies, Hall et al. (1993) found evidence of mind-body mediated influence on immunity in 18 of the 24 studies they reviewed.

In addition to the positive effects that mind-body practices can have on immunity, a significant downregulation of immunity has been demonstrated frequently with stressful life events, grief, and depression, all of which commonly accompany a cancer diagnosis (Glaser & Kiecolt-Glaser, 2005).

In addition to having patients imagine an effective immune response, we also encourage patients to imagine cutting off blood supply to tumors, or to imagine turning off the gene switches that stimulate tumor growth. Biofeedback research has shown repeatedly that people can alter blood flow patterns, and suggestion has been shown to reduce bleeding during surgery (Enqvist, et al., 1995; Lucas, 1975; Meurisse, et al., 1996). Altered genetic transcription responses in wounds have been shown to be part of a stress response (Roy, et al., 2005), and immune modulation is a result of upregulation of cytokines due to effects on regulatory genes.

While there is no evidence yet that a patient can specifically reduce blood flow to tumors, or turn off oncogenes, these images serve as autosuggestions representing other potential mechanisms of resisting or overcoming cancer. As long as they are not substituted for more definitive or effective treatment, clinically we feel it is ethical and reasonable to encourage patients to imagine healing in a way that has meaning for them.

REDUCING OR RELIEVING CANCER RELATED PAIN

Pain is both a physical sensation and an emotional experience. The way a patient manages stress, tension, and emotions can amplify or reduce pain. Not every cancer patient has pain, but many do at some point. Research shows that mind-body interventions can reduce or relieve pain in cancer patients, whether from the disease itself or from side effects of treatments.

Redd et al. (2001) reviewed 54 published studies of behavioral intervention methods in the control of aversive side effects of cancer treatments, and reported that hypnotic-like methods, involving relaxation, suggestion and distracting imagery, showed the greatest effects for pain management. Devine (2003) conducted a meta-analysis of the effect of psychoeducational interventions on pain in adults with cancer from 25 studies published between 1978 and 2001 and concluded that "reasonably strong evidence exists for relaxation-based cognitive-behavioral interventions, education about analgesic usage, and supportive counseling."

Dalton et al. (2004) showed in a randomized study of 131 cancer patients that a cognitive-behavioral therapy tailored to patient characteristics reduced pain and interference of pain with sleep, activities, walking, and relationships, and less confusion. Cutson (1998) reported that inclusion of nonpharmacologic treatments, including psychological, are important for effective management of cancer pain. Liossi et al. (2006) and Richardson et al. (2006) both report that hypnosis produced significant reductions in pain, anxiety, and distress in children with cancer undergoing lumbar punctures and other diagnostic and therapeutic procedures. Spiegel and Bloom (1983) showed that both group therapy and hypnosis reduced pain in a randomized study of 54 women with metastatic breast carcinoma. Both interventions reduced pain, and the combination worked better than each alone. Syrjala et al. (1995) found that relaxation and imagery training reduced pain levels in a study with 94 cancer patients receiving bone marrow transplants.

INFLUENCING THE PROGRESSION OR OUTCOME OF THE DIAGNOSIS

A nonintervention study by Cassileth et al. (1985) on patients with advanced metastatic disease showed no correlation at that time between psychosocial factors and survival. However, more recent studies suggest that there may be a survival advantage with psychosocial interventions.

The strongest evidence is a randomized, prospective study conducted at UCLA by Fawzy et al. (1993a) of newly diagnosed melanoma patients participating in a 6-week, 90-minute per week group that taught active behavioral coping skills, including relaxation, assertive communication, and emotional management. After 6 years, there were one-third fewer deaths and recurrences in the treatment group, along with improved immune and psychological functioning. Survival benefit weakened at 10 years but remained significant (Fawzy, Canada, & Fawzy, 2003). Studies by Richardson et al. (1990) and Shrock et al. (1999) also showed a survival advantage with supportive, educational program interventions. In a prospective, longitudinal study, Cunningham et al. (2000) concluded that there appears to be "a strong association between longer survival and psychological factors related to the involvement of cancer patients in psychological self-help activities."

Spiegel et al. (1989) reported a positive effect on survival with cancer in a group intervention with metastatic breast cancer patients. However, a careful replication of this study by Goodwin et al. (2001) demonstrated positive effects on psychological adjustment, mood, and pain perception, but not extended survival.

In a major review of mind-body medicine, Astin et al. (2003) concluded that "The debate regarding whether Mind-Body Therapies can influence survival among cancer patients remains unresolved." We agree with Astin, and also Dreher (1997), who stated that cancer patients should not be denied programs that improve quality of life and well-being simply because there is uncertainty about whether such programs might also lengthen life spans. Dreher cited a number of studies showing that quality of life measures can predict survival. Since we know that psychosocial interventions improve quality of life, and we know that quality of life can predict cancer survival, it is fully justified not only to intensify research into how psychological treatment can possibly extend life for cancer patients, but to make them widely available in clinical practice.

We concur that there is a scientific and moral imperative to provide cancer patients with support and skills that build strength, hope, and psychological resilience. Mind-body interventions offer clear benefits in quality of life, and may offer extended survival as well. Given the low cost, minimal risk, and significant benefits of such interventions, we feel they should be standard of care in cancer treatment.

Precautions and Contraindications to Using Mind-Body Approaches

While mind-body approaches are very safe, especially when compared to most medical and surgical interventions for cancer, there are some precautions to be taken.

First: We do not believe that the evidence warrants that mind-body techniques be offered as stand-alone treatment for any cancer, but that they be offered as ways that patients may be able to help themselves and complement medical care.

Second: Patients with mental illness, especially with a history of psychosis or diffuse dissociative disorders may be at risk for being overwhelmed by emotional content, especially if explorative techniques are used. Patients who have difficulty distinguishing outer reality from inner experience, should work with health professionals who understand these issues and are well-trained in both psychology and mind-body therapies.

Third: Our clinical experience has demonstrated that approximately 10% to 15% of patients have relaxation-induced anxiety and will become more anxious when asked to close their eyes, or as they begin to relax and do imagery work.

Mild cases can respond to reassurance and patience, but more severe cases are assisted best by a qualified health professional.

Fourth: If patients can help themselves by using mind-body approaches, it does not mean that they caused their disease by mind-body error or neglect. Mind-body approaches should offer patients an opportunity to participate in their efforts toward recovery or acceptance, and not be construed as "blaming the victim."

If these precautions are heeded, there is minimal risk and significant benefit to be had by providing mind-body training and support to people with cancer.

Mind-Body Resources for Patients and Physicians

Mind-body interventions often are taught and used as self-help tools, and resources for multimedia and audio teaching tools are listed in the following Resource Guide. Trained health professionals also are available to work with patients either in groups, classes, or individually, depending on the needs and willingness of the patient. Sources for referral are also listed.

RESOURCE GUIDE

Guided Imagery Self-Care Books and Tapes

The Healing Mind

Books and audio programs from Martin Rossman, MD (including book and CD home study program "Fighting Cancer from Within"), Jeanne Achterberg, PhD, Kenneth Pelletier, PhD, Rachel Remen, MD, Emmett Miller, MD, and more. Research reviews and professional community resources listed.
www.thehealingmind.org

Professional Training, Imagery Groups, and Referrals

Academy for Guided Imagery

Provides professional training and certification in Interactive Guided Imagery[sm] and referrals to certified practitioners.
www.acadgi.com

Center for Mind-Body Medicine

Provides training and referrals to Cancer Guides who can help patients survey and navigate their options for treatment.
www.cmbm.org

Simonton Cancer Center, Pacific Palisades, CA

Week-long retreats for cancer patients and support people for self-healing.
www.simontoncenter.com

Commonweal

Week-long retreats for cancer patients and support people for self-healing.
www.commonweal.org

BOOKS

1. Martin LR. (2003). *Fighting cancer from within*. NY: Owl Books.
2. Jeanne A, Barbara, Dossey RN, & Leslie KRN. (1994). *Rituals of healing: Using imagery for health and wellness*. NY: Bantam Doubleday Dell Pub.
3. Lawrence. (1999). *Cancer as a turning point: A handbook for people with cancer, their families, and health professionals*. Plume, NY: EP Dutton.
4. Marc Ian B. (1995). *The healing path: A soul approach to illness*. USA, Penguin.
5. Jean SB. (1998). *Close to the bone: Life-threatening illness and the search for meaning*. NY: Scribner, Touchstone Books.
6. Larry D. (1997). *Prayer is good medicine: How to reap the healing benefits of prayer*. San Francisco, CA: HarperCollins.
7. Dossey L. (1999). *Reinventing medicine*. NY: Harper Collins.
8. Deepak C. (1995). *Creating health: How to wake up the body's intelligence*. NY: Houghton Mifflin Co.
9. Emmett EM. (1997). *Deep healing: The essence of mind/body medicine*. Carlsbad, CA: Hay House.
10. O Carol S, Stephanie M-S, & James LC. (1992). *Getting well again*. NY: Bantam Books.
11. Bernie SS. (1990). *Peace, love and healing: Body-mind communication and the path to self-healing: An exploration*. NY: Harper Perennial Library& Row.
12. Rachel NR. (1997). *Kitchen table wisdom: Stories that heal*. NY: Riverhead Books.
13. Ernest R. (1993). *The psychobiology of mind-body healing: New concepts of therapeutic hypnosis*. NY: W.W. Norton revised Edition.
14. Andrew W. (1996). *Spontaneous healing: How to discover and enhance your body's natural ability to maintain and heal itself*. NY: Ballantine Books.
15. Dean S. (2000). *Doctor's orders: Go fishing*. State College, PA: First Publishers Group.
16. Martin R. (2000). *Guided imagery for self-healing*. Tiburon, CA: HJ Kramer/New World Library.

REFERENCES

Astin JA, Shapiro SL, Eisenberg DM, & Forys KL. (2003). Mind-body medicine: State of the science, implications for practice. *Journal of the American Board of Family Practice,* 16(2), 131–147.

Barsevick AM, Sweeney C, Haney E, & Chung EA. (2002). Systematic qualitative analysis of psychoeducational interventions for depression in patients with cancer. *Oncology Nursing Forum,* 29(1), 73–84.

Eller LS. (1999). Guided imagery interventions for symptom management. *Annual Review of Nursing Research,* 17, 57–84.

Fawzy FI, Kemeny ME, Fawzy NW, Elashoff R, Morton D, Cousins N, et al. (1993a). A structural psychiatric intervention for cancer patients.ii.changes over time in immunological measures. *Archives of General Psychiatry,* 47, 729–735.

Fawzy FI, Fawyz NW, Hyun CD, Elashoff R, Guthrie D, Fahey JL, et al. (1993b). Malignant melanoma: effects of an early structured psychiatric Intervention, coping, and affective state on recurrence and survival 6 years later. *Archives of General Psychiartry,* 50(9), 681–689.

Fawzy FI, Canada AL, & Fawzy NW. (2003). Malignant melanoma: Effects of a brief, structured psychiatric intervention on survival and recurrence at 10-year follow-up. *Archives of General Psychiatry,* 60(1), 100–103.

Goodwin PJ, Leszcz, M, Ennis M, Koopmans J, Vincent L, Guther H, et al. (2001). The effect of group psychosocial support on survival in metastatic breast cancer. *New England Journal of Medicine,* 345(24), 1719–1726.

Gruber BL, Hersh SP, Hall NR, Waletzky LR, Kunz JF, Carpenter JK, et al. (1993). immunological responses of breast cancer patients to behavioral interventions. *Biofeedback and Self Regulation,* 18(1), 1–22.

Hall H, Minness L, & Olness K. (1993). The psychophysiology of voluntary immunomodulation. *International Journal of Neuroscience,* 69(1–4), 221–234.

Mundy EA, DuHamel KN, & Montgomery GH. (2003). The efficacy of behavioral interventions for cancer treatment-related side effects. *Seminars in Clinical Neuropsychiatry,* 8(4), 253–275.

Redd WH, Montgomery GH, & DuHamel KN. (2001). Behavioral Intervention for Cancer Treatment Side Effects. *Journal of the National Cancer Institute,* 93(11), 810–823.

(A complete reference list for this chapter is available online at http://www.oup.com/us/ integrativemedicine).

13

Traditional and Modern Chinese Medicine

QING CAI ZHANG

KEY CONCEPTS

- In Chinese Medicine (CM), cancer is seen as a local manifestation of an underlying constitutional disease. Therefore, CM focuses on whole-body treatment, addressing the far-reaching effects of cancer which the localized treatment of Western Medicine (WM) can underestimate.
- The Chinese concept of cancer is a weakening of resistance in the body while the oncogenic factor grows. Therefore, treatment focuses on strengthening the body's resistance, rather than directly attacking the disease, which might also weaken the body as a whole.
- CM treatment aims to regulate body functions to maximize immunity, and mitigate the side effects, attenuate toxicity, and enhance the therapeutic effects of WM treatments.
- The goal of successful CM treatment is not to eliminate cancer totally, but to allow the patient to survive and maintain quality of life while coexisting with a stabilized cancer.
- Integrative CM combines zero-toxicity treatment with core WM cancer treatments to enhance the therapeutic effects of chemotherapy and radiation, while mitigating their side effects and improving quality of life.
- Cancer treatment is administered in four stages: (1) Initial diagnosis, including surgery, radiotherapy, and chemotherapy; (2) Recovery following aggressive treatment; (3) Additional rounds of treatment to eliminate residual cancer cells; and (4) Long-term recovery to prevent relapse and metastasis. Integration of CM and WM can benefit the patient at each stage.
- To improve postsurgical outcome, CM treatments are used presurgery to improve general health, following surgery to promote

recovery and relief from postsurgery symptoms, and following recovery to restore health and immunity.

- New CM cancer protocols have been developed that suppress cancer growth, promote cancer cell apoptosis, antiangiogenesis, and antimetastasis and prevent relapse.
- CM gives the cancer patient greater confidence and strength to combat illness by improving quality of life.

The theory, practice, and medications of Traditional Chinese Medicine (TCM) and modern Chinese medicine (MCM) for oncology differ significantly from those of Western medicine (WM). Cancer in CM is seen as a local manifestation of an underlying systemic disease occurring within the structure and functions of the body. There are various stages in the disease course, involving multiple body systems. Accordingly, treatment is based on the regulation of multiple targets in order to restore constitutional balance.

A theoretical and practical system of treating malignant diseases with CM herbology has been well established. New treatments are also being developed as an ongoing process of integrating CM and WM. Integrative WM and CM oncology treatment has been practiced for decades and has shown that CM is an excellent adjunct to WM cancer treatment (Yu, et al., 1985). In the area of theoretical research, CM explores various anticancer strategies, such as blocking the cancer cell–growth cycle, inducing cancer-cell differentiation; promoting apoptosis; facilitating antiangiogenesis, antirelapse, and antimetastasis; as well as prevention of cancer development in the first place. These studies have produced an important new concept—zero-toxicity anticancer treatment, which is under development at the Shanghai Traditional Chinese Medicine University and will be discussed later in this chapter (He, et al., 2005).

When combined with core WM treatments, CM is effective at mitigating the side effects and enhancing the therapeutic effects of chemotherapy and radiotherapy. CM can also aid in the preparation for and recovery from surgery, adjustment to biological response moderation (BRM), shrinking and stabilizing tumors, and improving quality of life and long-term prognosis.

However, it is still difficult to provide CM treatments for cancer patients in Western countries. Most oncologists do not want their patients to take any substances they do not prescribe—including dietary supplements—during treatment. Currently, acupuncture is the only accepted CM modality that can be utilized during WM oncology therapy. The mainstay of CM, however, lies in the application of botanical remedies, and it is important to explore how CM can be fully integrated with WM to enhance the effects of cancer treatments. This article is an introduction to the current integration of CM and WM in oncology as practiced and developed in China.

Overview of Integrative Chinese Medicine and Western Medicine Oncology

Integrative Chinese medicine and Western medicine oncology (ICWO) is the main method of modernizing TCM oncology so that CM and WM can be practiced in the same medical settings by the same doctors for the same patients. The modernization movement has also created new terminologies to interpret TCM concepts through the lenses of modern pathophysiology and phytopharmacology. Integrative oncology uses TCM principles for malignant diseases as a guideline and combines WM knowledge—cancer pathophysiology, diagnosis, and pharmacology—to formulate treatment protocols (Yu, et al., 1985). Integrative Chinese and Western oncology has been blending the best aspects of both medical systems and uses each system's understanding of cancer and the status of the individual patient to formulate a comprehensive treatment plan. The efficacy of integrative Chinese and Western oncology has proven to be better than TCM or WM used alone, as will be discussed further later (Yu, 1988; Yu, et al., 2005).

From five decades of development, ICWO has established the following basic precepts among Chinese oncologists:

1. Cancer is termed *zheng xu xie shi* (deficiency of genuine *Qi* and excess of pathogenic *Qi* [see glossary of Chinese terms at the end of chapter]), a chronic weakening of the body's resistance while malignant growth develops. The basic treatment strategy for managing cancer is *fu zheng qu xie* (strengthening the body's resistance to eliminate factors favoring tumor growth). Integrative Chinese and Western oncology studies attempt to explain the nature of *Zheng*, (also called *Zheng qi*, which can be translated as genuine *Qi* denoting life activity and host resistance, i.e., immunity) and *xie* (also called *Xie qi*, which can be any pathogenic factor or pathological damage in a broad sense) and the conflict between them (Yu, 1993).

Genuine *Qi* is responsible for the immune functions of the human body. When it becomes deficient, a favorable environment is created for cancer to occur. In Western terms, this is a deterioration of the immune surveillance function, which fails to discover cancerous mutations as they occur and suppress their growth. Genuine *Qi* is also damaged during the course of the core WM treatments, so CM treatment emphasizes *Fu Zheng* (supporting genuine *Qi*). Sun Yan of the Chinese Science Academy has been advocating Fu Zheng treatment for many decades and has significantly improved the outcome of Integrative Chinese and Western oncology treatments (Sun, 1995).

2. The disease course of cancer can be seen as a dynamic confrontation between genuine *Qi* and malignant growth. The course of treatment can be divided into four stages.

    a. Initial diagnosis, when oncogenesis is the predominant concern, should be followed by aggressive treatments such as surgery, chemotherapy, and radiation therapy, as well as anticancer herbs to eliminate cancer cells. At the same time, CM can be used to mitigate the toxicity of aggressive WM treatments and enhance their therapeutic effects.

    b. Recovery following aggressive treatments, after the cancer load has been dramatically reduced. Treatment is focused on maximizing recovery of the hematopoietic and immune functions of the bone marrow. CM treatment is used to restore general health by rebuilding zheng Qi.

    c. Additional rounds of anticancer treatment are used to eliminate residual cancer cells.

    d. Long-term recovery using supportive and adjuvant anticancer methods to prevent relapse and metastasis.

3. ICWO treatment should be based on WM's disease differentiation and CM's syndrome differentiation, the latter of which rationally addresses the relationship between the local lesion and systemic health and also the individualization of treatment. In CM, a syndrome is a summary of the patient's general health status, in which illness is seen as a result of functional imbalances caused by pathological changes in the context of the patient's internal constitution. The combination of systemic CM and cancer-focused WM treatments yields better efficacy than either modality used by itself.

4. The success of CM cancer treatment is not gauged by total elimination of the cancer. Instead, if malignancy cannot be eradicated, the objective is to allow the patient to survive and maintain quality of life while coexisting with the cancer. The purpose of Integrative Chinese and Western oncology cancer treatment is to prolong life and improve the quality of life. Thus, if the patient's condition can be stabilized, quality of life improved, and survival time prolonged while living with a stabilized cancer, the treatment efficacy should be considered to be better than if the cancer is reduced but the patient displays a

diminished quality of life and a reduced life span. The objective is to transform cancer into a chronic manageable disease (Yu, et al., 2005).

Integrating Chinese Medicine with Core Western Cancer Treatments

Following a diagnosis of cancer, all possible methods should be used to eliminate cancer cells. The main WM methods are surgery, chemotherapy, radiation therapy, biologic response modifiers, including targeted therapies. These treatments focus on the cancer itself and can quickly reduce tumor load. CM offers supportive treatments to regulate body functions to restore immunity, mitigate the side effects of WM treatments, attenuate toxicity, and enhance the therapeutic effects of WM methods. CM can act synergistically, sensitizing originally insensitive cancer cells to WM therapies, while attenuation of toxicity can make patients more tolerant of WM treatments (Yu, 1992).

Surgery and Chinese Medicine

Surgery is the first treatment choice in early- to mid-stage cancer, provided the cancer is localized and operable. The removed tissue can then be used for pathological and immunological examinations, as well as medication sensitivity tests.

Surgery, however, causes injury to the body and may promote metastasis and implantation to the surrounding tissues. Only those patients with lesions in situ or with diagnosis during the earliest stage can be cured by surgery alone. Surgery is most often combined with chemotherapy, radiotherapy, and biologic response modifiers. In China, surgery is routinely combined with CM treatments.

In order to improve long-term postsurgical outcomes, CM herbal treatments are used for three purposes:
- **Presurgery to prepare the patient by improving general health and the health of particular organs and systems, such as the liver and the cardiovascular system**
- **Immediately following surgery to promote recovery from surgical injury and anesthesia and to relieve postsurgery symptoms, such as low-grade fever and digestive disruptions, thereby preparing the patient for chemotherapy or radiotherapy**
- **Following recovery from surgery to restore general health and immunity to reduce the risk of recurrence and metastasis**

Before surgery, CM treatments can be used to reduce the risks of the procedure. Chinese oncologists have been using *sheng qi* (ginseng and *astragalus*) injection and administration of the polysaccharide fraction of *zhu ling* mushroom (*Polyporus umbellatus*) preoperatively to promote postsurgical recovery and improve immunity (Yu, et al., 2005) Presurgical use of anticancer herbal preparations such as 10% emulsion of *ya dan zi* (*Fructus bruceae*) strengthened immune reactions around the tumor as observed on pathology slides (Yu, et al., 2005). *Spleen qi-* (digestive function-) supportive herbs are used after surgery to promote recovery from the procedure itself (Yu, et al., 2005).

Both the cancer's direct effects and the trauma of anesthesia and surgery can suppress immune function. This, in turn, favors the escape of residual cancer cells from immune detection, increasing the possibility of recurrence and metastasis. CM treatment can help restore immune functions to reduce these risks (Yu, 1993).

Li Q et al. reported the immune-cell activities of 67 hepatocellular carcinoma (HCC) patients before and after surgery. Thirty patients were treated with CM herbal decoctions, consisting of the following substances:

- *Dang gui* (*Angelicae radix*)
- *Huang qi* (*Astragali radix*)
- *Bai ying* (*Solanum lyratum*)
- *Long guei* (*Solanum nigrum*)

Another 37 cases without herbal treatment acted as the control group. The results of immune cell counts before and after surgery are shown in Table 13.1. In the control group, the presurgery level was similar to the treatment group. Postsurgery levels of CD_3^+, CD_4^+, CD_4^+/CD_8^+, B cells, and natural killer (NK) cells were lower compared with presurgery levels. The postsurgery levels of

Table 13.1. Immune Cell Counts before and after Surgery for Hepatocellular Carcinoma.

Group	N	CD_3^+	CD_4^+	CD_8^+	CD_4^+/CD_8^+	B%	NK%
CM Rx	30	Presurgery 69.49 ± 9.10	47.72 ± 6.39	29.09 ± 6.39	1.64 ± 0.31	8.32 ± 2.69	23.68 ± 8.38
		Postsurgery 67.36 ± 2.88*	37.66 ± 1.53*	27.02 ± 1.73*	2.33 ± 0.98**	19.49 ± 11.10*	16.28 ± 11.30*
Control	37	Postsurgery 64.65 ± 1.16	36.31 ± 1.16	29.33 ± 0.58	1.54 ± 0.55	16.51 ± 9.56	9.40 ± 7.70

Compared with control group, * $P < 0.05$, ** $P < 0.01$.

the CM-treated group were significantly better than postsurgery levels of the control group. Among these figures, CD_4^+/CD_8^+ is especially interesting. The stability of this ratio maintains normal immune function. The cancer load, anesthesia, and the injury of the surgery all can suppress immunity and cause an imbalance in the ratio of T-cell subsets. The CM-treated group had significantly higher CD_4^+/CD_8^+ ratios compared with the control group. This may be related to the bone-marrow protective and immune regulatory effects of the herbal treatment. The immune-protective effects can help reduce the chance of postsurgery relapse and metastasis (Li, et al., 2005).

Rao XQ et al. reported that postsurgery CM treatment can improve the long-term survival of late-stage gastric cancer patients. In a study of 81 postsurgery stage III and IV gastric cancer patients, the CM herbal formula *shen xue tang* (hematopoiesis-promoting formula), combined with chemotherapy regimens (methotrexate, 5-fluorouracil, and vincristine [MFV], and mitomycin, 5-fluorouracil, and cisplatin [MFC]) extended survival compared to the control group. This was calculated according to the life table method and demonstrated that the survival time for the CM-plus-chemotherapy group was 3.2 years compared to 1.1 years for the chemotherapy-only group. The results are shown in Table 13.2 (Rao, et al., 1994).

Xu L et al. reported the metastasis rates of two groups of postsurgery lung cancer patients using the CM formula *Yi fei kang ai yin* (Lung nourishing anti-cancer decoction). One group was treated with CM combined with chemotherapy, while the control group was treated with stand-alone chemotherapy. They found that the CM-treated group had a significantly lower metastasis rate ($P < 0.01$). In addition, the CM-treated group showed greater activity levels of NK cells, OKT3, and OKT4 (Xu & Liu, 1997).

Li XR, et al. reported similar results in a study of 58 postsurgery lung cancer patients. When the CM herbal formula *Xiao liu ping* (Tumor-resolving formula) was combined with chemotherapy, the metastasis rate was 12.5%, and the relapse rate was 25%. In comparison, the rates in the stand-alone chemotherapy control group were 58.33% and 66.67%, respectively ($P < 0.05$) (Li, Zhou, Jiao, Ji, & Song, 2001). Clinical observations were done on the preventive treatment

Table 13.2. Survival Time of Late-Stage Stomach Cancer Patients Treated with Chinese Medicine (CM) and Chemotherapy and Stand-Alone Chemotherapy.

Group	Survival Time	3 Years Survival Rate	5 Years Survival Rate
CM + Chemo	3.188	54.8%	34.4%
Chemo	1.12	17.6%	5.9%

$P < 0.01$.

and treatment after cancer lesion therapy in lung cancer. These studies showed that TCM treatments were able to reduce the rate of relapse and metastasis (Liu, Lin, Biao, & Li, 2003).

Chemotherapy and Chinese Medicine

As the most important core WM systemic treatment, chemotherapy aims to kill cancer cells with cell-growth cycle-specific or nonspecific cytotoxic drugs. While suppressing metabolically active cancer cells, these drugs also suppress fast-growing normal tissues in the body, such as the bone marrow, causing considerable adverse effects. Damage to the bone marrow negatively affects hematopoietic functions, thus weakening immunity. Suppression of the epithelial lining of the gastrointestinal tract leads to digestive dysfunctions. Toxicity also affects liver, kidney, and cardiovascular functions.

CM herbal treatment during chemotherapy mitigates these side effects, enhances therapeutic effects, and improves QOL and long-term survival. Herbal treatment can also help patients better tolerate chemotherapy and complete the treatment plan.

Liu LM et al. reported the use of CM "heat-clearing, Qi-circulating, phlegm-resolving, and lump-dissolving" methods combined with chemotherapy in the treatment of pancreatic cancer. The comparison of the survival times between the CM-plus-chemotherapy group and chemotherapy-only group are listed in Table 13.3. The results showed that the CM-treated group survived significantly longer (Liu, 2004).

Liu J, et al. reported that postsurgery colon cancer patients treated with stand-alone chemotherapy fared worse than those patients treated with CM *jian pi huo xue* (strengthening digestion and promoting blood circulation) herbal treatment combined with chemotherapy: remission rates were 33.3% and 39.5%, respectively. In addition, digestive dysfunctions were improved in

Table 13.3. Survival Time of CM-Plus-Chemotherapy and Chemotherapy-Only Pancreatic Cancer Patients.

Group	1 Year %	2 Years %	3 Years %	5 Years %	Median Survival
CM + Chemo	53.37 ± 3.24	34.61 ± 16.31	25.96 ± 24.64	25.96 ± 24.64	16.3 months
Chemotherapy	21.95 ± 27.54	7.31 ± 27.54	0	0	7.5 months

$P < 0.01$.

the CM-treated group ($P < 0.01$), and adverse reactions to chemotherapy were significantly less in the CM-treated group ($P < 0.05$) (Liu, et al., 2005).

In the treatment of 60 stage III and IV non–small cell lung cancer patients, Zou et al. used Huang qi (*Astragalus*) injections combined with chemotherapy and compared the results with a stand-alone mitomycin-C, vindesine, and cisplatin chemotherapy protocol. The results of this randomized trial are listed in Table 13.4. *Astragalus* enhanced the effect of the chemotherapy and improved the patients' quality of life. The symptomatic improvement rate in the CM-plus-chemotherapy group was 80.4%, compared with the stand-alone chemotherapy group's 50% ($P < 0.01$). The quality of life improved in 13/30 (43%) of the CM-treated group compared to 7/30 (23%) of the control group ($P < 0.01$) (Zou &Liu, 2003). *Astragalus'* efficacy enhancing and toxicity reducing effects for chemotherapy have been seen in different clinical studies (Duan & Wnag, 2002).

Astragalus-based herbal treatment is the cornerstone of "Fu Zheng" therapy, which has been extensively used in China as an adjunct to chemotherapy. From 1978 to 2004, there were 1,305 articles published on treating non–small cell lung cancer with platinum-based chemotherapy combined with *astragalus*-based herbal treatment. McCulloch et al. performed a meta-analysis of 34 randomized studies representing 2,815 patients (McCulloch, et al., 2006). Twelve studies (n = 940) reported a reduced risk of death at 12 months (risk ratio [RR] = 0.67; 95% CI, 0.52 to 0.87). Thirty studies (n = 2,472) reported improved tumor response data (RR = 1.34; 95% CI, 1.24 to 1.46). In a subgroup analyses, herbal formula *Jin Fu Kang* used in two studies (n = 221) reduced risk of death at 24 months (RR = 0.58; 95% CI 0.49 to 0.68) and in three studies (n = 411) increased tumor response (RR = 1.76; 95% CI, 1.23 to 2.53). Another herbal *Ai Di* injection used in four studies (n = 257) reported stabilized or improved Karnofsky performance status (RR = 1.28; 95%cl, 1.12 to 1.46). The authors concluded that the *astragalus*-based Chinese herbal medicine may increase effectiveness of platinum-based chemotherapy when combined with chemotherapy. These results require confirmation with rigorously controlled trials.

Table 13.4. *Huang qi* Injection Combined with Chemotherapy and Stand-Alone Chemotherapy for Non–Small Cell Lung Cancer.

Group	N	PR NC PD	Average R	Median	1 Year	2 Years	3 Years
CM + chemo	30	14 14 4	5.4 months	11 months	46.7%	30.0%	16.7%
Chemo	30	11 11 5	3.3 months	7 months	13.3%	6.7%	6.7%
		$P > 0.05$	$P < 0.05$	$P < 0.05$	$P < 0.05$	$P > 0.05$	$P > 0.05$

CM's toxicity-attenuation and efficacy-potentiating effects on chemotherapy have been extensively tested in various animal models (Li, et al., 2004). In one study, the CM formula *Si jun zi tang* was given to mice implanted with bladder carcinoma. The results showed that the CM-treated group required a reduced drug dosage compared to the chemotherapy-only group in suppressing the same amount of cancer load (Li, et al., 2005).

Chinese Medicine for Western Medicine Treatment Toxicities

In WM, the toxic effects of chemotherapy on the gastrointestinal and immune systems can be treated with serotonin receptor antagonists and colony-stimulating factors; however, these treatments are costly. Xia AJ et al. treated toxic side effects with the CM herbal formula *Jia wei gui zhi ren shen tang* (Modified Cinnamon and Ginseng Combination) and found that the patients' white blood cell, platelet, T lymphocyte, and T-cell subsets after chemotherapy showed no significant change. The levels in the stand-alone chemotherapy group, however, were significantly worse post chemotherapy. The CM-treated group also experienced less nausea and vomiting. The effects of the herbal treatment were similar to the effects of antiemetics and colony-stimulating factors in mitigating the side effects of chemotherapy, but it was much less costly (Xia & Kuang, 2002).

Cisplatin has been used extensively as a broad-spectrum anticancer drug. Its anticancer effects have proven quite satisfactory. However, it is toxic to the kidneys and may cause kidney failure and even death. When cisplatin was used alone, kidney toxicity occurred in approximately 28% to 36% of patients (Williams & Hottendorf, 1985). In order to mitigate the toxic effects on the kidneys, large-volume intravenous drip hydration is used. This requires about 4,000 ml of fluids to be infused per day and is difficult for patients to tolerate. Even with hydration, about 10% to 20% of patients may still develop azotemia (Campbell, Kalman, & Jacobs, 1983).

Zheng JH et al. of Jiangxi Province Cancer Hospital designed the herbal formula *Jiang pi yi qi li shui tang* (spleen-nourishing, *Qi*-supporting, and diuresis-promoting formula) to treat kidney toxicity. This herbal treatment was much more effective than aggressive hydration in mitigating cisplatin's renal toxicity. It was observed that in 95 cases treated with cisplatin, the herbal formula showed a 93% efficacy rate. The CM-treated group showed much lower blood urea nitrogen and creatinine levels compared to the hydration group ($p < 0.05$ to $p < 0.01$). Also, the CM-treated group showed much lower levels of beta-2-microglobulin, urine N-acetyl-β-D-glucosamidase, and urine proteins indicating that the glomerular filtration and reabsorption rates were protected.

ed with chemotherapy, but actually the system...

With CM treatment, only one-third of usual amount of intravenous fluid was required.

Jiang pi yi qi li shui tang consists of following herbs:

- *Huang qi* (*Astragali radix*)
- *Bai zhu* (*Atractylodis macrocephalae rhizoma*)
- *Gui zhi* (*Cinnamomi ramulus*)
- *Fu ling* (*Polyporus, Poria*)
- *Dang shen* (*Codonopsis pilosulae radix*)
- *Ze xie* (*Alisma orientale*)
- *Zhu ling* (*Polyporus umbellatus*)
- *Gan cao* (*Glycyrrhiza uralensis*)

It is a modified form of the traditional formula *Wuling san* (Hoelen Five Herb Formula) (Zheng, et al., 1994).

The CM herbal formula *Wei chang an* (WCA), traditionally used for regulating the gastrointestinal system, has been used for postsurgery patients with progressive stages of gastric cancer. The composition of WCA is as follows:

- *Bai zhu* (*Atractylodis macrocephalae rhizoma*)
- *Fu ling* (*Polyporus*)
- *Xia ku cao* (*Prunellae spica*)
- *Hong teng* (*Sargentodoxae caulis*)

A clinical study evaluated three randomized groups of gastric-cancer patients: group 1 used stand-alone WCA, group 2 used stand-alone chemotherapy, and group 3 used a combination of WCA and chemotherapy. The short- and long-term survival rates and metastasis rates of these three groups are shown in Table 13.5.

The 1-, 2-, and 3-year survival rate differences between stand-alone WCA and combined WCA-and-chemotherapy groups were not significant. The

Table 13.5. Short- and Long-Term Survival Rates and Metastasis Rates of Gastric Cancer Patients.

Group	N	1 Year (%)	2 Years (%)	3 Years (%)	1 Year Metastasis (%)	2 Years Metastasis (%)	3 Years Metastasis (%)
WCA	59	93.23	79.34	71.78	15.25	28.81	33.90
Chemo	31	83.86	59.33	49.43	35.48	41.38	46.55
Chemo + WCA	58	89.51	69.77	55.76	15.52	45.16	51.61

differences in the stand-alone WCA and combined WCA-and-chemotherapy groups compared with stand-alone chemotherapy groups, however, were both statistically significant ($P < 0.05$). From the recorded metastasis rates, it was seen that stand-alone chemotherapy had a trend towards higher metastasis, while the WCA herbal treatment reduced metastasis (Yang, et al., 2003).

Upon completion of chemotherapy, herbal treatment can be used to prevent relapse and metastasis, and improve long-term prognosis.

Radiotherapy and Chinese Medicine

Radiotherapy is a localized treatment used in 60% to 70% of cancer patients. Radiation can directly kill cancer cells, but it can also damage surrounding normal cells. The main purposes in using CM treatment for patients undergoing radiotherapy are to enhance the anticancer effects of radiation therapy, reduce its side effects, restore general health, and prevent relapse and metastasis.

Radiation side effects include the suppression of bone marrow and disruption of gastrointestinal functions. According to CM syndrome diagnosis, this is seen as spleen and blood deficiency. The corresponding CM treatment principle is to nourish the blood and spleen. This treatment can also sensitize the cancer cells to the radiation. Yu EX, et al. used a modified *Si jun zi* decoction, a CM herbal formula to sensitize hepatocellular carcinoma, which is generally not sensitive to radiation therapy. This formula was combined with radiotherapy in treating 228 cases of mid-stage hepatocellular carcinoma. (In 1977 the Chinese National Cancer Prevention and Treatment Conference established three stages for hepatocellular carcinoma. In stage I there are no definite clinical symptoms and signs of hepatocellular carcinoma and in stage III there are definite dyscrasias, jaundice, ascites, or distant metastases. Mid-stage or stage II, is in between stages I and III). The 5-year survival rate was 43%, and the median survival time was 53.4 months. In comparison, the 5-year survival rate for stand-alone radiotherapy was 14.5%, and the median survival was 11.1 months ($P < 0.01$). Symptomatically, the CM-treated group exhibited fewer side effects and better appetite, and some patients even gained body weight. This observation suggests that *Si jun zi* decoction sensitized hepatocellular carcinoma to radiation (Yu, 1992).

Nasopharyngeal carcinoma patients treated by radiotherapy combined with CM formulas that promote blood circulation and remove stasis (PBCRS) required smaller doses of radiation than the control group. PBCRS treatment can improve the aerobic condition of the cancer and increase its sensitivity to radiation therapy. When the same dose of radiation was given, combined with CM, the elimination rate of the cancer was markedly higher than using radiotherapy alone, although the original manuscript does not quantitate this difference (Zhang, 1992).

CM considers radiation a form of "heat toxin" that can cause *yin xu huo wang* (hyperactivity of fire due to *yin* deficiency). The Beijing Sino-Japan Friendship Hospital reported that when "constitution-supportive, heat-clearing, and toxin-resolving" herbs were combined with radiation for lung cancer, the effectiveness rate was 70% in comparison with 41% for radiotherapy alone ($P < 0.05$). In addition, adverse reactions to radiation therapy were dramatically reduced (Zhang, et al., 1998).

Li DH, et al. reported that pallasone (Iq761-1), an active compound isolated from the seed of *Gris Pallasi Fisher*, enhanced the effect of radiation on HeLa cells in vitro and on breast cancer and transplanted human colon mucinous adenocarcinoma in mice. A clinical trial of 458 cases, including carcinoma of the lungs, esophagus, and head and neck, confirmed the radiation-enhancing effects of Iq761-1. Clinically, Iq761-1 prolonged the survival time of patients who received radiotherapy (Li, 1987).

Chinese Medicine for Radiotherapy-Related Reactions and Complications

Reactions to radiation, such as inflammation, mucous congestion, ulceration, and infections, can dramatically decrease the patient's QOL. The severity of radiation-induced injury increases with dosage and duration of treatment. CM treatments can help reduce symptoms, such as nasopharyngeal soreness caused by head and neck radiation, and prevent and treat acute radiation-induced pneumonitis, carditis, and esophagitis (Pan, Zhang, Yu, Yu, & Yu, 1992).

Yang et al. used CM formulas orally and topically on the skin and mucous membranes to treat radiation injuries. They observed 120 cases of head- and neck-cancer patients: 60 patients used combined CM and radiotherapy, the other 60 used stand-alone radiation. A topical aerosol spray was made from the extracts of following herbs:

- *Zhe bei mu (Fritillaria thunbergii)*
- *Xuan shen (Scrophularia ningpoensis)*
- *She gan (Belamcanda chinensis)*
- *Ban lan gen (Isatidis Radix)*
- *Sheng di (Rehmannia glutinosa)*
- *Gan cao (Glycyrrhiza uralensis)*
- *Bing pian (Borneolum syntheticum)*
- *Bo he nao (Mentholum)*

The aerosol was sprayed into the mouth and nose four to five times per day. The oral decoction was made from the following:

- *Dang shen (Codonopsis Pilosulae Radix)*
- *Huang qi (Astragali Radix)*
- *Bai zhu (Atractylodis Macrocephalae Rhizoma)*
- *Bei sha shen (Glehmia littoralis)*
- *Mai dong (Ophiopogon japonicus)*
- *Sheng di (Rehmannia glutinosa)*
- *Gan cao (Glycyrrhiza uralensis)*
- Xuan shen (*Scrophularia ningpoensis*)
- *Jin yin hua (Lonicerae Flos)*
- *Dang gui (Angelicae Radix)*
- *Dan shen (Salviae Miltiorrhziae Radix)*
- *Chuan xiong (Ligusticum chuanziong)*
- *Pang da hai (Steculia scaphigera)*

The decoction was given twice a day. The radiation dose and duration used for both groups were the same, and radiation reactions were evaluated according to the Acute Radiation Reaction Ranking System.

The acute mucositis reactions were ranked on a five-point scale: 0, no change; 1, congestion of mucous membrane and pain that did not require painkillers; 2, patchy mucus discharge with inflammation and moderate pain that required pain killers; 3, fused fibrotic mucus inflammation with severe pain that required analgesics; and 4, ulceration with bleeding. No patient in the group that used CM with radiotherapy needed to stop or interrupt the treatment. There were seven cases in the stand-alone radiation group that needed to interrupt treatment because of inability to tolerate the side effects. The results of the reaction rankings are presented in Table 13.6. The results show that CM treatments were able to reduce the severity of reactions to the radiation, facilitate the completion of radiotherapy course, and improve QOL (Yang, Zhong, & Liu, 2003).

Table 13.6. Comparison of Grade of Mucositis in Radiation Plus CM and Radiation Alone Groups.

Group	n	Rx Interruption	Grade I	Grade II	Grade III	Grade IV
CM + radiation	60	0	26	15	16	3
Radiation	60	7	4	14	27	15

$\chi^2 = 26.98$, $P < 0.01$.

Hu YR, et al. reported similar results with *Shen qi fang hou* formula for head and neck radiotherapy effects. They found that the oropharyngeal mucosa reaction, dryness in the mouth, and radiation-related dermatitis in the cervical region in the treated group were milder than in the control group. Moreover, radiation-induced side effects such as difficulty in opening the mouth were reduced in the treated group. Cervical muscular sclerosis was much less in the treated group, and the differences were significant ($P < 0.01$) (Hu, et al., 2005). They also used Shenling baizhu san (Ginseng and *Atractylodes* Formula) to treat postradiation colitis and found that, during the radiation, the treated group had fewer bowel movements per day and less stomach pain and mucus in the stool compared with the control group ($P < 0.05$). One year after the radiation, the severity and rate of radiation colitis were also less in the treated group ($P < 0.05$) (Hu, et al., 2004).

Biological Response Modifiers and Chinese Medicine

CM syndrome differentiation-based treatments can be considered a form of biologic response modification. The purpose of the treatment is to restore the body's general health and immunity. It is a multitarget regulatory treatment that aims to suppress the cancer by supporting and supplementing the body's innate defenses against malignant growth. CM attempts to regulate body functions on a wider scale, whereas biologic response modification focuses on the replacement or supplementation of one or a few molecules.

The immune status of a patient is the most important factor in determining the success or failure of cancer treatment. A weakened or dysfunctional immune system is a major predisposing factor to the initial occurrence of cancer. An escalating cancer load can further suppress immunity, which favors tumor spread. The three major WM treatments—surgery, chemotherapy, and radiotherapy—can all impact immunity, increasing the possibility of recurrence and metastasis after initial treatment. The major role of CM in the comprehensive treatment plan is to maintain immune function so that the benefits of WM treatments can be fully realized.

CM herbal anticancer treatments have a Fu zheng (genuine-Qi or immune-supportive) effect. Experimental studies found that herbs such as *Huang qi* (*astragali radix*) and Xiaochaihu decoction (*Minor bupleurum* combination) can enhance NK cell and lymphokine-activated killer (LAK) cell activities and increase the production of tumor necrosis factor. NK cells are able to kill cancer cells, both in vivo and in vitro; they are the body's first line of anticancer defence (Liu, et al., 2003).

Interleukin-2 (IL-2) is the T-cell-promoting factor that is the core material in the body's immune network. In cancer, the body's ability to produce and react to IL-2 decreases following surgery, chemotherapy, and radiotherapy. This form of immune deficiency can lead to infection, systemic inflammatory response syndrome, and multiple-organ dysfunction, as well as recurrence and metastasis.

Yu et al. treated postoperative gastric cancer patients with the *Jian pi tong li* (digestion-nourishing and bowel movement–facilitating) decoction as an intestinal drip.

The formula consists of

- *Huang qi* (*Astragali radix*)
- *Da huang* (*Rhei rhizoma*)
- *Bai zhu* (*Atractylodis macrocephalae rhizoma*)
- *Dang shen* (*Codonopsis pilosulae radix*)
- *Huang qin* (*Scutellariae radix*)
- *Hou pu* (*Magnoliae cortex*)
- *Zhi shi* (*Citri aurantii fructus*)
- *Dan shen* (*Salviae miltiorrhziae radix*)

The method entails twice-a-day installation of the herbal decoction via a nasogastric tube inserted into the intestine during surgery. A dose of 150 cc of the decoction, at a body temperature, was infused at a rate of 30 to 40 cc per minute. The control group received a similar drip of normal saline. The herbal decoction significantly improved the patients' IL-2, soluble IL-2 receptor, and IL-12 levels. The changes in immune markers are shown in Table 13.7. The results showed that early intra-intestinal administration of this decoction improved the immune markers of postoperative gastric cancer patients (Yu, et al., 2005).

Table 13.7. Immunity-Marker Changes in CM and Control Groups.

Group	Time	N	IL-2 (mg/L)	SIL-2R (U/mL)	IL-12 (ng/L)
Control	1 day presurgery	30	211.00 ± 44.45	341.75 ± 35.81	233.79 ± 38.46
	7 day postsurgery	28	216.29 ± 37.87	330.50 ± 48.17	244.71 ± 28.21
CM Rx	1 day Presurgery	30	209.97 ± 24.12	339.66 ± 37.60	230.79 ± 23.83
	7 day postsurgery	29	231.62 ± 29.37*	305.41 ± 49.37*	247.97 ± 31.48**

*Compared with presurgery in the same group, $P < 0.05$.

**Compared with postsurgery in control group, $P < 0.05$.

Cancer Prevention with Chinese Medicine

Chinese Medicine theory considers cancer a condition resulting from long-term influence of carcinogenic factors on the body. Generally, it takes decades for most cancer conditions to develop from a few cellular mutations to a clinically evident disease. A major internal environmental factor underlying cancer development is felt to be cellular ischemia and malnutrition. CMs promoting blood circulation and resolving stasis treatment can be used to relieve cellular ischemia and malnutrition by promoting microcirculation. The same type of treatment helps reduce the risk of metastasis by preventing cancer embolus formation in the bloodstream (Gan, Song, Wang, Wang, & Xu, 2003).

Some chronic inflammatory conditions can cause precancerous cell proliferation and malignancy. A study designed to interrupt severe esophageal epithelial hyperplasia with a modified CM formula called *Liu wei di huang* decoction in high-risk areas for esophageal carcinoma found that one ingredient of the modified formula, the herb *Bergenia purpurascens,* produced better anti-inflammatory and symptomatic therapeutic effects on esophageal epithelial hyperplasia than vitamin A (Liu, et al., 1983).

Han XH, et al. reported that CM treatment inhibited cancerous changes in chronic hepatitis patients with alpha-fetoprotein elevation. They treated 123 cases of alpha-fetoprotein-positive patients followed for 1 year and found only one case developed hepatocellular carcinoma compared with the control group without TCM treatment where there were 6 cases (Han, et al., 1991).

Human papillomavirus causes cervical cancer. The precancerous dysplasia is usually detected by a PAP smear. Treating premalignant mucous papules is important in the prevention of cervical cancer. WM treatment uses lasers, cryotherapy, and topical medications to remove the local lesions; however, relapse rates are high. CM herbal treatments combined with WM treatments can dramatically reduce relapse rates (Wu, Jiang, & Wang, 2003). In the Zhang Clinic, allitridi, a precursor of allicin, is used as a vaginal suppository for 2 to 3 weeks and, so far, dysplasia has receded in every single case.

The anticarcinogenic mechanisms of catechins (GTCs) in tea were first reported by Japanese scientists who found that people living in green tea–drinking areas showed much lower cancer-incidence rates than people in areas where green tea drinking was not as prevalent. This phenomenon was especially noticeable in cases of stomach and liver cancer. Bettuzzi et al. of the University of Parma in Italy studied the antiprostate cancer actions of green tea catechins and epigallocatechin gallate (ECGC). It was found that green tea catechins and EGCG inhibited cancer cell growth in laboratory animals (Bettuzzi, et al.,

2005). In a study of 64 men with high-grade prostate intraepithelial neoplasia, a lesion that often develops into prostate cancer within one year, 32 of these men were treated with 200 mg of green tea cathechins three times a day for one year while the remaining 32 men took identical placebo pills. One year later, only 1/32 (3%) of the treated group developed prostate cancer, compared to 9/32 (30%) of the placebo group. The difference was statistically significant, and no side effects were observed. This study showed that green tea cathechins could be a safe and effective preventive measure against the development of prostate cancer (Bettuzzi, et al., 2005).

Theoretical Studies of Chinese Medicine Oncology

CM has identified new anticancer agents that suppress cancer cells, promote cancer cell apoptosis, antiangiogenesis, antimetastasis, and improve quality of life. In the past 50 years, nearly 400 active herbal compounds have been found to have anticancer effects. The following have been used clinically in China as anticancer medications: arsenic trioxide (As_2O_3), bruceine, campto-thecine, catharanthine, cephalotaxine, coixenolide, ginsenoside Rg3, indirubin, matrine, rubescensin, taxol, tripterine, and vinblastine (Ji, et al., 1998; Jian & Yan, 1986).

Arsenic trioxide (As_2O_3) is called *Pi shuong* in Chinese and is a well-known TCM toxin. Its application in China for cancer dates back several hundred years. The TCM formulas *Qing huang san* and *Shi wei huan* have been used for treating cancer, and recent scientific analysis of their constituents found that the effective ingredient is arsenic trioxide. In 1992, Harbin Medical University first confirmed the therapeutic effect of As_2O_3 in treating acute promyelocytic leukemia and reported it in 1996 (Zhang, 1996). Chen et al. further confirmed its effects and also used As_2O_3 on leukemia patients resistant to all-trans retinoic acid. A high rate of complete remission with no bone-marrow suppression was achieved. Shen ZX et al. studied the mechanism of its actions on cytological and molecular levels (Shen, et al., 1997). The Chinese Food and Drug Administration approved arsenic trioxide as an anticancer medication in 1999. The U.S. Food and Drug Administration also approved its use as a treatment for acute promyelocytic leukemia.

Rubescensin is an active ingredient of *Dong ling cao* (*Rubdosia rebescens*). It strongly suppresses esophageal cancer cell CaEs-17 in vitro and showed obvious cytotoxicity. Cancer cell growth rate was suppressed by 75% at a concentration of 3 μg/mL. Rubescensin can kill human gastric adenocarcinoma cell line MGc80-3. It strongly suppresses hepatocellular carcinoma cell line BEL-7401 and esophageal cancer cell line 109. Clinically, it has been used for treating hepatocellular carcinoma, pancreatic cancer, breast cancer, rectal cancer, and thyroid cancer. When used as a slow intravenous infusion, side effects are mild and there is no marrow suppression (Li, et al., 1986).

Chinese Medicine Herbal Ingredients that Promote Cancer Cell Apoptosis

Many new cancer protocols are focused on promoting apoptosis of cancer cells. A number of active CM herbal ingredients have demonstrated this ability. The following are but a few examples.

The active ingredient of *Herba Artemisiae annuae* artemisinin as a nontoxic anticancer agent has been extensively studied at the University of Washington. Its derivative, artesunate, is a strong promoter of cancer-cell apoptosis (Efferth, 2002; Efferth, Dunstan, Sauerbrey, Miyachi, & Chitambar, 2001; Hu, 2000). In the Zhang Clinic, it has been used for hepatocellular carcinoma, chronic lymphatic leukemia, and breast cancer and has been found to keep cancer lesions stable.

Curcumin has marked inhibitory effects on the proliferation of the Raji cell, a strain of human non-Hodgkin's lymphoma. It can induce the apoptosis of Raji cells in time- and dose-dependent manners. Following curcumin treatment, the cell cycle of the Raji cell was blocked in the G0/G1 and G2/M phases and those in the S phase decreased proportionally. Curcumin did not show any cytotoxicity nor did it cause the apoptosis of normal mononuclear cells (Ma, et al., 1996; Sun, Liu, Chen, Liu, & Wang, 2004).

Mitosis disturbance and uncontrolled gene expression are the main characteristics of cancer development. Cell proliferation, apoptosis, differentiation, and aging are all cell mitosis cycle dependent. Therefore, the search for herbal substances that can disturb the cell cycle and at same time induce apoptosis is an exciting new approach to cancer treatment (Blagosklonny & Pardee, 2001).

Herbal Derivatives for Antiangiogenesis

Blood vessel formation in the cancerous mass can dramatically accelerate the expansion of the tumor. If the cancer mass becomes larger than 2 mm, the internal cells of the mass become ischemic, causing the secretion of cytokines, such as vascular endothelial growth factor (VEGF), to stimulate angiogenesis. In a metastatic cancer lesion, angiogenesis in the newly formed tumor provides oxygen and nutrition to promote growth as well as to provide additional pathways for metastasis. Therefore, suppressing angiogenesis is an important goal of cancer treatment. Many Chinese herbal derivatives have been studied for this effect, and some were found to be effective in suppressing angiogenesis.

Ginsenoside-Rg3 is an active component of *Ren shen* (*Ginseng radix*), which has shown definite antiangiogenesis effects and was approved by the Chinese FDA as a new anticancer drug. Tao et al. reported its effect on the growth of a metastatic mass of gastric cancer in SCID mice (Tao, Yao, Zou, Zhao & Qiu, 2002). Pan et al. reported its antiangiogenesis effects in immunodeficient mice implanted with human ovarian carcinoma (Pan, Ye, Xie, Chen, & Lu, 2002). When treated with Rg3, the cancer-implanted mice exhibited much smaller tumor masses, no ascites formation, and much lower levels of VEGF mRNA and VEGF protein compared to the untreated mice in the control group.

Gao Y, et al. studied *Hong Su* (tripterine), an active ingredient of *Lei gong teng* (*Tripterygium wilfordii*), and demonstrated its ability to suppress angiogenesis in vitro. Only a very minute dose, 0.1 μg/mL of tripterine, could inhibit 90% of blood vessel epithelial cell growth and microcapillary formation (Gao, et al., 1998).

Chinese Medicine Herbal Ingredients for Antimetastasis and Relapse

Cancer relapse and metastasis are the main causes of treatment failure and death. Metastasis occurs in the following steps: cancer cells detach from the primary lesion and enter the surrounding extracellular matrix. They then enter the blood or lymphatic system where they adhere to the epithelial lining of vessels and move out to extravascular tissues. Finally, they infiltrate distant tissues, stimulate new blood vessel proliferation, and form new lesions. Herbal components can suppress metastasis by interfering with one or more of these steps (Wang & Ling, 2004).

Suppression of the activity of proteolytic enzymes can prevent the degradation of basement membrane and extracellular matrix and prevent penetration by cancer cells. Cancer cells can secrete enzymes, such as cysteine protease, matrix metalloproteinases (MMPs), serine protease, and aspartic acid protease, to degrade the basement membranes and extracellular matrix. MMPs are the most important enzymes facilitating metastasis. Several compounds extracted from Chinese herbs that have shown suppressive effects on these enzymes. Emodin, an active ingredient of *Da huang* (*Rhei Rhizoma*), can suppress MMPs and inhibit the metastatic activities of large-cell lung cancer PG cell. PG cell is a line of lung cancer cells commonly used in China for in vitro studies. Treatment with emodin at concentrations of 40 μmol/L and 80 μmol/L for 24 hours lowered the invasion rate of the PG cells to 77% and 57% of the level of control group, respectively. At the same time, secretion of MMP-2 and MMP-9 was also reduced. This suggests that emodin can inhibit PG-cell metastasis by suppressing the activity of MMPs (Wang, et al., 2001).

Liu HY, et al. found that the extract of *Jin qiao mai* (*Fagopyrum cymosum meissn*) inhibited the metastatic potential of highly invasive melanoma tumor cell strain B16-Bl6 and suppressed the production of type IV collagenase in HT-1080 cells (Liu, et al., 1998).

Shao et al. found that curcumin exerted multiple suppressive effects on the invasive ability of human breast carcinoma cells in the MDA-MB-231 strain. This effect may be related to its upregulatory effect on tissue inhibitor of metalloproteinases (TIMP)-1 and downregulatory effect on MMP-2 (Shao, 2002). Lin et al. tested curcumin and found that it inhibits the invasion of SK-Hep-1 hepatocellular carcinoma cells in vitro and suppressed MMP-9 secretion. At a concentration of 10 mmol/L, curcumin suppressed metastases by 17% and invasion by 71%. The invasiveness of hepatocellular carcinoma is related to the activities of MMP-9 (Lin, Ke, Ko, & Lin, 1998).

Maeda et al. found that three tea polyphenols—epicatechin gallate, epigallocatechin-3-gallate, and theaflavin—can strongly suppress cancer-cell invasion and inhibit MMP-2 and MMP-9's activities in human fibrosarcoma HT-1080 cells (Dell' Aica, Donà, Sartor, Pezzato, & Garbisa, 2002; Maeda, 1999).

Urokinase-type plasminogen activator (u-PA) can degrade many proteins, including fibrin, fibronectin, and laminin. It has been considered one of the most important factors promoting cancer metastasis. Santibanez et al. found that genistein and curcumin can suppress u-PA expression, which was induced by growth factor TGF-beta 1, and can suppress the migratory and invasive phenotype in mouse epidermal keratinocytes (Santibanez, et al., 2000). Ishii et al. found that extracts from *Serenoa repens* suppressed the invasive activity of human urological cancer cells by inhibiting u-PA activator (Ishii, et al., 2001). The extract is one of the main components of the herb saw palmetto, commonly used for prostate and urinary-tract diseases.

Adhesion of cancer cells to the extracellular matrix is also an important step in metastasis. Cell adhesion molecules belong to the families of integrins, selectins, immunoglobulins, and cadherins. Decreasing the expression level of these cell adhesion molecules can reduce or suppress metastasis. Lin et al. found that the active components of two CM herbs—ligustrazine and matrine—can markedly inhibit the adhesion of endotheliocytes to cancer cell line PG and inhibit the expression of cell adhesion molecules CD44 and CD49 in vitro. They can also reduce the permeability of endotheliocytes and block adhesion to the extracellular matrix (Lin, et al., 1999).

The blood of cancer patients is often characterized by hyperviscosity and hypercoagulability, a condition termed "blood stasis" in CM. The changes in platelets and fibrin favor the formation of cancer emboli adhesion bridges between cancer cells and epithelial cells on the basement membrane of micro-capillaries. They can also protect cancer cells from immune detection, facilitating invasion and metastasis. CM promoting blood circulation and resolving-stasis treatment can improve blood quality, reduce clot formation, reduce adhesion between cancer cells and epithelial cells of the micro-capillaries, and decrease penetration of cancer cells into extravascular tissues, thereby suppressing metastasis (Zhang, Bei, Ji, & Biao, 1999).

Chen et al. examined the blood rheology of 25 advanced-stage lung-cancer patients and compared their lab markers to those of 26 healthy individuals. They found that the blood of the lung cancer patients showed hyperviscosity and hypercoagulability. The cancer patients were then treated with chuanxion-yzine (tetramethyl pyrazine), which is the active ingredient of Chuan xiong (*Ligusticum chuanziong*). After treatment, the adhesion and clustering of platelets and blood coagulating factors decreased significantly. It is one of the mechanisms by which chuanxionyzine can prevent cancer metastasis (Chen, Wang, Ying, Wu, & Wang, 1997).

Activator protein 1 (AP-1) is an important transmission channel and nuclear transfer factor. Activated AP-1 participates in metastatic activities, such as degradation of extracellular matrix, adhesion, and angiogenesis by regulating the expression of target genes. Mitani et al. found that berberine, an active ingredient of Huang lian (*Coptis chinensis Franch*), can inhibit spontaneous metastasis of Lewis lung carcinoma through lymph nodes in the mediastinal area and enhance the suppressive effects of irinotecan on growth of implanted tumor and metastasis via lymph nodes. The mechanism of this effect is related to the suppression of the activity and expression of AP-1 and u-PA by berberine, which lowered the penetrating ability of Lewis lung carcinoma (Mitani, Murakami, Yamaura, Ikeda, & Saiki, 2001).

Ichiki et al. found that curcumin, taken orally, can suppress Lewis lung carcinoma's metastasis to lymph nodes. Its mechanism is related to the downregulating effect on AP-1 and suppression of u-PA in the expression of its acceptor (u-PAR) mRNA (Ichiki, et al., 2000).

Most of the active components of these anticancer herbs are either nontoxic or very low in toxicity. They have been used at Shanghai Traditional Chinese Medicine University to develop *zero-toxicity* anticancer therapies, which aim to induce differentiation, promote apoptosis, suppress angiogenesis, prevent metastasis, and block the cancer cell mitosis cycle. Because most of these substances are benign, the treatment principle is in accord with the CM concept *wang dao* ("kingly way"; benevolent governing with a harmless therapeutic method) (He, et al., 2005).

Improving the Quality of Life of the Cancer Patient

Quality of life encompasses physical, psychological, and spiritual health. By improving the quality of life of the cancer patient, CM gives the patient greater confidence and strength to combat the illness. To treat cancer-induced symptoms is one of the most important measures to improve quality of life.

About 70% of late-stage cancer patients suffer from chronic pain, which is the most common and difficult symptom to control. The tumor mass may compress surrounding tissues and cause inflammation and pain that severely impacts quality of life. Treating pain is one of the four major cancer treatment goals of the World Health Organization. The "three-step pain controlling method" of the WHO is effective, but long-term use of analgesics can cause strong side effects, tolerance, and addiction. Wu et al. formulated *Aitonping* (cancer pain-releasing capsule) and administered it to 30 cancer patients who were compared with 30 other patients taking diclofenac. *Aitonping* contains the following herbs:

- Fu zi (*Radix Aconiti lateralis preparata*)
- Ru xiang (*Boswellia carterii*)
- Bi bo (*Piper Longum*)
- Yan hu suo (*Corydalis Yanhusao Rhizoma*)

Significant differences were shown in degree of pain relief, frequency of pain episodes, lessening of persistent and percussion pain, increase of plasma beta-endorphin, and decrease in cramping ($P < 0.05$ or $P < 0.01$) between the two groups. The results also showed that CM treatment was effective in ameliorating blood rheological features, such as the viscosity of the blood indexes and reducing the incidence of adverse reactions compared with the drug-treated group ($P < 0.05$ or $P < 0.01$) (Wu, Jiang, & Wang, 2005).

Acupuncture has been used for symptomatic control for cancer patients to improve quality of life quite effectively. Nausea, vomiting, and peripheral cytopenias are common side effects induced by WM core cancer treatments and contribute to the deterioration of quality of life in cancer patients. Acupuncture and moxibustion can help relieve pain and nausea and also help alleviate peripheral cytopenias caused by radiotherapy or chemotherapy and to improve immunity.

In 1997, the U.S. National Institutes of Health held a Consensus Development Conference on Acupuncture to evaluate its safety and efficacy. The 12-member panel concluded that promising research results showing the efficacy of acupuncture in certain conditions have emerged and that further research is likely to reveal additional areas in which acupuncture will be useful. The panel stated that "There is clear evidence that needle acupuncture treatment is effective for postoperative and chemotherapy-induced nausea and vomiting." It also stated that there are "a number of other pain-related conditions for which acupuncture may be effective as an adjunct therapy, an acceptable alternative, or as part of a comprehensive treatment program" (NIH, 1998). Acupuncture is used for individuals with cancer or cancer-related disorders, especially for pain management (Charlton, 1993; Sellick & Zaza, 1998) and chemotherapy-induced nausea and vomiting control (Xia, et al., 1986). It has also been used for other symptoms, such as anxiety, depression, insomnia, anorexia, weight loss, and diarrhea (Johnstone, Polston, Niemtzow, & Martin, 2002; Niemtzow, 2000). Theoretical studies to explore the mechanism of acupuncture for cancer treatment have been focusing on how acupuncture supports immune functions by increasing blood cell counts and enhancing lymphocyte and NK cell activity. So far, the major clinical observations and trials on acupuncture treatment for cancer patients have focused on symptom management to improve patient QOL. Convincing research data on the effects of acupuncture in cancer patients have emerged from studies of the management of chemotherapy-induced nausea and vomiting (National Cancer Institute, 2006).

For pain control, the acupuncture point prescription is derived from three selection methods.

1. Local points, also called "*Ah shih*" points, are nonfixed points chosen based on the location of the pain or tenderness on the body.
2. Symptomatic points are chosen based on the patient's symptoms and matched according to the traditional acupuncture points prescribed for such symptoms.
3. Channel point selection uses points along a particular organ channel that corresponds to a given symptom. For example, nausea and vomiting are usually treated by needling points along the digestive organ channels (Wang VZ, 1994).

Nausea and vomiting are the most common symptoms. The major points used for these symptoms are: Zusanli (ST36), Shangjuxu (ST37), Tianshu (ST25), Neiguan (PC6), and Zhongwan (CV12).

In China, acupuncture is usually conducted as part of the main treatment protocol for cancer patients undergoing radiation and chemotherapy. It is recognized as having a solid role in the comprehensive care of cancer therapy and has been demonstrated to improve the quality of life of patients. The degree of benefit from acupuncture treatment is dependent on various clinical factors such as presenting symptoms and clinical staging.

Summary

Integrative Chinese and Western medicine oncology has been developing in China for more than 50 years. In China it is routine to use both Western and Chinese medicine together to create a comprehensive treatment plan for cancer patients. This integration greatly improves clinical outcomes, quality of life, and survival.

Conventional Western oncology aims for complete eradication of the cancer cells, and the criterion for a cure is their total absence. Since most patients are diagnosed at a stage in which the cancer has already invaded surrounding tissue or has metastasized to distant locations, surgery, radiation, and chemotherapy cannot often achieve this aim. In the effort to eradicate cancer, overly aggressive treatment regimens are often employed, with resultant damage to patients' immunity, increased likelihood of recurrence and metastasis, and decreased quality of life.

In the practice of integrative Chinese and Western medicine oncology, complete eradication of cancer is not necessarily the aim. Rather, the goals are to extend survival time and enhance quality of life. Patients with strong defenses can coexist with stabilized cancers. Cancer can then be treated as a manageable chronic disease, not unlike insulin-dependent diabetes.

Appendix

GLOSSARY OF CHINESE TERMS

Aitonping. A pain-relieving capsule formulated to treat cancer by improving quality of life. It contains: *fu zi* (*Radix Aconiti lateralis preparata*), *ru xiang* (*Botswellia carterii*), *bi bo* (*Piper Longum*), and *yan hu suo* (*Corydalis Yanhusao Rhizoma*).

Chuan xiong. *Ligusticum chuanxiong* (Fig. 13.1). Active ingredient is chuanxionyzine (tetramethyl pyrazine); it is used to promote blood flow, remove blood stasis, promote flow of Qi and relieve pain.

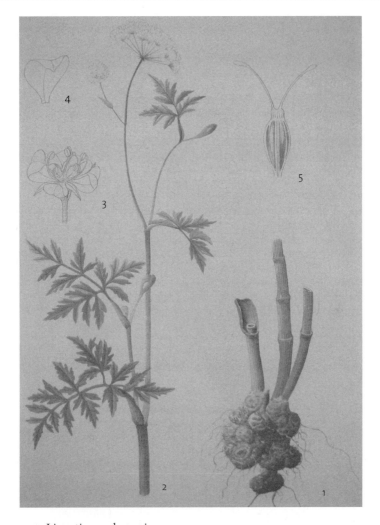

FIGURE 13.1. Ligusticum chuanxiong.
1. Lower part of the stem and the root, 2. Flower wood, 3. Flower, 4. Petal, 5. Fruit (not ripe).

Fu zheng. Strengthens the body's resistance. Support of immunity, or genuine *Qi*. The basis of Chinese cancer treatment is the emphasis on *fu zheng*.
Fu zheng qu xie. Strengthens the body's resistance to eliminate pathogenic factors. The basic Chinese treatment strategy for cancer; strengthening the body's resistance to eliminate oncogenic factors.
Genuine Qi. Zheng qi generally denotes the vital funtion, especially the body's resistance and regenerative capacity. This is the factor responsible for the immune functions in the body. When deficient, a favorable environment is created for cancer to occur.

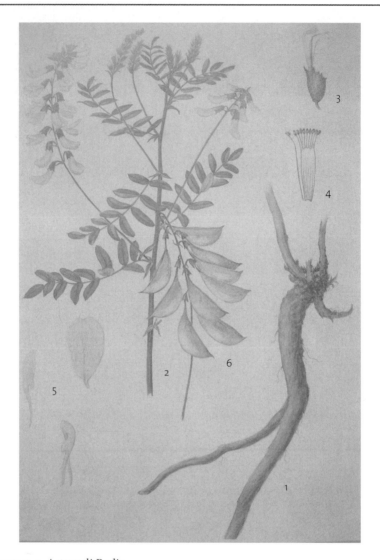

FIGURE 13.2. Astragali Radix.
1. Root 2. Flower wood 3. Calyx, stamen and pistil, 4. Stamen, 5. Petal, 6. Fruit.

Hong su. Tripterine. The active ingredient of *Lei gong teng* (Tripterygium wilfordii), a substance used to suppress angiogenesis.

Huang qi. Dried root of Astragalus (Astragali membranaceous Radix) (Fig. 13.2). It is used to replinish Qi and keep yang-qi ascending, to consolidate superficial resistance, to cause diuressis, and to promote pus discharge and tissue regeneration. A main component of fu zheng treatment. A common ingredient in anticancer formulas, including those used to enhance immunity, reduce toxicity, treat radiation injuries, and facilitate healthy digestion.

Jian pi huo xue. An herbal formula which strengthens digestion and promotes blood circulation. Used to lessen the adverse reactions to chemotherapy.

Jian pi tong li. An herbal decoction used to nourish digestion and facilitate bowel movement. It consists of huang qi (*Astragali radix*), *da huang* (*Rhei rhizoma*), bai zhu (*Astractylodis macrocephalae rhizoma*), dang shen (*Codonopsis pilosulae radix*), huang qin (*Scutellariae radix*), *hou pu* (*Magnoliae cortex*), *zhi shi* (*Citri aurantii fructis*), and dan shen (*Salviae miltiorrhziae radix*).

Jiang pi yi qi li shui tang. A spleen-nourishing, *Qi*-supporting and diuresis-promoting herbal formula used to treat kidney toxicity resulting from chemotherapy. It consists of huang qi (*Astragali radix*), bai zhu (*Atractylodis macrocephalae rhizoma*), gui zhi (*Cinnamoni ramalus*), fu ling (*Polyporus poria*), dang shen (*Codonopsis pilosulae radix*), ze xie (*Alisma orientale*), zhu ling (*Poliporus umbellatus*), and gan cao (*Glycyrrhiza uralensis*); a modified form of *wu ling san*.

Liu lei di huang wan. Bolus of Six Drugs including Rehmannia composed of Di Haung: (Rehmanniae radix), Shan zhu yu (Fructus corni), Fu Ling (Polyporus, Poria), Dan Pi (Moutan Radix Cortex), Shan Yao (Dioscoreae Batatis), and Ze Xie (Alisma orientale). Indicated for: syndrome due to deficiency of vital essence of the Liver and Kidney.

Pi shuong. Arsenic trioxide obtained by purifying crude, natural arsenic, used externally as aphagedenic agent to remove slough and orally (very small dose) as emetic, antirhematic. Atoxin also used as a cancer treatment.

Qi. The basic substance that comprises everything in the universe. In the human body, this refers to vital energy and generally denoting the physiological functions of the internal organs and tissues.

Ren shen. *Ginseng Radix* (Fig. 13.3). Dried root of Panax ginseng, used to reinforce Qi and restore from collapse, to tonify the lung and the spleen, to promote secretion of body fluid and relieve mental stress. One of its active ingredient Ginsenoside-Rg3 is an herbal cancer treatment promoting antiangiogenesis.

Si jun zi tang. Decoction of four Noble Drugs indicated for syndrome of deficiency of Qi of the Spleen and Stomach with symptoms such as dyspepsia, watery stool, lassitude of limbs, pale complexion, slow and weak pulse, or thready and weak pulse. An herbal formula used to decrease the reliance on drugs to combat chemotherapy toxicity and to sensitize HCC to radiation treatment.

Spleen qi. The functional activities of the Spleen includes transport, transformation, sending nutrients upward, and keeping blood flowing within the vessels. It often refers to the digestive function.

Wang dao. "Kingly way;" benevolent governing with a harmless therapeutic method. This is a primary treatment principle in Chinese Medicine.

Wei chang an. An herbal formula used for regulating the gastrointestinal system. Administered to postsurgical patients with gastric cancer in combination

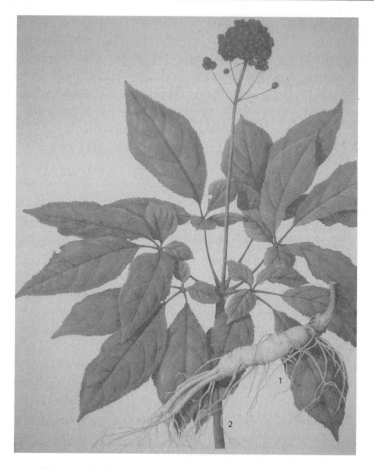

FIGURE 13.3. Ginseng Radix.
1. Root, 2. Branch bearing fruits.

with chemotherapy to promote recovery and reduce metastasis. It consists of bai zhu (*Atractylodis macrocephalae rhizoma*), fu ling (*Polyporus*), xia ku cao, (*Prunellae spica*) and hong teng (*Sargentodoxae caulis*).

Wu ling san. Powder of five Drugs with Poria. Indication: retention of fluid with exterior syndrome.

Xia ku cao. *Prunella spica* (Fig. 13.4). Dried spike of Prunella vulgaris, used to remove heat from the liver, resolve mass, and as an antihypertensive.

Xiao liu ping. An herbal formula used in combination with chemotherapy to resolve tumors and decrease metastasis.

Xie. Any pathogenic factor or pathogenic damage in a broad sense.

Yi fei kang ai yin. A lung-nourishing anticancer decoction, used in combination with chemotherapy.

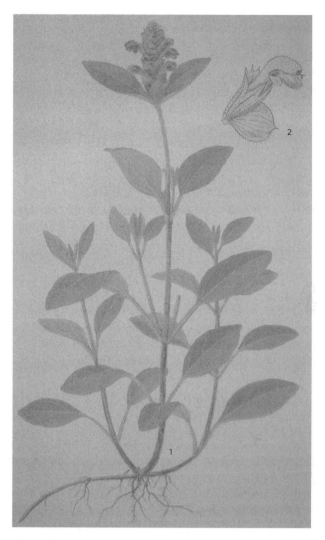

FIGURE 13.4. Prunella Spica.
1. Whole plant, 2. Flower.

Yin xu huo wang. Literally, hyperactivity of fire due to *yin* deficiency. A morbid state due to consumption of yin-essence, which leads to hyperactivity of asthenic fire. In radiotherapy, this is a condition brought on by radiation.
Zheng qi. Genuine *Qi* denoting the vital function and the body resistance, the immunity. Chinese cancer treatment focuses on the restoration of zheng qi.
Zheng xu xie shi. Body's resistance weakened while pathogenic factors prevailing. Chinese term for cancer, meaning a deficiency of genuine *Qi* and excess of pathogenic *Qi*.

REFERENCES

Efferth T, Dunstan H, Sauerbrey A, Miyachi H, & Chitambar CR. (2001). The anti-malarial artesunate is also active against cancer. *International Journal of Oncology,* 18, 767–773.

He YM, Gao YT, Li FJ, et al. (2005). Zero-toxicity anti-cancer treatment. In YM He (Ed.), Modern Chinese Medicine Oncology, (p. 134). Chinese Union Medical University Press, Beijing.

McCulloch M, See C, Shu X-J, Broffman M, Kramer A, Fan W-Y, et al. (2006). *Astragalus*-based Chinese herbs and platinum-based chemotherapy for advanced non-small-cell lung cancer: Meta-analysis of randomized trials. *Journal of Clinical Oncology,* 24(3), 419–430.

National Cancer Institute, Acupuncture (PDQ®) Health Professional Version, http://www.cancer.gov/cancertpiocs/pdq/cam/acupuncture/healthprofessional/, 10/11/2006

Shen ZX, Chen GQ, Ni JH, Li XS, Xiong SM, Qiu QY, et al. (1997). Use of arsenic trioxide (As_2O_3) in the treatment of acute myelogenous leukemia (APL): II. Clinical efficacy and pharmacokinetics in relapsed patients. *Blood,* 89(9), 3354–3360.

Sun Y. (1995). *Treating and preventing cancer with integrative Chinese and Western Medicine.* Beijing Medical University and Union Medical University Press: Beijing.

Wang X & Ling CQ. (2004). The progress of anti-metastasis studies on Chinese herbal active ingredients. *CJITWM,* 24(2), 178–181.

Yu EX et al. (1985). *The study of integrative Chinese and Western medicine on cancer treatments.* Shanghai: Shanghai Science and Technology Press.

Yu RC et al. (2005). The progress of treating and preventing cancer with integrative Chinese and Western medicine. In Sun Yan et al. (Eds.), *Advances in clinical oncology* (pp. 166–182). Chinese Union Medical University Press: Beijing.

Zhang DZ. (1992). A panel discussion on TCM's potentiation and attenuation effects on cancer radio- and chemotherapy. *CJITWM,* 12(3), 135–138.

(A complete reference list for this chapter is available online at http://www.oup.com/us/integrativemedicine).

14

Cancer: An Ayurvedic Perspective

ANAND DHRUVA, RAMESH NANAL, AND VILAS NANAL

KEY CONCEPTS

- *Ayus* means life and *veda* is knowledge or wisdom. Ayurveda is the wisdom or science of life.
- Ayurveda originated in ancient India with knowledge being passed through the oral tradition from teacher to student.
- The *Pancha Mahaabhootas* are the five great elements—air, fire, water, space, and earth.
- The qualities of these five great elements exist in varying proportions in all life in the universe.
- The qualities represented in the Pancha Mahaabhoota are present in all people in varying proportions to create each person's *Prakruti* or constitution.
- The Prakruti is defined in terms of the three *Doshas: Vaata, Pitta,* and *Kapha.*
- Vaata is a combination of air and space, Pitta is a combination of fire and water, and Kapha is a combination of earth and water.
- A balanced prakruti is the key to health.
- Ayurvedic therapy includes *shodhana, shamana,* and *rasayana.*
- Ayurvedic therapeutic modalities can be used for general wellness, which may lead to prevention of cancer and prevention of recurrence.
- Ayurvedic therapy may serve as a valuable form of supportive cancer care.

■

Ayurveda, an ancient Indian heritage science, is a holistic system of medicine with an emphasis on prevention. Ayurveda is often translated to mean the wisdom (veda) or science of life (ayus). It is related to other classical Indian schools of thought in a belief in a unifying force in the universe. It also espouses that health derives from a combination of harmony within, harmony in the universe, and harmony between the individual and the universe. In Ayurveda, a detailed code of daily and seasonal conduct ensures prevention of disease and a state of positive physical, mental, and spiritual health, in short, a general state of well being.[1]

A *Vaidya* (an Ayurvedic physician) of today is faced with a host of contemporary life-threatening diseases, such as cancer, which find no exact mention in the classic texts (*Samhitas*). She is supposed to diagnose them using the techniques laid down in the ancient texts.[2] On the basis of this diagnosis and state of the disease she is supposed to plan and execute her intervention. Many accomplished Ayurvedic physicians are successfully doing this today in their practice.

This chapter will review the principles of Ayurveda and present an Ayurvedic understanding of cancer.

Origin and Development of Ayurveda

Ayurveda has its origins many millennia ago before the written record when knowledge was transmitted through the oral tradition from guru (teacher) to student.

The story of the creation and propagation of Ayurveda may mirror the way in which Ayurveda actually developed. In particular, there may have been additions and interpretations to the classic texts to suit the needs of the times.

---

[1] *Sus`hruta Sootra Sthaana* 15/40 Edited by Chandrakanta Bhattacharya, Chaukhambha Surbharati Prakashana, Varanasi, 1999.
[2] *Charaka Chikitsaa Sthaana* 21/Visarpa Chikitsitam.

An ancient story of the origin of Ayurveda demonstrates the oral tradition and emphasizes that Ayurveda is a gift from the gods/universe/mother earth to all creatures:

> It is believed that Lord Brahma, creator of the universe, before creating any life, created Ayurveda from his memory. He wrote a text (Samhitaa) that contained 100,000 verses. This knowledge was passed on to the ruler Daksha Prajaapati who in his turn passed it over to the celestial twins Ashvinkumars, who classified it into medical and surgical branches and then passed it on to Lord Indra. Thus each received it and handed it over to his disciple. On earth humanity was suffering from various ailments that made it impossible for them to perform their daily regimens and occupations. Hence 44 sages gathered at the base of Himalaya to deliberate over the problem. It was decided that Lord Indra had a solution for the problem in the form of Ayurveda. Sage Bharadvaaja was deputed to visit him in the heavens and acquire it from him. Having gained the knowledge from Indra, he disseminated it to the assembly of sages, who took it upon themselves to spread it further through their disciples to all of humanity.

The origins of Ayurveda are rooted in the four Vedas (Rig Veda, Yajur Veda, Atharva Veda, and Sama Veda). The Vedas were the sacred texts of the Aryan tribes, who were thought to settle in northwestern India around 5000 BCE. Vedic literature is the most ancient and deals with exposition of a world of knowledge encompassing many branches such as *Jyotisha* (Astrology), *Vaidyaka* (Medicine), and *Gan`ita* (Mathematics). The science of life, Ayurveda, evolved from the hymns of the Atharva Veda and to a lesser extent the Rig Veda and Yajur Veda. It is believed that the knowledge contained in these Vedas were combined with indigenous medical knowledge to form the foundations of Ayurveda. The original texts of Ayurveda claim divine origin for the wisdom of life. These texts assert that the science of nature and healing is a divine gift to all life. In this context, the word divine may be interpreted as being from nature for the preservation of nature.

During the Classical period of Indian history beginning around the 3rd century BCE, there was significant development of the science of life. The major triad of *Samhitaas* (texts) called the *Brihat Trayee*, were written largely during this time. These texts, the *Charaka*, *Sus`hruta*, and *Vagbhatta*, dealt with both internal medicine and surgery. They contained both diagnostic and therapeutic recommendations in many areas, such as orthopedics (fracture management), toxicology, gastrointestinal surgery (suturing intestinal perforation and hernia repair), neurosurgical procedures (burr hole and rhinoplasty), neonatology, and pediatrics.

With the waning of the Classical period came waves of invasions including the Moghul and British colonization. During the 1000 years of these invasions, Ayurveda declined. With Indian independence in 1947, Ayurveda has had a resurgence both in India and around the world.

Principles of Ayurveda

Ayurveda shares many basic concepts with other ancient Indian sciences and in this sense is truly a culturally based healing tradition. However, while borrowing from other Indian traditions, it has treated the borrowed concepts with its own logic. Like all other ancient Indian sciences Ayurveda has a three-tier structure:

- *Tattva*—concepts
- *Shaastra*—scientific and systematic elaboration
- *Vyavahaara*—day-to-day application of *tattva* and *shaastra*, use of advancing technology judiciously, without compromising on the basic tenets, to further Ayurvedic science

Ayurveda by definition is knowledge about Life[3] in all its aspects from the moment of conception through birth, growth, procreation, aging, disease, degeneration, decay, and death.[4] Life according to Ayurveda consists of four parts:[5]

- *Shareera*—the physical body, the anatomical and physiological consideration
- *Indriya*—sensory motor apparatus
- *Manas*—the mind/psyche
- *Aatman*—the soul, spirit, consciousness

Ultimately, it is the inseparable allegiance of these four parts that ensures the integrity of life.

The physical body has multiple constituents and *Charaka* clearly states that every body is made of innumerable small particles known as *Shareera Paramaanu*.[6] *Shareera* is defined as the one that harbors the *Aatman*. *Manas* is derived from specific combination of the five primordial elements called *Pancha Mahaabhootas*.[7]

---

[3] *Charaka Samhitaa Sootrasthaana 1, Sootrasthaana 30, Sus'hruta Sootrasthaana 1.*
[4] *Charaka S'haareerasthaana 5/8.*
[5] *Charaka Sootrasthaana 1.*
[6] *Charaka S'haareerasthaana 7/17.*
[7] *Charaka S'haareerasthaana 6/4.*

Five Elements (Pancha Mahaabhoota)

The concept of the Pancha Mahaabhoota is found throughout ancient Indian thought systems and they are considered the basic causal entities.[8] It is the essence or quality of these five great elements (rather than their literal manifestation) that is meant by the Pancha Mahaabhoota. All things in the universe are a specific composition of these five primordial elements, each of which has a specific property and function, and therefore all things in the universe can be described according to their predominant elements. Human beings are also an assemblage of the Pancha Mahaabhoota in varying relative proportions [1].

- *Aakaasha* (space) is responsible for sound or the auditory perception and is also responsible for generating physical space, lightness, clarity, and differentiation within the internal environment. Its character is nonresistance (*Apratighaata*).[9]
- *Vaayu* (air) is responsible for movement and perception of tactile stimulus. It generates lightness, dryness, roughness, coldness, and subtlety in the internal milieu. Its character is mobility.[10]
- *Agni* (fire) is responsible for perception of visual stimulus and for generating heat, intensity, sharpness, and mobility in the internal environment. Its cardinal character is heat.[11]
- *Jala* (water) is responsible for perception of the gustatory stimulus and for generating moistness, fluidity, unctuousness, cold, satiety, suppleness, and mildness in the internal environment. Its cardinal character is fluidity.[12]
- *Prithvee* (earth) is responsible for perception of the olfactory stimulus and for generating hardness, heaviness, denseness, slowness, roughness, and imparting the basal matrix for formation of body constituents. Its cardinal character is roughness.[13] The basal matrix provided by earth is moistened by water to make it pliable, and the fire heats it to impart stability. The combined action of air and space is responsible for shape and space within the body.[14]

[8] *Charaka Sootra Sthaana* 1/48.
[9] *Charaka S`haareerasthaana* 4/12.
[10] *Charaka S`haareerasthaana* 4/12.
[11] *Charaka S`haareerasthaana* 4/12.
[12] *Charaka S`haareerasthaana* 4/12.
[13] *Charaka S`haareerasthaana* 4/12.
[14] *Asht`aanga Hridaya Sootrasthaana* 9/1–2 Chaukhambha Sanskrita Samsthaanna, Vaaraan`asee.

Three Doshas and Prakruti/Vikruti

Each of us is born with a particular constitution (called *Prakruti* in Sanskrit) that is derived from the Pancha Mahabhoota. The ancient texts define Prakruti as a *set of individual physical, sensory, motor, psychological and spiritual characteristics which are determined at the time of fertilization that remain unchanged throughout the lifespan of the individual.*[15]

There are seven types of Prakruti:

- Three of single Dosha predominance
- Three with two Dosha predominance
- One with three Doshas in equilibrium[16]

A substance that is capable of forming an individual's constitution (*Prakruti*) and is capable of initiating a disease process on its own is called a *Dosha*. The Doshas are invisible forces with physical manifestations that are actually waste products of the Pancha Mahabhootas. Therefore, proper flow and balance of the Doshas are essential to health [1]. The three Doshas are called Vaata, Pitta, and Kapha. All life is under their influence at all times. Within the Ayurvedic system of thought they are thought of as governing forces or energies.

Vaata is derived from the two Mahabhootas Aakaasha and Vaayu, and is responsible for all movements in the internal environment due to its properties of mobility, subtlety, dryness, coldness, lightness, clarity, and roughness. It is represented in gross movements like ambulation, intermediate movements like circulation, and subtle movements like positive and negative feedback. It is responsible for control of the mind, organogenesis, respiration, generation, and transmission of impulses such as hunger, thirst, urination, defecation, and ejaculation. Vaata is the transporter par excellence among the Doshas.[17]

Pitta is derived from Agni and Jala, therefore it contains opposite qualities such as fire and water. It is also characterized by mild unctuousness, mobility, intensity/sharpness, and softness. Its main function is digestion/processing. Primarily Pitta processes food and drink but also stimuli. Owing to its sharpness and heat it is capable of breaking down stimuli so that they can be assimilated by the body at a "cellular" level. It is responsible for digestion (and indigestion), vision (and blindness), optimal function of digestive fire (*Jaat`haraagni*) or lack

---

[15] *Charaka Vimaana Sthaana 8/95–100.*
[16] *Asht`aanga Samgraha Sootra Sthaana 1/26–27.*
[17] *Charaka Sootrasthaana 12/8.*

of it, normal skin color or lack of it, valor, anger, pleasure, indecision, and a sense of fulfilment.[18] Pitta is the transformer par excellence among the Doshas.

Kapha is derived from Jala and Prithvee. Vaata and Pitta are mobile, rough, dry, and intense therefore they can be degenerative. Kapha balances these effects through its binding qualities. Owing to its cold, heavy, dense, slow, mucilaginous, granular, and unctuous nature it exerts adhesive and cohesive forces. For example, it provides the basal matrix essential for organogenesis, retards aging, and controls fluidity in the internal environment. It is responsible for firmness or laxity, emaciation or corpulence, virility or impotence, knowledge or ignorance.[19]

Dhaatus and Aama

DHAATUS

There are other body constituents that take part in sustaining life called *Dhaatus*. There are seven Dhaatus:

- *Rasa*: first nutrient fluid, which is devoid of particulate matter responsible for maintaining fluid balance (analogous to plasma)
- *Rakta*: responsible for uninterrupted supply of *Praana* to the body constituents (analogous to blood)
- *Maamsa*: responsible for formation of tissue planes (and the skin) to maintain the natural shape and contractility (analogous to muscle tissue)
- *Meda*: responsible for supplying lubrication to counter the heat and dryness generated as a result of various physiologic processes in the internal environment (analogous to adipose tissue)
- *Asthi*: responsible for internal support (analogous to osseous tissue)
- *Majjaa*: responsible for nourishing the bones and controlling the higher center activity (analogous to bone marrow)
- *Shukra*: responsible for creating progeny and regenerative activity (analogous to reproductive tissue)[20]

The Doshas and Dhaatus can be thought of as operating at a cellular level. In this integrated Ayurvedic biomedical model, Kapha with Maamsa maintain

---

[18] *Charaka Sootrasthaana* 12/11.
[19] *Charaka Sootrasthaana* 12/12.
[20] *Asht`aanga Hridaya Sootrasthaana* 1/13 Hemadri commentary.

the elasticity of the cell wall, Vaayu with Pitta are responsible for generating pores in the cell wall through which the Rasa can move in and the waste products of metabolism can exude. Cell breakdown and regeneration is controlled by Vaata,[21] Pitta, and Shukra and is highly tissue specific. The generation and destruction of cells is controlled at the higher level of Aatman and Manas. These represent the spiritual power in this system.

The essential nutrients are supplied by Rasa, Praana is supplied by Rakta, contractility is supplied by Maamsa, and unctuousness is supplied by Meda. The Dhaatus function normally in health and abnormally in disease. Therefore in a disease such as cancer characterized by uncontrolled multiplication of cells, all parts of this model must be given consideration.

AAMA

Agni is the digestive capacity of an individual. It acts through the medium of Pitta.[22] Rasa[23], which nourishes the body, is created by the breakdown of food by Agni. Rasa has the quality of being fluid, warm and subtle, and it traverses the entire internal environment to nourish all cells.

If the function of Agni is errant the result is a toxic but transient metabolite called Aama.[24] Agni works at three levels, Jaat haraagni in the alimentary canal, Mahabhootagni, in which the Mahabhootas are converted to subtle nutrients/ energies at a cellular level, and Dhaatvagni, in which the Dhaatus are formed from nutrients/energies.[25] As Agni functions at three levels, production of Aama is also observed at these three levels. A unique characteristic of Aama is that it causes change in any substance that contacts it. For example, when Vaata contacts Aama, the treatments that normally control Vaata, such as application of oil, will instead aggravate Vaata.

All disease can be linked to the accumulation of Aama. The qualities of Aama are dense, cold, slimy, slow, immobile, and thick. Aama will accumulate at specific body sites due to faulty diet, trauma, or bad habits, and cause stagnation at these sites. Metabolism at these sites is altered and if uncorrected over time can lead to structural defects and eventually neoplasia.[26] Hence it is

---

[21] *Charaka S`haareera Sthaana 7/17.*

[22] *Charaka Sootrasthaana 12/11.*

[23] *Charaka Chikitsaa Sthaana 15/3–8.*

[24] *Asht`aanga Hridaya Sootra Sthaana 13/25, Asht`aanga Samgraha Sootrasthaan 11/19–21* Lalachandra S`haastree Vaidya, Shri Baidyanath Ayurveda Bhavan, Nagpur, 1996.

[25] Insight into Ayurveda—Vaidya Vilas Nanal, Nanal Softwares and Herbals, Pune, 2006.

[26] *Asht`aanga Hridaya Sootrasthaana 13/26–27* and *Sus`hruta Uttaratantra 66.*

imperative that one gives due consideration to the function of Agni and the presence and degree of Aama during diagnosis and in planning and executing an intervention.

Aama, as it is analogous to Rasa, has access to all the sites and routes of Rasa. As it accumulates, it can manifest as localized lesions (tumors or ulcers) or generalized conditions (leukemias).

> Clinical Note: Aama can be detected on inspection of the tongue. It appears as a coating on the surface of the tongue.

Since it is a product of malfunctioning Agni the main treatment modality for accumulating Aama is fasting. Fasting, which removes the burden of digesting food, improves Agni by essentially "resetting" the digestive system. A "reset" digestive system can then reduce accumulated Aama and increase nourishing Rasa.

Malas

There are four malas or waste products:

- *Pureesha* (fecal matter)
- *Moothra* (urine)
- *Sweda* (sweat)
- *Dhooshikadimala* (excretion from the eyes, ears, and nose)

The proper excretion of the Malas is essential to good health. Moothra is important for removing excess Kapha, Sweda for excess Pitta, and Pureesha for excess Vaata [1].

Rasas (tastes)

The tastes/essences of food have physiologic effects, and in particular Vipaka, tastes that are created through the process of digestion, have more powerful effects. The six tastes described by Ayurveda are as follows:

- *Lavan* (salty)
- *Madhura* (sweet)

- *Amla* (sour)
- *Katu* (bitter)
- *Tikta* (pungent)
- *Kasaya* (astringent)

Principles of Ayurvedic Treatment

All the Doshas, the state of Agni, and the condition of the Dhaatus can contribute to disease. To assess the role played by each of these in an individual and to plan management is a matter of skill and experience. Each case is distinct in the Ayurvedic view even though the allopathic diagnosis may be identical. A skilled and experienced Vaidya should be involved in administering these therapies.

Shamana and shodhana are the basic principles of disease management in Ayurveda. Shamana, meaning alleviation, aims to reduce the symptoms of disease, while shodhana, meaning elimination, aims to eliminate the causes of disease.

Treatment is planned in three stages:

- *Shodhana* is a class of cleansing therapies among which *Pancha Karma* is found.
- *Shamana* is palliative balancing therapy.
- *Rasaayana* is the treatment aimed at improving the immune status by bringing the Rasa to an optimal level ensuring remission. It is generally combined with Vaajeekarana, which improves the regenerative capacity of the tissues and Ojas (the vital energy of the body). The regenerative aspect rather than the aphrodisiac aspect of Vajeekarana is utilized.

PANCHA KARMA (SHODHANA)

Pancha Karma literally means the five actions. Pancha Karma is a set of cleansing therapies aimed at the cause of disease, which is doshic imbalance. Before Pancha Karma is initiated, two preparative procedures must be performed to elaborate toxins from points of stagnation.

- *Snehan*: oil massage
- *Svedana*: herbal sweat therapy

These preparative therapies are followed by the Pancha Karma.

- *Vamana* (emesis therapy)

Vamana is administered in conditions of Kapha predominance with secondary aggravation of Pitta. It is particularly good for upper respiratory infections, cough, and asthma. Herbs generally used to induce vomitting[27] include Madana (Randia dumettorum), Yasht`eemadhu (Glycerriza glabra), and Vachaa (Acorus calamus).

- *Virechan* (purgation)

Virechan is typically used for Pitta disorders. Virechan is particularly good for rash, acne, nausea, vomiting, and jaundice. Herbs generally used for purging[28] include Trivrit (Ipomea operculinum), Kat`ukaa (Pichrorriza kurroa), Aaragvadha (Cassia fistula), Eran`d`a (Ricinus communis), Mridveeka (Vitis vinifera), and Triphala (Three myrobalans).

- *Basti* (enema)

Basti, the per rectum administration of medication, is effective for Vaata disorders. Basti's potency lies in the fact that Vaata is often at the root of many conditions. Constipation, arthritis, and headaches are some conditions that often respond to Basti. The colon is the site of Vaata, and from this origination point Vaata performs its functions. The absorptive capacity is highest in the Pakvaas`haya (large intestine), which leads to generation of both Aahara Rasa and residual solid waste and flatus. The effect varies based on the substance chosen. It can be purifying (Nirooha Basti), palliative (Anuvaasan Basti), nourishing (Yaapana Basti),[29] or improve urinary and reproductive afflictions (Uttara Basti).

Herbs generally used for Nirooha Basti include Dash`amoola (group of ten herbs), Madanaphala (Randia dumetorum), Devadaaru (Cedrus deodara), and Eran`d`a (Ricinus communis). If done properly, Basti is effective in reducing the intensity of the aggravated Doshas, improving Agni function, Rasa production, reducing Aama, and strengthening the site of affliction so that the subsequent Rasaayana is more beneficial.[30]

- *Nasya* (nasal instillation of medication)

The life force, Prana, enters through the nose and governs mental activities. Deranged Prana can lead to disorder in any of the mental activities. Nasya is

---

[27] *Charaka Sootra Sthaana 4/13.*
[28] *Charaka Sootra Sthaana 4/13, Asht`aanga Hridaya Sootra Sthaana 18.*
[29] *Asht`aanga Hridaya Sootra Sthaana 19, Charaka Siddhi Sthaana 12 for Yaapana Basti.*
[30] *Asht`aanga Hridaya Sootra Sthaana 19/61.*

effective in treating these disorders of Prana. Since the nose is the only sense organ that is in direct contact with the central nervous system and contents of the cranium, medicine introduced in the nose is felt to be particularly potent.[31] Nasya is often used for anxiety, headaches, ear/eye disorders, congestion, and even brain tumors. The dose varies from 4 drops to 64 drops of a selected medication. For example, in anxiety or stress related disorders, dry powder of Vacha (*Acorus clamus*) and Maricha (*piper nigrum*) is blown in each nostril after proper preparation of the patient (Pradhamana Nasya).[32] This procedure induces sneezing and nasal discharge thereby reducing tension headache.

- *Rakta Moksha* (blood letting)

As Pitta and blood are closely related, Rakta Moksha is effective for Pitta disorders. Toxins from the gastrointestinal tract are absorbed into the blood and therefore are amenable to Rakta therapy. Skin, liver, and spleen disorders respond well to Rakta Moksha. Often only a small amount of blood is removed, and blood purifying herbs may also be used.

SHAMANA

Shamana is palliative management aimed at restoring the balance of doshas, improving the function of Agni, improving tissue metabolism, and therefore nullifying the damage done by the disease process. Diet and herbs are often used. Shamana is often used for those not strong enough to undergo shodhana.

RASAYANA

Rasayana therapy is aimed at rejuvenation. The role of Rasa in every disease is crucial as nourishment reaches the body through Rasa. The doshas move in the internal milieu through Rasa.[33] Therefore no treatment is complete without administration of appropriate Rasaayana. Since cancer is a disease characterized by uncontrolled growth of cells and aggravation of all three Doshas, disruption of Agni, and involvement of multiple body constituents, the Rasaayana utilized is of equally broad spectrum. Some commonly used Rasayanas include

---

[31] *Asht`aanga Hridayam Sootra Sthaana* 20/1.
[32] *Charaka Siddhi* 9/89–92.
[33] *Charaka Sootra Sthaana* 28/47.

Bhallataka (*Semicarpus anacardium*), Chyavanapraasha (an herb blend that includes amalaki), and Ashwagandha.

Many Rasaayanas (such as Ashwagandha) have demonstrated anti-cancer properties in the laboratory setting.

Ayurveda and Diet

Dietary therapy is an important part of an Ayurvedic treatment plan. A person's Prakruti advises what a person should eat for good health. The five great elements can be used to describe food. For example, nuts represent earth element, fruits with high water content such as grapes or watermelon represent water, fire element is represented by spices such as black pepper, foods that produce gas such as broccoli or cabbage represent air element, and intoxicants represent space element. In Ayurveda, food has specific qualities such as hot or cold, oily or dry, and heavy and light to name a few. The quality of the food is important to the physiologic effects of the food. The taste or rasa of the food is also important in its physiologic effects [2]. All of these qualities of food may be used to construct a diet to soothe an aggravated dosha and to keep one's Prakruti in balance. Dietary therapy is most effective after shodhana.

Often in Integrative Oncology, dietary recommendation from many Western diets may seemingly conflict with Ayurvedic dietary advice. However, many of the Ayurvedic dietary recommendations can be slightly modified to allow foods that may normally aggravate a dosha. For example, cruciferous vegetables, which are often an important part of a Western "anticancer" diet, may aggravate Vaata. However, if they are taken with ginger, which soothes Vaata, then they may be included as part of a Vaata pacifying diet. Proper collaboration between a skilled nutritionist and Vaidya can make much of this possible.

Ayurveda and Oncology

Ayurveda is a complex medical system in which multiple modalities operate together to achieve their health maintaining and therapeutic ends. Within this system, it is somewhat counter-intuitive to use single modalities. However, for the purpose of presenting the biomedical research that has been completed on these individual modalities, a deconstructed approach is taken for this section.

A pilot clinical study using a whole systems approach to Ayurveda for the management of diabetes mellitus type 2 showed some benefits in glucose control [3]. This study is unique in its complete approach to Ayurveda including diet, botanicals, exercise, and lifestyle therapies.

TURMERIC (HALDI)

Curcuma longa, turmeric, is a member of the ginger family. The rhizome of the plant is boiled and then dried to produce the yellow powder that is used for culinary and medicinal purposes. Curcumin, a polyphenol, is thought to be one of the active medicinal components. Haldi has a long history of use within Ayurvedic medicine. Within Ayurveda, haldi is felt to have pungent, bitter, and astringent properties. Although it is felt to have heating effects, it may be used by all doshas. It is good for digestion, and it has been used for millenia as an antiseptic for cuts, as an antibacterial agent, for cough, and burns [2].

A detailed review of both preclinical and clinical studies of turmeric is found in Chapter 6.

ASHWAGANDHA

Ashwagandha, *Withania somnifera*, is a plant in the Solanaceae family and is native to India, Pakistan, and Sri Lanka. The root of this shrub is commonly used for its medicinal properties. Ayurveda considers Ashwagandha to be bitter, astringent, and sweet. Although it reduces Vaata and Kapha, in excess it can aggravate Pitta and even produce Aama. It is an adaptogen and is therefore used for states of debility. It also has aphrodisiac properties. It calms and clarifies the mind and promotes restful sleep through its sedative properties. However, it also has rejuvenating effects on the body and is therefore used for states of exhaustion. The fruit and the seed of the plant have diuretic effects and the seed specifically is felt to have hypnotic effects. An infusion made with the leaves of the plant is used to treat fevers [1].

This herb has been well-studied in the preclinical arena in both laboratory and animal experiments. Details of the preclinical data can be found in
Chapter 6. Interested readers can also read Marie Winters excellent review on
the uses of Ashwagandha in the oncology setting [4]. Definitive clinical trials
of this Ayurvedic botanical have not yet been conducted.

YOGA

For many serious practitioners of yoga, it is a way of life rather than an exercise. Yoga practice includes asanas (physical postures with putative physiologic
effects), pranayama (regulated breathing practices), and meditation.

Yoga has been studied as a modality to improve quality of life in breast cancer
patients. A recently published study [5] investigated the effects of a multi-modality
yoga approach that included asanas, pranayama, and meditation. In this study, 128
patients with breast cancer were randomized to yoga or a wait-list control. Using
an intent-to-treat analysis, the investigators found that yoga was associated with
beneficial effects on social functioning and a sense of enhanced emotional well-
being and mood. However, due to problems of study design, including poor compliance with the study treatment, the investigators were not able to demonstrate
improvements in many of the quality of life parameters included in the study.

A randomized controlled clinical trial by Cohen and colleagues [6] investigated the effects of a Tibetan yoga intervention that included controlled breathing, visualization, mindfulness, and low-impact asanas. Thirty-nine patients
with lymphoma were randomized to treatment or wait-list control. Among the
treatment group 58% of the patients were able to complete five of the seven
prescribed weekly yoga sessions. The intervention group was superior for the
sleep endpoints, but was not different for the anxiety, depression, or fatigue
endpoints compared to control. However, compliance with study treatment
may be an important confounder to their results.

A randomized controlled pilot study of a pure yoga asana intervention in a
population of breast cancer survivors [7] showed improvements in psychosocial variables such as global quality of life compared to control subjects.

A randomized controlled study by Cohen and colleagues showed that a program of yoga exercises and pranayama improved quality of life in women with
breast cancer getting radiation therapy [8].

An uncontrolled study of a multimodality yoga approach in metastatic
breast cancer patients [9] demonstrated that the participants experienced less
pain, fatigue and greater invigoration, acceptance, and relaxation the day after
yoga practice. Though these results are interesting, the study sample was small,
including only 13 patients.

PRANAYAMA/BREATHWORK

In Sanskrit, Prana is the life force and breath, and yama means expansion, control, or regulation. Pranayama is the regulation and expansion of breath. The importance of breath is seen in many cultures and traditions of medicine throughout history. In Western medicine, breathing is a bridge between the conscious and unconscious mind as it is controlled by both, and is a connection between mind and body.

There are a number of studies demonstrating the effects of pranayama on human physiology. A study in asthmatics suggested that pranayama improved clinical symptoms of asthma and reduced bronchodilator use [10].

A study by Pal and colleagues demonstrated that slow pranayama breathing increased parasympathetic and decreased sympathetic activity in normal volunteers [11]. Increases in parasympathetic activity may translate into balancing or anxiety relieving effects.

Two small studies have investigated the effects of pranayama on oxidation. Bhattacharya and colleagues found that subjects performing pranayama had reduced the levels of free radicals but no change in superoxide dismutase levels compared to control subjects [12]. Yadav and colleagues found that a yoga-based lifestyle modification program that included pranayama reduced oxidative stress [13].

An interesting study by Chaya and colleagues investigated the effects of a yoga-based lifestyle program, including yoga asanas, pranayama, and meditation, and found that this program reduced study patient's basal metabolic rate compared to the no treatment controls [14].

A specific program of pranayama, called Sudarshan Kriya Yoga, was studied for its antidepressant effects and found to have effects similar to imipramine, a pharmacologic antidepressant [15]. A randomized study by Wood showed that normal subjects who performed pranayama had improved perceptions of both physical and mental energy while also having less nervousness [16].

A controlled clinical study by Raju and colleagues investigated the effects of pranayama on athletic performance and found that it increased the work rate and reduced the oxygen consumption [17].

Two small studies by Kim and colleagues [18,19] evaluated the effects of a physical exercise and deep breathing exercise that resembled pranayama in patients who had undergone allogenic stem cell transplant and found improvements in symptoms of fatigue, anxiety, and depression.

The effects of pranayama on immune function have begun to be studied. Kochupillai and colleagues demonstrated that NK cells increased in numbers in cancer patients who practiced pranayama [20].

Breathing through a particular nostril can have specific physiologic effects. Left nostril breathing is thought to have calming effects and right nostril breathing to have activating effects. Although a study comparing these to alternate nostril breathing did not show any differences in oxygen consumption between the groups, it did show that the left nostril group had a reduction in sympathetic activity [21]. Another study of right nostril breathing showed that it may have a sympathetic stimulating effect [22]. It is interesting that pranayama practice does not affect arterial blood gas values [23], suggesting that another mechanism besides improved oxygenation is causing the physiologic changes.

Although pranayama has not yet been well studied in the oncology setting, the studies presented in this section speak to the great potential of pranayama for symptom management and palliative care in oncology.

Integrating Ayurveda

INTEGRATING AYURVEDIC CONCEPTS INTO CANCER CARE

Ayurveda is a "whole system" of medicine and therefore should ideally be utilized in its complete form under the care of an experienced Vaidya. An initial consultation with a Vaidya may lay the foundation for integrating Ayurvedic concepts over the course of a Western allopathic treatment plan. Ayurveda is a system of medicine with a strong emphasis on prevention and therefore it is a system that intuitively would be ideal for cancer prevention among both high risk individuals and the general public. Because of its emphasis on healing, well being, and prevention, Ayurveda may be ideally suited for maintaining remission in cancer survivors. The modalities of yoga and pranayama can be utilized for supportive care during cancer chemotherapy. There is some evidence that they may improve certain quality of life parameters [5,18,19]. Studies are needed to evaluate the effects of Ayurveda for prevention of cancer and recurrence.

Conclusions

Ayurveda is a holistic system of medicine with ancient roots and contemporary vibrancy. A belief in unifying forces in the universe and a corresponding affinity towards wholeness are important features of Ayurveda. As a system of medicine that emphasizes wellness, healing, and prevention, it has many possible applications for cancer care. These applications include cancer prevention, supportive care, and among survivors prevention of recurrence. Although Ayurveda comes with thousands of years of experiential evidence on best practices, which can be a very valuable form of evidence, it has not yet been well studied by

Western research paradigms. Though such investigations are perilous due to the many differences in conceptual framework between Ayurveda and allopathic medicine, future studies will be important to guide the application of Ayurveda to modern conditions. In the end, Ayurveda and Western medicine are bound together in their common aim to alleviate human suffering.

REFERENCES

1. Svoboda RE. (1992). *Ayurveda: Life, health, and longevity.* Penguin Books Ltd.
2. Lad ULaV. (2002). *Ayurvedic cooking for self-healing, 2nd edition* (p. 254). Albuquerque, NM: The Ayurvedic Press.
3. Elder C, Aickin M, Bauer V, Cairns J, & Vuckovic N. (2006). Randomized trial of a whole-system ayurvedic protocol for type 2 diabetes. *Alternative Therapies in Health and Medicine,* 12(5), 24–30.
4. Winters M. (2006). Ancient medicine, modern use: Withania somnifera and its potential role in integrative oncology. *Alternative Medicine Review,* 11(4), 269–277.
5. Moadel AB, Shah C, Wylie-Rosett J, Harris MS, Patel SR, & Hall CB. (2007). Randomized controlled trial of yoga among a multiethnic sample of breast cancer patients: Effects on quality of life. *Journal of Clinical Oncology,* 4, 4.
6. Cohen, L, Warneke C, Fouladi RT, Rodriguez MA, & Chaoul-Reich A. (2004). Psychological adjustment and sleep quality in a randomized trial of the effects of a Tibetan yoga intervention in patients with lymphoma. *Cancer,* 100(10), 2253–2260.
9. Carson JW & Porter LS. (2007). Yoga for women with metastatic breast cancer: results from a pilot study. *Journal of Pain and Symptom Management,* 33(3), 331–341.
18. Kim SD & Kim HS. (2005). Effects of a relaxation breathing exercise on fatigue in haemopoietic stem cell transplantation patients. *Journal of Clinical Nursing,* 14(1), 51–55.
19. Kim SD & Kim HS. (2005). Effects of a relaxation breathing exercise on anxiety, depression, and leukocyte in hemopoietic stem cell transplantation patients. *Cancer Nursing,* 28(1), 79–83.
22. Telles S, Nagarathna R, & Nagendra HR. (1996). Physiological measures of right nostril breathing. *Journal of Alternative and Complementary Medicine (New York, NY),* 2(4), 479–484.

(A complete reference list for this chapter is available online at http://www.oup.com/us/ integrativemedicine).

15

Homeopathy for Primary and Adjunctive Cancer Therapy*

DANA ULLMAN, MENACHEM OBERBAUM, IRIS BELL, AND SHEPHERD ROEE SINGER

KEY CONCEPTS

- Homeopathy is a medical specialty that recognizes symptoms as adaptive responses of the organism to endogenous and exogenous factors. This system of medicine utilizes drugs that have undergone a specific pharmaceutical process of serial dilution with vigorous shaking, which homeopaths have found stimulates the healing process. Each drug is selected according to the "law of similars," with the intention of initiating a healing process by stimulating the body's own adaptive capacities.
- Clinical research exists to support the biological activity of homeopathic preparations, as well as their efficacy, in a number of clinical indications. However, this research often lacks sufficient replication or corroboration, and thus must be considered as yet inconclusive.
- Individual studies have shown that homeopathic medicines can be used to mitigate the adverse effects of chemotherapy and radiation treatment, though this research also requires replication and corroboration. However, due to the widely recognized safety of homeopathic medicines, there appears little risk in employing these drugs in conjunction with conventional anticancer treatment.
- The historical and international experience with homeopathic medicines in a wide variety of acute and chronic illnesses, combined with a growing body of scientific evidence and a benign

*Supported in part by NIH/NCCAM grant K24 AT00057 (IRB).

safety profile, would suggest a place for homeopathic treatment in an integrated medical approach to cancer treatment.

■

Though far from conclusive, much headway has been made in homeopathic cancer research in recent years. The bulk of this effort resides in the realm of basic science; however, anecdotal evidence and limited clinical trials offer hope that homeopathy may indeed be of value in cancer prevention, treatment, mitigation of conventional cancer therapy side effects, and in palliative care. Some case reports and case series even claim cancer cures. Independent replication of the more exceptional claims is notably lacking. In spite of these encouraging preliminary findings, existing evidence and ethical considerations place homeopathy at this point as an adjunct to conventional cancer therapy, not in its lieu, save where conventional therapy is ineffective or futile. With these caveats in mind, we proceed to review "the best in homeopathic anticancer research."

Homeopathy employs an entirely novel paradigm and therapeutic arsenal in comparison with conventional medicine. The approach to cancer treatment illustrates this philosophical rift. Western medicine tends to view cancers as a localized disease (which may metastasize and develop systemic properties), while homeopathy views cancer (and other diseases with seemingly local manifestations) as a local expression of underlying system-wide illness or "disorder." Conventional medical treatments, including surgery, radiation, and

Definitions

Homeopathic medicine: Homeopathic medicine is the application of specially prepared nanodoses (described in the following paragraphs) of a plant, mineral, animal, or chemical substance to treat the similar syndrome of symptoms that it is known to cause in overdose.

Homeopathic medicines, also termed "remedies" are made through a process of serial dilution with vigorous shaking in between each dilution. Water soluble medicines are repeatedly diluted by a factor of 1:10, 1:100, or 1:50,000, in double-distilled water in glass vials. Mineral substances are initially triturated and diluted with lactose powder. In most countries, homeopathic medicines are recognized as drugs—usually over-the-counter—that have a long history of safety, thereby permitting their use without a doctor's prescription.

When a medicine has been diluted 1:10 six times, it is termed 6X (X = Roman numeral for 10). When it is diluted 1:100, it is termed 6C. According to Avogadro's number, in all probability, there should be no remaining molecules of the original medicinal substance after it has been diluted 1:10 twenty-four times (24X) or 1:100 twelve times (12C). Homeopathic medicines include both pre-Avogadro number doses and post-Avogadro number doses.

Nanodoses: The prefix nano derives from Latin and means dwarf; today, the prefix is used in nanotechnology or the nanosciences, which explore the use of extremely small technologies or processes, at least one-billionth of a unit, designated as 10^{-9}, though our use of the word nanopharmacology and nanodose draws from its modern usage, suggesting "very small and very powerful."

Hormesis: Hormesis is the term for generally favorable biological responses to low exposures to toxins and other stressors. The wide variety of scientific researchers who have experimented with and explored hormetic effects have only evaluated the effects the pre-Avogadro number doses (Calabrese, 2005).

chemotherapy, seek to exterminate the rogue cancer cells. By contrast, homeopathic medicines, along with other holistic approaches, purport to augment the individual's resistance and empower the body to reestablish its own health.

The Homeopathic Approach to Cancer

Homeopathy is a branch of holistic medicine first conceived by the German physician, translator, and chemist Dr. Samuel Hahnemann at the turn of the 19th century. The central tenet and basis for this form of medicine is the *law of similars*. This purported law of nature dictates that a patient with a given syndrome of disease can be effectively treated by giving a medicine that would *create* a similar syndrome in a healthy individual (Hahnemann, Organon §26).

The premise underlying the law of similars is that symptoms of illness are adaptations and defenses of the entire organism—mind and body—in response to stress, infection, or toxic exposures. Rather than using pharmaceutical agents to inhibit or suppress specific symptoms or biochemical processes, homeopathic medicines (remedies) are tailored to the unique body–mind syndrome of the patients.

This principle of using "like to treat like" is both ancient and modern. Hippocrates asserted that, "By similar things disease is produced, and by similar things, administered to the sick, they are healed of their diseases." More recently, the principle of similars may be observed in the modern medical applications of immunization and allergy desensitization, though homeopaths use much smaller doses of medicines and prescribe these medicines with greater individualization of treatment. Homeopaths assert that it is no coincidence that radiation causes cancer, and many chemotherapeutic drugs are themselves carcinogenic.

Though the law of similars is the *sine qua non* of homeopathy, the field is actually best known for its use of submolecular doses. While a widely accepted explanation for such activity is still lacking, nonlinear dose–response relationships are well documented in conventional pharmacology–toxicology literature as the phenomenon of hormesis (Calabrese & Baldwin, 2001; Calabrese, 2005). In this response, an agent, which may be radiation, a toxin, or chemotherapeutic drug, causes an effect at a given dose but attenuates or reverses that effect at a different dose. Though hormesis is more likely to occur at doses below the lowest observed adverse effect level for a given agent, homeopaths use even smaller, more potentized doses. Homeopathic medicines may include dilutions in which no material amount of the original medicinal substance remains, and which are prepared through a well-defined process of serial dilution and succussion.

Of additional relevance to biological homeopathic remedy effects are animal and in vitro data demonstrating experimentally measurable effects of increasing duration from homeopathic remedies administered at increasingly higher, ultra-dilute doses (potencies) (Sukul, Bala, & Bhattacharyya, 1986; Witt, et al., 2007). As noted earlier, a tenet of homeopathy is state dependency. That is, the direction of response to a given remedy depends on the condition of the host at the time of taking the medicine (a remedy can cause symptoms in a healthy individual, but relieve the same symptoms in a sick individual). Consistent with this claim, Bertani et al. (1999) showed in animals that a homeopathically prepared mixture of mineral remedies worsened carrageenan-induced paw edema when given prior to the experimentally induced injury but attenuated the edema when given after the injury had been established (Bertani, Lussignoli, Andrioli, Bellavite, & Conforti, 1999).

The use of extremely small, often submolecular, doses in homeopathic medicine, was in fact an afterthought of Hahnemann's, in an effort to minimize the side effects of "physiological" doses. For over 20 years after Hahnemann developed the system of homeopathy, he only used material doses of medicines, until he and his colleagues began experimenting with even higher dilutions of their medicines and discovered more longlasting results requiring less frequent dosing. While not common in homeopathic practice, the possibility of employing "crude" doses is not inconsistent with homeopathic theory. Basic science studies increasingly indicate that succussion (vigorous shaking), juxtaposed with serial dilution, is essential to the preparation of active homeopathic remedies, and is key to activating persistent measurable changes in the physical chemistry and material science solvent properties (Elia & Niccoli, 1999, 2004; Elia,

Napoli, & Germano, 2007; Rao, Roy, & Hoover, 2007; Rey 2003; Roy, Tiller, Bell, & Hoover, 2005).

Hahnemann practiced medicine in the early 1800s, but had a deep and radical understanding of cancer causation. He recognized that there was a genetic component to cancer, and understood the contribution of diet and chronic poisoning to the development of many cancers. However, Hahnemann also attributed great importance to past experience and mental and emotional states in the development of cancerous and precancerous conditions (Hahnemann, 1828). Indeed, most homeopaths today accept the centrality of mental symptoms to selection of the best-acting homeopathic medicine and their use in evaluation of the healing process.

In recent years, many environmental exposures have been associated with cancer. That smoking is a pervasive carcinogen can now be doubted by only the most cynical. Likewise, the carcinogenic effects of certain environmental pollutants are no longer subject to serious debate (asbestos, diethylstilbestrol (DES), radon). The carcinogenic effects of additional environmental exposures are now the subject of heated debate (dietary pesticides, low-frequency electromagnetic fields). However, homeopathic theory adds to this debate the concept of individual susceptibility. Indeed, for many if not most cancers, no environmental exposure is implicated, and the person is left with his/her genetic disposition (eg., breast cancer and BRCA-1). Though unproven, homeopathy aspires to decrease individual susceptibility, be it from genetic, environmental, or other causes.

Concurrent with his general abhorrence of local and cursory therapies, Hahnemann invoked the term "suppression" to describe yet another possible factor contributing to deep pathologies. Homeopathy theorizes that symptoms of acute illnesses represent the organism's innate "best choice" defense mechanism and that suppression of this response, by strong pharmaceuticals or other means, reduces the overall integrity of the defenses, risking transmuting minor ailments into deeper and more serious pathologies, including cancers.

Modern complex systems and network science offers a rational basis for the concept of suppression. That is, every body part plays some role within the larger system; the organism as a whole. Systems biologists view the human being holistically as an indivisible, integrated, interdependent, and interactive complex system or network of component parts (http://www.systemsbiology.org/Intro_to_ISB_and_Systems_Biology/Systems_Biology_-_the_21st_Century_Science, accessed November 24, 2007). As numerous conventional (Barabasi & Bonabeau, 2003; Coffey, 1998; Goldberger et al., 2002) and CAM researchers (Ahn, Tewari, Poon, & Phillips, 2006; Bell, et al., 2002b; Bell & Koithan, 2006; Hyland & Lewith, 2002) have noted, because of the indivisibility and interconnectedness of subsystems within the person as a network, change in one local subsystem or part necessarily leads to changes distally throughout the rest of the network across levels of organizational scale (Vasquez, et al., 2004).

The nature of the change is nonlinear (i.e., the size of the output is disproportionate to the size of the input) and multiscale (i.e., manifest across different levels of organizational scale, large or global and small or local). The degree to which other parts of a network (organism) will change their behavior depends in a complex manner on the initial state of the organism (thereby accommodating the potential for state-dependent, bidirectional effects of the same agent), the role of the initially affected part within the organism as a whole (e.g., brain is more crucial to survival than a toe), and the strength of the functional interrelationships it has with remaining parts of the system (Brandt, Dellen, & Wessel, 2006). Endogenous (genetic, biochemical, nutritional, age, sex, biorhythm) and environmental individual difference factors that interact with the organism will affect whatever changes actually manifest.

In a biological system, treatments that effectively block functioning at one level of scale, that is, suppress expression of function (dysfunction) at a specific body part or local subsystem level, will have multiple hard-to-predict distal effects on other functions throughout the rest of the organism both globally (organism level) and locally (other body part or subsystem levels). The rest of the larger system must and will adapt to changes in the ability of any one of the parts to perform its customary role.

Thus, in systems biology, suppressive local treatment must inevitably produce major or minor clinical consequences by imbalancing other functions to a greater or lesser extent in the rest of the organism. Empirically, there are documented examples suggesting that the nature of the adaptations that the rest of the organism makes in response to effective local suppression may lead to serious emergent adverse clinical outcomes in other, arguably more important body parts, for example, increased risk of cardiac disease in certain patients treated with Cox-2 inhibitor drugs or lymphoma in patients treated with tumor necrosis factor alpha suppressing drugs for local inflammation of arthritic joints; type II diabetes mellitus in certain patients treated with newer generation antipsychotic drugs; or Clostridium difficile-associated diarrhea in patients treated with antibiotics and proton pump inhibitor drugs.

To understand the homeopathic approach to cancer treatment, we must first clarify that homeopathy does not purport to treat "cancer," but rather "people with cancer." This is not mere sophistry. Homeopathy aspires to affect an inanimate "vital force," (the homeopaths' term for the organism's overall immune and defense system), by prescribing for the totality of symptoms (Hahnemann Organon, Aphorism 7), of which the cancer is but a part (see also Milgrom, 2002). Some consider homeopathy the ultimate "holistic" medicine, because it involves all levels of the individual—local, physical-general, emotional, and mental—in treating all maladies. In addition to this broad biologic approach, homeopaths also assess the person's social and physical environment in search of "obstacles to cure." Prescription is based upon the totality of a person's physical and psychological characteristics, with the aim of inducing a curative reaction.

It would be prudent to reiterate that cancer is a deep and serious pathology, and no rigorous proof replicated by multiple independent researchers currently exists to support the contention that homeopathy alone can cure cancer. However, based upon our own professional experience, we believe it is reasonable to recommend homeopathy as an adjunct to conventional medical treatment for cancer, particularly in cases for which the efficacy of conventional treatment is limited, and as treatment for side effects and peripheral issues that arise during conventional cancer treatment.

Homeopathic Mechanisms of Action-1

Scientists at several universities and hospitals in France and Belgium have discovered that the vigorous shaking of the water in glass bottles causes extremely small amounts of silica fragments or chips to fall into the water (Demangeat, et al., 2004). These silica fragments or chips may help store the information in the water or possibly change the structure of the water, with each medicine that is initially placed in the water creating its own effect on water structure (Anick & Ives, 2007).

Homeopathic Mechanisms of Action-2

Microbubbles that are created by vigorous shaking may burst and thereby produce microenvironments of higher temperature and pressure. Several studies by chemists and physicists have revealed increased release of heat from water in which homeopathic medicines are prepared, even when the repeated process of dilutions should suggest that there are no molecules remaining of the original medicinal substance (Elia & Niccoli, 1999; Elia, et al., 2007; Rey, 2003).

Homeopathic Mechanisms of Action-3

Recent spectroscopic analyses have successfully differentiated one homeopathic medicine from another and one sub-Avogadro homeopathic potency from another (Rao, et al., 2007).

The Homeopathic Treatment of Cancer Patients

The evidence in support of the use of homeopathy as a primary treatment for cancer patients is generally weak, often conflicting, and inconclusive. Milazzo et al. (2006) recently reviewed the efficacy of homeopathic treatment in cancer and concluded that there was insufficient evidence to support the clinical efficacy of homeopathic therapy in cancer care. We proceed to present some of the more promising homeopathic research.

Curing Cancer

A remarkable study on Indian patients with brain tumors was performed in conjunction with the M.D. Anderson Cancer Center at the University of Texas. Fifteen patients diagnosed with intracranial tumors, nine of which were gliomas, were treated orally with *Ruta graveolens* (garden rue) diluted to 1/10^{12} (6C) and *Calcarea phosphorica* (Calcium phosphate) 1/10^3 (3D)[1]. Eight of nine glioma patients showed complete regression of tumors. These patients were receiving no conventional anticancer therapy (Pathak, Multani, Banerji, & Banerji, 2003).

Four articles appearing in a single edition of *Integrative Cancer Therapies* demonstrate intriguing results of homeopathic treatment of prostate cancer. *Sabal serrulata* (saw palmetto) is the most popular complementary treatment for prostate pathology ranging from benign hyperplasia to carcinoma.

Jonas et al. (2006) injected 100 Copenhagen mice with a standardized dose of MAT-LyLu rat prostate cancer cells. From day 2, animals were given 100 µL daily of one of four homeopathic remedies in rotation (*Thuja occidentalis 1000C, Conium maculatum 1000C, and Sabal serrulata 200C, and Carcinosin 1000C*) or control water by oral gavage. Tumor volume was measured every 4 days. Animals treated homeopathically had a 23% decrease in tumor incidence, and significantly longer overall and tumor-free survival, as compared with controls. Tumor volume among tumor-bearing animals was 38% lower in the homeopathically treated group, and tumor weight was 13% lower than in the control group. In an attempt to elucidate mechanisms for

[1] Homeopathic potencies in common use are serially diluted by a factor of 1/10 ("D," decimal potencies) or 1/100 ("C," centesimal potencies). Thus, the 2D potency is the initial substance diluted by ten, and then again by ten for a concentration of 1/100 or 10^{-2} of the original solution. A 30C potency is serially diluted 30 times by a factor of 1/100 for a final concentration of 1/100^{30} or 1/10^{60}, far beyond Avogadro's number, 6.022x 10^{23}.

this phenomenon, proliferating cell nuclear antigen (PCNA) was measured in tumor tissues of the two groups. There was a 6% reduction in PCNA-positive cells in the homeopathy-treated group as compared to control. Terminal deoxynucleotidyl transferase mediated D-uridine triphosphate nick end labeling (TUNEL) assay of tumor tissues demonstrated a significant 19% increase in apoptotic positive nuclei in the homeopathy-treated group as compared to control. Cell viability and apoptosis gene expression were not affected, as measured by MTT assay and rAPO-1 multiprobe, respectively. The authors concluded that, in this model, homeopathy slowed progression of cancer and reduced cancer incidence and mortality. However, the mechanism remains obscure.

Whereas this study did not elucidate specific antitumor activities of any one of the remedies under study, MacLaughlin et al. (2006) went on to investigate the specific activity of the individual homeopathic components. They assessed the in vivo antiproliferative effects of homeopathic preparations of *Sabal serrulata, Thuja occidentalis, Conium maculatum,* and *Carcinosin,* in nude mouse xenografts, and in vitro, on human prostate cancer as well as human breast cancer cell lines. Mice were inoculated subcutaneously with either PC-3 human prostate or MDA-MB-231 human breast cancer cell lines on both sides of the abdomen, and then treated daily for 5 weeks with either homeopathic *Sabal serrulata* (SS 200 CH) or homeopathic multitreatment (MT) including all four aforementioned remedies in series. Two control groups were employed, one without treatment and one with homeopathically prepared water. Tumors were measured with a caliper and mice were weighed weekly. Prostate tumor xenograft size was significantly reduced in *Sabal serrulata*–treated mice compared to untreated controls ($P = 0.012$). No effect was observed on breast tumor growth. Additionally, homeopathic multitreatment did not affect tumor size.

In the in vitro part of this experiment, androgen receptor–negative human prostate cancers DU-145 and PC-3, and human breast cancer MDA-MB-231 cell lines were treated with a variety of treatment regimens and potencies and measured for cell proliferation using crystal violet protein stain and for cell viability using MTT both at 24 and 72 hours after treatment. Treatment with *Sabal serrulata* in vitro resulted in a 33% decrease of PC-3 cell proliferation at 72 hours and a 23% reduction of DU-145 cell proliferation at 24 hours ($P < 0.01$). However a range of potencies of *Sabal serrulata* had no effect on breast cancer cell lines, suggesting the specificity of *Sabal serrulata* for prostate cancer cells. These findings remained robust after correcting for multiple comparisons (Amri H, personal communication).

In two studies directed at elucidating the cellular mechanism of these apparent anticancer effects, Thangapazham (2006a, 2006b) investigated the effect of various homeopathic medicines (including *Sabal serrulata*) on cell proliferation using the MTT assay, and on mRNA levels for apoptotic genes using RiboQuant multiprobe set rAPO-1. Homeopathic medicines showed no significant effect on growth and viability in three cell lines. These results would appear to conflict with the findings of MacLaughlin et al. (2006).

Symptom Management and Quality of Life in Cancer Patients

Homeopathy is frequently employed adjunctively to improve quality of life in cancer patients. To evaluate the efficacy of homeopathy in symptom control and its impact on mood and quality of life in cancer patients, Thompson and Reilly (2003) studied 100 consecutive patients at a cancer research clinic in the United Kingdom. Of 100 patients enrolled in the study, 81 had breast cancer, 39 had metastatic disease, and 9 had refused conventional cancer treatment. Patients were given a 60-minute consultation and a homeopathic prescription, followed by four to six follow-up visits over a period of 3 to 12 months (mean—6.7 months.) Up to three symptoms characterized by the patient as problematic were chosen as basis for comparison. As a baseline measure, the patients were asked about the effect of these symptoms on daily life and their overall sense of well being. Additionally, patients completed the Hospital Anxiety and Depression Scale, as well as the European Organization for Research and Treatment in Cancer Quality of Life Questionnaire (Core 30). These measures were taken again at follow-up visits. At conclusion of the study, patients completed a final assessment questionnaire asking about satisfaction with the homeopathic approach. Fifty-two patients completed the protocol. Satisfaction with treatment in this group was high, with 75% of these patients scoring 7 or higher on a 0–10 scale. Symptom scores for fatigue and hot flushes improved significantly during the study, as did the three primary symptoms the patients experienced. Further, the mean depression and anxiety scores also improved significantly, while the pain index showed a trend towards improvement. The study also found that 59% of the patients who completed the study measured an improved quality of life.

This study's major limitations are its high drop-out rate and lack of a control group. However, it does seem to indicate a high level of satisfaction with homeopathic treatment and impressive rates of improvement in fatigue and hot flushes, at least among the 52% of patients who completed the study.

The same researchers conducted an observational study of 45 women with breast cancer who were being treated with homeopathic medicines as they were being withdrawn from estrogen usage (Thompson & Reilly, 2003). The most common presenting symptoms were hot flushes (38), joint pain (12), and fatigue (16). Each woman was prescribed an individually chosen homeopathic medicine. Forty women (89%) completed the study. The effect on "daily living scores" (the primary end-point of this study) showed significant improvement ($P = 0.001$). Significant improvements in anxiety ($P = 0.013$), depression ($P = 0.039$), and quality of life ($P = 0.05$) were also demonstrated, as were hot flushes, fatigue, and mood disturbance scores. It should be noted that 49% of the referrals came from the local oncology center, that 32 (55%) of the women were taking tamoxifen, and that 21 (48%) had undergone adjuvant chemotherapy. Twenty (44%) of the women were on other medications (11 on antidepressants and 3 on clonidine).

In a similar study, Jacobs et al. (2005) compared the efficacy of homeopathy treatment (both individualized remedies and a homeopathic "complex[2]") with placebo in the treatment of hot flushes in menopausal breast cancer survivors. They found no difference in the hot flush severity score (primary outcome), but did find a statistically significant improvement in general health score (SF-36) in both homeopathy groups ($P < 0.05$) at 1 year.

Certain homeopathic medicines may be of use in reducing the side effects of radiation treatment. Clinical research suggests that homeopathic remedies may be beneficial in providing protection from side effects of radiation. To study the effect of homeopathic treatment on radiation-induced dermatitis, Balzarini et al. (2000) randomized 66 women undergoing post-surgical radiation therapy to either *Belladonna* 7C and *X-ray* 15C or placebo. Outcome was measured using a composite index of total severity score. This score evaluates breast skin color, warmth, swelling, and pigmentation. They found homeopathy superior to placebo in improving total severity during recovery, as measured by a composite score. There was a trend toward improvement during treatment, but this did not reach statistical significance.

The herbal and homeopathic ointment *Calendula officinalis* (marigold) was found significantly better than triethanolamine salicylate (Trolamine, the current standard of care) in preventing radiation-induced dermatitis. (Pommier, 2004) Two hundred fifty-four women receiving postoperative radiation treatment for breast cancer were randomized in a single-blind manner to receive either *Calendula* ointment or Trolamine. *Calendula* is commonly used in homeopathy, and in this study was given at herbal (crude) dosages. The ointments were applied to the breast after the first radiation session and twice or more daily, depending on the occurrence of dermatitis and pain. The incidence of acute dermatitis of grade 2 or higher was significantly lower (41% vs. 63%; $P < 0.001$) in the *Calendula* group. Patients given *Calendula* had fewer

---

[2] A homeopathic "complex" remedy is a fixed, and often patented, mixture of homeopathic medicines, each considered partially effective for a common indication, and marketed OTC for that indication. (e.g., "Allergy") "complex".

interruptions of radiotherapy because of skin toxicity (9 vs. 12 patients), and they had less radiation-induced pain ($P = 0.03$). *Calendula* was slightly more difficult to apply, but the overall satisfaction with its use was greater than with Trolamine.

Schlappack (2004) studied 25 patients who were treated homeopathically for radiation-induced itching. Fourteen of these patients had developed itching during postoperative radiation and 11 after completion of radiotherapy. A single dose of an individually selected homeopathic medicine diluted to $1/10^{60}$ (30CH) was given in the clinic. Patients used a visual analogue scale (VAS) of severity of itching at baseline and at follow-up. Patients were evaluated at a median of 3 days (range: 1–27 days) after administration of the homeopathic medicine. In total, 14 of the 25 patients (56%) responded to the intervention. Nine of the remaining patients were prescribed a second medicine, to which seven responded. Altogether 21 of 25 (84%) patients improved under homeopathic treatment. The VAS measurements before and after homeopathic treatment showed a reduction from a median of 64 mm (range: 20–100 mm) to 34 mm (range: 0–84 mm). The most frequently effective medicine was fluoric acid in homeopathic dilution (Schlappack, 2004). This study lacked a control group; however, the prescription and represcription design of the study reflects the real-life trial and error conditions under which many homeopathic prescriptions are made.

Stomatitis is another troublesome and often treatment-limiting side effect of cancer therapy. It has been purported that the homeopathic medication *Traumeel S* may reduce the severity and duration of chemotherapy-induced stomatitis in patients undergoing bone marrow transplantation. Thirty patients between the ages of 3 and 25 years who had undergone allogeneic (n = 15) or autologous (n = 15) stem cell transplantation were randomly assigned to receive either *Traumeel S* or an indistinguishable placebo. Patients were instructed to rinse their mouths with their allocated medication five times daily for a minimum of 14 days or until all signs of stomatitis were absent for at least 2 days. At treatment conclusion, mean stomatitis scores were lower in the homeopathy group than in the placebo group ($P < 0.01$). Five patients (33%) in the *Traumeel S* group did not develop stomatitis at all, as compared to one patient (7%) in the placebo group ($P = 0.01$). Stomatitis worsened in only seven patients (47%) in the *Traumeel S* group compared with 14 patients (93%) in the placebo group ($P = 0.001$) (Oberbaum, 2001). This study suggests that a homeopathic medication is superior to placebo in preventing and treating stomatitis in stem cell transplantation patients.

In addition to clinical studies testing the efficacy of *Traumeel S* in humans, laboratory research also indicates that this homeopathic medicine may affect the behavior of immune cells, lending credence to *Traumeel*'s anti-inflammatory effects. T cells, monocytes, and gut epithelial cells were treated with *Traumeel* S and exposed to PHA-, PMA- or TNF. Secretion of IL-1β, TNF-α, and IL-8 was measured over a period of 24 to 72 hours. *Traumeel* S was found to inhibit pro-inflammatory mediators IL-1β, TNF-α, and IL-8 by 54% to 70% as compared with untreated cells. The effect was paradoxically inversely dose related, countering claims that the effects of this remedy may be cytotoxic in nature (Porozov, 2004).

Conclusion

Until recently, most clinical studies relating to the homeopathic treatment of cancer patients had been of low quality and relegated to publications outside the mainstream medical literature. Recent years have seen a quantum leap in both the quantity and quality of research. Despite this fact, a critical mass of research has not been reached that would allow firm conclusions to be drawn. Judging the state of homeopathic cancer-related research against the hierarchy of study methods for clinical decision making (Guyatt, et al., 2000), we conclude that homeopathic research still has a long way to go. Most of the research we present is at the level of basic science, with promising, though not definitive, evidence in favor of homeopathic remedies in certain animal and cell models of cancer. The observational and controlled study data are also encouraging, though not universally positive, in support of homeopathic remedies as adjunctive cancer care and for palliation. Randomized and blinded clinical trials exist demonstrating the efficacy of homeopathy in treating side effects of cancer therapy, but to date these suffer from either small sample sizes, inadequate controls, or borderline statistical significance. One small but remarkable study demonstrated apparent cure of glioma in eight of nine cases using homeopathy alone (Pathak, et al., 2003). We would await indubitable reproduction of these results before drawing overly optimistic conclusions.

The field of homeopathic research in cancer treatment requires independent replication studies with larger sample sizes, as well as investigation of individual variations in responsiveness to distinguish potentially good versus poor responders, a pressing concern for much of complementary and alternative medicine (CAM) research (Bell, Baldwin, & Schwartz, 2002a; Caspi & Bell 2004a, 2004b). Until further evidence of the efficacy of homeopathy in cancer treatment becomes available, patients should be warned of the danger of opting for homeopathic treatment in lieu of proven conventional therapies. However, homeopathy may be a useful adjunct in treating cancer treatment side effects, and may improve patients' moods and quality of life. Many homeopaths balk at prescribing homeopathically for patients receiving conventional cancer therapies, particularly those as aggressive as radiation or chemotherapy. However, we believe integration of these therapies should be encouraged. Homeopathy may be of benefit to cancer patients, even in conjunction with aggressive cancer protocols. Moreover, homeopathic remedies historically do not interact adversely from a pharmacodynamic or pharmacokinetic perspective with conventional cancer treatment drugs, in contrast to some nutritional and botanical supplements.

In summary, the literature we have reviewed does not offer convincing evidence to support the contention that homeopathy is currently a reasonable alternative to conventional cancer therapy. However, from an integrative medicine perspective, the evidence favors further testing of homeopathy as one component in an overall cancer treatment program, including prevention or mitigation of chemotherapy and radiation therapy side effects and support of patient well-being during these stressful life events. Until the body of researchers allows different conclusions, we believe homeopathy's place in cancer therapy must be as an adjuvant, rather than alternative, to conventional cancer therapies.

REFERENCES

Balzarini A, Felisi E, Martini A, & De Conno F. (2000). Efficacy of homeopathic treatment of skin reactions during radiotherapy for breast cancer: A randomised, double-blind clinical trial. *British Homeopathic Journal,* 89, 8–12.

Caulfield T & DeBow S. (2005). A systematic review of how homeopathy is represented in conventional and CAM peer reviewed journals. *BMC Complementary and Alternative Medicine [Electronic Resource],* 5(1), 12.

MacLaughlin BW, Gutsmuths B, Pretner E, Jonas WB, Ives J, Kulawardane DV, et al. (2006). Effects of homeopathic preparations on human prostate cancer growth in cellular and animal models. *Integrative Cancer Therapies,* 5, 362–372.

Milazzo S, Russell N, & Ernst E. (2006). Efficacy of homeopathic therapy in cancer treatment. *European Journal of Cancer (Oxford, England,* 42(3), 282–289.

Oberbaum M, Yaniv I, Ben-Gal Y, et al. (2001). A randomized, controlled clinical trial of the homeopathic medication Traumeel S® in the treatment of chemotherapy-induced stomatitis in children undergoing stem cell transplantation. *Cancer,* 92(3), 684–690.

Pathak S, Multani AS, Banerji P, & Banerji P. (2003). Ruta 6 selectively induces cell death in brain cancer cells but proliferation in normal peripheral blood lymphocytes: A novel treatment for human brain cancer. *International Journal of Oncology,* 23(4), 975–982.

Pommier, P, et al. (2004) Phase II randomized trial of calendula officinalis compared with trolamine for the prevention of acute dermatitis during irradiation for breast cancer, *Journal of Clinical Oncology,* 22, 1147–1453.

Porozov S, Chalon L, Weiser M, et al. (2004). Inhibition of IL-1beta and TNF-alpha secretion from resting and activated human immuncytes by the homeopathic medication traumeel S. *Clinical & Developmental Immunology*, 11(2), 143–149.

Schlappack O. (2004). Homeopathic treatment of radiation-induced itching in breast cancer patients. A prospective observational study. *Homeopathy: The Journal of the Faculty of Homeopathy*, 93(4), 210–215.

Thangapazham RL, Rajeshkumar NV, Sharma A, Warren J, Singh AK, Ives JA, et al. (2006b). Effect of homeopathic treatment on gene expression in Copenhagen rat tumor tissues. *Integrative Cancer Therapies*, 5, 350–355.

Thompson EA & Reilly, D. (2002). The homeopathic approach to symptom control in the cancer patient: a prospective observational study. *Palliative Medicine*, 16(3), 227–233.

16

Anthroposophic Medicine, Integrative Oncology, and Mistletoe Therapy of Cancer

PETER HEUSSER AND GUNVER SOPHIA KIENLE

KEY CONCEPTS

ANTHROPOSOPHIC MEDICINE AND INTEGRATIVE ONCOLOGY

- Anthroposophic medicine (AM) is a holistic form of integrative medicine.
- AM uses a comprehensive multimodal therapy concept that simultaneously addresses specific processes and interactions of the physical body, life functions, soul, and spirit.
- In oncology, AM integrates conventional tumor therapy, mistletoe and other plant or mineral medications, art therapy (painting, modeling, music, poetry recitation), eurythmy (a movement therapy), and psycho-oncological and spiritual care.
- Quality of life (QoL) studies show significant improvements of global, physical, emotional, cognitive, spiritual, and social QoL after holistic AM treatment in advanced cancer.

MISTLETOE TREATMENT OF CANCER

- Mistletoe treatment of cancer originates in AM, but has advanced to one of the most extensively used and investigated complementary cancer treatments in Central Europe.
- In preclinical in vitro and animal models, mistletoe preparations and their isolated constituents such as lectins, viscotoxins, oligo- and polysaccharides have induced apoptosis, cytotoxicity, tumor inhibition, immunomodulation (e.g. activation of macrophages/

monocytes, granulocytes, killer cells, T cells), DNA stabilization, and DNA repair.

- As to clinical effectiveness, to date 20 randomized, 15 non-randomized trials, and 12 prospective single-arm cohort studies, and 4 pharmacoepidemiologic retrolective cohort studies were conducted with varying methodology and quality. Most of them describe substantial clinical effects in disease-free survival, reduction of side effects of conventional treatments, and quality of life.

■

Anthroposophic Medicine: An Academic Form of Integrative Medicine

Anthroposophic medicine (AM) is an occidental and academic form of integrated medicine [1]. AM is practiced on all continents, with its densest distribution in central European countries like Germany, Switzerland, The Netherlands, and Austria. Historically, AM dates back to the cooperation of Rudolf Steiner (1861–1925) and Ita Wegman (1876–1943) in the 1920s [2]. Steiner had studied mathematics, natural sciences, and philosophy; held a Ph.D. in epistemology; and had worked as the editor of Goethe's natural scientific work [3]. Later he became known as the founder of anthroposophy, an empirical yet holistic scientific approach to the human being and its relation to the world (Greek: "anthropos" the human being, "sophia", wisdom or science). Based on philosophical, psychological, and medical reasons, anthroposophy as a holistic scientific discipline had already been proposed and outlined in the 19th century at Central European universities by professors such as Ignaz Paul Vital Troxler (1780–1866) and Immanuel Hermann Fichte (1796–1879) [4,5], and it is implicit already in Goethe's natural scientific work [6]. Rudolf Steiner then worked out the epistemological, methodological, and practical basis for anthroposophy and its many possible fields of application such as natural sciences, psychology, medicine, pedagogy, agriculture, arts, and social sciences [7,8]. In congruence with the principle of natural science as developed in the occident since Aristotle, anthroposophy relies on an *empirical* cognitive approach to the human being and nature, based on observation and logical thinking [9]. However, in contrast to the reductionist method of restricting science to external observations and the realm of matter only, anthroposophy *extends* it to the fields of inner observation and the phenomena of life, soul, and spirit [7,10]. In medicine, this results in a *rational* form of holism in theory and practice that is compatible with conventional medicine and forms an extension thereof [2,11].

As a consequence, AM is fairly well integrated with mainstream academic medicine in European countries like Germany and Switzerland. AM is practiced by physicians who are university-trained MDs with usual specializations in general or internal medicine, oncology, pediatrics, gynecology, psychiatry, and others, and who have completed an additional complementary postgraduate training in AM. The certification for AM is acknowledged in Switzerland by the Swiss Medical Associations and in Germany by the Anthroposophic Medical Association. Anthroposophic hospitals are conventionally equipped but provide additional holistic treatments (Fig. 16.1). AM hospitals are state-approved private hospitals whose services are reimbursed by the compulsory health insurance system. They are licensed for the postgraduate internship training of young doctors by the German and Swiss Medical Associations and for clerkships of medical students of Swiss and German universities. AM education is delivered with lectures and in outpatient facilities at several university hospitals. Research programs are carried out in cooperation with other university institutes. Recently, a comprehensive health technology assessment report on AM has been published within the framework of the Swiss National Program for the Evaluation of Complementary Medicine [12].

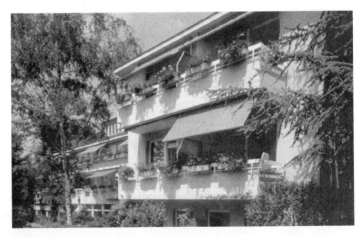

FIGURE 16.1. The Lukas Klinik in Arlesheim. Switzerland, an anthroposophic hospital specialized in oncology.

Apart from AM hospitals and integration of AM in academic research settings, AM is largely practiced by general practitioners in central Europe and worldwide. Most AM GPs participate in the regular regional or national ambulatory patient care systems, and some of them work together with other GPs, nurses, massage, art, and eurythmy therapists in larger group practices called "therapeutica." Nurses and therapists in AM have regular professional trainings and licenses supplemented by additional specific trainings and certifications in AM.

Anthroposophic Medicine, a Humanistic and Holistic Form of Integrative Medicine

Conceptually, AM constitutes a differentiated humanistic form of holism [1,2,11], one of the most basic aspects of which is schematically depicted in Table 16.1.

The four realms of nature can be distinguished by the four main discernible levels of properties they exhibit. Minerals, plants, animals, and human beings all consist of matter; and after death the bodies of plants, animals, and humans even dissolve into the mineral realm. While living, however, the opposite happens: they suppress the increase of entropy in forming and maintaining high-order structures through the typical functions that constitute life such as growth, autopoiesis, metamorphosis, metabolism, nutrition, respiration, self-healing, self-defense (including immunologic processes), reproduction, and others. In animals and humans, an additional third set of properties arises, which is classically attributed to a soul and necessitates states of consciousness:

Table 16.1. Emergent Properties of the Four Realms of Nature.

Minerals	Plants	Animals	Humans	Emergent Properties
			Spirit	Self-consciousness ("I"), rational thinking, free will, self-control, coping, meaning, morality, spirituality
		Soul	Soul	Consciousness, sensations, pain, lust, emotions, desires, instincts, intentions, movement
	Life	Life	Life	Growth, metamorphosis, autopoiesis, nutrition, respiration, metabolism, self-healing, self-defense
Matter	Matter	Matter	Matter	Physicochemical properties, functions and structures, chemical reactions

sensation, pain, lust, emotions, desires, intentions, locomotion, and others. Additionally, the human being can be distinguished from the animal through its faculty of self-consciousness, rational thinking, free will, self-control, search for meaning, morality, spirituality, and so on. This is due to the innermost self of the soul, the individual spirit or "I" ("Ich", "Ego") that is hierarchically higher than the soul. An example for this is an ability that plays an important role in cancer: *coping*. No animal can "cope" with pain or fear or can cognitively control emotional aspects of its disease. This is only possible when another, higher agency within the soul can exert active influence or power on the soul, that is, the human "I" or spirit.

Reductionism tries to causally explain the three higher-order property levels from a knowledge of their underlying physicochemical processes. But the latter are but the *conditions* for the realization of the former. The properties of the higher levels are *emergent* from the respective lower ones, they are enacted by their own laws (the whole is "more and something else" than an aggregate or sum of its parts). For this reason, in AM life, soul and spirit are not considered as epiphenomena of the physical body, but as *real organizations* of their own right, which in their mutual integration and unity with the physical body, constitute the human being as a "whole" [1,2,11].

Consequently, this view leads to extended concepts of health and disease. In this sense, health and disease are not only due to normal or abnormal interactions of molecules but also due to harmonious or disharmonious interactions of processes in the physical, life, soul, or spirit organizations of the individual. And causally not only bottom-up, but also top-down processes between the four systems of body, life, soul, and spirit are responsible for what appears as processes of health and disease. This view can be practically applied in anamnesis, diagnosis, and therapy within a systematic and integrative approach to medicine, especially in oncology.

Table 16.2 schematically depicts this approach as practiced in AM. A multimodal array of measures is tailored to the individual needs of patients in such a way that active principles on all systemic levels are accounted for: (a) structures and functions of the physical body, (b) regulation of life functions, (c) processes within the soul, and (d) activity of the spirit, as well as causal interactions between these four levels of organization within the human being as a whole. This approach applies to all possible fields of medicine. In oncology, for example, all therapeutic measures, conventional as well as unconventional, are aimed at contributing to an overall combat of cancer, symptom control, therapy of comorbidities, and prevention of side effects within a rational overall therapy plan, the elements of which correspond to the four levels indicated in Table 16.2. In this respect, the singular treatment modalities are targeted at specific factors of these levels. For example, surgery, radiotherapy, and cytotoxic chemotherapy

Table 16.2. Holistic Multimodal Integrative Therapy
in Anthroposophic Medicine.

Humans	Therapeutic Approach
Spirit ⇕	⇐ **Activation of cognitive and spiritual forces:** cognitive coping strategies, biography work, meditation, spirituality, meaning, destiny (karma), religion
Soul ⇕	⇐ **Improvement of emotional functions:** art therapy (e.g. music, painting, poetry recitation), psychotherapy, empathy, dedication
Life ⇕	⇐ **Improvement of health related life functions:** hormones, mistletoe therapy, phytotherapy, homeopathy, therapeutic eurythmy, rhythmic massage
Matter	⇐ **Elimination of pathological structures:** surgery, radiotherapy, chemotherapy **Improvement of physical functions:** physiotherapy

are primarily aimed at the *physical* elimination of tumor tissue, and physiotherapy serves to improve physical strength, functions, and structures of the musculoscletal system. Treatments primarily aimed at the system of *life* processes are mistletoe therapy to enhance the body's own self-defense and regeneration through immunologic processes, gene repair, and gene protection [12–14]; phytotherapeutic or homeopathic preparations to improve various organ functions such as liver detoxification, kidney excretion etc.; or therapeutic eurythmy, a movement therapy with specific effects on inner life functions and on the re-integration of body, soul, and spirit. Therapies primarily affecting emotional processes of the *soul* are music, painting, poetry recitation, or direct psychotherapy; but personal empathy and dedication of physicians, therapists, and nurses also work in this direction. Therapies primarily directed at the *spirit* are cognitive coping strategies, biography work, meditation and forms of counseling responding to questions of spirituality, meaning, life after death, religion, and others. Depending on concrete patient needs, individualized compositions of such multilevel treatment elements are applied, resulting in the holistic and integrative treatment approach that characterizes AM.

What effects does this integrative strategy have in practice? Within a Swiss National Science Foundation Research Program a quality-of-life (QoL) study with 144 inpatients with advanced cancers was carried out at the Lukas Klinik in Arlesheim, Switzerland, an internationally known hospital specialized in anthroposophically extended oncology. Validated instruments were utilized so that QoL could be extensively assessed on all systemic levels of the human wholeness addressed. Patients received individualized AM integrative palliative cancer treatment for 3 weeks on average, including conventional and anthroposophic medication, mistletoe therapy with Iscador (the most frequently used and most widely researched mistletoe preparation for cancer treatment), art, and eurythmy therapy, massage, baths and compresses, biography work, and counseling, including issues of meaning and spirituality. As a result, QoL improvements were observed in all 20 assessed QoL parameters, 12 of which were statistically significant ($P < 0.0025$). This concerned all major QoL domains: global health status and QoL, physical tumor symptoms and QoL, and emotional, cognitive, spiritual, and social QoL. At follow-up after 4 months a partial persistence of these effects could be found, and the subjectively perceived benefits from AM confirmed that integrative AM cancer treatment was experienced as intended: humanistic and holistic [15,16].

A Swedish study compared QoL of breast cancer patients treated in an AM hospital for 2 weeks on average or in a conventional medical setting. A prospective matched-pair design was chosen because a randomized clinical trial was not feasible. While AM patients had significantly worse QoL and disease coping before AM treatment at study entrance, both QoL and coping significantly improved during AM therapy and, after 1 year, were superior compared to conventionally treated patients who showed no significant change in QoL [17,18]. In addition, qualitative studies showed impressively that a treatment reaching all levels—physical, emotional, and spiritual—results in gains of patients' self-confidence, experience of strength, life perspectives, relationships, and meaning, whereas treating mind and body as separate was perceived by the patients as additional violation that increased their suffering [19–21].

Mistletoe Therapy of Cancer

Mistletoe extract, an old herbal remedy for various indications, was first introduced for cancer treatment in the context of AM by Steiner and Wegman in 1920[22]. Today mistletoe therapy is the most popular and most frequently prescribed complementary cancer therapy in Central Europe [23,24]. AM mistletoe preparations—Abnobaviscum, Helixor, Iscador (labelled as "Iscar" in the US), Iscucin, Isorel—are extracts from defined parts of the European mistletoe, *Viscum album* L. (VAE), that is, fresh leafy shoots and berries. The mistletoe plant is a parasite, growing on a variety of host trees (Fig. 16.2). Preparations are available from different host trees such as fir (*Abies*, A), oak (*Quercus*, Q), apple tree (*Malus*, M), pine (*Pinus*, P), elm (*Ulmus*, U), and others. Route of application and dosage are varied individually, depending on the patient's reaction and stage of disease. AM mistletoe is used in all stages of disease, either alone (when

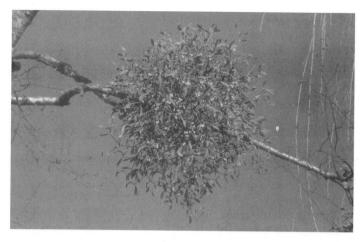

FIGURE 16.2. European mistletoe (Viscum album L.) plant, growing on a birch tree branch.

conventional therapy is not feasible) or in combination with chemotherapy, radiation therapy, or hormone therapy.

Biological and pharmacological properties of VAE have been subject to extended scientific investigations (overview in [13,14]). Several pharmacologically active compounds have been isolated, such as mistletoe lectins (ML I, II and III) [25], viscotoxins [26,27], oligo- and polysaccharides [28,29], lipophilic extracts [30], and several others [13,14]. The most prominent properties of VAE are their cytotoxic and immunomodulating effects. Cytotoxic and growth-inhibiting effects on a variety of human tumor cell lines, lymphocytes, and fibroblasts have been well investigated in vitro [13,14]. The cytotoxic effects of VAE are mainly due to the mistletoe lectins, which induce apoptosis and inhibit protein synthesis by inactivating ribosomes [31–33], while the viscotoxins induce necrotic cell death by membrane destruction [33,34]. In vivo, these cytotoxic effects play a role mainly in the intratumoral and intracavitary application of higher VAE dosages such as intrapleural, intraperitoneal or intravesical instillations ([35–38] (see also table 16.5). VAE are also recognized for their immunomodulating activity. Immunomodulation can be found in lower and medium dose ranges when applied by the subcutaneous, intravenous, or intracavitary route. In vitro and in vivo studies have demonstrated activation of monocytes/macrophages, granulocytes, natural killer (NK) cells, T cells (especially T-helper cells), and the induction of various cytokines [14]. VAE also possesses DNA stabilizing and DNA repairing properties [39–42]. In animals, VAE displays potent antitumoral effects when administered either directly into the tumor or systemically [13,14].

Numerous clinical studies have been conducted on clinical efficacy and effectiveness of anthroposophic mistletoe preparations [12,13,43,44]. These investigated clinical benefit, immunmodulation or safety. Sixteen randomized (RCT, see Table 16.3), 9 non-randomized (N-RCT, see Table 16.4) prospective controlled trials, 12 prospective single-arm cohort studies (see Table 16.5), and 2 elaborate retrolective[1] controlled studies have been conducted evaluating effectiveness [43,44].

Cancer types studied included breast, lung, gastrointestinal, melanoma, genital, head and neck, brain, kidney, follicular non–Hodgkin lymphoma, and malignant effusions. Nineteen of the controlled studies investigated survival and half of them reported a statistically significant benefit. Eight studies investigated reduction of side effects of chemotherapy, radiation, or surgery, and all reported a benefit. Quality of life was investigated in 11 trials, 7 of which found a statistically significant benefit. Influence on tumor behavior remained inconclusive in controlled trials, while single-arm studies reported substantial remissions (see Table 16.5). Methodological quality of the controlled trials varied considerably; some had major limitations while others were reasonably well conducted. Only a few of the trials were blinded. As blinded mistletoe application is easily unblinded because of the local reaction at the injection site [45,79], blinding procedure is questionable. Quality of reporting in cohort studies was reasonably good in most cases.

Altogether, with regard to quality of studies and consistency of results, the best evidence concerning efficacy of mistletoe therapy seems to exist for improvement of QoL and reduction of side effects of cytoreductive therapies—limited by the fact that the interventions are not blinded, and cannot be reliably blinded. Survival benefit is possible: conventional RCTs on this issue had varying results and best evidence relies on studies using epidemiological methodology unfamiliar to most scientists and less widely accepted [51,80,81]. Tumor remission in cohort studies is best described in the reviewed single-arm cohort studies, often using high dosage and local application. The largest controlled studies that show survival benefit used a mistletoe application that recommends an individually adapted and rhythmically alternated dosage schedule [43,44].

Mistletoe therapy is generally well tolerated and safe. The yearly use of the most frequently applied preparation, Iscador, amounts to 4 million ampoules, accounting for about 33,000 patients treated per year [82]. Two

---

[1] The term retrolective was suggested by Alvan Feinstein (Clinical Epidemiology, 1985) and is used today for elaborate studies, with both retrospective and prospective elements—when clinical outcomes have already occurred and have been documented in medical records or other sources, and when the prospective data collection from medical records and the data analysis follows a study protocol and the rules of good epidemiological practice.

Table 16.3. Randomized Controlled Trials on Mistletoe Treatment in Cancer.

Author, Year	Site	Stage	Intervention (Evaluable Patients)	Survival		Tumor		Other Outcomes
Auerbach 2005 [45]	Breast	T1–2, N0–1, M0	CMF, radiation, Helixor A (11) CMF, radiation, placebo (9)					CMF-induced NK-cell decrease ↓*, SCE-increase ↓, QoL, other immune markers: no difference
Enesel 2005 [46][†]	Gastrointestinal	II–III	Surgery, Isorel (40) Surgery (30)					Surgery-induced lymphocyte reduction ↓, KPI ↑‡, anxiety ↓‡
Kleeberg 2004 [47]	Melanoma	High-risk primary (≥3 mm) or LN+	Surgery, Iscador M (102) Surgery, IFN-α (240) Surgery, IFN-γ (244) Surgery (244/102)	Overall survival (hazard ratio)	1.21 (0.84–1.75) 0.96 (0.76–1.21) 0.87 (0.69–1.10)	Disease-free interval (hazard-ratio)	1.32 (0.93–1.87) 1.04 (0.84–1.30) 0.96 (0.77–1.2)	QoL: not stated
Piao 2004 [48]	Breast, ovary, lung (NSCLC)	T1–4, N0–3, M0–1	Chemotherapy‡‡, Helixor A (115) Chemotherapy‡‡, Lentinan (109)					FLIC ↑ (9 vs. 4,7)* TCM ↑ (−1 vs. 0)* KPI ↑ (50 vs. 32% of patients)* Chemotherapy-induced AEs ↓ (28 vs. 77)

(continued)

Table 16.3. (Continued)

Author, Year	Site	Stage	Intervention (Evaluable Patients)	Survival		Tumor	Other Outcomes
Cazacu 2003 [49]	Colon, rectum	Dukes C and D	Surgery, 5-FU, Isorel A (29) Surgery, 5-FU (21) Surgery (14)	Median/mean survival (months)	Dukes C | D 25* | 17* 18 | 7 17 | 15		5-FU side effects (% of patients) 0% 19% QoL: ↑, no data shown
Borrelli 2001 [50]	Breast	IV	Iscador spezial (20) Placebo (10)				QoL (Spitzer) ↑*
Grossarth 2001 [51]	Breast	IIIA–IIIB	Iscador (17) None (17)	Mean survival (months)	57.5* 28.9		Psychosomatic selfregulation ↑
Grossarth 2001 [51]	Breast, lung, colon, rectum, stomach	All stages	Iscador (39) None (39)	Mean survival (months)	42* 29		Psychosomatic selfregulation ↑*
Kim 1999 [38]	Pleural effusion	Advanced	Helixor (11) Doxycyclin, Meperidin, Lidocain (15)			Complete response | partial response[††] 81% | 9% 40% | 26%	

Study	Cancer	Stage	Treatment (n)	Survival		Complete response | overall regress[††]	Patients subjectively improved
Dold 1991 [52]	Lung	All stages	Iscador U or Qu, c.Hg. (114) / Placebo (vitamin B) (113) / Polyerga (110)	Median survival (months)	9.1 / 7.6 / 9.0	4% | 26% / 3% | 20% / 2% | 19%	59%* / 45% / 43%
Salzer 1991 [53]	Lung	I–IV	Surgery, Iscador (87) / Surgery (96)	Median survival (months)	33 / 31	Recurrence 50% / 55%	
Gutsch 1988 [54]	Breast	T1–3, N0–3, M0	Surgery, radiation,*** Helixor (192) / Surgery, radiation*** (274) / Surgery, radiation*** CMF (177)	5-year survival	69.1%* / 59.7% / 67.7%*		
Salzer 1987 [55]	Lung	I (II)	Surgery, Iscador (12) / Surgery (14)	Median survival (months)	117 / 34.5		
Douwes 1986 [56]	Colon, rectum	Advanced	5FU/FA, Helixor (20) / 5FU/FA (20) / 5FU/FA, Ney Tumorin (20)	Mean survival (months) Responder | n-Resp	27 | 12 / 14 | 5 / 24 | 12	Complete response | partial response 15% | 35% / 15% | 30% / 15% | 25%	Reduction of side effects of chemotherapy (no data shown)

(continued)

Table 16.3. (Continued)

Author, Year	Site	Stage	Intervention (Evaluable Patients)	Survival		Tumor	Other Outcomes
Lange 1985 [57]	Lung, head and neck, ovary	Inoperable	Radiation, cisplatin, ifosfamide, Helixor (23) Radiation, cisplatin, ifosfamide (21)				KPI ↑,‡ Nausea ↓,* vomiting ↓,* depression of myelopoiesis ↓*
Salzer 1979, 1983 [58–60]	Stomach	II–III	Surgery, Iscador (62) Surgery (75)	Mean survival (months)	Lymph node +/– 25*|55 18|45		

* Statistically significant superiority compared to comparison-group.
† Statistical significance of pre-post-difference within the group.
‡ Essential information in a supplementary statement.
** Chemotherapy: breast cancer: CAP, CAF; ovarian cancer: CP, IcP; NSCLC: VP, MViP. Cyclophosphamide (C), Adriamycin (A), cisplatin (P), 5-fluorouracil (F), vinore-lbine (V), mitomycin (M), ifosfamide (I), vindesine (Vi), carboplatin (cP).
†† Side effects in Helixor and doxycyclin group: pain in 3 and 6, burning sensation in 0 and 5 patients, respectively; difference statistically significant.
‡‡ Not corresponding to WHO definition of tumour response
*** Co-intervention (i.e, radiation) applied to part of the group.

AE, adverse effect; CMF, cyclophosphamide, methotrexate, 5FU; FLIC, functional living index—cancer; 5FU, 5-fluorouracil; FA, folic acid; KPI, karnofsky performance index; NSCLC, non–small cell lung cancer; QoL, quality of life; SCE, sister chromatid exchange; TCM, traditional chinese medicine index.

Table 16.4. Nonrandomized Controlled Clinical Trials on Mistletoe Treatment in Cancer.

Author, Year	Site	Stage	Intervention (Evaluable Patients)	Survival		Tumor Response, Other Outcomes	Design/Control for Confounding
Von Hagens 2005 [61]	Breast	I–II	Surgery, CMF/EC, Iscador (33) Surgery, CMF/EC (33)			CMF/EC-induced nausea/vomiting ↓*, and general side effects ↓*; platelets ↑*	Self-selected treatment group; no difference in reported baseline data
Büssing 2005 [62]	Breast (suspected)		Surgery, Iscador M spezial (47) Surgery (51)			Surgery-associated inhibition of granulocyte function ↓*	Comparison of two different hospitals. Pair-matching for analysis
Grossarth 2001 [51]	Breast, lung, colon, rectum, stomach	All stages	Iscador (396) None (396)	Mean survival (months)	50,8* 36,6		Prospective pair matching
Schuppli 1990 [63]	Melanoma	Not specified	Surgery, Iscador P c. Hg (84) Surgery, BCG (114)	5-year survival	~86% ~72%		Penalty, prognostic disadvantage for mistletoe group
Douwes 1988 [64]	Colon, rectum	Advanced	5FU/FA, Helixor (19) 5FU/FA (20)	Mean survival (months)	26 14	Complete | partial | minimal response 16% | 37% | 26%* 0% | 30% | 20%	Planned as an RCT; however, computer error occurred

(continued)

Table 16.4. (Continued)

Author, Year	Site	Stage	Intervention (Evaluable Patients)	Survival		Tumor Response, Other Outcomes		Design/Control for Confounding
Salzer 1987 [55]	Breast	I–III	Surgery, Iscador, (76) Surgery, radiation, hormone (79)	Alive 1985 (after 11–14 years)	29% 24%			Alternating treatment allocation
Salzer 1978 [65]	Lung	I–III	Surgery, Iscador (37) Surgery (40)	6-year survival		38%* 15%		Treatment allocation by type of hospital referring the patient to surgery
Fellmer 1966 [66]	Cervix	I–III	Radiation, Iscador (81) Radiation (709)	5-year survival	83%* 69%			Treatment allocation by indifferent attending physician
Majewski 1963[67]	Genital	All stages	Surgery[†], radiation[†], Iscador (155) Surgery[†], radiation[†] (ns)	Disease-specific survival partly improved				Alternating treatment allocation

* Statistically significant superiority compared to comparison-group.

[†] Co-intervention (i.e. radiation) applied to part of the group

EC, epirubicin cyclophosphamide; ns, not shown; CMF, cyclophosphamide, methotrexate, 5FU; 5FU; 5-fluorouracil; FA, folic acid; ns, not shown.

Table 16.5. Prospective Single-Arm Cohort Studies (e.g. Phase II Trials) on Mistletoe Treatment in Cancer.

Author, Year	Treatment[I]					Site[II]	Result[III]					n[IV]
	Preparation	Injection Site	Dosage	Escalating Dosage	Duration		CR	PR	NC	PD	QoL	
Solid tumors or lymphoma												
Kuehn 2005 [68]	Iscador P (M, Qu occasionally)	sc	0.01–30mg	Yes	mean 24 months	Follicular lymphoma	17% [IIIa]	25 % [IIIa]	–	38%		24
Matthes 2005 [69]	Helixor M	it[Ia]	300–1000 mg	Yes	Repeatedly	Pancreas	8%	50%	33%	8%	↗	12
Bar-Sela 2004 [70]	Abnobaviscum Qu	sc	3 × 0.15–15 mg/w	Yes	med. 14 w	Colon, Rectum	0	0	84%	16%	↗ [IIIb]	25
Mabed 2004 [71]	Viscum fraxini	sc	1 × 30 mg/w	No	med. 17 w	HCC	13%	9%	(39%)[IIIc]	39%		23
Mahfouz 1999 [72]	Viscum fraxini	sc or it	1 × 45 mg/w	No	18–136 w	Breast	8%	54%	35%	4%	↗	26
Mahfouz 1998 [73]	Abnobaviscum Fr	sc	1 × 45 mg/w	No	17 w	Breast, Brain	27%	27%	27%	20%	↗	15
Kjaer 1989 [74]	Iscador Qu or M, c.Cu	sc	Varying	Yes	med. 13/47 w	Kidney	0	0	14%	86%	↘	14

(continued)

Table 16.5. (Continued)

Author, Year	Treatment[I]					Site[II]	Result[III]					n^{IV}
	Preparation	Injection site	Dosage	Escalating dosage	Duration		CR	PR	NC	PD	QoL	
CIN												
Portalupi 1995 [75]	Iscador M	sc	2 x 1 ng MLI/kg bw/w	No	16 w	CIN I–III	41%	27%	27%	5%		27
Malignant effusion												
Bar Sela 2006 [37]	Iscador M	ipe	10 mg	No	Repeatedly	Ascites	Increase of interval between two successive paracenteses from 7 to 12 days, $P = 0.001$[IIId]				↗[IIIe]	23
Werner 1999 [76]	Abnobaviscum Fr	ip	1 x 75 mg/w	No	3–8 w	Pleural effus.	88%				↗	32
Stumpf 1994 [77]	Helixor A, M or P	ip	100–1000 mg each	Yes	Repeatedly	Pleural effus.	61%	11%	22%			18
Friedrichson 1985 [78]	Helixor	ipe	100–1000 mg each	Yes	Repeatedly	Ascites	70%				↗	12

[I] sc: subcutaneous, it: intratumoural, ip: intrapleural, ipe: intraperitoneal, w: week, med.: median. [Ia] Endoscopic ultrasound-guided fine-needle injection.

[II] HCC: hepatocellular carcinoma, CIN: cervical intraepithelial neoplasia, effus.: effusion (malignant). Stage: advanced, except CIN; plural effusion and ascites indicates treatment site.

[III] CR: complete, PR: partial remission, NC: no change, PD: progredient disease, QoL: quality of life, ↗: improved, ↘ impaired; [IIIa] responses under mistletoe monotherapy, without concomitant oncologic cytoreductive therapies; [IIIb] symptomatic relief (40% of patients); [IIIc] undetermined response due to early death; [IIId] median values, comparable abdominal circumference and symptom score or drained fluid before or during each paracentesis, respectively; [IIIe] Trend improvement in symptom score, especially abdominal pain, abdominal pressure, and waking up at night due to shortness of breath.

pharmacoepidemiologic studies found systemic adverse reactions of Iscador treatment in 0.8%–3.3%; they were non-specific and of predominantly mild-to-intermediate severity (WHO/CTC grade 1–2) [80,81]. Frequent are minor dose-dependent reactions at the injection site (swelling, induration, erythema, pruritus, local pain), that subside spontaneously. Occasionally, allergic reactions can occur, but serious adverse events (including anaphylactic reactions) are very rare (<0.01%) [12,13,82,83]. High-dose mistletoe therapy ([71–73], see also Table 16.5) was reported to be safe; nevertheless, as only a few of these patients have been carefully documented, application should be cautious. Currently, an NCCAM/NCI phase I study is investigating safety, toxicity, and drug interactions between mistletoe extract and gemcitabine [84]. A first interim report suggested good tolerability, with neither dose-limiting toxicity of the mistletoe extract nor any effects on the plasma concentration of gemcitabine [85].

Recently, a list of serious side effects of mistletoe therapy was published [86,87], but this turned out to be erroneous interpretations of reports not referring to mistletoe therapy (for details see [12 or 88]). Enhancement of brain metastases was discussed in preliminary reports [89] from a melanoma trial, but the data were not confirmed in the final publication [47] and may have resulted from detection bias [43,90]. Still, they gave rise to an elaborate retrolective multicenter pharmacoepidemiologic study: No tumor enhancement could be observed in mistletoe-treated patients, and the incidence of brain metastases, brain metastases–free survival, disease-free survival, and overall survival were all statistically significant in favor of the mistletoe group [80].

Altogether, the anthroposophic concept of mistletoe therapy has turned out as a reasonably well-founded hypothesis. In preclinical investigations, mistletoe extracts show various antitumor, immunmodulating, DNA stabilizing, and DNA repairing properties in mononuclear cells that clinically correspond to reduction of side effects of cytoreductive therapies, improvement of QoL, tumor remissions (with appropriate application), and possibly prolongation of survival. Mistletoe extracts are well tolerated but can occasionally induce allergic reactions. Adverse interactions with conventional anticancer therapies are currently unknown. In vitro and in animals, mistletoe extracts tend to enhance cytotoxic effects of conventional cancer drugs [91,92]. Further investigation of its clinical benefits should be encouraged.

Addendum

After completion of this chapter the following clinical studies have been published: two retrolective pharmacoepidemiological studies on pancreatic carcinoma and colorectal carcinoma [93,94]; four randomized matched-pair studies on early breast cancer, on cervical cancer, and on ovarian cancer [95–97]; five prospective non-randomized matched-pair studies on early breast cancer, cervical cancer with and without metastases, and ovarian cancer [95–97]. All of these studies indicate positive effects of mistletoe therapy (survival, disease-free interval, quality of life, reduction of side effects of conventional oncological treatments).

REFERENCES

2. Steiner R & Ita W. (1996). *Extending practical medicine (1925). 2nd Edition.* London: Rudolf Steiner Press.

7. Steiner R. (1984.) *A Theory of knowledge - implicit in Goethe's world conception. 3rd Edition.* Spring Valley NY: Anthroposophic Press, 1984.

12. Kienle GS, Kiene H, & Hans UA. (2006). *Anthroposophic Medicine: Effectiveness, Utility, Costs, Safety.* Stuttgart, NewYork: Schattauer Verlag.

13. Kienle GS & Helmut K. (2003). *Die Mistel in der Onkologie - Fakten und konzeptionelle Grundlagen.* Stuttgart, New York: Schattauer Verlag.

14. Büssing A. (Ed.). (2000). *Mistletoe. The Genus Viscum.* Amsterdam: Hardwood Academic Publishers.

15. Heusser P, Berger BS, Ziegler R, Bertschy M, Helwig S, van Wegberg B, et al. (2006). Palliative in-patient cancer treatment in an anthroposophic hospital: I. Treatment patterns and compliance with anthroposophic medicine. *Forschende Komplementärmedizin,* 13, 94–100.

16. Heusser P, Berger BS, Bertschy M, Burkhard R, Ziegler R, Helwig S, et al. (2006). Palliative in-patient cancer treatment in an anthroposophical hospital II: Global, physical, emotional, cognitive-spiritual, and social quality of life during and after stationary treatment, and subjectively perceived treatment benefits. *Forschende Komplementärmedizin,* 13, 156–166.

17. Carlsson M, Arman M, Backman M, Flatters U, Hatschek K, & Elisabeth H. (2004). Evaluation of quality of life/life satisfaction in women with breast cancer in complementary and conventional care. *Acta Oncologica,* 43, 27–34.

43. Kienle GS, Berrino F, Büssing A, Portalupi E, Rosenzweig S, & Helmut K. (2003). Mistletoe in cancer – a systematic review on controlled clinical trials. *European Journal of Medical Research,* 8, 109–119.

44. Kienle GS, & Helmut K. (2007). Complementary Cancer Therapy: A Systematic Review of Prospective Clinical Trials on Anthroposophic Mistletoe Extracts. *European Journal of Medical Research,* 12, 103–19.

(*A complete reference list for this chapter is available online at http://www.oup.com/us/integrativemedicine*).

17

Energy Medicine and Cancer

SUSAN K. LUTGENDORF AND ELIZABETH MULLEN

KEY CONCEPTS

- Energy medicine is a complementary and alternative medicine (CAM) modality whose practitioners purport to restore the flow of energy fields associated with the human body for symptom relief, disease prevention, and health restoration.
- Experimental evidence of the health benefits of energy medicine has been mixed, with many studies suffering from methodological weaknesses.
- Preclinical trials suggest that energy medicine may enhance immunity and decrease both growth and activity of cancer cells.
- Clinical trials have reported evidence of improved mood, quality of life, and immune parameters such as natural killer cell activity and leukocyte number; however, these results have not always been replicable in later studies.
- Larger energy medicine clinical trials with stronger methodology are needed to address both the effectiveness and mechanisms of action, as well as factors influencing replication of these effects.
- The majority of patients using energy medicine do not automatically inform their physicians of CAM use. Medical practitioners are advised to ask their patients whether they are utilizing energy medicine treatments or other CAM modalities.

■

Use of Energy Medicine in Oncology Settings

Complementary and alternative medicine (CAM) therapies are commonly used by cancer patients, with reports of CAM use among cancer patients varying from 30% (Fouladbakhsh, Stommel, Given, & Given, 2005; Markovic, Lenore, Natalie, & Michael, 2006) to 66.7% (Boon, et al., 2000). Cancer patients using CAM therapies are more often female, are undergoing surgery or chemotherapy, are experiencing substantial symptoms (Fouladbakhsh, et al., 2005), are well educated, and report higher income (Alferi, Antoni, Kilbourn, & Carver, 2001). Energy-based therapies are among the CAM therapies sought out by cancer patients (Fouladbakhsh, et al., 2005; Hann, et al., 2005; Markovic, et al., 2006; Molassiotis, et al., 2005; Sparber, et al., 2000). However, there is little data establishing the efficacy, effectiveness, and putative mechanisms of these therapies. This chapter examines the use of energy therapies in oncology settings and the state of the evidence-based literature on preclinical and clinical findings. Although there is substantial literature on the effects of long-distance healing and prayer (Astin, Harkness, & Ernst, 2000; Benson, et al., 2006; Sicher, Targ, Moore, & Smith, 1998), the focus of the present chapter is on energy therapies used at close proximity to the patient.

National Institutes of Health Definition and Assumptions of Energy Medicine

According to the National Center for Complementary and Alternative Medicine (NCCAM), energy medicine deals with two types of energy fields—those that can be measured (called *veritable*) and those that have yet to be measured (called *putative*) (see Table 17.1 for a summary of NCCAM Classified Energy Therapies). Veritable energy fields include measurable vibrations such as sound, visible light, laser beams, and rays from the electromagnetic spectrum. Measurement of putative energy fields is more controversial. It has been proposed that energy emanating from healers may actually incorporate both types of energies. Energy therapies conceptualize the physical body as an energy field suffused with a "life force." This life force is called different names according to the culture such as *prana* in Ayurvedic medicine and *Qi* in Traditional Chinese Medicine and flows through pathways such as meridians in the traditional Chinese system or *nadis* and *chakras* in the Ayurvedic system. Free flow of this "life force" through the body is thought to support health, whereas disturbances or blockages in the flow of this energy are thought to cause impaired function in organs and tissues, and ultimately illness. Potential illness is described as visible

Table 17.1. Brief Description of NCCAM Classified Energy Therapies.

Name	Description
External Qi Therapy (Qigong therapy) (Shannon, 2003)	• Formalized within the last century, external Qi therapy is based on Qigong, 2,000-year-old Chinese mind–body exercises. *Qi* means breathing and vital energy, according to Traditional Chinese Medicine and *Gong* means power. • This is described as a "body strengthening technique of cultivating the primordial Qi." • Intentional transfer of Qi-energy from one person to another. • Several general forms exist: (1) as part of a touch therapy such as massage, (2) without touching but in close proximity, or (3) from a great distance. • There are many different types of Qigong and Qigong traditions. • No formal organizational structures regulate the teaching and certification of practitioners. • Qigong can also be used as a system of exercises that a patient can do to strengthen flow of Qi within the body and decrease energy congestion.
Reiki (IARP, 2006; Miles & True, 2003)	• This healing method was created in Japan by Mikao Usui in the early 1900s. • Compared to "laying on of hands" in many spiritual traditions, Reiki is purported to increase health by accessing universal life energy and connecting this with the body's own innate healing abilities via hands-on healing. • Formalized Reiki training exists, in which a Reiki master transfers the healing ability to a student through a process called "attunement," and formalized levels of training have been developed.
Johrei (Laidlaw, et al., 2003; Taft, et al., 2005)	• Founded in Japan by Mokichi Okada, this modality was brought to the United States in 1953. • It involves a nontouch transfer of life energy. Healing ability is thought to develop through a life of spiritual practice, not formal training. • Practitioners direct energy from their hands toward the recipient. The practitioner visualizes healing light entering their own body and directs it via an outstretched hand to the recipient in a spirit of goodwill.
Polarity Therapy (Wilson, 2007)	• Developed by Randolph Stone, D.C., D.O., N.D. in the 1940s. • Energy conduction through hands-on touch to resolve energy blocks and restore a smooth flow of energy. • Part of a larger health system including diet, exercises, and increased self-awareness.

(continued)

Table 17.2. (Continued)

Name	Description
Therapeutic Touch (Krieger, 1979; Mathúna, 2000)	• A system formalized by Dora Kunz and Dolores Krieger, R.N., Ph.D. in the 1970s, it is used in many health care settings. • TT utilizes nontouch energy transfer to restore balance and self-healing capacity. • Posits that living organisms have energy fields which interact with information from the environment. • Practices include centering, assessment, unruffling, modulation of energy, and closure. • Advanced practitioner status is achieved through a certification process
Pranic Healing (Sui, 1999)	• Originating in China thousands of years ago, it was reformulated more recently by Master Choa Kok Sui, based in the Philippines. • Healers are said to manipulate patient ki by perceiving "auras" of color around the human body, and projecting corrective colors in to the aura to bring a state of balance and health.
Healing Touch (Mentgen, 2001; Mentgen Bulbrook, 2002)	• Developed by Janet Mentgen, B.S.N., R.N., and Dorothea Hover-Kramer, Ed.D., R.N., in the 1980s, HT integrates techniques of many prominent healers as well as indigenous healing techniques. • It uses a noninvasive therapeutic approach to healing that uses gentle touch to restore harmony and balance the patient's energy system to assist the patient to self-heal. • Practitioners place their hands above and on the patient's body to determine areas of energy imbalance, unblock energy, and promote physical healing and emotional, mental, and spiritual balance. • Over 30 specific techniques are taught as part of this process. These include techniques that address specific problem areas (mind clearing, pain, and lymphatic drain) as well as specific pathologies (arthritis, back pain) • There is a standardized HT curriculum offered through Healing Touch International and endorsed by the American Holistic Nurse's Association. Formal certification for practitioners who have completed five levels of HT training and required supervision hours is coordinated by Healing Touch International.

in the energy system before physical signs appear. Modulation of a patient's energy field to recreate flow and balance is thought to relieve certain symptoms of illness, as well as to prevent emergence of illness (Mentgen & Bulbrook, 2002; NCCAM, 2004).

Veritable electromagnetic fields. Measurable (veritable) electromagnetic fields have had substantial use in medicine. Both static and pulsing electromagnetic fields have been used for the diagnosis and treatment of a variety of illnesses in current medical practice. For example, pulsed electromagnetic fields (PEMFs), using waves of approximately 15 Hz, have been shown to enhance healing of bone fractures, to stimulate bone formation, and are commonly utilized in medical practice (Fredericks, Nepola, Baker, Abbott, & Simon, 2000; McLeod & Rubin, 1992; Rubin, Donahue, Rubin, & McLeod, 1993). The effect of magnetic fields for treatment of cancer has been examined, though much of this work is still in preclinical stages. Pulsating magnetic fields have been used to inhibit tumor growth in animal models (Salvatore & Markov, 2004) and to inhibit tumor angiogenesis (Markov, Williams, Cameron, Hardman, & Salvatore, 2004; Williams & Markov, 2001; Williams, Markov, Hardman, & Cameron, 2001). Some reports, however, have indicated that EMF can enhance tumor growth (Hannan, Liang, Allison, & Searle, 1994; Watson, Parrish, & Rinehart, 1998). Electromagnetic fields have also been used to reverse resistance of tumor cells to chemotherapy and to enhance the effects of chemotherapy. These experiments have been successful in both in vitro and animal models and have the potential of ultimately decreasing the amount of chemotherapy required and providing alternative means of dealing with resistance to chemotherapy (Cadossi, et al., 1991; Salvatore & Markov, 2004; Zucchini, et al., 1991). Some phase I work has also established safety and minimal toxicity of static magnetic fields accompanying antineoplastic chemotherapy in humans (Salvatore, Harrington, & Kummet, 2003).

Measurement and properties of putative energy fields. The concept of the presence of electromagnetic fields underlying the pattern and organization of biological systems is not new (Burr, 1972; Tiller, 1977) and has been a basic tenet of medical systems such as Traditional Chinese Medicine and Ayurvedic medicine for centuries (NCCAM, 2004). Various attempts have been made to empirically validate these putative energy fields. From 1916 to the mid 1950s, Harold Saxton Burr, Professor of Anatomy at Yale University School of Medicine, made pioneering efforts in this field and devoted his career to mapping the energy fields of living organisms, publishing more than 93 scientific papers and several books. Burr proposed that electrodynamic fields, which he called "fields of life" or "L-fields," were the organizing matrix of all living organisms and determined the relative state of health or illness of the organism. He developed a methodology of measuring and mapping these fields with standard voltmeters, and using this technology he demonstrated that changes in the electrical potential of the L-field preceded changes in the health of the organism. Some of his experiments, examining changes in L-fields with various trees on the Yale campus, spanned decades and demonstrated effects of lunar changes and sunspots on the L-fields (Burr, 1972).

Burr's voltmeter technology was extended to cancer populations in two publications that were reported in the mainstream journals *American Journal of Obstetrics and Gynecology* and *Science* in the late 1940s and early 1950s (Langman & Burr, 1947, 1949). He was part of a team from Bellevue and New York University hospitals that measured voltage differences between the tip of the cervix and the ventral abdominal wall in 428 patients with gynecologic cancers and healthy controls. A reversal of these polarities was noted in almost 99% of patients as compared to the controls, a pattern subsequently replicated in 860 women (Langman, 1972; Langman & Burr, 1947, 1949). The authors suggested that such electromagnetic patterns may allow for atypical cell growth in patients (Langman, 1972). Later in his life, Burr's work received strong criticism, and this line of work does not appear to have been continued in cancer patients. In the 1960s and 1970s his student, Leonard Ravitz, showed that L-fields are strongly influenced by emotional stimuli and that the L-field disappears shortly before death (Ravitz, 1950; http://en.allexperts.com/e/l/l/l-field.htm; March 27, 2007).

To date, the putative role of electromagnetic patterns or fields in maintaining health has been poorly characterized. However, there is some documentation that the physiological processes of a living system such as plant growth, enzyme activation, or hemoglobin production can be positively influenced by nontouch influences thought to work by "exchange of energy" (Byrd, 1988; Grad, 1963, 1964; Grad, Cadoret, & Paul, 1961; Krieger, 1972; Smith, 1972; Smith, 1973). Since these effects occurred without actual physical contact, they have been used to support the interpretation that these effects were induced by means of an energy transfer from the healer to the recipient.

Effects of energy therapies are hypothesized to occur through alteration of "biomagnetic fields" (Chen & Liu, 2004; Kiang, Marotta, Wirkus, Wirkus, & Jonas, 2002; Oschman, 2000; Wirth, Brenlan, Levine, & Rodriguez, 1993; Wirth & Cram, 1993) by practitioners of various energy therapies including therapeutic touch (TT) and Qigong (Berden, Jerman, & Skarja, 1997; Grad, 1963, 1964; NCCAM, 2004; Zimmerman, 1990). In an experiment to determine the types of wavelengths that were emitted during biofield healing, a group at the University of Pennsylvania examined waves emanating from the hands of a Japanese "Ki-expert" (healer using Qi energy) and studied the effect on cellular mitochondria function. His treatment appeared to protect mitochondria from oxidative stress (discussed in more detail in the following paragraphs). Examination of materials that could block these effects suggested that the emitted energy involved a wavelength near the infrared spectrum, with a size of approximately 0.8–2.7 μm (Ohnishi, Ohnishi, Nishino, Tsurusaki, & Yamaguchi, 2005). Other studies have implicated γ radiation as being fundamental to energy therapy. Researchers from the University of Arizona have now found that reliable alterations in amplitude in the extra low frequency range can be detected to be emanating from hands of healers who were "running energy" (Connor, Schwartz, & Tau, 2006).

An extremely sensitive magnetometer (device used to detect magnetic fields) known as the *SQUID* (*superconducting quantum interference device*) has been able to detect pulsing magnetic fields from the hands of therapeutic touch practitioners during treatments, as well as from the hands of practitioners of yoga, meditation, and Qigong (Benford, 2001). These fields were of extremely low frequency, from approximately 21 to 50 Hz, but interestingly, they were similar to the fields being tested for accelerating healing in tissues in various medical experiments (Benford, 2001). However, with a few exceptions (Berden, et al., 1997), testing of the hypothesis of energy transfer has been largely absent (Quinn, 1989).

In vitro studies of Energy Medicine and Cancer

In vitro studies have been used as experimental models to examine the effects of energy medicine without the placebo effect confounds seen in human trials. In general, in vitro studies of biofield medicine have shown effects both in enhancing immunity and in decreasing growth and activity of cancer cells, although the findings have been mixed and often attempts at replication have not been successful. Many of these experiments have been plagued by lack of proper controls and problems in design. A number of the most well-designed studies are presented in the following paragraphs. Readers are also referred to Kevin Chen's review of Qigong studies on cancer in China (Chen & Yeung, 2002). It is thought that CAM approaches may affect both the signaling and transcriptional level of cellular homeostasis (Ventura, 2005).

Ohnishi and colleagues reported that 5- to 10-minute treatments of cultured human liver carcinoma cells by a Japanese Ki-expert decreased cancer cell numbers by 30.3% at 5 minutes and by 40.6% at 10 minutes and also increased protein content/cell (Ohnishi, et al., 2005). RT-PCR analyses indicated that the mRNA expression for *c-myc*, a tumor stimulator gene, was decreased, whereas that for regucalcin, a suppressor of DNA synthesis, was increased. Levels of *p53* did not change with the Ki-intervention. The authors suggest that the Ki-energy suppressed proliferation of these cells by influencing gene expression in the nucleus. These effects were blocked when either aluminum foil or black acrylic plates were placed between the healer and the cells but were not blocked by a clear plastic plate. As noted earlier, the authors suggested that the emanated Ki-energy may be a form of electromagnetic wave in the spectrum of infrared radiation that is blocked by the acrylic but not by the plastic.

Yan and colleagues (2006) treated BxPC3 pancreatic cancer cells with external Qigong for 5 minutes and examined its effects on pathways relevant to survival, proliferation, and resistance to apoptosis (Akt and extracellular signal–regulated kinase pathways). External Qi differentially regulated the survival pathways in cancer versus normal fibroblast cells. In the pancreatic cancer cells, inhibition of pathways critical to cell growth, including Akt, epidermal growth factor (EGF), and nuclear factor kappa-B (NF-κB), were observed. A 5-minute external Qi treatment also induced apoptosis and DNA fragmentation, and prolonged treatment caused rapid lysis of these cells. In marked contrast, external Qi treatment of normal fibroblasts did not have a cytotoxic effect and induced transient activation of pathways described earlier. These intriguing findings indicate that external Qi may have differential effects on the survival of cancer cells as opposed to normal cells and that cytotoxic effects of Qi may be seen specifically in cancer cells. In another work by these same authors, cytotoxic effects of external Qi were seen in breast cancer, pancreatic cancer, and glioma cells, whereas fibroblasts and human umbilical vein endothelial cells were unaffected. Molecular pathways (Akt and ERK) were differentially activated in cancer versus normal cells by energy healing (Yan, et al., 2006).

Kiang and colleagues (2005) reported that a 15-minute treatment of Jurkat T cells by a biofield healer increased intracellular calcium by approximately 22%, an effect that lasted 2 hours. This outcome was indicative of improved cellular functioning as intracellular free calcium stimulates many key cellular functions such as metabolism, proliferation, gene expression, and movement. Interestingly, a blunted version of this effect (11% increase in calcium) was observed when cells were placed in an area where the biofield experiments had previously been performed. This contextual effect disappeared after 24 hours. Externally applied bioenergy was also able to decrease cellular responses to heat stress, without induction of heat shock protein-72 (HSP-72), which is known to be calcium dependent.

A recent study by Gronowicz's group at the University of Connecticut (Jhaveri et al, 2008) showed differential effects between the effects of TT on healthy human osteoblasts (HOB) and on an osteosarcoma-derived cell line (SaOs-2). Cells received TT twice weekly for 10 minutes over the course of 2 weeks. TT significantly increased mineralization in HOB cells and decreased mineralization in SaOs-2 cells as compared to no-treatment controls. Additionally, TT induced an increase in mRNA expression for

Type I collagen, bone sialoprotein, and alkaline phosphatase in HOB cells whereas these bone markers decreased in SaOs-2 cells. Two weeks of TT treatment significantly increased DNA synthesis in HOB but not in SaOs-2 cells. These effects were not seen at 1 week. These findings highlight differential effects of TT in healthy and cancer cells. TT appears to increase DNA synthesis, differentiation, and mineralization in healthy human osteoblast cells, whereas differentiation and mineralization are decreased in bone cancer cells.

In contrast to these successful demonstrations of cellular changes following applications of biofield energy, a considerable number of in vitro studies have shown no effects of biofield energies. Yount and colleagues performed three double-blinded studies to determine the ability of both energy medicine practitioners and nonpractitioner controls to distinguish cancer cells from culture medium or sterile water. Participants performed at the level expected by chance in all studies (Yount et al., 2004). Yount and colleagues also showed a significant increase in the proliferation of cultured normal human brain cells following external Qigong treatment by practitioners under controlled conditions, but this effect was not observed in a replication study (Yount, et al., 2004). These researchers also found that healing treatments by six highly experienced healers to normal brain cells that had been damaged by oxidative stress did not alter cell death rates as compared to normal control cells (Mager et al., 2007).

Zachariae and colleagues conducted three controlled in vitro experiments with three different biofield healers with the goal of reducing the proliferation and viability of two cancer cell lines (an adherent human breast cancer cell line [MCF-7] and a nonadherent mouse B-lymphoid cell line [HB-94]). Five different doses of healing or control were used. No differences between the treated and control cells were found on a number of markers of growth and viability (Zachariae, et al., 2005). Taft and colleagues (2005) performed experiments in which Johrei treatment was delivered to human brain cancer cells (glioblastoma multiforme SF188GBM) by practitioners who participated in teams of two, alternating every half hour, for a total of 4 hours of treatment. Proliferation and cell death were documented by computerized time-lapse microscopy before, during, and after Johrei experiments and were compared to similar parameters of control cells observed under identical conditions. No differences were seen in cell death and proliferation rates of cultured human cancer cells.

These findings, taken together, illustrate the equivocal nature of some of the best in vitro studies of energy medicine with cancer cell cultures. Although there are some very strong positive in vitro studies, with well-characterized molecular endpoints, there are multiple studies with negative or equivocal findings.

Animal Models

Preclinical models afford the ability to examine biofield effects on cancer cells within an animal model, but without placebo effects. There is some debate on how representative animal models of cancer are of the human setting. Chen and colleagues studied 30 mice injected intravenously with lymphoma cells that localize and aggressively grow into lymphoid tissues. Mice were treated with Qigong from a Qigong healer, with sham Qigong from an untrained individual, or were not provided any treatment. Qigong treatment significantly decreased the tumor growth in lymph nodes as compared to sham-treated or control mice; however, in a replication study, although the same pattern was seen, the results did not reach statistical significance, secondary to large variability in all groups in this study (Chen, et al., 2002). Bengston and Krinsley (2000) reported an intriguing set of experiments in which skeptical individuals apprenticed in "techniques alleged to reproduce a healing effect" were the healers. Five experimental mice were injected with a mammary adenocarcinoma that usually causes death within 14 to 27 days and were then treated for an hour a day for 1 month. "Tumors developed a 'blackened area', then ulcerated, imploded, and closed, and the mice lived their normal lifespans." The experiment was repeated three times and produced an overall cure rate of 88% in 33 experimental animals. Interestingly, control mice with adenocarcinoma that were given no healing experienced an enhanced rate of total remissions over the four experiments as well. In contrast, control mice with adenocarcinoma and no healing housed in another lab in another city died within the expected time frame. Although this experiment implies the possibility of (a) biofield healing of the experimental mice and (b) contextual transfer of the healing effect to the control mice, similar laboratory conditions may underlie the longer survival of the experimental and control mice as opposed to the distant mice—thus a replication of this type of experiment is necessary before any conclusions are drawn. Table 17.2 provides a summary of preclinical trials in energy medicine.

Clinical Studies

There is a paucity of clinical studies on energy medicine in cancer. The few that have been done, with some exceptions, have certain methodological weaknesses such as low sample size and statistical concerns. To a certain extent this area of research has been hampered by inadequate funding for conducting clinical

Table 17.2. Summary of Preclinical Trials in Energy Medicine.

References	Treatment Modality	Type of Cancer / Biological Marker	Method	Results
Bengston & Krinsley, (2000). The effect of the "laying on of hands" on transplanted breast cancer in mice. *Journal of Scientific Exploration, 14,* 353–364.	Laying on of hands	Mice injected with mammary adenocarcinoma (H2712)	*Experimental condition:* Mice treated by "skeptical" healers apprenticed to laying on of hands. *Two control conditions:* • Mice not treated but housed on-site • Mice not treated and housed off-site Four replications of experiment	*Experimental mouse:* tumors imploded and healed and mice lived a normal span and showed resistance to future carcinoma injection. *Control mice:* • On-site evidenced enhanced remission and survival • Off-site died within predicted time frame (14 to 27 days). Investigators suggest belief in treatment not necessary for effectiveness.
Chen, et al., (2002). A preliminary study of the effect of external Qigong on lymphoma growth in mice. *The Journal of Alternative and Complementary Medicine, 8,* 615–621.	Qigong	Lymphoma	*S/L/J mice:* Randomized, dual blind (research director, assistants and statistician were blinded to procedure; Qigong healer was not). *3 groups:* Treated with Qigong, sham treatment (not described) and no-treatment group. *Study 1:* Qigong group receives treatment 10 minutes every other day for 5 sessions. Mice injected with lymphoma cells 24 hours after first treatment. *Study 2:* Qigong group receives treatment 10 minutes every day for 5 days.	*Study 1:* Day 9 sacrifice: Qigong showed less tumor in lymph but not spleen than either other group. Day 11 sacrifice: Qigong group exhibited less tumor growth in lymph nodes and spleen than control but not sham group. *Study 2:* No significant differences. Larger standard deviations than study 1. Study differences may be due to greater handling stress of control mice in study 1.

(continued)

Table 17.2. (Continued)

References	Treatment Modality	Type of Cancer / Biological Marker	Method	Results
Fukushima, et al., (2001). Evidence of Qigong energy and its biological effects on the enhancement of the phagocytic activity of the human polymorphonuclear leukocytes. *The American Journal of Chinese Medicine, 29*, 1–16.	Qigong	Human peripheral blood leukocytes	External Qigong applied to saline solution (PBS) vs. no-treatment control. Experimental condition of PBS was masked, and either treated or untreated PBS added to leukocyte suspensions and phagocytic activity measured. Repeated for 10 trials. Subset of samples exposed to rotated microwave treatment and autoclave treatment. Another subset of samples exposed first to unrotated microwave and then to pulsed laser treatments.	Qi-treated samples demonstrated greater phagocytic activity. Rotated microwave but not autoclave treatments decreased this effect. Unrotated microwave and laser irradiation produced similar effects as Qi-treatment.
Hall, et al., (2006). Radiation response of cultured human cells is unaffected by Johrei. *Evidence-based Complementary and Alternative Medicine, 4*, 191–194.	Johrei	Cultured human brain cells	Cultured human brain cells exposed to incrementally greater concentrations of ionizing radiation to stimulate cell death. Cell proliferation and death quantified by computerized time-lapse microscopy. Cultures randomly assigned to experimental or control conditions. Johrei practitioners directed healing toward experimental cultures for 30 minutes from a distance of 20 cm. Control cultures had no treatment. Cell proliferation and death calculated every 30 minutes before, during, and after treatment for a total of 22.5 hours.	Few cell deaths were observed, thus data were pooled from entire observation to estimate death rate. Treatment groups did not differ in rates of cell division or death.

Jhaveri, et al. (2008)	Therapeutic Touch	Human Osteoblasts (HOB) and human-osteosarcoma cell lines (SaOs-2)	Division rates estimated for each 30 minutes and averaged over the eight experiments. Experimental condition: TT applied twice weekly for 10 minutes for 2 weeks Control Condition: No TT treatment but identical lab conditions. Placebo control: Hand movements by untrained individual counting backward from 1000.	TT increased DNA synthesis, differentiation and mineralization in HOB cells compared to controls. TT decreased differentiation and mineralization in SaOs-2 cells compared to controls. Placebo-treated cultures did not differ from controls in proliferation or mineralization.
Kiang, et al., (2005). External bioenergy-induced increases in intracellular free calcium concentrations are mediated by Na^+ / Ca^{2+} exchanger and L-type calcium channel. *Molecular and Cellular Biochemistry, 271*, 51–59.	External bioenergy (EBE)	T cells	*Experimental condition:* • bioenergy specialist emitted external bioenergy (EBE) toward tubes of cultured Jurkat T cells for 15 minutes. • Intracellular calcium levels measured at baseline, for 4 minutes during treatment, and immediately post treatment. • In a subset of samples, EBE treatment applied at varying distances and/or time intervals. • In one experiment, untreated cells were placed in the site of previous EBE treatment for 15 minutes. • External calcium and sodium were depleted from some samples before EBE Sham condition: samples with no EBE treatment.	• EBE treatment increased intracellular free calcium concentrations by 30% at 3 inches; sham treatment did not increase intracellular free calcium. • Distance from healer did not diminish results. • Number of treatments did not change results. • Intracellular free calcium increases were seen in samples exposed to the site where EBE treatment had previously occurred, suggesting contextual effects. • EBE effects were not seen in samples depleted of external calcium and sodium. Authors suggest that sodium/calcium exchange is a mechanism of EBE-related intracellular free calcium increases.

(*continued*)

Table 17.2. (Continued)

References	Treatment Modality	Type of Cancer / Biological Marker	Method	Results
Lee, et al., (2001). Effects of emitted Qi on in vitro natural killer cell cytotoxic activity. American Journal of Chinese Medicine, 29, 17–22.	Qi therapy	NK and leukemia cells from cell lines	Blood collected from six men and five women without history of neurohormonal or immunological disease. NK cells isolated and mixed with K562 chronic myelogenous leukemia cells. Each sample divided into one experimental and one control sample. Experimental received various lengths of Qi treatment between 30 and 300 seconds.	NK cell activity increased in the Qi treated cells only; no change in control cells.
Mager, et al., (2007). Evaluating biofield treatment in a cell culture model of oxidative stress. EXPLORE: The Journal of Science and Healing, 3, 386–390.	Six practitioners including two Qigong, two Johrei and two "Biofield Healers," using techniques similar to Qigong and Johrei	Cultured human brain cells	Cultured human brain cells exposed to incrementally greater concentrations of hydrogen peroxide to stimulate cell death. Biofield practitioners delivered treatment for 30 minutes to four cell lines, one at a time. Treatment applied before and after hydrogen peroxide application. Nontreated cell cultures served as controls. Cell death quantified by computerized time-lapse microscopy. Samples blinded for outcome measures.	Cell death did not differ significantly between cell lines in treatment and control conditions.
Ohnishi, et al., (2006). Ki-energy (Life-energy) protects isolated rat liver mitochondria from oxidative injury.	Ki-energy	mitochondria of rat liver	Rat liver mitochondria either exposed 5 to 10 minutes of Ki-energy or not.	Ki-energy improved respiration ratios in nonheated mitochondria.

Evidence-Based Complementary and Alternative Medicine, 3, 475–482.		A portion of these mitochondria then exposed to a 10 minute heat treatment (39 °C).	Lipid peroxidation was reduced in the heat treated mitochondria when Ki was applied, suggesting Ki protected it from oxidative stress.
Ohnishi, et al., (2005). Growth inhibition of cultured human liver carcinoma cells by Ki-energy (life energy): Scientific evidence for ki-effects on cancer cells. *Evidence Based Complementary and Alternative Medicine, 2,* 387–393.	Ki-energy	Human cultured liver carcinoma cells, HepG2	Cells either exposed to 0, 5, or 10 minutes of Ki-energy by a Japanese "Ki-expert" or handled by non–Ki expert for 5 or 10 minutes. Blocking experiments were also done.	• Significant decrease in cell numbers and increase in protein content per cell seen in Ki condition. In non–Ki handling condition, no changes seen. • Non–Ki handled cultures also had significantly less growth post treatment. • Covering cultures with aluminum foil, and acrylic, blocked changes induced by Ki-expert but polysterene did not block changes.
Rubik, et al., (2006). *In Vitro* effect of Reiki treatment on bacterial cultures: Role of experimental context and practitioner well-being. *The Journal of Alternative and Complementary Medicine, 12,* 7–13.	Reiki	*E. coli* K12 cultures	*E. coli* samples heat-shocked, then each Reiki practitioner applied treatment to 5 samples. • In 2 samples, Reiki first applied to a patient with a sprained ankle (healing context), in 3 samples no prior healing was performed (nonhealing context). • Well-being self-report of Reiki practitioners assessed pre-post all sessions. • Outcome measure: *E. coli* growth. (hypothesized to be increased with Reiki)	In the nonhealing context: • No difference between Reiki and controls • In practitioners with diminished well-being bacteria counts were less than control • Practitioners with high well-being, bacteria counts higher than control In healing context, • Reiki-treated cultures had more bacteria counts than controls, suggesting augmenting effect of prior treatment. • Mood × treatment effect: In practitioners with lower mood, bacteria counts were less than controls.

(continued)

Table 17.2. (Continued)

References	Treatment Modality	Type of Cancer / Biological Marker	Method	Results
Taft, et al., (2005). Time-lapse analysis of potential cellular responsiveness to Johrei, a Japanese healing technique. *BMC Complementary and Alternative Medicine,* 5. Retrieved January 30, 2007, from http://www.biomedcentral.com/1472–6882/5/2	Johrei	Brain tumor cell line: glioblastoma multiforme	Johrei treated cultures: treated for 4 hours each, with 2 healers assigned to each culture, alternating every half hour. Time-lapse microscopy used to quantify tumor cell death, proliferation, and cellular emigration	No evidence of response to Johrei treatment
Yan, et al., (2006). External Qi of Yan Xin Qigong differentially regulates the Akt and extracellular signal-regulated kinase pathways and is cytotoxic to cancer cells but not normal cells. *The International Journal of Biochemistry & Cell Biology,* 38, 2102–2113.	Qigong	Pancreatic cancer cells (BxPC3)	Cells treated with external Qi for 5 minutes, then harvested and analyzed 10 minutes post treatment. • Subset of cells received three 5 minute treatments. • Subset of cells serum-starved 48 hours before treatment, then stimulated 10 minutes after treatment and harvested. • Fibroblast cells serum-starved 24 hours pretreatment, then harvested at various time points post treatment.	Differentially regulated survival pathways in cancer versus normal cells. • Qi treatment of cancer cells inhibited cell growth mechanisms (Akt, epidermal growth factor, nuclear factor kappa B), induced apoptosis and DNA fragmentation. • Prolonged treatment of cancer cells led to rapid cell lysis. • For fibroblasts: transient activation of pathways above but did not show cytotoxic effect.

Reference	Biofield	Cell type	Method	Results
Yount, et al., (2004). Biofield perception: A series of pilot studies with cultured human cells. *The Journal of Alternative and Complementary Medicine*, 10, 463–467.	Biofield Perception	Glioblastoma cells	Three double-blinded studies to determine ability of participants to distinguish cancer cells from culture medium or sterile water: • Study 1: Participants given 2 flasks and asked whether they perceived cells inside. Repeated 34 times • Study 2: Repeat of study 1, but labeled samples of both targets given as comparison • Study 3: Participants asked which 1 of 10 samples contained live cells	Participants performed at level expected by chance in all studies
Yount, et al., (2004). In vitro test of external Qigong. *BMC Complementary and Alternative Medicine*, 4. Retrieved January 30, 2007, from http://www.biomedcentral.com/1472–6882/4/5	Qigong—external	Normal brain cells	Series of three studies (96 total experiments between these studies) involving 20-minute external Qigong treatment or no treatment. Brain cells cultured and examined for colony-forming efficiency (CFE).	*Study 1:* No significant difference in cell duplication between Qigong treated and control cells. *Study 2:* Qigong-treated cells duplicate significantly more than control *Study 3:* Cell duplication did not differ between Qigong treated and sham cells.

For a summary of Qigong research in China, the reader is also referred to Chen & Yeung, (2002). Exploratory studies of Qigong therapy for cancer in China. *Integrative Cancer Therapies*, 1(4), 345–370.

This chart includes several additional studies which are not contained in the text because they did not directly deal with cancer.

trials, and thus opportunities for large scale trials and physiological outcome measures have been limited. There are several good reviews of Healing Touch and TT in noncancer settings (Astin, et al., 2000; Wardell & Weymouth, 2004); thus, the findings presented here will be limited to cancer patients.

Post-White and colleagues (2003) prospectively studied 230 heterogeneous cancer patients (including breast, gynecological, gastrointestinal, hematological, lung, genitourinary, or other) at all stages during chemotherapy. Patients were divided into three groups: massage (MT), healing touch (HT), or "caring presence" (P). Patients received four weekly 45-minute sessions of their assigned intervention and four weekly 45-minute sessions of a standard care control, with the order of intervention or control randomized. Session 1 started prior to the next scheduled day of chemotherapy. Care providers for MT and HT were nurses credentialed in their modality. In comparison with standard care and presence, both MT and HT significantly reduced heart rate (approximately 7 bpm) systolic blood pressure, and self-rated pain within-session. Over the 4-week intervention period, HT significantly reduced total distress and fatigue as assessed by a validated questionnaire, the Profile of Mood States, whereas massage reduced total distress and anxiety. Patients receiving massage, but not those receiving HT, showed a decrease in medication use (non-steroidal anti-inflammatory drugs) over the intervention period. There was no change in nausea over time in the intervention groups. Although there was a relatively high dropout rate (29%), likely due to the lengthy commitment to this study among sick patients (44% of whom had Stage III disease), findings of this study indicate that during the course of a HT session in cancer patients undergoing chemotherapy, HT induced relaxation as assessed by decreases in blood pressure, heart rate, and pain. Over time, patients receiving HT showed sustained decreases in distress and fatigue. This study was methodologically sound, had a good sample size, and used adequate statistics.

Olson and colleagues (2003) compared pain, quality of life, and use of analgesic medications in 24 advanced stage cancer patients with pain who were randomized to receive Reiki plus standard opioid management or standard opioid management alone. Following their first afternoon analgesic dose on days 1 and 4 of the study, participants either rested or received Reiki for 1.5 hours. Participants receiving Reiki reported less pain as measured by visual analog scales (VAS) on days 1 and 4 following treatment. These patients also experienced significant drops in heart rate and diastolic blood pressure on day 1 and improved quality of life from days 1 to 7. There was no reduction in opioid use. The research assistant was present for both rest and Reiki, but because the patients in the Reiki arm had the additional presence of the Reiki practitioner, it is not known whether the pain reduction was due to the Reiki or due to nonspecific aspects of the treatment such as the mere presence of another person. Patients report that the effect of a Reiki treatment lasts approximately 2 to 3 days—thus ratings that include days 1 to 7 might well be subject to the bias of retrospective report. The trial ended prematurely when patients became unwilling to accept random assignment to the control condition.

Cook and colleagues (2004) conducted a single-blind randomized clinical trial examining the effectiveness of HT versus mock HT among gynecological and breast cancer patients receiving radiation treatment for their cancers. Seventy-eight patients were randomized to receive six 30-minute weekly sessions of either HT or mock treatment, which commenced during the first third of their radiation treatment. Approximately 20% of patients dropped out of the study before completing, leaving a final sample of 62. The study had a number of methodological strengths, including the fact that patients were separated from providers by an opaque screen placed between their head and body so they could not determine whether they were receiving HT or mock treatment and thus were blind to condition. In the mock therapy group, providers walked around the lower portion of the massage table with their hands at their sides, performing mathematical calculations silently in their heads. A random subset of mock treatment and HT sessions were videotaped to ensure the integrity of the interventions. Providers had a standard level of HT certification and used a standard protocol, although the specific HT techniques used were not specified. At the end of the study, HT participants demonstrated higher overall quality of life scores (SF-36) and showed specific gains in mental health, emotional role functioning, and health transition. At the end of the study, the HT group also showed significantly better outcomes in physical functioning, pain, and vitality compared to the mock HT. The mock treatment group did not have increased overall quality of life but did show significant increases in physical role functioning and health transition. However, the experimental and control groups were not evaluated in the same statistical model over time due to power considerations. Thus, the inadequate statistics prevent drawing robust conclusions from this otherwise well-designed study.

This study also brings to light some of the difficulties involved in selecting an adequate control group. For example, many HT practitioners use techniques involving points around the head (such as "mind clearing") in their work with cancer patients. Such techniques are thought to be valuable for helping the patient develop a calm frame of mind and also for clarity of thought. A design involving HT treatments only below the neck to provide for an adequate control group may actually have blunted the efficacy of the HT treatments. On the other hand, developing an adequate control strategy is one of the most difficult challenges in clinical research with energy medicine.

Laidlaw and colleagues (Laidlaw, Bennett, Dwivedi, Naito, & Gruzelier, 2005) found improvements in quality of life and mood over 3 months in a small pilot study of self-hypnosis versus Johrei versus wait-list control among metastatic breast cancer patients. The self-hypnosis intervention used breathing training to control acute anxiety, suggestions for immune enhancement such as visualization to see "sharks" cleaning up the bloodstream, creation of personal scenarios, and ego strengthening suggestions. The Johrei intervention utilized training in directing Johrei to others and to oneself, and Johrei principles such as the importance of fresh organic food, finding beauty in one's life, and sensitivity to nature were also taught. The interventions were practiced daily for 3 months with diary monitoring of compliance. Although 37 women were randomized, only 16 completed the study, largely due to death and deteriorating health of the noncompleters. Adequate statistical analyses could not be conducted because of the small number of patients in the study. However, interesting patterns emerged, even in this small sample, with Johrei patients showing less hostility and less anxiety than controls, and hypnosis patients showing less anxiety, less fatigue, and less overall distress than the Johrei patients. Notably, these effects were observed over the 3-month study period. Compliance with the experimental interventions was not reported, a factor that would be important in interpreting these findings. Ziembroski and colleagues conducted an uncontrolled study of 21 patients who had received HT while in hospice care and found improvements in mood, relaxation, and pain relief. As no statistical analyses were performed, the results should be interpreted with caution (Ziembroski, Gilbert, Bossarte, & Guldberg, 2003).

Roscoe and colleagues examined effects of polarity therapy in reducing fatigue induced by radiation therapy in a small study of 15 breast cancer patients who were randomized to receive 0, 1, or 2 polarity treatments during their radiation treatment. In the 10 patients who received a treatment, there was a decrease in fatigue and an increase in health-related quality of life as compared to the control patients. In addition, there was a dose–response effect, with the five patients who received two treatments having a more pronounced alleviation of symptoms than the two other groups. These preliminary findings in a small sample suggest a positive effect on fatigue in this group of patients and suggest the possibility of energy therapies on fatigue as a possible fruitful area of study in the future (Roscoe, Matteson, Mustian, Padmanaban, & Morrow, 2005).

One intriguing case study has been published (Lee, Yang, Lee, & Moon, 2005) in which effects of external Qigong (specifically Korean Chun Soo Energy Healing) were examined on cancer symptoms of a 35-year-old man with Stage IV lung cancer with metastases to the stomach, lung, and bone, and with complications such as diabetes and hypertension. He had received radiation and chemotherapy 6 months previously and at the time of the study was receiving opioid medication (120 mg/day oxycodone) for pain but no other treatment. At the start of the study his Karnofsky Performance Scale (Schag, Heinrich, & Ganz, 1984) score was 40, indicating that over the past month he was disabled and required special care and assistance. Over the course of 16 days, the patient received eight 20-minute Qi therapy sessions performed on alternate days at the hospital. Daily VAS were used to assess symptoms such as pain, vomiting, and fatigue. At baseline the patient reported that his pain was 8 on a 10 point scale. Following the first treatment, the patient discontinued oxycodone, and following the second treatment, his pain further decreased to 2 on a 10 point scale. For the 2 weeks of assessment following treatment, his pain increased slightly to 4 on a 10 point scale, still without medication. The patient, who reported moderately high levels of vomiting at the start of the study, reported no vomiting after the fifth Qi session, an improvement that was sustained throughout the follow-up. Dramatic improvements were reported for anorexia, fatigue, insomnia, and peace of mind, and were maintained through follow-up. His Karnofsky score improved to 70 after the fourth session (indicating that he was in bed less than 50% of the time and was able to care for self) and was maintained at the 2-week follow-up. This study suggests positive effects of intensive treatments.

Practicing Qigong has also been associated with improvements in physiological markers in several studies. Many of these studies from China have been discussed in Chen's review (Chen & Yeung, 2002) with the conclusion that the Qigong recipients had better survival rates or more improvement than controls. In one study in the United States, Qigong was taught to 19 healthy volunteers aged 27 to 55 who practiced daily for 14 weeks, and were assessed after 3, 7, and 14 weeks. Following practice, PHA-stimulated interferon gamma (IFN-γ)-secreting cells increased and interleukin-10 (IL-10)-secreting cells decreased, resulting in a shift in balance toward the type 1 cytokine. IFN-γ supports the cellular immune response that is important in cancer control. In contrast, IL-10 suppresses cell-mediated immunity. Although this study was uncontrolled, these findings suggest the potential relevance of examining the effects of Qigong practice among cancer patients to see whether similar patterns can be reproduced (Jones, 2001).

Along the same lines, immunologic profiles of six adults who had practiced Falun Gong (a type of Qigong) for 1 to 5 years were compared against those of normal healthy controls. The Falun Gong practitioners showed enhanced neutrophil phagocytosis and accelerated cell death in inflammatory neutrophils, as compared to normal neutrophils whose lifespans were longer than expected (Li, Li, Garcia, Johnson, & Feng, 2005). Lee and colleagues found that 1 hour of Qi training increased growth hormone (GH) and insulin-like growth factor-1

(IGF-1) levels and O^{2-} production of neutrophils as compared to the basal state among 16 healthy young men (Lee, Kim & Ryu, 2005). Many of these parameters indicate a healthier immune response and would be of relevance to cancer prevention and control.

Taken together these studies suggest that energy healing may have clinically relevant effects on mood, fatigue, and quality of life in cancer patients. Sustained effects of energy treatments appear to be most robust for distress and fatigue, but with the exception of the Post-White study, small sample sizes and statistical considerations limit the generalizations that can be made from this data. The data indicating physiological changes in individuals who practice Johrei or Qigong also point to possibilities of people increasing their own physical health without an energy medicine practitioner, although most of this data has been generated by small samples of healthy individuals.

Cancer patients use energy medicine for many indications, including dealing with the nausea and fatigue induced by cancer treatments, as well as the hope that energy practice can prolong survival. To date data that test the question of whether energy medicine supports immune function or retards tumor growth in cancer patients are not available, and physiological data from non-cancer patients are still at an early stage. Well-controlled, adequately powered studies are critically needed to examine questions of whether energy medicine applications can serve to support physiology and prolong survival in cancer patients.

Several studies have examined potential psychophysiological mediators of changes induced by energy healing in healthy individuals. A subset of these is presented here to help clarify possible mechanisms that underlie the effects of energy medicine that may be investigated in clinical studies. Wardell and colleagues examined physiological effects before and after 30 minutes of Reiki in 23 healthy subjects. There was no control group in this study. During the session there were significant reductions in systolic blood pressure and anxiety accompanied by nonsignificant decreases in muscle tension as measured by electromyography and in galvanic skin response and a nonsignificant increase in skin temperature. There was no significant change in salivary cortisol (Wardell & Engebretson, 2001). In a second study of 45 healthy individuals, measures of autonomic nervous system function were examined before, during, and after a 30-minute Reiki treatment by an experienced Reiki practitioner versus a rest-only control, versus a placebo Reiki treatment. Cardiac monitoring was done with instrumentation which recorded all parameters continuously. Both Reiki and placebo Reiki groups had significant reduction in heart rate accompanied by increases in cardiac vagal tone and in cardiac sensitivity to baroreflex. This constellation suggests an increase in parasympathetic activity. Both of these groups also had significantly decreased respiration. Additionally, the Reiki group had significant decreases in diastolic blood pressure and mean blood pressure that were not seen in either the placebo or the control group. The drops in heart rate and diastolic blood pressure in the Reiki group were significantly different from the findings in the placebo group. There were no changes in any of these autonomic parameters in the control group. These findings suggest that Reiki may have some effect on the autonomic nervous system over and above a placebo control, although effects were limited to blood pressure changes (Mackay, Hansen, & McFarlane, 2004). These studies suggest possible directions for future examination of psychophysiological mediators of energy healing. Table 17.3 summarizes the results of published clinical trials in energy medicine.

Several ongoing National Institutes of Health (NIH)-funded studies with cancer patients may provide clarification on some of these issues in the future. Larkey and colleagues at the Arizona Cancer Center are examining Medical Qigong exercises versus restful movement stretches based on the Lebed method of rehabilitation and lymphedema-preventative exercises for breast cancer patients in 60 Stage I or II breast cancer survivors who are 6 months to 5 years beyond treatment for breast cancer and report persistent fatigue and cognitive dysfunction. Examination of fatigue and objective measures of cognitive performance are used to assess whether medical Qigong will improve fatigue and cognitive function in breast cancer survivors. Physiological mechanisms that may be associated with effects of Qigong including inflammatory cytokines are also being examined (Larkey, 2006–2009).

Fox and colleagues at the Cleveland Clinic are examining Reiki versus sham Reiki versus no treatment for prostate cancer patients for 4 weeks during the 6- to 8-week period between their initial diagnosis and radical prostatectomy. Effects of these treatments are being assessed by evaluating PSA levels, self-reported anxiety, and the stress hormones cortisol and DHEA (Fox, 2007).

Lutgendorf and colleagues at the University of Iowa are examining effects of HT versus relaxation versus standard care in 64 cervical cancer patients undergoing a standard 6-week course of chemotherapy and daily radiation treatment. HT and relaxation sessions (approximately 20 to 30 minutes) are given immediately following radiation 4 days a week (days on which the patient does not receive chemotherapy). The relaxation group was designed to provide a credible active control group using an intervention that is known to reduce stress and enhance the immune response. Primary outcomes include measures of cellular immunity, distress, and side effects. (Lutgendorf, 2008; Prestwood, 2008). Lutgendorf and colleagues also are conducting a study examining the effects of daily HT versus standard care on fatigue and inflammatory mechanisms that may underlie fatigue in 44 early-stage breast cancer patients during their radiation therapy treatment (Lutgendorf, 2007)

Jain and colleagues at the University of California at San Diego are examining the effectiveness of short-term energy healing versus mock healing for fatigued breast cancer survivors. Outcome measures include inflammatory immune markers that are thought to be relevant for fatigue, cortisol, as well as assessments of fatigue, depression, and quality of life. This study utilizes a crossover design. During a 1 week period, 50 participants will receive either three energy healing sessions or three mock energy healing sessions and then will crossover to the opposite condition for three sessions during a separate 1-week period. The study also examines whether specific patients (e.g., those with a more holistic world view) are more likely to benefit from treatment. (Jain, 2008).

Health Beliefs of Patients Using Energy Medicine

Critical to the understanding of patients' use of energy medicine is an appreciation of why patients choose to use CAM treatments such as energy medicine. Several studies have indicated that patients most likely to use complementary medicine have health beliefs, indicating that cancer etiology involves external factors such as diet, stress, and environment (Gawler, 2001; Maskarinec, Gotay, Tatsumura, Shumay, & Kakai, 2001; Plant, 2002).

In a recent study of Australian gynecologic cancer patients, specific health beliefs about cancer leading to the use of complementary therapies and energy therapies were assessed. Patients who used complementary therapies did so for four major reasons (Markovic, et al., 2006):

- Belief in alternative theories of cancer etiology (e.g., cancer was caused by stress, diet, environment, and energy imbalances). These patients sought complementary therapies to minimize risks of cancer recurrence and were most likely to engage in changes in diet and life style, energy healing, or yoga.
- Belief in the efficacy of complementary treatments to reduce the side effects of biomedical treatments. These patients predominantly used meditation, acupuncture, Reiki, or vitamins.
- Belief in the efficacy of biomedical treatments combined with interest in maximizing their overall health. These patients tended to use exercise and diet as CAM therapies.
- Exploratory users, some of whom turned to CAM treatments as a last resort after their cancer had metastasized or in the absence of effective biomedical treatments for their stage of cancer. Use of energy treatments in this group was low.

Table 17.3. Summary of Clinical Trials in Energy Medicine.

References	Treatment Modality	Type of Cancer / Biological Marker and no. of Participants	Method	Results
Cook, et al., (2004). Healing Touch and quality of life in women receiving radiation treatment for cancer: A randomized controlled trial. *Alternative Therapies, 10,* 34–41.	HT	Gynecological or breast N = 62	Patients received six 30-minute weekly sessions of either HT or mock treatment. Quality of life measured pre and post treatment. Attitude toward HT measured pretreatment. Participants blind to condition.	HT recipients demonstrated higher outcome quality of life scores on all subscales compared to mock HT. Within group analyses: HT recipients reported significant gains in total, emotional, mental, and health transition quality of life dimensions during treatment. Mock treatment participants improved significantly on physical and health transition quality of life.
Jones, (2001). Changes in cytokine production in healthy subjects practicing Guolin Qigong: A pilot study. *BMC Complementary and Alternative Medicine, 1.* Retrieved January 30, 2007, from http://www.biomedcentral.com/1472-6882/1/8	Qigong—Guolin (exercise type)	Cytokine production N = 19	Participants engaged in 14 week Qigong training program. IFN-γ, IL-4, IL-6, IL-10, IL-12, TNF-α and cortisol in peripheral blood as well as blood pressure and pulse rate measured at baseline and weeks 3, 7 and 14.	Changes in blood pressure and pulse were not found. Cortisol was reduced at weeks 3 and 14, although not at week 7. Increases in IFN-γ and IL-6 and reductions in IL-10 were found. No changes were found on IL-12 or IL4. TNF increased at weeks 3 and 7 but returned to normal by week 14. Qigong may alter cytokine production in healthy subjects in the direction of Type 1 (cellular) immune responses and lower the stress hormone cortisol, although responses were not consistent.

(continued)

Table 17.3. (Continued)

References	Treatment Modality	Type of Cancer / Biological Marker and no. of Participants	Method	Results
Kelly, et al., (2004). Therapeutic touch, quiet time, and dialogue: Perceptions of women with breast cancer. *Oncology Nursing Forum*, 31, 625–631.	Therapeutic touch	Early-stage breast cancer N = 18	3 conditions: Therapeutic Touch (TT) (10 min), quiet time (10 min), both including dialogue with nurse (20 minutes); conditions administered twice, pre and post operatively. Telephone interview of women's perceptions of the interventions	Few differences between conditions in participant perceptions of treatment.
Lee, et al., (2001). Psychneuroimmunological effects of Qi-therapy: Preliminary study on the changes of level of anxiety, mood, cortisol and melatonin and cellular function of neutrophil and natural killer cells. *Stress and Health*, 17, 17–24.	Qi therapy	Neutrophil, NK cells, cortisol, melatonin N = 20 healthy men	10 participants received Qi treatment for 10 minutes, with 5 minutes of rest pre and post tx. Mood measures and blood samples drawn before tx, and again 5 minutes and 1 hour post treatment. 10 control participants followed same protocol without receiving Qi treatment.	Mood, melatonin, superoxide generation, and NK cytotoxicity were significantly better post tx in the Qi treatment group.
Lee, et al., (2003). Effects of Qigong on immune cells. *The American Journal of Chinese Medicine*, 31, 327–335.	Qigong: both training and therapy	Lymphocyte, monocyte, neutrophils N = 11	Experimental group participated in either 1 hour of movement Qigong and training to manipulate Qi or 10 minutes of Qigong treatment. Controls participated in either movement Qigong (without Qi manipulation training) or sham Qi treatment.	*Qi training*: Leukocytes and lymphocytes increased significantly in 2 hours in Qi training but not sham groups. Monocytes increased immediately post both Qi training and sham. NK cell numbers decreased significantly with both Qi training and sham.

Citation	Intervention	Measures	Methods	Results
			Immune cells measured pre intervention, and postintervention immediate, 1 and 2 hours.	*Qi-therapy:* Monocytes and lymphocytes increased in Qi but not sham group. Neutrophils did not change in either group.
Lee, et al., (2005). Qi-training (Qigong) enhanced immune functions: What is the underlying mechanism? *Journal of International Neuroscience, 115*, 1099–1104.	Qigong training	Growth hormone (GH) and Superoxide free radical (O_2^-) metabolism by neutrophils $N = 10$	Elderly men completed Qigong exercise training for 1 hour. • Blood samples taken pre- and post-training and incubated with neutrophils from young subjects. • Neutrophils treated with GH-antibody and pre- and post-blood samples added, then O_2^- generation measured • Neutrophils treated with genistein, then pre- and post- blood samples were added, O_2^- generation measured	• Posttraining, significant increases in GH, O_2^- neutrophil production. • No increases in GH-depleted samples • Suggests that endogenous GH released during and after Qi training mediates neutrophil function
Lee, et al., (2005). Effects of Qi therapy (external Qigong) on symptoms of advanced cancer: A single case study. *European Journal of Cancer Care, 14*, 457–462.	Qigong therapy	Lung (metastatic) $N = 1$	6 days of preassessment, 8 treatment sessions on alternate days over 16 days, 2 week follow up. Assessments: cancer symptoms using visual analog scale	Reductions in pain, vomiting, dyspnoea, fatigue, anorexia, insomnia, and increases in daily activity and calmness both immediately and 2 weeks post Qi therapy.

(continued)

Table 17.3. (Continued)

References	Treatment Modality	Type of Cancer / Biological Marker and no. of Participants	Method	Results
Li, et al., (2005). Genomic profiling of neutrophil transcripts in Asian Qigong practitioners: A pilot study in gene regulation by mind-body interface. *The Journal of Alternative and Complementary Medicine*, 11, 29–39.	Qigong	Gene profiling in blood of healthy individuals N = 12	Genetic profiling including phenotypic changes in gene expression compared in six Qigong practitioners and six healthy controls. Neutrophils isolated from blood samples and assayed for gene expression, function and survival.	Qigong practitioner cells demonstrated enhanced immunity, downregulation of cellular metabolism, more rapid response to inflammation, prolonged lifespan of normal neutrophils, accelerated death of inflammatory neutrophils, and enhanced phagocytosis compared to controls.
MacKay, et al., (2004). Autonomic nervous system changes during Reiki treatment: A preliminary study. *The Journal of Alternative and Complementary Medicine*, 10, 1077–1081.	Reiki	Heart rate, cardiac vagal tone, blood pressure, cardiac sensitivity to baroreflex, breathing activity N = 45	15-minute rest period followed by 30-minute Reiki treatment and then 10-minute rest period. Groups: Reiki, sham Reiki, rest-only control	True and sham Reiki groups demonstrated greater decreases in heart rate, increase in vagal tone, and increase in cardiac sensitivity to baroreflex and decreased respiration compared with rest-control. True Reiki had decreases in diastolic blood pressure and mean blood pressure compared with either placebo group.
Olson, et al., (2003). A phase II trial of Reiki for the management of pain in advanced cancer patients. *Journal of pain and symptom management*, 26, 990–997.	Reiki	Advanced cancers, site not specified N = 24	Participants completed a 1.5 hour treatment, either rest or Reiki, on days 1 and 4. Participants not blinded to condition. Patients also received opioid medication as usual. Edmonton Staging System for cancer pain administered on day 1.	Reiki group reported less pain on days 1 and 4 and improved quality of life. No differences were found in opioid use. Trial ended prematurely when patients became unwilling to accept random assignment to control condition.

| Post-White, et al., (2003). Therapeutic massage and HT improve symptoms in cancer. *Integrative Cancer Therapies, 2,* 332–344. | HT vs. Therapeutic Massage vs. presence | Breast, gynecological, gastrointestinal, hematological, lung, genitourinary, or other; stages unstaged–IV
N = 230 | Visual analog scales of pain collected pre and post treatments, and daily at home at mealtime. Participants recorded all opioid use.

Patients randomly assigned to one of three interventions: HT, Massage, or simple presence of a healer.

Patients received four weekly sessions of one intervention as well as standard care control condition, and within-subject order of condition randomly assigned.

Outcome variables included:
• Pre and post session: heart rate, respiratory rate, blood pressure, self-reported nausea, and pain.
• Days 1 and 4 of each condition: anxiety, mood, fatigue, and satisfaction with overall care.
• Day 4 of intervention condition: satisfaction with intervention.
• Weekly: diaries of analgesic and antiemetic use. | Pre–post intervention effects (within session over 4 weeks):
• Greater reduction in pain, respiratory, and heart rate and blood pressure in both Massage and HT than in standard care control
• Greater reduction in heart rate, systolic blood pressure, and pain in both HT and Massage than in presence of healer.

Change from week 1 to week 4:
• Both Massage and HT reduced total mood disturbance and anxiety more than standard care
• Overall satisfaction with care similar between groups |

(continued)

Table 17.3. (Continued)

References	Treatment Modality	Type of Cancer / Biological Marker and no. of Participants	Method	Results
Roscoe, et al., (2005). Treatment of radiotherapy-induced fatigue through a nonpharmacological approach. *Integrative Cancer Therapies, 4,* 8–13.	Polarity therapy	Breast cancer N = 15	Women receiving radiation therapy randomized to either standard care or to receive either 1 or 2 sessions of polarity treatment. In 2 session groups, treatments were separated by 1 week. Fatigue and health-related quality of life (QOL) were assessed at baseline (pretreatment) and 3 days after each treatment.	After the first week of treatment, both treatment groups reported less fatigue and greater QOL than those in standard care. • After the second treatment, there was a significant difference in both outcome measures between all three groups, with the 2-session group reporting greatest adjustment, and the 1-session group reporting greater adjustment than standard care. Study suggests that polarity therapy may reduce fatigue and increase health-related QOL in a dose-response manner in breast cancer patients undergoing radiation.
Wardell & Engebretson, (2001). Biological correlates of Reiki Touch healing. *Journal of Advanced Nursing, 33,* 439–445.	Reiki	Salivary IgA, cortisol, SBP, skin temperature, EMG N = 23	30 minutes of Reiki applied with pre and post measures of anxiety, salivary IgA, blood pressure, galvanic skin response, muscle tension, and skin temperature	Significant: IgA rose, anxiety reduced, drop in SBP in Reiki group. No change in cortisol. Insignificant trend toward increase in skin temp and decrease in EMG in Reiki group.

These charts include several additional papers not included in text because they did not directly deal with cancer.

Patients tend to have explanatory or "common sense" beliefs about the etiology, chronicity, and treatment of their illness (Leventhal, Nerenz, & Steele, 1984; Martin, et al., 2004). These beliefs may or may not be consistent with the beliefs of their health care providers. For example, we have recently found that 46% of gynecologic cancer patients feel that their disease has been caused by stress, and 39% think it was an act of God (Costanzo, Lutgendorf, Bradley, Rose, & Anderson, 2005). Because common sense beliefs of patients are critical factors in compliance with traditional medical care and in seeking out alternative care (Leventhal, et al., 1984; Markovic, et al., 2006), patients' health beliefs should be addressed by practitioners.

Recommendations for Physicians and Health Care Practitioners

- Ask patients if they are using CAM therapies, including energy medicine. Usually only about 30% to 40% of patients tell their physician that they are using CAM treatments (Boon, et al., 2000).
- Find out what your patient thinks about the CAM therapies they are using. Is their use of energy medicine an experiment or is it fundamentally related to how the patient understands sickness and health?
- Familiarize yourself with emerging research on energy medicine to facilitate a supportive discussion based on evidence.
- Find out whether your patient's practitioner is certified, or what kind of training the practitioner has had.

Design Issues

Specific methodology issues need to be considered in clinical studies examining energy medicine. Many of these have been outlined in a text edited by Jonas and Crawford (2003). What constitutes an adequate "dose" of a particular treatment, how often should it be repeated, how long do treatment effects last, and the adequate treatment length or intensity to produce the required dose have not been well characterized. Patients are treated weekly in most studies; however, anecdotal reports from the healers in our research indicate that daily treatment increases the ability of patients to "hold" the new energy patterns. In many studies with energy modalities, sessions have been short and/or time-limited and limited in number, designs that may contribute to minimizing an intervention effect by not providing an adequate "dose" of treatment. In some therapeutic touch studies, patients have received single treatments for as short as 5 minutes, a time span thought by practitioners to be inadequate

(Winstead-Fry & Kijek, 1999). Studies allowing the practitioner to individualize the biofield treatment so as to deliver an "adequate dose" of the treatment have shown greater effects (Winstead-Fry & Kijek, 1999). More treatment sessions have tended to produce stronger results (Turner, Clark, Gauthier, & Williams, 1998). However, individual differences among healers exist, and the relative "dose" and application of energy derived from any particular healer may vary substantially (Connor, et al., 2006). Furthermore, the state of well-being of the practitioner on a given day has been shown to have effects on the efficacy of healing in vitro (Rubik, Brooks, & Schwartz, 2006). This is an important variable in energy research, as well as clinically.

For biofield treatments designed to reduce the side effects of radiation or chemotherapy, no clear understanding exists on how soon after chemotherapy or radiation therapy energy treatments should be given, so as to not interfere with the desired effects of the chemotherapy or radiation. Our research designs call for a 24-hour delay between chemotherapy and energy treatment to allow the drugs to have an opportunity to work in the body before any toxic effects are "cleared" from the liver. Based on recommendations from radiation oncologists, our group has used energy treatments immediately after radiation therapy, but it is not known whether energy treatments also "clear" the desired effects of radiation from the body. This is an empirical question that needs to be tested for optimal trial design.

Assessment of expectancy or placebo effects has also been recommended. To address whether expectancy or belief in the treatment accounted for outcomes, several researchers have administered questions on the extent to which subjects believed in the logic or the efficacy of the treatments they were receiving (Gagne & Toye, 1994; Turner, et al., 1998). Interestingly, in at least one study, reported belief in the treatment (or sham treatment) has not correlated with outcomes (Turner, et al., 1998). Demographics have also not been correlated with outcomes (Spence & Olson, 1997).

Recommendations for the use of energy medicine research include (1) treatments that are tailored to the patient and gauged as being adequate by the healer, (2) examining the number and frequency of treatments needed for effective outcomes, (3) examining the effects over time when appropriate (e.g., with chronic illness), (4) using study designs in which the healer is not the investigator so that they are not attached to outcomes, (5) using patients with chronic illness rather than healthy individuals, and (6) using experienced practitioners who can describe their practice (Astin, et al., 2000; Winstead-Fry & Kijek, 1999). Several reviews suggested the need to compare energy therapies to other analgesic or relaxation techniques as a way of more adequately specifying mechanisms (Quinn & Strelkauskas, 1993; Samarel, Fawcett, Davis, & Ryan, 1998; Spence & Olson, 1997). This field very much needs to move to understanding mechanisms, replication of effects, and conditions underlying failure to replicate. Clinical trials need to be larger, contain objective outcome markers (physician assessment, biomarkers), and have adequate randomization and control groups.

Future Research

There are more unanswered than answered questions in this field. There are multiple domains of cancer research that would be relevant for energy medicine research. These include effects of energy healing on presurgical preparation, postsurgical recovery (nausea and vomiting, removal of effects of anesthesia, pain reduction, wound healing), effectiveness of clearing undesired side effects of chemotherapy and radiation from the body, minimizing cognitive deficits from chemotherapy, minimizing fatigue and depression, minimizing radiation burns, increasing well-being, posttreatment health maintenance, and promotion of survival. Use of energy medicine, or energy-based practices such as Qigong, to promote health maintenance after a definitive treatment or after recurrence, for assistance with pain management and palliative care, or in bone marrow transplant would also present important domains for future work. Understanding individual differences in response (personality, stage or disease, belief in treatment) is also an important research question.

Possible Mechanisms of Action of Biofield Therapies for Cancer

The clinical outcome studies have not addressed to date whether energy medicine therapies can actually affect the course of disease. This is often the hope of cancer patients who use this modality. There are several possible mechanisms, both direct and indirect, by which effects on disease course might occur. The in vitro research, although equivocal, suggests that some types of energy therapies can directly impair the growth of cancer cells. There have been some very promising results, but replication has been difficult. Indirect mechanisms include induction of relaxation with subsequent downregulation of the neuroendocrine stress response that may have downstream effects on tumor growth and on the immune response. To the extent that energy therapies can provide social support, instill hope, and induce the relaxation response, they are likely to modulate the sympathetic nervous system and neuroendocrine stress responses. The findings of Post-White and colleagues indicate that HT was able to decrease autonomic activity in heterogeneous cancer patients.

Several ongoing studies are currently addressing the issue of the extent to which cortisol and other stress hormones are affected by HT. Stress hormones, particularly norepinephrine and epinephrine, are known to promote tumor growth by processes including increased tumor angiogenesis and invasiveness (Antoni, et al., 2006; Sood, et al., 2006; Thaker, et al., 2006). The immune response can also be impaired with chronic life stress (Antoni, et al., 2006). Thus to the extent that the neuroendocrine stress response can be blunted by energy therapies, these cancer growth processes may be retarded. A third possibility includes mechanisms not mediated by the neuroendocrine stress response, such as the possibility that energy therapy unblocks obstacles to free flow of energy within the patient. This allows for freer circulation of "life energy" through the patient, supporting greater resistance to disease, higher levels of energy, and less side effects of treatment by effecting multiple physiological systems. There may also be cellular receptors sensitive to energy dynamics. Any or all of these mechanisms could also work together.

How are possible effects of energy healing understood? Bell and colleagues propose that models from complex systems and network science are necessary for understanding the types of effects noted here (Bell, Baldwin, & Schwartz, 2002). It has been suggested that conceptual frameworks based on Newtonian physics, molecular biology, and biochemistry are not adequate to address the phenomenology reported in energy healing (Liboff, 2004). This is particularly true of long-distance healing and spontaneous remissions. Rather quantum physics, post-quantum physics, and a model of the organism as an electromagnetic system are proposed as being integral to an understanding of the phenomenology of energy healing (Liboff, 2004; Tiller, 2002).

Because Newtonian physics and the biomedical model are part of the "common sense" model of the laws of nature for most people, and particularly health care practitioners, there has been substantial resistance to accepting a more inclusive alternative. In a similar vein, 35 years ago, the concept that the mind could influence the immune system was seen as being outrageous. Robert Ader, Professor of Psychology at the University of Rochester and one of the early pioneers of the field of psychoneuroimmunology, stumbled upon findings demonstrating that the immune response could be conditioned (Ader, 1995). He was severely criticized for this work—but over the last 35 years, pathways of communication between the central nervous system and the immune system have been well characterized and central nervous system involvement in modulation of the immune response is now widely accepted (Ader, 2007). It was only after the data was replicated and mechanisms delineated that a new understanding of the bi-directional communication between the brain and immune system emerged and became accepted.

Similarly, an acceptance of energy medicine will require a paradigm shift by the public and the scientific community. Because understanding this field may involve the use of a novel scientific paradigm, there has been substantial resistance. The promising but equivocal data presented herein support the necessity for rigorous preclinical and clinical research to address some of the fundamental questions delineated in the preceding text. Energy medicine may present an important adjunct in cancer treatment; however, much more needs to be known.

ACKNOWLEDGMENTS

Work on this chapter was partially supported by grants R21CA102515, R01CA104825, and R21AT0095801 from NIH to S.L. and the grant P20AT75601 from NIH (Karen Prestwood, P.I.) We are grateful to Gary Schwartz, Melinda Connor, and Aliza Weinrib for helpful comments on the chapter.

REFERENCES

Antoni M, Lutgendorf S, Cole S, Dhabar F, Sephton S, Green McDonald P, et al. (2006). The influences of biobehavioral factors on tumor biology: Pathways and mechanisms. *Nature Reviews Cancer, 6*, 240–248.

Astin J, Harkness E, & Ernst E. (2000). The efficacy of distant healing: A systematic review of randomized trials. *Ann Intern Med, 132*(11), 903–910.

Burr HS. (1972). *The fields of life*. New York: Ballantine Books.

Chen K & Yeung R. (2002). Exploratory studies of Qigong therapy for cancer in China. *Integrative Cancer Therapies, 1*(4), 345–370.

Cook CAL, Guerrerio JF, & Slater VE. (2004). Healing Touch and quality of life in women receiving radiation treatment for cancer: a randomized controlled trial. *Alternative Therapies, 10*(3), 34–41.

Jhaveri A, Walsh SJ, Wang Y, McCarthy MB, & Gronowicz G. (2008). Therapeutic touch affects DNA synthesis and mineralization of human osteoblasts in culture. *Journal of Orthopedic Research*. Epub ahead of print. (www.interscience.wiley.com).

Kiang JG, Ives JA, & Jonas WB. (2005). External bioenergy-induced increases in intracellular free calcium concentrations are mediated by Na^+/Ca^{2+} exchanger and L-type calcium channel. *Molecular and Cellular Biochemistry, 271*, 51–29.

Krieger D. (1979). *The therapeutic touch: How to use your hands to help or heal*. NJ: Prentice Hall.

Mentgen J & Bulbrook M. (2002). Healing Touch *level I notebook*. (Revised Edition). Carrboro, NC, North Carolina Center for Healing Touch.

Oschman JL. (2000). *Energy medicine: The scientific basis*. New York: NY: Churchill Livingstone.

Post-White J, Kinney ME, Savik K, Gau JB, Wilcox C, & Lerner I. (2003). Therapeutic massage and Healing Touch improve symptoms in cancer. *Integrative Cancer Therapies,* 2(4), 332–344.

Yan X, Shen H, Jiang H, Zhang C, Hu D, Wang J, et al. (2006). External Qi of Yan Xin Qigong differentially regulates the Akt and extracellular signal-regulated kinase pathways and is cytotoxic to cancer cells but not to normal cells. *The International Journal of Biochemistry & Cell Biology,* 38, 2102–2113.

(*A complete reference list for this chapter is available online at http://www.oup.com/us/ integrativemedicine*).

18

Tending the Spirit in Cancer

RACHEL NAOMI REMEN

Perhaps it is useful to say that spirit is accessed as often through life experience as it is through formal religion. Falling in love, marriage, the birth of a child; these moments may initiate a revolution in personal values and spiritual perspective. The spiritual is really a human birthright; it is the dimension of our being that is the meeting place which underlies human diversity and which creates a genuine connection among all people. Religion attempts to make this real for us through community, practice, and belief, and may become a bridge to the spiritual; but the lived experience of spiritual realities lies beyond all beliefs and practices; it is the all-inclusive ground of being.

Very often a spiritual path does not look like what it is at its beginning but only reveals itself later on. In fact, much genuine spiritual growth is initiated by loss, by suffering, by what might be conventionally called bad luck....or even by significant illness.

After 30 years of working as a physician and therapist to people with cancer and listening to their stories it seems to me that a significant illness such as cancer almost always has a spiritual dimension; and the physical changes of cancer are accompanied by spiritual movement. In some people this movement is small and subtle and in others profound enough to divert the course of the remainder of their lives, but some change is almost always present. This capacity in people to grow in spiritual perspective is perhaps the currency, which will enable them to fully recover their lives after cancer, to live more deeply, more meaningfully and more passionately in a body that has been altered by surgery or diminished by disease. The challenge to us as providers of care is not to initiate this movement but to recognize it and tend it and strengthen it as it often allows people the opportunity of living a deeper and more meaningful life.

Cancer takes us out of our usual way of life, our way of defining our familiar activities and ourselves. It removes the hooks on which we have hung our accustomed identity: I am an engineer, a runner, a tough guy and leaves us adrift in open space and open time. As painful as it is, this shift in habitual identification may ultimately offer spiritual possibilities. After years of observing people engage in this process I have come to wonder if there is something innate about the experiences of a life-threatening disease such as cancer that opens people to the larger possibilities in life, even those who have never considered such matters before.

In the process of recovering from kidney cancer, one of my patients underwent a transformation from a hard driving CEO to a volunteer and supporter of many good causes. He told me of the experience, which had changed his way of moving through the world. As a child of atheistic and intellectual parents, he had no religious upbringing or spiritual inclination and had immersed himself in the world of competition and business with much success. While formerly his business had been the focus of his life; now his cancer and its treatment required him to be away from the multitasking demands and pressures of his work and instead to spend several months in the quiet of his living room.

At first this had been frightening and deeply disorienting but then as the fatigue of his chemotherapy took hold, he had simply surrendered to this silence and spent hours on his couch dozing in the company of his cat. One afternoon as he lay drifting in and out of sleep he found himself looking at a bookshelf on the opposite wall and it seemed to him that one of the books stood out from the others in an odd way. Getting up for a closer look he saw that it was the very same Bible that the clergy who had performed his marriage years ago had given to him and his wife. Taking it back to the couch he opened it for the first time and started to read the story of the beginning of the world. He was surprised to feel a deep response to the simple words, how real and familiar and terrifying the formlessness and darkness felt to him and how it seemed to be somehow connected to the terrible recent events in his life. And then he encountered the statement with which the world begins: "LET THERE BE LIGHT." He lay there for a time feeling the great power in these four words wash over him.

As he ruminated about this, the words suddenly shifted their meaning and he realized that they were addressed to him personally; that he personally was able to choose to act in ways that increased the light in the world. He had never considered this possibility before but over the next days and weeks it became a more and more compelling thought, until he recognized it as a deep yearning in himself to live in a certain way. That perhaps the purpose of life was not to become wealthy or succeed in business or to leave a financial inheritance to his children as he had thought. Perhaps his life had been given back to him so he might have the chance to fulfill the real purpose of life…which is to bring more light into the world. Perhaps this was the inheritance he could leave to his children.

Spiritual growth is often the outcome of a spontaneous shift in perspective, which enables us to live beyond our previous ways of life and free ourselves from beliefs and limitations that have held us hostage for decades. As serious illness wrests control from us and exposes us to new experiences we may develop new eyes. Another patient of mine who had carried the diagnosis of obsessive compulsive disorder was seemingly unresponsive to therapy. A card-carrying perfectionist, she had kept her home perfectly organized for years, right down to the rows of socks in her sock drawer as well as the bureau drawers of her children and husband. She insisted her children have play dates at the homes of their friends instead of their own home and avoided entertaining because the presence of others disturbed the way she had arranged the house. But cancer changed all this. When she became so ill from her chemotherapy that she could not leave her bed, neighbors and friends, oblivious to the house rules, brought food and did laundry, rearranging years of careful order in the process. Prayers written by the classmates of her children were taped to the walls. The dog was allowed to sleep on the bed. Somehow this did not trouble her as it once had. When I asked her about this she laughed, "I would never go back to the way I was before my cancer Rachel," she told me. "I drove everyone crazy. I resented them because they disturbed the order I had assigned to the world. Maintaining order was the most important thing in my life. I left no room for life to touch me or for anyone else to touch me either. I had been lonely for years and I did not even know it. Now my life is full of friends and kittens and puppies and children learning things and making messes. Lots of messes. Real life is so much more important than a perfectly clean kitchen floor."

Life-threatening illness can shuffle our values like a deck of cards. Sometimes a card we carried at the bottom of our deck turns out to be the top card, the thing that really matters. Having watched people play their hand in the presence of cancer for many years I would say that rarely is the top card perfection or possessions or even power. Most often the top card is the greatest of the spiritual values . . . which is love.

Often a shift in values and perspective is a slow process and is achieved before we even fully realize that we have been changed by our experience. But sometimes it can happen all at once in a setting that is highly unlikely. A few years ago, one of the most powerful physicians in our community required cancer surgery. He prepared himself for this experience by reading the current literature thoroughly, and researching the best and most skillful surgeons through his many connections. He ended up traveling to another city to avail himself of the best care. "I was determined that this experience would not change my life," he told me. "I fully expected to go back to work in a few weeks. As a matter of fact no one knew why I had taken a brief leave. If anyone thought much about it they would have assumed that I was completing a chapter or preparing a paper for submission." But despite his careful planning, his life changed anyway.

When he awoke in the recovery room; he was in pain more terrible than he had ever known. "I was 53 years old and I had no idea that my body could cause me this sort of pain. I was just stunned by it," he told me. "I did not think I could endure it…but as I lay there I slowly became aware of a sort of a split in my experience. A part of me was in agony but at the same time I was also filled with a sense of absolute peace, more profound than anything I could have previously imagined. It was a peace so absolute that it was like some sort of a promise, a trust of life, no matter what. I lay there and suddenly a phrase from my childhood returned to me, 'The peace that passeth all understanding.' What if this was what I was experiencing? I felt a sense of profound gratitude for being shown this, for just being able to experience it. I had never experienced anything like it before." He and I sat in silence together thinking about this. Then he looked at me, slightly embarrassed. "That's when everything changed," he said quietly. "I had this insight into my work and the rest of my life. Actually it was not really an insight, it was a knowing. What if my work wasn't as I had thought? What if it was not about being better than all the others at what I do, or making my department the most profitable in the hospital or winning the most teaching and research awards? What if my work was really about cultivating this experience of peace and deep trust of life and bringing it with me into places of fear and suffering and despair. Holding it in myself so strong and so steady that in the midst of their suffering others might be able to feel it too and take refuge in it just as I was taking refuge in it now." We sat together for a while longer. Then he smiled. "We can't fix the suffering Rachel." He told me. "There is always more suffering. Healing is different than fixing the suffering."

Experiences of healing and spiritual connection are not rare; and our response as a healthcare professional or friend or family member does not require that we have answers or explanations. What it does require is our presence and our willingness to wonder. The simple act of sharing these stories enables people to find a deeper meaning in both their suffering and their lives.

It has been argued that spiritual care is not the concern of the health professions; that those who tend the sick lack the proper training to engage with issues of the soul or of first order causality and need to leave such matters to others. But perhaps the world cannot be divided up in quite so tidy a way. As healthcare professionals, we participate in the spiritual growth of our patients whether we are aware of it or not and indeed may even become an agent of such growth without ever knowing it. I suspect this has happened to many of us. Spirit is omnipresent and does not wait on expertise; it uses whoever is present to point to itself. Spiritual movement occurs at the moment of readiness and whoever is privileged to be there may be used to facilitate change just exactly as they are. Often spiritual growth is initiated by an unexpected kindness, or the ordinary tasks of showing a patient to their bed, or cleaning and straightening their room, taking a blood pressure, offering medications or even in the process of performing highly technical procedures and testing.

My patient Susan was a highly educated woman with a reputation for being judgmental and impatient. On discovering that she had colon cancer, she withdrew into an angry silence, rejecting the concern and support of others. She succeeded in alienating her friends and family and many of her health professionals as well. The night before her surgery when she was admitted to the hospital, an aide had come to her room to shave her abdomen in preparation for the procedure. Susan had greeted her rudely, answering the aide's friendly overtures with a monosyllabic response or a cold silence. But the aide did not respond as many others had. As she continued with her task of shaving Susan's belly she asked her about tomorrow's surgery. In a superior and dismissive tone, Susan described in detail the invasive procedure, which was planned, including a description of the colostomy, which would become permanent part of her life. Irritated by the calm with which this information was received, Susan had become intensely angry. "And how would YOU feel if they were going to do this to you tomorrow?" she demanded. The aide looked at her for a long and thoughtful moment. "Why if I needed it, I would be grateful for the help," she replied. Susan was shocked into silence. "I had been responding as if I had been taken off the street and made to have this procedure," she told me afterward. "The idea that I needed help and that others might be there for me, might have prepared for years to be there for me, might have committed their lives to learn the skills that could save mine had just not crossed my mind. I had denied that I needed help because I had thought I was alone. She allowed me to see that I was in trouble and to know that others were with me. I began to cry and she just held me for a long time. What a blessing she was, Rachel. And I am deeply grateful for so many things now, including the gift of my life. I hope to use it well."

Simply listening to the experience of others validates its importance and weaves it more deeply into their lives. Most of us do not recognize the power of our attention and few of us can listen generously. As we listen we become busy considering things that concern us: do we agree with what is being said or not? do we believe it? We listen competitively: what does this say about the person who is speaking and what does it say about me? Is this person more educated than I am? Smarter? More fortunate? More competent? And of course if we are health professionals we listen to diagnose and to fix. But this is not the sort of listening that spiritual experience requires. Sharing a spiritual experience is always an act of trust and when someone trusts us with a story we need to listen not in order to agree or even understand but simply to know what is true for this other person. In witnessing it we give it value and we make it more real for them and perhaps for ourselves as well.

This is especially true of the experiences of a spiritual nature which are shared by the elderly and the dying. Such experiences may take the form of dreams, voices, or even visions. The daughter of an elderly woman discovered that her mother, who is 96, often "saw" her husband and her brother, both long dead, walking through her home deep in conversation. She told her daughter that she was troubled not by the presence of these two beloved men but by the fact that she was unable to get their attention. She would follow after them from room to room until they would suddenly disappear, leaving her with a deep curiosity and the question "Where did they go?" The daughter, a doctor herself, responded not by attempting to talk her mother out of her experience or dismissing it as a hallucination but by sharing the question with her and wondering together with her mother about the realm of the mysterious and the possibility of larger realities. This conversation became deeply comforting to both of them, as her elderly mother approached the close of her life.

Medicine is often a front row seat on spiritual reality; and yet many of us sit in this seat with our eyes closed. Much in our training discourages us from bringing to the table the part of ourselves that can appreciate spiritual realities and indeed can experience them. After years of professional training, bringing your full humanity to your work may feel risky. My own training valued the intellect. While this was never explicitly said, the hidden curriculum made it clear that other parts of my humanity were somewhat of a liability, almost a professional weakness. Yet our ability to make a difference in the lives of others goes far beyond our ability to analyze and cure. If we become present in our work not only intellectually but also as whole people, we have the opportunity to become fellow travelers, to accompany our patients on their path, to share their insights and experiences and at the same time to deepen the quality of our own lives. A diagnosis of cancer is a confrontation with the unknown. Meeting our patients right there in that unknown place may heal us both.

For many health professionals, engaging with the spiritual dimension of their work is often a deliberate choice. Being present not as an expert but as a human being requires us to move beyond our training and become willing to wonder and to appreciate. This is not an area of right or wrong but an area of intimacy best approached with humility and an openness to learning. Often a conversation of deep meaning can begin with a single question. The questions I ask my patients are very simple: "Your recovery is important to us both, but besides this, what really matters to you now?" Or, "I am impressed by the way you handle this difficult time in your life....what do you call upon for your strength?" or, "Have you had any experiences or even dreams during the time that you have been ill that make you wonder?"

It was in response to this last question that I discovered that one of my patients with breast cancer had a recurring dream of a woman in a blue veil that visited her nightly and laid her right hand gently on her forehead. Speaking of this aloud enabled her to recognize the touch as a blessing. Another of my patients, a nurse with ovarian cancer, told me that she had periods of "heightened gratitude" which at first had caused her to wonder if they were the prodromata of a seizure, times when she was suddenly and acutely aware of little things—a perfectly sharpened pencil, the sparkling clean of the dishes in the dish washer, the growth of the new grass in her yard. Things she usually did not notice which now gave her so powerful a sense of personal grace that she would find tears in her eyes. Yet another patient was startled to smell Chanel Number 5, the perfume his mother had worn throughout his childhood, drifting through the radiation suite as he lay on the table. After carefully enquiring about it, and discovering that none of the young women on staff wore it or had ever heard of it, he had simply accepted it as the mystery it was and taken deep comfort in it.

A discussion about religious beliefs and doctrine may require expertise and training; but a dialogue about spiritual experience is a common human interaction between people who share what has meaning and value to them and what it is like to listen deeply and respectfully to one another. What is needed is simply a willingness to bear witness to the insights and experiences of others and to strengthen and validate them. Both the telling and the listening stirs up wonder about the nature of the world and is an opening for the movement of spirit, which is an essential need of human nature.

These experiences and insights have deep meaning for many people. Over the years people have told me with regret that their sense of wider perspective has attenuated over time. They would not want to repeat their cancer experience but still wish they could see things in the way that they saw them when they were ill. It may be important not only to witness the spiritual movement in people but also to encourage them to make their insights part of their way of life. This may not require making large changes in lifestyle, or it may; but even the smallest action to move in the direction of their new perspective stabilizes the change in their lives. Cancer is often a doorway that enables people to experience a deeper connection to themselves and to others and to larger realities. People may emerge more able to feel empathy, embody compassion, or enter deeply into relationship with others who suffer, without fear. Often the intention to use these hard won capacities in the service of others anchors them in people's lives and becomes the final step in their healing. As a young patient told me many years ago, "I've paid for my ticket. I might as well take the trip."

Integrative medicine has been described as the "Medicine of the Whole Person" and conceptualized as a medicine that addresses the full range of a patient's needs; and yet there are wider implications to this new approach. To practice integrative medicine is to invite life in its wholeness into our hospitals, our clinics, and our workplaces and to be willing to meet it there. This may require us to change the way we think about our work and about ourselves; to uproot and revise the very notion of our role as a healthcare professional. Having the courage to do this may reward us with a new awareness of the meaning of our work and a far deeper satisfaction in our service than we had imagined possible.

19

The Role of Spirituality

MARY JO KREITZER AND ANN MARIE DOSE

KEY CONCEPTS

- Spirituality: Spirituality has been defined in a multitude of ways and is generally understood to be related to but distinct from religiosity. In the broadest sense, spirituality is focused on purpose, meaning and connectedness with self, others and a higher power. Spirituality is recognized as an integral part of being human that is interconnected with health and well-being.
- Spiritual Assessment: A spiritual assessment or screening can be conducted by a physician, nurse, spiritual care provider, or other health professional as a routine part of providing care. It is common for screening questions to be incorporated into standard health history interviews and forms.
- Spiritual Issues: Grief, loss, pain, suffering, shock, denial, fear, hopelessness, spiritual distress, despair, isolation, and survivor guilt are examples of spiritual issues faced by patients with cancer and their families. These issues may differ in their occurrence and intensity at different phases along the cancer continuum, such as new diagnosis, periods of remission, recurrence, long-term survival and/or at the end of life.
- Spiritual Practices: Commonly used spiritual practices include prayer, meditation, journaling, labyrinth walking, and interacting with nature.

In a book titled *"Close to the Bone"*, psychiatrist Jean Shinoda Bolen writes about the impact of a serious illness such as cancer in a person's life. "A life threatening illness" she writes, "has the impact of a stone hitting the still surface of a lake, sending concentric rings of disturbance out, as feelings, thoughts and reactions radiate out from this center. It impacts relationships, it stirs the depths of others, and it potentially brings the patient and those who are affected 'close to the bone' " (Bolen, 1996). A diagnosis of cancer provokes a spiritual crisis in the lives of many patients and their families. Feelings of anger, grief, loss, despair, and hopelessness accompany questions that include "why me?", "why now?" and "what is the meaning of this?" This chapter will explore the topic of spirituality through examining definitions of spirituality, the relationship between spirituality and health outcomes, ways to assess the spiritual needs of patients, commonly used spiritual interventions and practices, and the role of the health-care professional in meeting the spiritual needs of patients and their families.

Throughout history, and across all cultures, spiritual beliefs and practices have been expressed in a myriad of ways. The word spirit comes from the Hebrew work "ruah" which means wind, breath or air, that which gives life (Golberg, 1998). Greeks viewed the spirit in opposition to the body and any material reality. In Chinese, spirit means *chi* or vital energy (Chiu, 2000). The Latin, *spiritus*, means breath. Spirituality, in its broadest sense, is recognized as an integral part of being human that is interconnected with health and well-being.

The healing professions of nursing and medicine, from their earliest beginnings, were grounded in spirituality. In ancient societies, the connection between spirituality and healing was so close that the roles of priest, shaman, and healer were one and the same. Hildegaard of Bingen, a 12th century Christian mystic was well known for her use of herbs, art, music, and prayer. The first hospitals were founded by religious orders, and missionary movements across the centuries and continents have recognized the need for spiritual healing alongside physical healing.

It was only since the time of the scientific revolution and the advent of dualism in the 17th century that a wall of separation divided the care of people into mutually exclusive and often antagonistic camps. Medicine was charged with caring for the body, and later the mind, while religion was left with care and feeding of the soul. Contemporary Western science including the disciplines of medicine and nursing have often dealt poorly with the spiritual side of human nature by ignoring it and viewing these needs as being beyond the scope of their professional practice.

Over the past 20 years, there has been a growing interest in the topic of spirituality and its impact on health and well-being in both the lay press and professional literature. Consumers are demanding care that is holistic and attentive to the whole person—mind, body, and spirit. Clinicians are beginning to recognize the importance of both assessing and addressing spiritual needs of patients and researchers are establishing a link between spirituality and spiritual interventions and health outcomes.

Defining Spirituality

Spirituality is a multidimensional construct that has been defined in a multitude of ways and is generally understood to be related to but distinct from religiosity (Albaugh, 2003; Ameling & Povilonis, 2001; Chiu, Emblen, VonHofwegen, Sawatzky, & Meyerhoff, 2004; Fry, 1998; Narayanasamy, 1999; Tanyi, 2002). Religious beliefs are associated with a particular faith tradition. Participation or commitment to a religion may involve adherence to certain beliefs (ideology), religious practices (prayer, sacraments, and rituals), religious proscriptions (dietary modifications or avoidance of tobacco, alcohol, and drugs) and participation in a religious community. Spirituality is understood to be a broader concept that includes many dimensions. Murray and Zentner (1989) define spirituality as a quality that goes beyond religious affiliation and that strives for inspiration, reverence, awe, meaning and purpose, even in those who do not believe in God. The spiritual dimension, they suggest, is in harmony with the universe, strives for answers about the infinite, and comes into focus when the person faces emotional stress, physical illness, or death. Spirituality has also been described as a process and sacred journey (Mische, 1982), the essence or life principle of a person (Colliton, 1981), an experience of the radical truth of things (Legere, 1984), and the propensity to make meaning (Reed, 1992). Waldfogel (1997) notes that the experiences of joy, love, forgiveness, and acceptance all depend on, and are manifestations of, optimal spiritual well-being. Cohen (1993) adds that spirituality involves finding deep meaning in everything including illness and death and living life according to a set of values. Chiu et al. (2004) describe spirituality as a power, force, or energy that stimulates creativity, motivation, or a striving for inspiration. The simplest and most straightforward definition is from Pargament (1997), who coined spirituality as the "search for the sacred." Table 19.1 lists characteristics commonly associated with spirituality.

Relationship between Spirituality and Health Outcomes

Spiritual and religious beliefs and practices are prevalent in contemporary American society. According to the Gallup Poll that has tracked US religious beliefs for over 50 years, 95% of Americans believe in God, and 92%

Table 19.1. Characteristics of Spirituality.

Connectedness/relationships with self, others, Higher Power, nature

Meaning and purpose in life

Transcendence

Love/compassion

Wholeness

Energy

express a particular religious denomination (Gallup, 1998). In another survey (Yankelovich, 1996), researchers reported that 82% of Americans believe in the healing power of personal prayer and 73% believe that praying for someone else can cure their illness. Interest in spiritual matters is not limited to a particular age-group. In a national study conducted by the Higher Education Research Institute at the University of California, Los Angeles, CA (2005) of over 112,000 college freshmen, 74% of the students reported that they experience a connection with God or a higher power that transcends their personal self, four out of five indicated an "interest" in spirituality and nearly two-thirds reported spirituality to be a source of joy in their lives.

Studies of health professionals have also documented their perceptions of the importance of spiritual and religious beliefs and practices. A survey of family physicians revealed that 99% believe in the ability of religious beliefs to contribute positively to medical treatment. (Yankelovich, 1996). Eighty-seven percent of nurses reported the high importance of paying attention to patient's spiritual needs (Strang, Strang, & Ternestedt, 2002), 71% felt they identified spiritual needs in their practice (McSherry, 1998), yet both groups felt they fell short in meeting those needs. When asked about their attitudes toward spirituality and healing, 94% of HMO executives indicated that they believe that personal prayer, meditation, or other spiritual and religious practices can speed or help the medical treatment of people who are ill. (Yankelovich, 1997). The Joint Commission on Accreditation of Healthcare Organizations (JCAHO) has added spiritual care to the criteria for accreditation (JCAHO, 2000). Hospitals are now required to establish guidelines for the documentation of assessments of spiritual beliefs and practices, pastoral care must be available for patients who request it, and hospitals must meet the spiritual needs of dying patients and their families.

A number of studies report findings that suggest that spiritual and religious beliefs contribute to positive health benefits including stress reduction and an increased sense of well-being (Larson, et al., 1992). A meta-analysis of 29 studies by McCullough et al. (2000) revealed that the odds of survival were significantly greater for people who scored higher on measures of religious involvement than for people who scored lower, even after controlling for a variety of social and health-related variables.

While there is no evidence that religion or spirituality can impact cancer progression or mortality (Stefanek, McDonald, & Hess, 2004), a substantial number of studies have found a link between spirituality and quality of life, adjustment and symptom management. Spiritual well-being is significantly associated with the ability of cancer patients to enjoy life despite high levels of pain or fatigue (Brady, Peterman, Fitchett, Mo, & Cella, 1999). A study of 95 cancer patients diagnosed within the past 5 years found that spirituality was associated with less distress and better quality of life regardless of perceived life threat. In this study, existential well-being rather than religious well-being was the major contributor to positive health outcome (Laubmeier, Zakowski, &Bair, 2004). Existential well-being was found to have a strong negative correlation with depression (Nelson, Rosenfeld, Breitbart, & Galietta, 2002), whereas existential distress has been associated with loss of autonomy, lowered self-esteem, and a sense of hopelessness (Morita, Tsunoda, Inoue, & Chihara, 2000). In a longitudinal study of cancer pain and depression, spirituality and well-being were found to be inversely related to depression (O'Mahony, et al., 2005). Cancer survivors who draw on spiritual resources reported substantial personal growth related to the trauma associated with their diagnosis of cancer (Carpenter, Brockopp, & Andrykowski, 1999). Spiritual struggle, on the other hand, is associated with poorer quality of life and life satisfaction (Hills, Paice, Cameron, & Shott, 2005) and emotional adjustment (Manning-Walsh, 2005). Spiritual well-being has been found to be a contributor to overall quality of life at the end of life (Tang, Aaronson, & Forbes, 2004; Thomson, 2000).

Assessing Spirituality

A spiritual assessment or screening can be conducted by a physician, nurse, spiritual care provider or other health professional as a routine part of providing care. It is common for screening questions to be incorporated into standard health history interviews and forms. Table 19.2 provides an example of questions that may help to detect a spiritual need or issue.

The FICA interview guide (Puchalski & Romer Anna, 2000) is frequently used to obtain a spiritual history in clinical settings. FICA is an acronym that

Table 19.2. Spiritual Screening Questions.

What are your sources of hope, strength, comfort, and peace?

Are you part of a religious or spiritual community?

What spiritual practices do you find most helpful to you personally?

Are there any specific practices or restrictions I should know about in providing your health care?

SOURCE: Leonard, Barbara and Carlson, David. Spirituality in Healthcare (2003). www.csh.umn.edu/modules/index.html (accessed December 16, 2006).

stands for faith, importance/influence, community and address. Within each of there four areas, there are a set of questions: "What is your faith?" "How important is your faith?" "Are you part of a religious community?" "How would you like spiritual issues addressed in your care?" A tool called *Hope* developed by Anadarajah et al. (2001) taps into four similar domains. Examples of questions in the interview guide include the following:

- H stands for sources of hope, meaning, comfort, strength, peace, love and connection.
  - What do you hold onto in difficult times?
  - What sustains you and keeps you going?
- O stands for organized religion.
  - Are you part of a spiritual or religious community?
  - What aspects of your religion are helpful or not so helpful to you?
- P stands for personal spirituality and practices.
  - Do you have personal spiritual beliefs that are independent of your religion?
  - What spiritual practices do you find most helpful to you personally?
- E stands for effects on medical care and end-of-life issues.
  - Has being sick affected your ability to do things that usually help you spiritually?

Beyond these tools, there are a growing number of standardized measures developed to assess spiritual and religious beliefs and practices for the purpose of research and evaluation. The Spiritual Well-Being Scale (SWBS), developed by Paloutzian and Ellison (1982), measures both religious and existential well-being. Religious well-being refers to one's relationship with God or some higher power and existential well-being refers to a sense of purpose in life and satisfaction with life. The Functional Assessment of Chronic Illness Therapy—Spiritual Well-Being (FACIT-Sp) tool (Brady, et al., 1999; Peterman, Fitchett, Brady, Hernandez, & Cella, 2002) is part of the widely used Functional Assessment of

Cancer Therapy (FACT) quality-of-life battery (Cella, et al., 1993). It taps into both traditional religiousness dimensions (faith factor) and spiritual dimensions (meaning and peace factor). The Serenity Scale, developed by Roberts and Aspy (1993), focuses on a dimension of spirituality called serenity. *Serenity* is defined as being a spiritual experience of inner peace that is independent of external events.

Addressing Spiritual Issues

Grief, loss, pain, suffering, shock, denial, fear, hopelessness, spiritual distress, despair, isolation, and survivor guilt are examples of spiritual issues faced by patients with cancer and their families. These issues may differ in their occurrence and intensity at different phases along the cancer continuum, such as new diagnosis, periods of remission, recurrence, long-term survival and/or at the end of life. Being diagnosed with cancer brings the patient to a full and acute awareness of personal mortality and vulnerability. A heightened sense of one's spirituality may accompany this awareness. Reed (1986) found that people diagnosed with cancer had significantly higher levels of religiousness than healthy matched controls and later found greater spiritual perspective among hospitalized terminally ill patients compared with other hospitalized patients (Reed, 1987). Johnston Taylor (1997) described more intense experiences of spirituality as death becomes more imminent and identified two fundamental end-of-life questions: "How shall I die?" and "How shall I live before I die?" Experiences of loss and change may manifest spiritually as a search for meaning, she writes, while isolation or loneliness may prompt efforts toward loving others and strengthening relationships. Feelings of guilt or shame may lead to a search for forgiveness and acceptance by others.

The National Cancer Institute, in a document titled "*Spirituality in Cancer Care*" (NCI, 2006) identified intervention strategies that are appropriate to consider in addressing the spiritual concerns of patients. These interventions include the following:

- The health-care provider may choose to explore the spiritual concerns of the patients within the context of usual medical care.
- The patient may be encouraged to seek assistance from their own clergy or spiritual care provider.
- A referral may be made to a chaplain or religious or faith-based therapist.
- A referral may be made to a support group that is known to address spiritual issues.

To be effective in assessing and addressing the spiritual needs of patients, health-care providers need skills in the following areas:

- Listening: Careful listening enables the health care provider to be alert for meanings, connections, and yearnings reflected in conversations. It is important to listen to both what is said as well as what is not said. Authenticity is critically important. Patients can sense when the listener is distracted or not really interested.
- Seeing: Observing the nonverbal messages that accompany the client's spoken words may reveal thoughts and feelings that the client is unable to verbalize.
- Presence: When we are truly present to another human being, we are intentionally choosing to be with another in a healing way. It requires more than just physical presence. In the western culture, there is a strong bias for action. Health-care providers too often feel that they are not effective unless they are doing something. Presence requires being, not doing. This may be especially challenging for providers during times of expressions of anger or anguish by patients and/or families during their cancer journeys.
- Touching: The healing power of touch, which can range from the informal touch provided in usual care to that accompanied by healing intentions, is well established. Healing and therapeutic touch have emerged from the discipline of nursing over the past 25 years and gained varying levels of acceptance by patients and providers. There is a more ancient tradition called "*laying on of hands*" that has been associated with many faith traditions and healing ministries for centuries.

In addition to these skills, health-care providers also need information and ongoing education on commonly used spiritual practices.

- Prayer: There are many forms of prayer. Prayer may be offered in words, song, sighs, cries, gestures, or silence. Prayer may be individual or communal, public, or private. Prayers may be petitions, requests for healing, for peace, for safety, for acceptance, for strength to continue, as well as for courage. Prayer is a means of reaching out and connecting with a Higher Power.
- Meditation: Meditation is a self-directed practice for relaxing the body and calming the mind that has been used by people in many cultures since ancient times. Kabat-Zinn (2005) emphasizes that meditation is best thought of as a way of being rather than a collection of techniques. Mindfulness expands the capacity for awareness and for self-knowing.

When a mindful state is cultivated, it frees people from routinized thought patterns, routinized senses, and routinized relationships and destructive mind states and emotions that accompany them. When people are able to escape from highly conditioned, reactive, and habitual thinking, they are able to respond in more effective and authentic ways.

- Music, art, and nature: The arts are powerful healing tools that can help people explore feelings, gain new insights and perspectives, and enhance other spiritual practices. For some, being in nature is a powerful spiritual experience.

- Journaling: Journaling is both a way to record experiences and way to get in touch with inner thoughts and feelings. People who journal on a regular basis often find it to be a way to measure progress in self-growth and attain a broader perspective on life and relationships.

- Walking a labyrinth: A labyrinth is a circuitous path that leads to a center. It is different from a maze that has twists, turns, and blind alleys. A labyrinth has only one way in to the center and one way out. When people walk the labyrinth, they may pray, meditate, listen to music, or just observe nature. People report that when they walk the labyrinth, they gain insight or perspective. For some people, walking the labyrinth is both an actual physical experience as well as a metaphor for life's journey.

- Spiritual direction or counseling: Spiritual directors or counselors accompany people on their spiritual journeys. They help people explore such spiritual issues as grief, loss, anger, and abandonment as well as life challenges. They may offer guidance in prayer, journaling, and reading of sacred texts. Spiritual directors may also help explore how God or the Divine is present and active in one's life. Spiritual directors are listeners and companions. Like other forms of counseling, spiritual directors do not give answers but assist individuals in exploring questions, issues, and concerns in their lives. Spiritual directors are found at retreat centers and in private practice and may be employed by health care institutions or faith communities.

A task force (Lo, et al., 2002) of physicians and end-of-life specialists offers several guidelines for health-care providers as they respond to patients' spiritual concerns. Respect the patient's views and follow the patient's lead. It is not appropriate to impose one's own beliefs and practices on the patient. Identify common goals for care and health care decisions. Mobilize other resources of support for the patient such as referring the patient to a chaplain or other spiritual care provider.

Summary

Although the terms spirituality and religion are often used interchangeably, they hold different meanings in people's lives and are expressed in a myriad of ways. Health-care providers need to remain mindful of these individualities, respect them, and factor them into care. There is a growing body of literature that has documented the relationships between spirituality, religious beliefs and practices, and health outcomes. Given this connection and the expectation that patients have that their spiritual needs should be addressed, health-care providers and hospitals are developing the competencies and capacities to respond to spiritual issues and concerns. Spirituality can no longer be ignored in the provision of holistic care.

People whose lives have been touched by cancer either as a patient or as a family member commonly experience spiritual distress which may be expressed as grief, loss, pain, suffering, shock, denial, fear, hopelessness, despair, isolation, and survivor guilt. Spiritual interventions offered by health professional or spiritual care providers may both address these issues and contribute to overall health and well-being. This may help lessen the ripple effect of cancer on the patient and family as described by Bolen. This can perhaps be accomplished by strengthening relationships and promoting a sense of meaning and purpose as individuals struggle with the existential questions of "Why me, why us, why now?"

REFERENCES

Chiu L, Emblen J, Van Hofwegen D, Lynn S, Rick, & Meyerhoff H. (2004). An integrative review of the concept of spirituality in the health sciences. *Western Journal of Nursing Research,* 26(4), 405–428.

Hills J, Paice JA, Cameron JR, & Shott S. (2005). Spirituality and distress in palliative care consultation. *Journal of Palliative Medicine,* 8, 782–788.

Laubmeier KK, Zakowski SG, & Bair JP. (2004). The role of spirituality in the psychological adjustment to cancer: A test of the transactional model of stress and coping. *International Journal of Behavioral Medicine,* 11, 48–55.

Leonard B & Carlson D. (2006). Spirituality in healthcare (2003). www.csh.umn.edu/modules/index.html.

Manning-Walsh J. (2005). Spiritual struggle: Effect on quality of life and life satisfaction in women with breast cancer. *Journal of Holistic Nursing,* 23, 120–144.

National Cancer Institute. (2006). Spirituality in Cancer Care: Health Professional Version. Online. Available at: http://www.cancer.gov.

Peterman AH, Fitchett G, Brady MJ, Hernandez L, & Cella D. (2002). Measuring spiritual well-being in people with cancer: The functional assessment of chronic illness therapy—Spiritual Well-Being Scale (FACIT-Sp). *Annals of Behavioral Medicine, 24,* 49–58.

Puchalski C & Romer A L (2000). Taking a spiritual history allows clinicians to understand patients more fully. *Journal of Palliative Medicine, 3,* 129–137.

Reed PG. (1992). An emerging paradigm for the investigation of spirituality in nursing. *Research in Nursing & Health, 15,* 349–357.

Tanyi RA. (2002). Towards clarification of the meaning of spirituality. *Journal of Advanced Nursing, 39,* 500–509.

(A complete reference list for this chapter is available online at http://www.oup.com/us/ integrativemedicine).

20

Integrative Medicine and Breast Cancer

DEBU TRIPATHY

KEY CONCEPTS

- Many forms of complementary and alternative medicine (CAM) are widely used in breast cancer.
- Very few controlled clinical trials have been performed to evaluate the safety and effectiveness of CAM for either symptom management or the prevention and treatment of breast cancer.
- A low-fat diet with ample vegetable and fruit and a high level of physical activity shows the most promise in improving recurrence and mortality for early-stage breast cancer in retrospective and prospective trials.
- Group support and mind–body approaches appear to improve quality of life and emotional state but improvements in survival have not been shown.
- Acupuncture is effective in controlling pain, nausea, and fatigue.
- Herbal and botanical agents have significant potential as bioactive agents that can affect cellular pathways involved in breast cancer, but may also cause side effects and drug interactions. Further study is needed and cautions should be excercised when used with other treatments.
- Some approaches such as Essiac tea, Laetril, hydrazine sulfate, high-dose oral vitamin C, and shark cartilage have been tested and found to be ineffective in advanced breast and other cancers.

The fields of breast cancer and integrative medicine have a long and complicated relationship for numerous reasons. The interest level in alternative and complimentary approaches is high, with documented use of these approaches in part because of the demographics of breast cancer, affecting women of younger age and higher socioeconomic strata and hence a higher level of education, awareness, and activism. The role of environment and lifestyle in breast cancer, while still poorly understood, has contributed to the scientific study and public interest in modifiable factors in these domains. Multicultural and natural approaches to health have become desirable alternatives or adjuncts to diseases for which limited benefits are seen with conventional medicine. Exponential growth in the availability and exchange of information via the Internet, journals, support groups, and other means have encouraged patients to consider a more holistic approach to breast cancer prevention and treatment (Tripathy, 1998). While advances have clearly been made in earlier detection and better outcomes for early-stage breast cancer, these have come at the cost of significant side effects due to therapies that typically include surgery, radiation therapy, chemotherapy, and hormonal therapy. (Berry, et al., 2005; EBCTG, 2005). Additionally, the prognosis for advanced breast cancer remains bleak, even though modest improvements in survival have been achieved with these standard therapies as well as newer targeted biological therapies.

Physicians and patients alike appreciate the optimism engendered by advances in biotechnology, but remain concerned about the slow and incremental advances and the lack of attention to the patients as an individual. Moreover, the diagnosis of breast cancer is increasingly recognized as affecting the psychological, emotional, and spiritual balance, leading many to question whether these dimensions can also be addressed therapeutically by integrative modalities. The Oriental medicine concept of achieving "balance" in the homeostatic mechanisms whose disturbance leads to disease finds many corollaries in Western medicine as more relationships of altered biological pathways in breast cancer are discovered and found to be important in treating disease. Interestingly, the more modern tenets of stressing the use of therapeutic combinations that are customized to proteomic and gene expression signatures are beginning to resemble the centuries-old practice of individualized Oriental medicine. Unfortunately, the professional and ideological separation between "Western conventional" and "alternative" forms of medicine has led to parallel systems of care with some degree of distrust and noncommunication as opposed to collaboration, cross-education, and the development of an integrated body of knowledge that would offer patients a well-rounded and safe comprehensive treatment plan.

The use of complementary modalities is well-documented in patients with breast cancer, with a multiethnic study in San Francisco showing that about half of women who were recently diagnosed received CAM (Lee, Lin, Wrensch, Adler, & Eisenberg, 2000). The most popular approaches included diet, herbal, spiritual/mental, and physical methods, but conventional therapy, in particular surgery, was undertaken by nearly all patients (Table 20.1). A larger survey from over 2000 breast cancer survivors in the Harvard Nurse's Cohort Study showed CAM was used by 62%, with utilization correlating with worse quality of life (QOL) scores and younger age, although yoga use was associated with better QOL scores (Beuttner, et al., 2006). In some surveys, the proportion of breast cancer patients who reported CAM use to their physician was much

Table 20.1. Forms of Therapy Used by Patients Recently Diagnosed with Breast Cancer (Lee, et al., 2000).

	Ethnicity				
	White	Black	Latino	Chinese	All
Number or Respondents	97	100	100	82	379
Treatment Modality	% Usage				
*Conventional**					
Surgery	100	100	88	95	98.4
Chemotherapy	27	53	52	41	43.5
Radiation Therapy	50	46	42	40	44.7
Hormonal Therapy	21	23	44	17	26.6
Complementary					
Dietary†	35	18	30	23	26.6
Herbal/Homeopathy‡	8	9	15	23	13.5
Mental/Spiritual**	35	40	31	11	30.1
Physical Methods††	21	7	17	12	14.2
≥1 Complementary Modality	54	45	52	42	48.3
≥2 Complementary Modalities	38	27	37	28	32.6

* Choices are likely to be stage dependent; stage information not provided.

† Includes macrobiotic diet, megavitamins, antioxidants.

‡ Includes Chinese herbs, nonfood botanicals and homeopathy (very dilute substances).

** Includes meditation, relaxation, guided imagery, visualization, hypnosis, prayer, biofeedback.

†† Includes acupuncture, acupressure, massage therapy, body work, yoga, Tai-Chi, Chi-Gong.

higher than that has been reported in general, and specific modalities chosen depended on the type of conventional breast cancer therapy and symptoms experienced (Ashikaga, Bosompra, O'Brien, & Nelson, 2002; Beuttner, et al., 2006; Gray, Fitch, Goel, Franssen, & Labrecque, 2003; Nahleh & Tabbara, 2003; Richardson, Sanders, Palmer, Greisinger, & Singletary, 2000). Users of integrative modalities are more likely to be younger, well-educated, more concerned about harms of therapy or risks of cancer, and under more emotional stress or with depression (Ashikaga, et al., 2002; Boon, et al., 2000; Burstein, Gelber, Guadagnoli, & Weeks, 1999; Henderson & Donatelle, 2004; Lee, et al., 2000; Montazeri, Sajadian, Ebrahimi, Haghighat, & Harirchi, 2005; Moschen, et al., 2001; Navo, et al., 2004; Rakovitch, et al., 2005; Shen, et al., 2002). However, these generalizations belie the fact that integrative medicine is extremely heterogeneous and its use is motivated by diverse reasons that differ according to demographic factors.

This chapter will focus on integrative approaches that involve lifestyle (exercise and diet), nutritional supplements, acupuncture, Oriental medicine/herbal medicine, mind-body approaches, and other complementary and alternative therapies. Most of the data available are from patients who incorporate these modalities with conventional treatment. Integrative therapy is composed of a broad array of interventions so the goals of therapy range from improving physical and emotional well-being to attempting to treat or cure cancer. Most integrative disciplines advocate a combination of therapies that are highly individualized. Thus, with the exception of dietary and group support trials, most clinical data on integrative medicine are derived from experiential observations, cohort/case–control, or small pilot prospective studies.

A literature review of all CAM breast cancer trials found that of 1000 citations in the English language biomedical literature from 1980 to 1997, 51 met the criteria of prospective clinical research and only 17 were randomized trials (Jacobson, Workman, & Kronenberg, 2000). None showed clear impact on breast cancer endpoints, but some were useful in symptom management such as acupuncture for nausea. A more recent review of CAM studies for early breast cancer also concluded that this field of research is still immature with few prospective trials and multiple methodological problems including vague end points, nonreproducible treatments, and limited sample sizes (Gerber, Scholz, Reimer, Briese, & Janni, 2006). The nature of integrative medicine poses difficulties in trial design, and the chasm between biomedical sciences and CAM research dictates that recommendations in this area be based on the best available data and a balance of potential benefits and harms of specific therapies for defined situations.

The Role of Exercise and Diet in Breast Cancer

Many cell growth, signaling, and inflammation pathways that are aberrant in cancer are mediated by fatty acid derivatives, oxidative stress, amino acid balance, and vitamin cofactors. These factors are influenced by diet and activity. Overall energy balance of caloric intake and expenditure affect estrogen as well as insulin, insulin-like growth factor, inflammation, and immune pathways, many of which are implicated in breast cancer risk (Borugian, et al., 2004; Hankinson, 2005–2006). Body mass index is linked to breast cancer, particularly in postmenopausal women, and overall weight gain raises the risk of breast cancer and mortality after a diagnosis of breast cancer (Irwin, et al., 2005; van den Brandt, et al., 2000).

Physical activity and exercise over one's lifetime, particularly early in life, have been associated with a lower risk of developing breast cancer (Bernstein, et al., 2005; Tehard, Friedenreich, Oppert, & Clavel-Chapelon, 2006). In women with breast cancer, overall physical activity after diagnosis exhibited a linear relationship with improved survival at 10 years (Holmes, Chen, Feskanich, Kroenke, & Colditz, 2005). Pilot trials of exercise in breast cancer have shown that it is feasible, safe, and associated with improvements in fitness and fatigue as well as reduced markers of hormonal signaling and inflammation (Fairey, et al., 2003; Fairey, et al., 2005; Schmitz, et al., 2005). Two overviews of randomized exercise trials for early-stage breast cancer showed improvements in physical fitness and quality of life, but none of the trials were designed to assess survival (Markes, Brockow, & Resch, 2006; McNeely, et al., 2006). Moreover, exercise has not been shown to exacerbate the risk of postoperative lymphedema (Ahmed, Thomas, Yee, & Schmitz, 2006). While large definitive trials assessing breast cancer recurrence and survival have not been done, it seems reasonable to recommend an activity regimen for both general disease prevention and survivorship.

Diet has a clear role in many diseases, although the relationship of specific dietary components to the risk of breast cancer development or progression is not well understood (Holmes & Willett, 2004). Retrospective studies of overall diet have yielded mixed and inconsistent effects on survival or recurrence after a diagnosis of breast cancer, with some showing improved outcome with lower fat and higher fruit, vegetable, and fiber intake or avoiding dietary extremes (Fink, et al., 2006; Goodwin, et al., 2003; Holmes, et al., 1999; Ingram, 1994; Jain, Miller, & To, 1994; McEligot, Largent, Ziogas, Peel, & Anton-Culver, 2006; Rock & Demark-Wahnefried, 2002; Zhang, Folsom, Sellers, Kushi, & Potter, 1995). Two prospective randomized studies of diet have been conducted in healthy women and in women with breast cancer. The Women's Health Initiative study compared a 20%-fat diet supplemented with fruits, grains, and vegetables to normal diet in healthy individuals and found a nonstatistically significant decrease in breast cancer development over an average of 8 years, but longer follow-up is needed for definitive conclusions (Prentice, et al., 2006). In women with a diagnosis of early-stage breast cancer, a low-fat diet was associated with less weight gain and fewer recurrences (Chlebowski, et al., 2005). Longer follow-up from this study as well as another trial still awaiting analysis may provide firmer recommendations in the future.

Specific dietary components could potentially modulate breast cancer with defined compound in different foods listed in Table 20.2. However, no single component has been found to clearly influence breast cancer development or outcome, with primarily retrospective studies available. Studies with omega-3-fatty acid, based on the principle that fatty acid structure influences cell signaling, have not shown a clear clinical association in breast cancer risk despite abundant preclinical data against cancer, but prospective controlled clinical trials in breast cancer are lacking (Hardman, 2004; Maclean, et al., 2006). With the exception of a marginal improvement with vitamin A and C, no cohort studies have shown any vitamin supplementation to influence breast cancer risk (Rohan, Howe, Friedenreich, Jain, & Miller, 1993, reviewed in Holmes & Willett, 2004). In a subset of the Harvard Nurse's Study,

Table 20.2. Nutritional Sources
of Bioactive Compounds.

Food	Compound
Cruciferous vegetables	Isothiocyanates, indole-3-carbinol
Turmeric	Curcumin
Soy	Isoflavones
Pineapple	Bromelain
Grapes	Resveratrol
Green tea	Catechins
Ginger	Gingerols
Cayenne pepper	Capsaicin
Multiple foods	Quercitin
Citrus fruits	Limonene
Berries	Anthocyanidins
Garlic	Organosulfur compounds

premenopausal women with a positive family history of breast cancer had an inverse breast cancer risk with α and β-carotene, lutein/zeaxanthin, total vitamin A and C consumption (Zhang, et al., 1999). Other studies have shown lower recurrence risk with higher β-carotene, vitamin C intake, and higher serum carotenoid levels (Jain, et al., 1994; Rock, et al., 2005). However, a large prospective trial of β-carotene for breast cancer prevention was halted early after reports that this supplementation increased lung cancer among smokers, so this supplement is not likely to be studied further in breast cancer (Omenn, et al., 1996).

Antioxidants and Breast Cancer

Many vitamins and other cofactors have antioxidant properties that have protective effects on genomic and membrane damage in the laboratory. Therefore, the use of antioxidants has been popular in CAM, particularly naturopathic medicine, both as long-term therapy as well as to minimize side effects of chemotherapy, particularly neuro- and cardiotoxicity. The use of vitamin C has also been popular given its antioxidant effects (even though there may be oxidative effects) on the basis of case reports of response in advanced cancer. Two blinded controlled trials of intravenous vitamin C in patients with advanced cancer did not show any difference in survival or symptoms, but combinations with vitamin C with chemotherapy has not been formally tested (Creagan, et al., 1979; Moertel, et al., 1985). Few studies have examined the use of antioxidants in patients after a diagnosis of breast cancer. A randomized study of fenretinide, a synthetic vitamin A analog, in patients with early-stage breast cancer showed no reduction in second breast cancers overall, but did in premenopausal patients (Veronesi, et al., 2006). An overview of trials examining selenium, an essential trace element with antioxidant properties, to alleviate side effects of surgery, radiotherapy, and chemotherapy did not show clear effects (Denner & Horneber, 2006). A cohort study of patients using numerous vitamin and antioxidant supplements showed an outcome no different to a matched population-based cohort (Lesperance, et al., 2002). Coenzyme Q-10 has been of interest in both potentiating the effects of tamoxifen and lowering anthracycline cardiotoxicity, but the available clinical data are again scant (Folkers, 1996; Takimoto, et al., 1982). Concurrent use of antioxidants with chemotherapy or radiotherapy remains controversial as some argue that it may actually counteract the anticancer effect of conventional therapy, while others argue that the preclinical data actually supports a favorable effect with chemotherapy and anecdotal clinical experience also suggests benefits (D'Andrea, 2005; Labriola & Livingston, 1999; Saintot, et al., 2002). To date, the literature lacks well-done prospective trials, with a review of observational and interventional trials negative for clear effects on cancer outcomes (Ladas, et al., 2004). A reasonable recommendation based on current data would be to avoid high-dose antioxidants, particularly during chemotherapy and radiation therapy, but to consider them more long-term at either lower and more physiological doses, or ideally, through a balanced diet rich in vegetables and whole grains.

Soy and Other Phytoestrogens

Several food products contain phytoestrogens, so named because of binding to the estrogen receptor (ER). However, signaling via ER is complex, and phytoestrogens have shown both stimulation and inhibition of these pathways in the laboratory, such that the ultimate effects of these compounds must be evaluated in prospective clinical studies (An, Tzagarakis-Foster, Scharschmidt, Lomri, & Leitman, 2001). Phytoestrogens can be classified as isoflavones found in soy, lignans in seeds and nuts, and coumestans in red clover and bean spouts. Epidemiological studies of soy intake have not shown a clear association with breast cancer risk, with one study showing usage at young age and in high amounts associated with lower risk (Ingram, Sanders, Kolybaba, & Lopez, 1997; Peeters, Keinan-Boker, van der Schouw, & Grobbee, 2003). Based on their hormonal effects, soy and other phytoestrogens have been studied for their ability to alleviate hot flashes and other menopausal effects, especially in breast cancer patients, where estrogen is contraindicated. A review of placebo-controlled phytoestrogens trials for hot flashes did find that one of six studies with red clover and 3 of 11 with soy isoflavones showed effectiveness, while the largest single soy study did not (Nelson, et al., 2006; Quella, et al., 2000). A large randomized cross-over trial of black cohosh (also known as Remifemin) showed no effect although smaller studies have demonstrated reduction of hot flashes (Pockaj, et al., 2006). A small randomized study showed that 25 g of lignan-containing flaxseed for 1 month lowered cell proliferation, increased apoptosis (programmed cell death), and reduced HER2 oncogene expression in breast cancers before surgery but no data exist on the use of phytoestrogens for prevention or treatment of breast cancer (Thompson, Chen, Li, Strasser-Weippl, & Goss, 2005). Several pilot studies assessing soy for breast cancer prevention, or intermediate/surrogate end points, such as reducing mammographic breast density, are ongoing.

Immunostimulants

Several products that are known to activate the immune system and modulate inflammation include mushrooms and mistletoe extract. Mushrooms, including maitake, shiitake, reishi, and turkeytail (trametes versicolor) and their contents including polysaccharopeptides (β-glucans), glycoproteins, sterols, and terpenoids, as well as components like PSK and lentinan can augment immune parameters and downregulate estrogen response (Grube, Eng, Kao, Kwon, & Chen, 2001; Jiang, Slivova, & Sliva, 2006). Protein bound polysaccharide (PSK and PSP) have been tested extensively in the laboratory and clinic, and are known to stimulate cytotoxic T cells. In randomized clinical trials, PSK has shown mixed results in improving disease-free survival when added to chemo- and/or endocrine therapy (Morimoto, et al., 1996; Toi, et al., 1992). However, the Oxford Overview of randomized trials involving immunotherapy in 6000 patients, heavily represented by PSK, did not show an advantage (EBCTG, 1992).

Mistletoe extract and fermented preparations such as Iscador contain the lectin viscumin, that also activates the immune system and this has been studied extensively in Germany and Switzerland as a part of anthroposophical medicine. It is primarily used as adjuvant therapy for several cancers, given by subcutaneous or intratumoral injection. While there are immune and antitumor effects against breast cancer in preclinical models, prospective randomized trials have had significant design limitations although some have shown improvements in immune function, QOL, and survival (Grossarth-Maticek & Ziegler, 2006; Kaegi, 1998a; Semiglasov, Stepula, Dudov, Schnitker, & Mengs, 2006). An overview of 23 studies concluded that the quality of these trials were suboptimal as placebo, double-blind methodology was not generally used (Kienle, et al., 2003).

Acupuncture, Manipulative and Body-Based Methods

Acupuncture modulates nervous pathways and neurotransmitters, and has even been shown to affect immune function, yet mechanisms of action are still not known and its application is empirically based on experience and modifications over generations. This modality has been studied systematically in high-quality randomized trials, primarily for management of symptoms, with sufficient benefits demonstrating that the NIH issued a consensus statement in support of its use for cancer-related symptoms of pain, fatigue, and nausea (NIH Consensus Statement on Acupuncture 2006). In breast and other cancers, some but not all small randomized studies have shown improvements in pain, nausea, and fatigue, but not dyspnea (Cohen, Menter, & Hale, 2005; Vickers, Feinstein, Deng, & Cassileth, 2005). An overview of point stimulation for nausea showed that electroacupuncture reduced first-day vomiting, but manual acupuncture did not (Ezzo, et al., 2006). Acupressure reduced first-day nausea, but was not effective on later days, while acupressure showed no benefit for vomiting, and electrical stimulation on the skin was not effective. A randomized trial of auricular acupuncture for cancer-related pain with about half the patients having breast cancer showed a benefit (Alimi, et al., 2003). Studies of menopausal symptoms have also shown benefit, but most of these are small and limited to studies in the Chinese literature (Tagliaferri, Cohen, & Tripathy, 2002).

Acupressure in the form of pressured wrist bands appear to alleviate chemotherapy-induced nausea in patients at high risk of symptoms (Roscoe, et al., 2006). Massage therapy can provide relaxation and may also help with certain cases of postoperative arm lymphedema (McNeely, et al., 2004; Williams, Vadgama, Franks, & Mortimer, 2002). While other forms of body-based therapies are being increasingly used in medical centers and by breast cancer patients, they are generally viewed as soothing and safe, so formal measures of benefit from randomized trials are not available (Cassileth & Vickers, 2004).

Oriental Medicine—Chinese, Ayurvedic, and Tibetan

It is difficult to formally study Oriental medicine given its highly individualized application and the diagnostic criteria for which they are applied. This form of medicine uses botanical and animal products, trace elements, diet and activity modifications. Controlled studies using Chinese medicine are mostly represented by acupuncture, although small studies, primarily in the Chinese literature have suggested improvements in immune function, symptoms, and in some cases, even disease-free survival with the use of herbal medicine, usually in combination with acupuncture and dietary modifications (Tagliaferri, Cohen, & Tripathy, 2001; Tagliaferri, et al., 2002; Wong, Sagar, & Sagar, 2001). Botanical agents used in Oriental medicine are bioactive and can cause hepatic, renal, and hematological side effects and can interfere with the metabolism of other drugs (Sparreboom, Cox, Acharya, & Figg, 2004). However, several Chinese herbal agents historically used against cancer do possess in vitro and in vivo activity against human breast cancer cell lines (Campbell, et al., 2002). One herb, Ban Zhi Lian (Latin name *Herba Scutellaria Barbatae*) has been shown to have proapoptotic properties, and in a phase I study in patients with advanced metastatic breast cancer, was found to be safe and, while formal responses were not seen, minimal responses were observed (Rugo, et al., 2006).

Very little clinical data are available for specific herbs, although the use of green tea has been of interest as numerous compounds including polyphenols, particularly catechins, have shown antineoplastic, or cancer prevention potential in laboratory models (Kaegi, 1998b). An overview of cohort and case-controlled studies of green and black tea did show a lowered risk of breast cancer with green tea but interestingly, a slight increase in risk with black tea (Sun, Yuan, Koh, & Yu, 2006).

Ayurvedic medicine has not been formally evaluated in breast cancer with prospective trials, but herbs commonly used like triphala and amooranin do possess in vitro activity against breast cancer cell lines (Sandhya & shra, 2006; Rabi, et al., 2003). Similarly, Tibetan medicine being highly individualized with alternate diagnostic categories that do not exclusively address cancer, is not easily amenable to clinical investigation. One pilot study that allowed individualization of Tibetan herbs as sole therapy for advanced breast cancer showed that this therapy was feasible, safe, and associated with one partial response out of nine evaluable patients (Leeman, et al., 2001). Clearly there is a large potential to test natural botanicals in defined situations—the problems of individualized therapy and implications on trial design must be addressed.

Other Alternative Systems

Homeopathy is based on the premise that very dilute versions of pathogenic materials can induce a correction in pathology (Milazzo, Russell, & Ernst, 2006; Shang, et al., 2005). In the area of breast cancer, few reports exist—one double-blind, placebo-controlled trial of individualized homeopathy for breast cancer patients with estrogen withdrawal symptoms showed no benefit (Thompson, Montgomery, Douglas, & Reilly, 2005). Naturopathic medicine includes a large array of diet, natural products as well as special blood diagnostic and imaging tests, and the discipline provides for training and certification for independent care provision. Many of the principles involve similar themes as seen in Oriental medicine, but with modern adaptations. A survey of naturopathic physicians caring for breast cancer showed that the modalities utilized included dietary counseling (94%), botanical medicines (88%), antioxidants (84%), and supplemental nutrition (84%), and the most common specific treatments were vitamin C (39%), coenzyme Q-10 (34%), and Hoxsey formula (29%) (Standish, Greene, Greenlee, Kim, & Grosshans, 2002). No trials comparing Western-only medicine to either naturopathic or homeopathic therapy, or the addition of these systems to standard therapy, have ever been reported, although some are in progress. More recent off-shoots of alternative systems such as chelation, cleansing/detoxification, and enzyme therapy are being studied in small pilot trials, but no definitive or suggestive data are available that would form the basis for recommendations in breast cancer.

Mind-Body Approaches

Mind–body medicine is generally considered to be any maneuver that involves mental, psychological, or behavioral methods either in a highly structured environment or more loosely self-applied. The neurological axis can induce physiologic and possible immunological changes that can affect the disease course, but emotional improvement alone is an important goal in breast cancer (Bakke, Purtzer, & Newton, 2002). The early observation that breast cancer patients in support groups lived longer raised interest in this approach (Spiegel, Bloom, Kraemer, & Gottheil, 1989). A randomized trial involving 235 patients with metastatic breast cancer and testing supportive–expressive group therapy did not show a survival advantage, but did show enhanced mood and decreased pain perception in the intervention arm (Goodwin, et al., 2001). Four other randomized trials of group support in patients with metastatic breast cancer have been reported and none have shown a survival advantage, but other improvements were noted as outlined in Table 20.3 (Classen, et al., 2001; Edelman, Bell, & Kidman, 1999; Edmonds, Lockwood, & Cunningham, 1999). A randomized cognitive–existential support trial in early-stage breast cancer

Table 20.3. Randomized Trials of Group Support in Advanced Breast Cancer.

Number of Patients	Group Support Type	Survival Effect	Other Effects	Reference
86	Supportive-expressive	Positive 36.6 vs. 18.9 months $P < 0.0001$	Lower mood disturbances maladaptive coping, phobias	Spiegel, et al., 1989
66	Supportive-cognitive	Negative $P = 0.35$	Increased anxiety, better coping	Edmonds, et al., 1999
124	Cognitive-behavioral	Negative $P > 0.1$	Less depression, mood disturbance	Edelman, et al., 1999
235	Supportive-expressive	Negative $P = 0.72$	Improved mood, less pain	Goodwin, et al., 2001
125	Supportive-expressive	None reported	Improved mood, less stress	Classen, et al., 2001

also failed to show a survival advantage but improvements in anxiety and satisfaction with therapy were noted (Kissane, et al., 2004). Another study addressing insomnia also showed a benefit (Savard, Simard, Ivers, & Morin, 2005). Few studies have attempted to compare different forms of group support. One randomized trial comparing cognitive-behavioral to affirmation, imagery, meditation, and ritual demonstrated improvements from baseline in both group, but only subtle differences in multiple psychological and spiritual domains (Targ & Levine, 2002).

Other forms of psychological therapy, such as mindfulness, that incorporates relaxation, meditation, and yoga can have effects on cortisol and neurotransmitters such as melatonin (Carlson, Speca, Patel, & Goodey, 2004). A small controlled study of yoga in breast cancer survivors yielded improvements in global quality of life, emotional function, and diarrhea (Culos-Reed, Carlson, & Hately-Aldous, 2006). In one small randomized trial in early-stage breast cancer patients, art therapy led to improvements in coping skills (Oster, et al., 2006). Music has the potential to reduce anxiety although other QOL index changes have not been seen (Bozcuk, et al., 2006; Haun, Mainous, & Looney, 2001). A small randomized cross-over trial of dance and movement showed significant improvements in quality of life, range of motion, and body image in breast cancer survivors (Sandel, et al., 2005). A pilot study of journaling suggested that the writings of patients with breast cancer may provide some insight into levels of distress and anxiety (Smith, Anderson-Hanley, Langrock, & Compas, 2005). Hypnosis may affect psychological and physiologic parameters, and studies for treatment of hot flashes have shown encouraging benefits, but these studies need confirmatory follow-up controlled trials (Bakke, et al., 2002; Elkins, Marcus, Palamara, & Stearns, 2004). Meditation may also help with anxiety and depression (Hidderley & Holt, 2004). Guided imagery has been useful in alleviating side effects of chemotherapy, particularly nausea, depression, and anxiety (Cameron, Booth, Schlatter, Ziginskas, & Harman, 2006; Rossman, 2002; Yoo, Ahn, Kim, Kim, & Han, 2005). Similarly, aromatherapy has been found to reduce anxiety and depression (Kite, et al., 1998). All these modalities involve neural cortical and primitive pathways that are relatively unstudied, but may secondarily affect physiological responses, and with further study, could represent safe and valuable adjuncts to breast cancer care.

Alternative Approaches Shown to be Ineffective for Breast Cancer

One can ask at what point a series of studies should convincingly reject a given modality. In some cases, very little data are available. This is the case for energy, bioenergetic/magnetic, and related therapies. In the case of certain biological therapies, trials have been performed to assess anticancer activity, especially in those therapies that are commonly sought to the exclusion of conventional therapy (Vickers, 2004). Shark cartilage therapy became popular with early reports of antiangiogenic and antitumor activity, yet a clinical trial of 60 patients with various cancers, including breast cancer, yielded no responses (Miller, Anderson, Stark, Granick, & Richardson, 1998). The chemically modified camphor-based substance 714-X is believed to interfere with microcycles of somatids that are felt to be visible by dark-field microscopy of the blood, yet this compound was not felt to be substantiated in animal studies or based on any available human experience (Kaegi, 1998c). Other substances including Essiac tea, laetrile, and hydrazine sulfate have been found to be ineffective in randomized or Phase II clinical trials (Kaegi, 1998d; Loprinzi, et al., 1994; Moertel, et al., 1982).

Moving toward Integrative Breast Cancer Care: Current Recommendations and the Role of Research and Advocacy

Integrative and holistic medicine represents the art of judgment and individualization in addressing the whole person, while adhering to the accepted scientific methods of scientific inquiry. Limitations in trial design must be taken into account when interpreting data—these include the wrong patient population, incorrect application of the modality, inappropriate endpoint measures, and limited sample size and follow-up time. However, oncology professionals must prioritize a myriad of approaches that have different safety profiles and theoretical underpinnings, and that are applied for different indications in breast cancer in the absence of the type of data that is available for more conventional care.

A prioritization for integrative therapy in the prevention and treatment of breast cancer should follow the same paradigm used in all of medicine—balancing potential benefits and risks using the best available data. A schematic for the deployment of an integrative medical system that combines conventional and complementary therapies is shown in Table 20.4. Dietary and physical activity measures for prevention of breast cancer and other diseases should receive a high priority, given the safety of the interventions and the strong epidemiological data. For example, recommendations recently proposed by the American Cancer Society Nutritional and Physical Activity Guidelines Advisory Committee would represent a comprehensive starting point (Kushi, et al., 2006). Dietary components are best obtained through a

Table 20.4. Prioritization of Integrative Modalities for Breast Cancer.

Integrative	Conventional
Prevention/Early Detection	
Diet (low fat, whole grain, fruits, vegetables, low refined carbohydrates)	Mammographic screening
Exercise/activity regimen	Tamoxifen/"chemoprevention" in selected cases
Early-Stage Breast Cancer	
Group therapy, meditation, stress management, movement therapy, dance, art journaling	Surgery, hormonal therapy, chemotherapy, trastuzumab as indicated to maximize risks benefit
Acupuncture for symptoms	Clinical trials (Phase III agents)
Advanced Breast Cancer	
Same modalities as for early stage	Systemic therapies whose benefits (response/delay of progression) outweigh side effects
Experimental approaches, botanical therapies in the context of a clinical trial or an experienced practitioner working in concert with oncologist	Clinical trials of Phase I/II agents
Survivorship and Ongoing Care	
Massage, music, art, journaling, aromatherapy – these are generally safe with quality of life benefits, but need more study for disease-related outcomes	Routine medical follow-up, assessment of risk factors
Avoidance of high-dose supplements and antioxidants during therapy, but consideration of low dose vitamin/antioxidant supplements long term, or ideally via a balanced diet	Review of ongoing concomitant mediations, minimizing overall medications and patients education regarding risks and interactions

Note that the center dashed line represents intercommunication and coordination by the two "sides."

Note that clinical trials are needed for specific supplements like antioxidants with chemotherapy, botanical/herbal agents, and mind–body approaches that could have physiological effects.

balanced diet and apart from calcium for bone health, no specific supplementation can be uniformly recommended. Symptom management using modalities that have shown benefits, including acupuncture and group therapy/relaxation/meditative techniques, should also be considered along with conventional therapies whose effectiveness and side effect profile merit side-by-side therapy. Herbal products are powerful and potentially useful agents that merit more study, but when used with little experience or communication between care providers, could produce deleterious effects and interfere with other medications. Unorthodox techniques without a physiologic basis or clinical track record should be avoided.

It is clear that advocacy and survivorship involvement in policy-making and participation in the clinical research process is critical. Research tools need to be adapted to study individualized integrative modalities while preserving the fundamental tenets of scientific research. Broad participation in clinical trials and multidisciplinary input into study design are urgently needed. More communication across disciplines is required; indeed, a new generation of cross-trained practitioners and researchers must lead the field of breast cancer to a new model that capitalizes on the knowledge explosion in the biomedical sciences but preserves individual identity and diverse cultures and traditions of medicine.

REFERENCES

Bernstein L, Patel AV, Ursin G, Sullivan-Halley J, Press MF, Deapen D, et al. (2005). Lifetime recreational exercise activity and breast cancer risk among black women and white women. *Journal of the National Cancer Institute*, 97, 1671–1679.

Beuttner C, Kroenke CM, Phillips RS, Davis RB, Eisenberg DM, & Holmes MD. (2006). Correlates of use of different types of complementary and alternative medicine by breast cancer survivors in the nurses' health study. *Breast Cancer Research and Treatment*, 100, 219–227.

Campbell MJ, Hamilton B, Shoemaker M, Tagliaferri M, Cohen I, & Tripathy D. (2002). Antiproliferative activity of Chinese medicinal herbs on breast cancer cells in vitro. *Anticancer Research*, 22, 3843–3852.

Cassileth BR & Vickers AJ. (2004). Massage therapy for symptom control: Outcome study at a major cancer center. *Journal of Pain and Symptom Management*, 28, 244–249.

Goodwin PJ, Leszcz M, Ennis M, Koopmans J, Vincent L, Guther H, et al. (2001). The effect of group psychosocial support on survival in metastatic breast cancer. *The New England Journal of Medicine*, 345, 1719–1726.

Jacobson JS, Workman SB, & Kronenberg F. (2000). Research on complementary/alternative medicine for breast cancer: A review of the biomedical literature. *Journal of Clinical Oncology*, 18, 668–683.

Ladas EJ, Jacobson JS, Kennedy DD, Teel K, Fleischauer A, & Kelly KM. (2004). Antioxidants and cancer therapy: A systematic review. *Journal of Clinical Oncology*, 22, 517–528.

Lee M, Lin SS, Wrensch MM, Adler SR, & Eisenberg D. (2000). Alternative therapies used by women with breast cancer in four ethnic populations. *Journal of the National Cancer Institute*, 92, 42–47.

Nelson HD, Vesco KK, Haney E, Fu R, Nedrow A, Miller J, et al. (2006). Nonhormonal therapies for menopausal hot flashes: Systematic review and meta-analysis. *JAMA*, 295, 2057–2071.

Richardson MA, Sanders T, Palmer JL, Greisinger A, & Singletary SE. (2000). Complementary/alternative medicine use in a comprehensive cancer center and the implications for oncology. *Journal of Clinical Oncology*, 18, 2505–2514.

(A complete reference list for this chapter is available online at http://www.oup.com/us/integrativemedicine).

21

Prostate Cancer: An Integrative Approach

MARK A. MOYAD

KEY CONCEPTS

- Cardiovascular disease is still the leading cause of death in men in the developed world. In general, what is heart healthy is also good for the prostate!
- Fitness and overall health should be emphasized first, and not weight loss, by encouraging patients to get approximately 30 minutes of physical activity a day and to lift weights or perform resistance exercises several times a week. Aerobic and resistance exercise should be emphasized equally, not one more than the other.
- There is no ideal weight loss diet or intervention for patients. Choose a diet, lifestyle change, or other interventions that are tailored to the specific personality of the patient.
- Reducing the intake of unhealthy dietary fat such as saturated, trans-fatty acids, and even dietary cholesterol, should be encouraged and the unhealthy fat replaced by more healthy types of monounsaturated or polyunsaturated fat (omega-3 fatty acids).
- Patients should be encouraged to consume a diversity of fruits and vegetables and not just tomato products, lycopene, or pomegranate juice!
- Patients should be encouraged to incorporate moderate amounts of traditional dietary soy and other "plant estrogen" products (flaxseed for example) into their diet because they also contain much more than just phytoestrogens. This is another method of replacing unhealthy high caloric foods with healthy low-calorie foods.
- Encourage patients to incorporate moderate weekly intakes of a variety of canned, broiled, baked, and even raw/smoked fish in their diet while avoiding fried fish. Other healthy sources of omega-3 fatty acids—a variety of nuts and plant-based cooking oils—should also be encouraged because many of these

also contain other healthy compounds such as vitamin D and selenium.

- It is the sum of what patients can do in *moderation* that has the highest probability of impacting health compared to just one or several lifestyle changes in extreme.

◼

S implistic and practical observations from numerous research studies need mentioning to place lifestyle recommendations in their appropriate perspective. Cardiovascular disease (CVD) is the number one cause of death in the United States and in other industrialized countries [1]. CVD is currently the primary cause of death worldwide. CVD, according to the World Health Organization (WHO), is the number one cause of death in every region of the world with the exception of sub-Saharan Africa, and it is predicted that this disease will become the number one cause of death in that specific region, replacing infectious diseases, within the next decade [2–5].

Media stories have been recently replete with reports that cancer has now surpassed coronary heart disease (CHD) as the leading cause of death in Americans [6]. This was an intriguing new discovery, but it was not entirely accurate. For example, in 2002, the latest year for which complete mortality data were available, cancer was responsible for 478,082 deaths and CHD was responsible for 446,727 deaths in individuals younger than 85 years. Thus, cancer was reported as the number one killer for Americans younger than 85 years. If this age consideration was not included, then CHD is still the number one killer of Americans. In 2002, 696,947 individuals in the United States died of CHD versus 557,271 deaths from cancer. CHD is the number one cause of mortality in those aged 85 and above. In this older age-group, CHD was responsible for three times more deaths (greater than 250,000) compared to cancer (approximately 80,000 deaths) in 2002.

If one actually compares CVD (heart disease and diseases of the blood vessels, including strokes and vascular diseases) to cancer, an entirely different situation is revealed. CVD is responsible for 38% of all deaths and for more deaths than the next five leading causes of death combined. Why some information sources utilized comparisons of one disease entity (CHD) to an entire spectrum of organ-specific diseases (cancer) seems more promotional than educational. Why not compare the entire spectrum of CVD to that of cancer, which is more of an apples-to-apples approach? When this is done, again the burden of CVD is more accurately portrayed. The bottom line is that CVD is and has been the number one cause of death in the United States every single year since 1900, with the exception of 1918, which was the year of the great influenza pandemic [1].

The good news for patients is that death rates from all cancers combined have been slowly declining over the past decade (1.5% per year since 1993 for men and 0.8% per year for women since 1992). However, the death rate from CHD has been falling for a greater period of time, since the mid-1970s. Therefore, even in 1999, cancer deaths outnumbered CHD deaths in individuals younger than age 85. Even in individuals over the age of 85, CHD deaths have declined compared to cancer. The major improvements in mortality rates for both prevalent diseases apparently were partially due to a decrease in smoking rates in the United States. For example, in men, the death rate has also continued to fall for the three most commonly diagnosed cancers (colorectal, lung, and prostate). Still, it is of enormous interest to health-care professionals and patients that one of the most dramatic reductions in mortality rates in US history for CVD and cancer was through a common behavioral change (smoking cessation) that had such a profound simultaneous impact on the rates of both diseases.

Several of the largest US cancer prevention trials and cancer screening studies exemplify the need for a more proper perspective. For example, results of the Prostate Cancer Prevention Trial (PCPT) seem to have generated a lot of interest and controversy regarding the use of finasteride (Proscar, Merck, Whitehouse Station, NJ) daily versus placebo to reduce the risk of prostate cancer [7–9]. Finasteride was responsible for a significant 25% reduction in the number of prostate cancer cases during 7 years of study, but an apparent higher risk of aggressive prostate cancer was also found in the finasteride arm of the trial. The debate over the advantages and disadvantages of finasteride will continue, but several important observations from this trial have not received adequate attention in the medical literature. Over 18,000 men were included in this randomized trial. Five men died from prostate cancer in the finasteride arm and 5 men died of prostate cancer in the placebo arm, but 1123 men died during this trial. Thus, prostate cancer was responsible for less than 1% of the deaths, while the majority of the overall deaths were apparently due to CVD and other causes. Therefore, the results of the first large-scale prostate cancer prevention trial demonstrated that another disease is indeed the primary cause of death in men. This finding does not reduce the seriousness or impact of prostate cancer prevention utilizing a prostate-specific chemoprevention agent, but again it places the overall risk of mortality in its proper perspective. Men inquiring about the benefits and detriments of finasteride for prostate cancer prevention need to be reminded that the number one risk to them in general is CVD; the potential prostate cancer risk-specific consultation should occur after the first more relevant point is discussed and emphasized.

The well-known selenium supplementation randomized trial that noted a significant reduction in the number of prostate cancer cases with the use of 200 μg of yeast-based selenium daily versus placebo seems to have generated attention in utilizing selenium supplements to reduce the risk of prostate cancer. However, despite men in this trial having a higher mean risk of cancer, the number one cause of death in this randomized trial was still CVD [10]. Selenium supplementation did not significantly reduce the impact of CVD.

Past and recent observations from a variety of studies have also found that the primary or secondary cause of death in patients with prostate cancer seems to be CVD [11,12], which continues to emphasize that clinicians and patients need to give more attention to the impact of CVD on overall mortality. Heart disease seems to be the primary cause of death within 10 years after localized treatment for prostate cancer. Also, a study of the macrophage scavenging receptor gene 1 (*MSR1*) demonstrated that a mutation in this gene not only increases the risk of atherosclerosis, but it also appears to increase the risk of prostate cancer [13]. Thus, some of the potential pathophysiologic mechanisms involved in increasing a person's risk for heart disease may also increase his risk for prostate cancer [14,15], and other chronic disease risks may also be increased with an abnormal cardiovascular risk [16,17] or lipid mutation [18]. If the clinician were to highlight lifestyle changes that may impact one or, ideally, both conditions (CVD and cancer) favorably, this would seem to be the wisest, most practical, and realistic approach for the individual before being diagnosed with prostate cancer and after being diagnosed or treated for this or any other urologic condition [19].

It is important to reiterate that these findings are not mentioned to belittle the seriousness of prostate cancer, but it places the average risk of mortality for a person in its proper perspective. Dietary or lifestyle changes to reduce the risk of CVD just make sense when examining the larger overall mortality picture. A so-called "forest over the tree" approach seems most appropriate when discussing options with men. Clinicians should not solely emphasize a prostate cancer-specific diet or prostate-specific lifestyle change only because this would ignore the previous important but seemingly unstressed findings from the past studies of prostate cancer. Heart health seems tantamount to prostate health, and this should be constantly and consistently reiterated and emphasized to the individual concerned about prostate cancer.

Probability-based education is needed for patients, which means knowing their lipid profiles, blood pressure values, and other cardiovascular markers as well as prostate-specific antigen (PSA) values is paramount to providing excellent comprehensive care. Stories about patients bringing in hundreds of pages of Internet material, and even graphs that specifically followed their PSA values over numerous years abound. Currently, this is such a common practice in my opinion that clinicians are almost expecting this type of patient on a regular basis after a diagnosis of prostate cancer. What has been interesting is not that such patients are so common today but rather the lack of general health knowledge despite an impressive and obsessive need-to-know position concerning prostate health. Most men seem to be well aware of their past PSA values, but have either never had a cholesterol test, or are unaware of their latest values or how to correctly construe these values. This finding seems initially frustrating, because again the first and second cause of death in these patients is CVD [1,7,10,11].

> Our institution along with the National Prostate Cancer Coalition (NPCC) conducted two large PSA screenings of African American men in 2004 in two large metropolitan areas [34]. Previously, these screenings only offered PSA testing. However, we also offered cholesterol and other types of screenings in these settings and we were surprised to find that although PSA abnormalities were observed in less than 10% of these men, the rate of dyslipidemia was over 50% at both sites! Again, this drives home the thought that more comprehensive screening and education seems to be a better approach for individuals concerned about prostate or urologic disease.

Fitness First!

Fitness and overall health should be emphasized first, and not weight loss, by encouraging patients to get approximately 30 minutes of physical activity a day on average or more depending on individual need, and to lift weights or perform resistance exercises several times/week. Aerobic and resistance exercise should be emphasized equally; one is not more important than the other. An extensive review of the epidemiologic evidence pointed toward a "probable" reduction in risk of prostate cancer with regular physical activity and a potential impact on the progression of disease [59]. More recently, higher levels of physical activity defined as at least 3 hours of vigorous exercise weekly were associated with an approximate 70% lower risk of an aggressive prostate cancer, advanced disease, and a potential for improved survival in the Health Professionals Follow-up Study [60]. Over 47,000 men were included in this study with a mean follow-up period of 14 years. The largest correlation was found for men aged 65 years or older; minimal to no association was found for younger men. Researchers theorized that since many of the fatal prostate cancers in younger men probably have a strong genetic component, it would be difficult to impact with physical activity. However, a large number of sporadic cancers may occur in older men so the influence of hormonal factors may have a stronger role in these men. Reducing levels of insulin-like growth factor 1 (IGF-1), leptin, insulin, and testosterone could occur with vigorous activity, and this may be one of the many reasons elderly men tend to garner a greater benefit. The investigators from this study appropriately concluded their publication by recommending 30 minutes a day of physical activity to all individuals because of the overall health benefits of this intervention.

Results of the first randomized study of resistance exercise or weight lifting for men receiving androgen deprivation therapy (ADT) or luteinizing hormone–releasing hormone (LHRH) therapy for prostate cancer were compelling [66]. The trial was 12 weeks in duration. One hundred and fifty-five men were randomized to either lift weights three times a week or they were assigned to a non-lifting group. No change in body composition occurred during this short study as expected, but a significant reduction in fatigue and improved quality of life occurred in the weight-lifting group. This trial should be the impetus to begin emphasizing this standard lifestyle change for men with prostate cancer, especially those receiving ADT. Men with bone metastasis should be told to consult with their primary physicians to receive the approval of a resistance program because of the theoretical possibility of an increased risk for fracture with bone lesions.

Physical activity may reduce the risk of other urologic conditions such as benign prostatic hyperplasia (BPH) [67] and erectile dysfunction [68]. A unique and recent 2-year randomized trial from Italy of vigorous exercise to improve erectile dysfunction also needs to receive more clinical attention [69]. One-third of the obese men reporting erectile dysfunction regained normal function in this trial, but the majority of men experienced at least some improvement in function and a simultaneous reduction in the risk of common CVD markers [68]. Also, the potential to impact the risk of several major cancers, such as colorectal carcinoma, should make exercise a lifelong priority for most men [70].

The Impact of Excess Body Weight

The adverse impact of being overweight or obese on overall health and longevity is well known. Less known is the impact of weight on prostate cancer risk, but it seems that its impact may be just as detrimental [35]. Body mass index (BMI) is a moderately reliable and rapid method to determine who may be overweight or obese [36]. BMI is defined as the weight (in kilograms) divided by the square of the height in meters (kilograms per square meter). Another method to calculate the BMI is to take weight in pounds and divide it by the height in inches squared and to multiply this number by 704 (pounds/ inches^2 × 704). A BMI<25 is considered normal by the Word Health Organization (WHO), whereas 25 to 29 is overweight, >30 is defined as obese, and 35 or more is considered morbidly obese. Several large recent random- ized trials have demonstrated that most individuals in these studies are indeed overweight at baseline [37], and this includes dietary trials to prevent prostate cancer or reduce PSA [38]. In other words, it has become so common to be overweight or obese that only a minority of the participants in clinical trials had a BMI in the healthy range.

The body mass index (BMI) should not be routinely used anymore; instead, the waist-to-hip ratio (WHR) or especially waist circumference (WC) mea- surement should become a regular part of patient clinical record. WHR may be another simple measurement to determine obesity [36]. Individuals must stand during the entire measurement of WHR. WHR more precisely measures abdominal adipose circumference or tissue and fat distribution. The waist is defined as the abdominal circumference midway between the costal margin and the iliac crest. The hip is defined as the largest circumference just below the iliac crest. For men, a WHR >0.90, is a fairly accurate indicator of an increased risk for obesity-related conditions independent of BMI. Regardless, serial measurements on a specific prostate cancer patient are more valuable than comparing his value to a national standard. In other words, patients should attempt to lower their values and compete with themselves and not with some ideal standardized measurement.

Waist circumference (WC) is perhaps the simplest and fastest method to currently access obesity, and is my current personal preference in men because "belly fat" seems to have the best predictive value of CVD risk among all the other measurements. WC is actually rapidly gaining acceptance as one of the best predictors of a future cardiovascular event, regardless of the ethnic group studied [39]. Recent evidence also suggests that it may be a better pre- dictor of early mortality from prostate cancer compared to other methods of weight measurement [40]. Regardless, WC has been one of the criteria to access metabolic syndrome. WC of 35 inches or more has been suggested as "overweight" and 40 or more is considered obese. Interestingly, a WC of 40 or more is also one of the five specific criteria of metabolic syndrome. WC has an important advantage over BMI, which can be appreciated after a patient com- mits to resistance exercise or weight training. An increase in muscle mass from resistance exercise can actually cause an increase in BMI, which is frustrating to the patient and clinician. However, this does not occur when utilizing the WHR or WC measurement.

Dual energy X-ray absorptometry (DEXA) has become the gold standard of measuring bone mineral density and determining the future risk of fracture in women and men [41]. However, in the future, this or another safe low-radiation imaging device may be one of the most accurate predictors of overall body and belly fat. This is due to the fact that there are two types of belly fat, the subcutaneous form, which can be removed by liposuction but has no impact on lipid parameters, and the deep visceral fat that surrounds organ systems and has a significant impact on health measurements. So, ideally a cheap and safe device that can accurately discriminate between the two belly fat types should be a future clinical tool utilized in urology. In the meantime, WC and WHR work well, and a summary of the meaning of the BMI and WC values are listed in Table 21.1 [36,39].

Clinicians need to keep in mind once again that ultimately the meaning of these numbers compared to the rest of the population is not what is important because the individual should only be competing with himself. In other words, a patient with a BMI of 35 and a WC of 40 inches is not what I personally find concerning, but a lack of fitness and not being able to lower this value over time is more of an issue.

Table 21.1. A Summary of the Body Mass Index (BMI) and Waist Circumference (WC) Values and Their Meaning for Patient Discussions.

BMI Number	What Does This Mean to the Patient?
Less than 25	Normal weight
25–29	Overweight
30 or more	Obese
WC Number	What Does This Mean to the Patient?
Less than 35 inches (or 89 centimeters) in men	Normal
35 to 39 inches (or 89 to 100 centimeters) in men	Overweight
40 or more inches (101 or more centimeters) in men	Obese
Less than 32.5 inches (or 83 centimeters) in women	Normal
32.5 to 36 inches (or 83 to 93 centimeters) in women	Overweight
37 or more inches (94 or more centimeters) in women	Obese

Investigations of weight and prostate cancer are preliminary and far from conclusive [42], but some of the largest studies to date suggest a potentially serious negative impact, especially if men are obese over a long period. A large-scale cohort study by Andersson et al. followed 135,000 Swedish construction workers [43]. It included one of the largest numbers of prostate cancer cases (2368), prostate cancer deaths (708), and one of the longest follow-up periods to date (18 years). All of the anthropometric measurements were correlated with the risk of prostate cancer, but there was a stronger relation to mortality rather than incidence. The risk of mortality from prostate cancer demonstrated statistical significance in all of the BMI subsets above the reference. This investigation represented a young cohort because >50% of these men were younger than 40 years at entry into this investigation.

The Netherlands Cohort Study was one of the largest prospective studies to evaluate diet and lifestyle and the risk of prostate cancer [44]. No associations between larger intakes of overall dietary fat and prostate cancer incidence were found [45]. A total of 58,279 men aged 55 to 69 were enrolled and a total of 681 new cases of prostate cancer were diagnosed during 6.3 years of follow-up. However, there was a moderate correlation observed for BMI and prostate cancer (RR = 1.33) if a person was obese at a younger age, which was stronger for localized cancers than for advanced cancer.

One of the few large-scale randomized trials to report on obesity and prostate cancer risk was a study whose primary endpoint was lung cancer incidence after taking low-dose vitamin E, β-carotene, both, or neither [46,47]. Prostate cancer incidence and mortality was a secondary endpoint of the trial. This study was known as the "Alpha-Tocopherol Beta-Carotene" Trial (ATBC), and it documented 579 cases of prostate cancer with an 11-year follow-up. No correlation between prostate cancer risk and BMI was noted in the moderate to overweight BMI ranges [46]. Researchers discovered later that men in the highest weight and BMI category had a 40% increased risk of developing prostate cancer compared to men with a normal BMI [47]. This was an interesting later discovery of the trial, because it was this same study that found that men consuming 50 mg of vitamin E daily as a supplement had a 32% reduction in prostate cancer risk [46]. The vitamin E results seemed to garner the most publicity in most major media outlets. Yet, another way of interpreting the results of this study was that the potential negative impact of being obese was greater than the positive impact of taking a vitamin E supplement, though few if any media sources seemed to extract this finding from the trial. Men were not only obese but smoked a mean of 20 cigarettes daily over several decades. The negative synergism of being obese and having a chronic heavy smoking history, or having other significant unhealthy habits, may lead to a greater risk and progression of prostate cancer. Clinicians need to explain to men that two of the largest dietary and supplement studies to analyze the risk of prostate cancer essentially both arrived at the same conclusion that obesity can negatively impact prostate cancer risk or progression. This seems to provide a convincing argument that men need to maintain a healthy weight before or after a prostate cancer diagnosis, which obviously is similar to the recommendation before or after a diagnosis of CVD.

One of the largest prospective epidemiologic investigations to evaluate the impact of obesity on cancer mortality involved more than 900,000 U.S. adults (404,576 men) who did not have cancer in 1982 at baseline and were then followed up for 16 years [48]. Higher cancer mortality rates were correlated with increasing BMIs and this included prostate cancer mortality. A significant ($P < 0.001$) increased risk of prostate cancer mortality was associated with an increasing BMI from 25 to 29.9 (RR = 1.08), 30 to 34.9 (RR = 1.20), and 35 to 39.9 (RR = 1.34) for the 4004 documented deaths from prostate carcinoma.

Postdiagnosis studies of the effect of excess body weight are also concerning because two large retrospective pooled multi-institutional analyses arrived at nearly identical conclusions after evaluating patients following radical prostatectomy [49,50]. The first study of 3162 patients found that a higher BMI was a significant independent predictor of a higher Gleason score and a higher BMI was significantly associated with a higher risk of biochemical recurrence [49]. The second study compared 1106 men treated with radical prostatectomy from 1998 to 2002. A BMI >35 was correlated with a significant risk of biochemical recurrence after treatment even when controlling for surgical margin status [50]. Obesity was associated with higher-grade prostate cancers, a trend toward an increased risk of positive surgical margins and higher biochemical failure rates.

The Health Professionals Follow-Up Study (HPFS) is one of the largest and most comprehensive ongoing prospective epidemiologic studies. HPFS has published incidence but not mortality data from prostate cancer and found a significantly lower risk of prostate cancer in men with higher BMIs if they were younger (<60 years old) or had a family history of this disease [51]. However, men with more sporadic cancers seemed to have a higher risk of prostate cancer with an increasing BMI. This finding led researchers of this study to hypothesize that since obesity is associated with lower testosterone levels and higher estrogen levels or partial androgen suppression, this could theoretically have resulted in a reduced risk of prostate cancer in the early-onset or hereditary prostate cancers in these men compared to the more sporadic cancers. Obese men could theoretically harbor prostate tumors but have lower PSA levels by a dilution effect, which could lead to the clinician falsely considering these men to be cancer free, and this may explain why some have been identified to have more advanced disease at the time of diagnosis and treatment

[49,50]. Clinicians may soon have to lower PSA biopsy threshold values for obese individuals.

The proper perspective should be constantly emphasized to patients even if these recent alternative findings are accurate. Prostate cancer recurrence and mortality, and especially early mortality, have been highly correlated with an increasing BMI. Whether obesity impacts prostate cancer incidence should not be the primary focus for any person because this observation simply fails to see the forest over the single tree when discussing the overall effect of obesity on the general health status of an individual [35]. For example, two of the largest prospective epidemiologic studies examining the issue of BMI and overall mortality had similar findings [52,53]. Both studies utilized data from the American Cancer Society (ACS). The first investigation was the ACS Cancer Prevention Study I [52]. Over 62,000 men with no smoking history, no history of heart disease, stroke, or cancer (other than skin carcinoma) and no history of recent involuntary weight loss at baseline were included. Overall mortality was measured over a 12-year period. The second study was the Cancer Prevention Study II [53]. This was a study of 457,000 men observed for 14 years. Both studies documented that men with a BMI of approximately 25 to 30 had an increased mortality of 10% to 25% [52,53]. Individuals with a BMI of 30 or more had a 50% to 100% increased mortality compared with those with a BMI less than 25. The second study not only included more men but also looked at general cancer mortality [53]. The men within the highest BMI category (>35) had a 40% to 80% increased risk of mortality from cancer, and no evidence of any increased risk was found among the leanest individuals (BMI<20). Past studies completed in the United States indicate that only a minority of adults (less than 8%) have a BMI<20, and >50% of men in the United States have a BMI >25 [54].

Clinicians need to let their patients know that maintaining a healthy weight should be one of the primary goals. For example, placing a BMI chart in the clinic office and always making BMI or WHR or WC a part of the individual clinical record should be a goal for every patient regardless of his specific disease risk because early mortality from all causes is associated with increasing BMI. Clinicians should also refer patients on a regular basis to nutritionists, therapists, and a variety of professional weight loss programs, and to become familiar with local weight loss resources. Clinicians should be able to provide the name and number of these individuals and organizations to the patient at the time of the appointment to improve compliance, convey enthusiasm, and the immediacy or importance of this lifestyle change. Also, clinicians need to begin to carry and utilize tape measures that can rapidly assess WC, and I often argue that this is as important as a stethoscope to the individual working in the field of urologic disease.

There is no ideal weight loss diet or intervention for patients. Choose a diet, lifestyle change, or other interventions that are tailored to the specific personality of the patient. Low-fat, low-carbohydrate, high-protein diet, drug therapy, surgery, and so on—the list of potential methods to impact weight continues to abound, confuse, motivate, and frustrate patients [36]. The diversity of approaches needs to be embraced and not discouraged. Some dietary interventions involving men with prostate cancer, such as reducing total dietary fat have been beneficial in terms of a PSA response [75], while other longer randomized trials have not demonstrated a benefit for men without prostate cancer [38]. Low-carbohydrate diets have provided some sustained weight loss in recent randomized trials, but compliance rates only approach 50% in the first year and more PSA and prostate cancer risk data are needed [76,77]. Higher insulin or glucose levels from a variety of etiologies such as diet and obesity have been preliminarily associated with a higher prostate cancer risk, mortality, as well as overall mortality [78–81].

One of the better designed and implemented randomized trials comparing the effects of a variety of fad diets on weight loss and cardiovascular risk should provide the impetus for any clinician dealing with patients attempting to reduce weight with a more practical perspective on weight loss itself. A total of 160 overweight individuals (mean BMI = 35) were randomized to one of the following diets for 1 year: low-carbohydrate (Atkins), low-fat (Ornish), low–glycemic load (Zone), or a calorie-restricted and support-group enhanced (Weight Watchers) dietary program [82]. All of the diets were associated with weight loss and a reduced risk of coronary heart disease from Framingham risk scores in participants that were able to adhere to their respective allocated dietary regimens. However, the drop-out rates were 48% with the Atkins diet, 50% with the Ornish diet, 35% for the Zone diet, and 35% for Weight Watchers. Compliance is difficult, but for those who can adhere to these diets, the benefits may outweigh the risks when considering the impact of obesity on all-cause mortality. All of these so-called "fad" diets carry consistent themes such as reducing overall caloric intake, increasing physical activity levels, and becoming more adept at reading basic nutrition labels. The consistent simple mantra of overall caloric restriction combined with increasing physical activity should be emphasized.

Food and beverage sizes have increased in recent years with obesity rates, and greater portion sizes and fast food availability appear to at least encourage greater caloric or energy intake [83,84]. Preliminary research suggests an increased risk of prostate cancer in men with higher caloric intakes over time regardless of whether these calories are mostly derived from fat, protein, or carbohydrate [85]. Simple caloric control may be one method of effective weight loss, and the research derived from the centenarians and schoolchildren on the island of Okinawa (Japan) have been a model for the benefits of caloric restriction and its potential impact on all-cause mortality [86]. Restricting total fat intake cannot be the only viable, realistic, or even practical approach and the effectiveness of this method over just caloric restriction has been questioned recently in a meta-analysis [87], especially since greater caloric concentrations can now be found in a variety of carbohydrate sources, for example [88].

> Diet should indeed fit the personality of the patient. Patients who like to learn about dietary change in solitude have many options such as the South Beach Diet, but for those patients that tend to do better with social support, a program such as Weight Watchers may be more ideal. The common clinician goal should not be to extinguish enthusiasm, but rather to foster it. A patient inquiring and enthusiastic about weight loss and at least willing to engage in a fad diet is at least a "glass is half-full" situation for the clinician dealing with this individual.

One of the most extensive animal studies to date examining the correlation between prostate cancer and fat and energy intakes may have revealed the best insight on energy restriction and cancer progression [89]. Researchers utilized transplanted androgen-sensitive prostate tumors from donor rats, transplanted them to other rats, and fed them either fat-restricted or carbohydrate-restricted diets. Severe combined immunodeficient mice (SCID) were injected with LNCaP human prostate cancer cells to promote tumor growth and then ingested similar diets. Researchers restricted energy intakes by reducing energy from fat or carbohydrate, or simply reducing total energy from all sources, while at all times keeping other nutrients constant. Tumor growth was observed to be independent of the percentage of fat in the diet, as long as the total energy was restricted. The reduction in cancer growth was identical in all types of energy-restricted laboratory animals. The findings suggest that a reduction in overall caloric intake, and not just fat, reduced the risk or progression of prostate cancer [89,90].

Reducing unhealthy dietary fat intake such as saturated, trans-fatty acids, and even dietary cholesterol should be encouraged and replaced by more healthy types of monounsaturated or polyunsaturated fat (omega-3 fatty acids). Post-treatment lifestyle changes or dietary fat intake and the impact on the progression of prostate cancer have been well reviewed elsewhere and again the data support heart-healthy changes which seem to be tantamount to urologic health [96]. A Canadian prospective study of men with prostate cancer observed a total of 384 men for a median of 5.2 years [97]. Compared with the men consuming the lowest levels of saturated fat, those consuming the highest amount had a significant increase in risk of mortality from prostate cancer (RR, 3.1). Total fat and other subtypes of fat (except saturated) did not show any correlation between prostate cancer and mortality.

Reducing all saturated fat in an individual's diet is not necessarily a practical or healthy dietary lifestyle change. The current cardiovascular goal of obtaining less than 7% of calories from saturated fat seems almost ideal from past studies because getting little to no calories from saturated fat not only seems too excessive but also actually reduces levels of HDL [99]. In fact, one of the most consistent drawbacks of a nonfat diet has been the dramatic reduction in HDL that occurs in these situations. In addition, reducing all saturated fat intakes implies that all types of these specific fats are unhealthy, which is simply not the case. Therefore, the old adage "everything in moderation" applies to this lifestyle recommendation.

The association of trans-fat with cancer is unknown because epidemiologic studies have not found an association [44,116], but interestingly some other recent studies have suggested that these fatty acids may encourage cancer growth [117–119] and increase the risk of prostate cancer. Thus, the simple rule of what is heart healthy/unhealthy is also prostate healthy/unhealthy may also be applicable to these specific types of fatty acids. The observation that trans-fat is heart unhealthy makes the recommendation to reduce the intake of these fatty acids a priority.

The simple past suggestion of just reducing overall dietary fat intake, instead of subtypes of fat has not been supported recently in the prostate cancer or CVD literature [38,122,123], especially in regard to mortality data [123]. Clinicians need to emphasize that the types of fat ingested seem to influence disease risk overall more than just dietary fat intake. In the worst case scenario, this tends to change the lipid profile favorably and reduce the risk of CVD, which is why this recommendation makes the most practical sense to any individual concerned about prostate cancer.

Cholesterol from dietary sources increase serum cholesterol, but not as significantly as saturated fat. A total of 100 mg of dietary cholesterol increases serum cholesterol by approximately 10 mg/dL per 1000 kcal [21]. Daily mean cholesterol intake is greater for men in the United States (331 mg) compared to women (213 mg). Foods high in cholesterol include eggs, animal and dairy products, poultry, and shellfish. Sterols or the marine equivalent of cholesterol in shellfish and shrimp do not greatly impact human serum cholesterol unless cooked in butter, fried, or consumed in high quantities [124,125]. Dietary cholesterol ingestion should be encouraged to be less than 200 mg/day to impact or lower LDL cholesterol [21]. The impact of dietary cholesterol on prostate cancer is unknown, but it is known that prostate cancer cells tend to utilize large amounts of cholesterol in their cellular membranes [126], and this is especially

Table 21.2. A Partial Review of the Types of Dietary Fat Available to Patients, the Sources of These Fats, and Their Impact on Lipid Levels.

Type of Dietary Fat	Where Is It Commonly Found?	Good or Bad Fat, and Impact on Cholesterol Versus Carbohydrates (Sugars)
Monounsaturated fat	Health cooking oils (canola, olive), nuts	Good Lowers LDL Increases LDL
Polyunsaturated fat (includes omega-3 fatty acids)	Healthy cooking oils (canola, safflower, soybean), flaxseed, fish, nuts, soybeans	Good Lowers LDL Increases HDL
Saturated fat (also known as hydrogenated fat)	Non-lean meat, high-fat dairy, some fast food	Mostly bad Increases LDL Increases HDL
Trans-fat (also known as partially hydrogenated fat)	Some margarines, fast food, snack foods, deep-fried foods	Bad Increases LDL Lowers HDL

notable with a greater extent or progression (metastases) of the disease itself [127]. Reducing dietary cholesterol just makes practical sense from a cardiovascular risk standpoint, but may impact other urologic type conditions. Recent evidence also demonstrates a potential significant benefit of changing prostate cancer progression and mortality rates with significant healthy lipid changes [128–130]. A review of healthy versus unhealthy fat intakes advice that can be given to patients is found in Table 21.2.

Not Just Lycopene

Patients should be encouraged to consume a diversity of fruits and vegetables and not just tomato products, lycopene, or pomegranate juice. Clinicians need to also forewarn patients that although some specific fruits and vegetables will receive more media attention than others for prostate cancer from time to time, they should remain calm and committed to consuming a diversity of fruits and vegetables. Dietary supplements that claim to substitute for fruit and vegetable consumption should not be recommended.

The compound known as "lycopene" seems to be synonymous with prostate health in a variety of media and commercial sources. Few topics in prostate cancer prevention have enjoyed as much attention as lycopene, tomato products, and their potential benefits. Numerous epidemiologic studies support the intake of tomatoes and tomato products, but numerous other investigations have not found a positive relationship. For example, a well-referenced analysis of over 80 epidemiologic studies on tomatoes and cancer risk was published several years ago [131]. Half of the studies analyzed support the consumption of tomato products at least once a day to reduce the risk of a variety of cancers including prostate cancer, but a large number of studies in this same analysis failed to detect a correlation. Another important finding was that no investigations to date have indicated that a greater consumption of tomato products significantly increases the risk of cancer, but the overall recommendation of the author of the meta-analysis was to increase the consumption of a diversity of fruits and vegetables and not just tomato products.

The ongoing research of tomatoes and lycopene continues to support a potential that is moderate at best for these products to impact prostate cancer risk or progression [132–134]. Lycopene, tomato powder, or a calorie-restricted diet were utilized in one of the larger animal studies, and the results seem to have some clinical applications [135]. Tomato powder consumption, but not lycopene, inhibited prostate carcinogenesis, which suggests that tomato products contain compounds in addition to lycopene that can potentially inhibit the growth of prostate cancers.

A recent dietary case–control study from China that observed one of the largest reductions in prostate cancer risk in the literature (odds ratio = 0.18) found that watermelon consumption may have been partially responsible, but the impact of pumpkin, spinach, tomatoes, and citrus intake was also notable even after adjusting for a variety of confounders such as fat and total caloric intake [137]. The preliminary and ongoing interest in lycopene and its sources may actually be the result of a potential reduced risk of CVD with a greater intake of this compound from dietary sources [138–141]. Again, CVD prevention seems to at least promote prostate health.

Fruits and vegetables, in general, have been associated with a reduced risk of prostate cancer [142]. For example, the Brassica vegetable group is diverse and includes broccoli, brussels sprouts, cabbage, cauliflower, kale, watercress, and many others that may reduce the risk of prostate cancer [143]. The Allium vegetables have also been associated with a reduced risk, and this group includes chives, garlic, leeks, onions, scallions, and so on [144]. Fruits and vegetables have combined unique and shared anticancer and antiheart disease compounds that may contribute to improved overall health [142]. The sum of the epidemiololgic data continues to support the increased consumption of a diversity of fruits and vegetables to potentially impact urologic disease, but the overall data currently supports a far greater potential reduction in CVD risk and mortality.

Interestingly, some of the largest prospective epidemiologic studies have not found a correlation between the increased consumption of fruits and vegetables and a reduced risk of most cancers or mortality from cancer [145–149], and this includes prostate and other urologic cancers. Clinicians need to encourage an objective and honest discussion with patients about this data and explain that currently at least a CVD risk reduction may occur, but the data is not nearly as profound in cancer or survival from cancer.

Shifting focus from one fruit or vegetable to another with each passing day and news story seems more likely than ever before. Clinicians need to explain to patients that this does not necessarily represent any major breakthrough but rather supports the ongoing and past research that consuming a diversity of fruits and vegetables is the most practical and logical approach currently and in the future. One of many potential recent examples of this controversy is the recent research concerning pomegranate juice. A small trial (n = 48) of men with a rising PSA after localized therapy for prostate cancer demonstrated that those consuming 8 ounces of pomegranate juice daily for 2 years experienced an increase in PSA doubling time [150], which preliminarily suggests that this juice may favorably impact prostate cancer. This was interesting, but it did not include a placebo group or another group of men who consumed another type of healthy juice product. It is also important to keep in mind that larger intakes of healthy juices can contain a significant amount of calories. Many brands of pomegranate juice contain at least 140 calories per 8 ounce serving, which translates into more calories than most commercial regular soft drinks (about 100 calories). Many of these juices are also very expensive and it is of concern that our low-income patients cannot afford them. Finally drug and juice interactions are still being researched, which is important since grapefruit juice studies has provided a paradigm of medication interactions [136].

The data on pomegranate juice is interesting and researchers should be commended for completing such a unique study and for suggesting that a phase III study is still needed [150], but again this preliminary trial seems to continue to emphasize that a variety of fruits and vegetables may offer a potential benefit to an individual concerned about urologic disease. Other recent studies on avocados [151] and cranberries [152] and prostate disease have also added to the ongoing long list of healthy foods that may benefit individuals with and without urologic conditions. Long-term data on lycopene dietary supplements are simply lacking, and these supplements can be expensive. A recent 1-year pilot trial of small to large (15–120 mg/day) intakes of lycopene pills for rising PSA following failed local conventional therapy in 36 men also did not demonstrate any initial PSA kinetic or clinical benefits [153]. Despite the dosage utilized during the study, all doses eventually demonstrated a similar serum saturation or threshold. This recent study is a disappointment because older preliminary studies utilizing the same form of lycopene supplement, at lower doses, and for a limited amount of time suggested a potential benefit [154,155]. It is difficult to remember when a dietary component or compound formulated as a pill was ever able to substitute for a fruit or vegetable in terms of prevention data, except for folic acid and the prevention of neural tube defects in pregnant women. Again, daily intake of lycopene from dietary sources at this time continues to remain the wisest, cheapest, and evidenced-based choice.

> Another personal clinical observation needs to provoke some thought when encouraging fruit and vegetable consumption. In my experience, when a patient begins to rely on a pill instead on a lifestyle change, the potential for seeking other nonlifestyle changes to be substituted for pills increases [136]. In other words, when a patient begins to exercise there is an increased potential to seek other healthy behavioral changes such as eating better or quitting smoking. However, this momentum effect also works in a negative direction, so the patient who takes fruit and vegetable compounded pills such as lycopene, will reduce overall fruit and vegetable consumption and look for other pills (cholesterol, blood pressure, weight loss) to substitute for healthy behavioral changes.

The consumption of more total dietary fiber (20–30 g/day) from food and even supplements for overall health advantages should be encouraged, especially viscous ("soluble") fiber, but insoluble fiber is also beneficial. The impact of dietary fiber on PSA levels has not been thoroughly evaluated, but a randomized trial of a combination of a low-fat and high-fiber diet over a 4-year period failed to demonstrate a reduction in PSA and prostate cancer risk in Caucasians and African American men [176,177]. A large case–control study published from Europe found a moderate reduced risk of prostate cancer with increased consumption of dietary fiber, especially soluble fiber, cellulose, and vegetable fiber [178]. One of the only clinical studies of soluble fiber compared to insoluble fiber only for PSA reduction was published several years ago [179]. This small investigation (n = 14) of short duration (4 months) included men with hyperlipidemia and without cancer. A small but statistically lower PSA level in men consuming soluble fiber compared to those consuming insoluble fiber (25–30 grams per 1000 kcal) was documented. However, the results could have been confounded by a lower caloric intake in the soluble fiber arm. Costly commercial products or dietary supplements that contain modified citrus pectin (MCP) are popular with some patients with prostate cancer because some laboratory studies [181,182], and a small (n = 13) and short clinical study have suggested that this compound may inhibit the growth of a variety of cancers and may increase PSA doubling time after recurrent prostate cancer [183].

The vast majority of the MCP is composed of fiber, especially soluble fiber. Increasing amounts of soluble, insoluble, and total fiber from food or cheaper supplements, for example, psyllium, seems to be more practical and less costly for patients than recommending MCP. Other cheaper food choices, such as flaxseed (see following text) have garnered a good deal of initial positive clinical research for prostate health, but it is important to keep in mind that flaxseed also contains an unusually high amount of healthy compounds including soluble fiber [136]. A variety of low-cost high-fiber bars with a low amount of total calories (less than 150–200 calories) are now commercially available and I have started to mention these products to patients who spend far too much money on protein bars with minimal to no fiber.

The Soy Story

Patients should be encouraged to incorporate moderate amounts of traditional cheap dietary soy and other so-called low-cost "plant estrogen" products (flaxseed, for example) into their diet because they also contain much more than just phytoestrogens. This is another simple method of replacing unhealthy high caloric foods with healthy low-calorie foods. Cardiovascular disease (CVD) reductions have been associated with a higher consumption of traditional soy products. International comparison studies have observed a reduced CVD rate in Asian countries along with a higher consumption of traditional soy products compared to Western countries [184]. This correlation is likely to be confounded by other dietary and lifestyle factors, such as a lower overall intake of saturated fat, more physical activity, and a variety of other healthy additions, but laboratory and clinical studies have been fairly consistent in supporting the cardiovascular benefits of soy [185–190]. Soy protein may promote LDL uptake and elimination and increase the activity of hydroxy-methylglutaryl-coenzyme A reductase and cholesterol 7-α-hydroxylase, which further reduces the concentration of cholesterol in bile acids. Soy may contain added benefits beyond its protein and phytoestrogen content, such as an adequate concentration of omega-fatty acids (healthy omega-6 and omega-3), fiber, natural vitamin E, and no trans-fat [191].

Meta-analysis of clinical studies suggests that two to three servings a day of soy protein (approximately 25 grams) or greater may be sufficient to significantly reduce cholesterol levels in men and women, especially in individuals with higher cholesterol levels [192,193]. The U.S. Food and Drug Administration (FDA) has supported this observation from clinical studies, but it is important to understand that the benefits of soy were enhanced when soy protein consumption was increased and saturated fat consumption was decreased because otherwise the beneficial effects may not be tangible. The FDA did not provide support for the plant estrogen content of soy and cardiovascular protection because the majority of the evidence demonstrated that the soy protein content was more closely related to cholesterol reduction.

A genistein precursor known as biochanin A and genistein itself have demonstrated an ability to inhibit the proliferation of both hormone-responsive and hormone-insensitive cancer cell lines [194,194], and both compounds have reduced PSA levels of LNCaP cells in vitro [195]. Genistein may inhibit the growth of prostate cancer through a variety of mechanisms such as interfering with tyrosine kinase growth factor and other similar growth factors and receptors [196–199]; affecting topoisomerase II [200]; inhibiting angiogenesis [201]; and encouraging apoptosis [202]. Significant consistent reductions in testosterone have not been observed in Japanese men consuming these products [203]. Perhaps partial suppression of a variety of hormones such as testosterone over several months, years, or even decades may be sufficient to delay the onset of clinically significant prostate cancer or a recurrence [204]. Additional potential benefits of genistein and other soy compounds may occur because of their estrogenic activity, the ability to inhibit 5- α-reductase and/or the aromatase enzyme, and overall antioxidant free radical scavenger properties [205]. Clinical trials utilizing soy, its various isolated compounds, such as genistein, at a variety of dosages are needed to determine if the in vitro and epidemiologic data correlate to an actual significant clinical response. Numerous clinical studies are currently being conducted with soy products [206,207]. Early results from some small pilot trials have observed some minor benefits for genistein pill supplementation in men with prostate cancer undergoing watchful waiting, but not as an adjunct to, or after, conventional treatment [208]. Another smaller randomized trial did not find a significant impact with soy isoflavones on PSA, but increasing dosages of soy protein was not studied [209].

A unique randomized trial of men after being diagnosed with prostate cancer undergoing a combination lifestyle change (vegan diet, physical activity, stress reduction) and supplement (vitamin E, vitamin C, selenium, and fish oil) regimen versus controls included one daily serving of tofu and 58 grams of a fortified soy protein powdered beverage in the intervention group. After 1 year of study the results have been encouraging in men with lower Gleason scores (6 or less; well-differentiated tumors) [210]. A small but significant PSA reduction in the intervention group compared to controls was noted, but a significant 30-point reduction in "bad cholesterol" or LDL also occurred. This trial also serves as a potential teaching point to encourage numerous moderate changes over any one or multiple changes in extreme. Men in this trial walked 30 minutes a day and consumed 10% or less of their total calories from fat. This may also be part of the explanation why men in the intervention group experienced a significant ($P <$0.001) 5-point average reduction in HDL despite favorable changes in LDL. This reiterates the importance of moderate to strenuous regular physical activity (not just walking in healthy patients) and healthy fat consumption, which can increase levels of HDL independently of each other.

The cardiovascular benefits of soy seem adequate to recommend these products to the majority of urologic patients. The cholesterol-lowering benefits of incorporating soy products in the diet seem reason enough to promote their consumption, along with saturated fat reduction [211]. Clinicians should recommend products that are high in soy protein or that represent one of the many traditional Asian soy products such as soybeans, tofu, tempeh, soy protein powder, soy oil, soy nuts, and soy milk that are low in saturated fats, low in sodium, and simply heart healthy [136,212,213]. Soy protein bars are popular, but most contain too many calories (200–300 calories) and little to no fiber; therefore, most of these products should be avoided. It is interesting again that some of the cheapest soy products have the most to offer in terms of nutritional value.

There is another simple concern with soy dietary supplement pills because they have not demonstrated a consistent ability to reduce hot flashes [214], which may be an indicator of poor potency, and/or they do not contain the numerous other beneficial compounds available in the traditional dietary sources of soy [136]. In my opinion, patients often try one traditional soy product and are frustrated by the lack of an appealing taste, and they begin to associate most soy products with this one experience. Patients need to be instructed that soy products are a diverse group with a diverse potential for taste, so if one is not appealing another product should be tried. For example, just because one is not excited about the taste of tofu, this should not in any way discourage the use of soy beans or soy protein powder in a drink, or soybean oil, which in my experience patients seem to enjoy. For example, when tofu is cooked in something with flavor such as a soup or sauce the tofu itself absorbs the flavor of its milieu, making it surprisingly palatable, and this is similar to how tofu is utilized in traditional Asian cooking methods. Still, clinical research and recommendations should not be limited to soy because of the potential benefit of numerous other cheap sources of phytoestrogens and other compounds in the food supply.

Lignans, another type of plant estrogen, are found in unusually high concentrations in flaxseed, and these compounds and others in flaxseed (ALA) have demonstrated anticancer properties in laboratory studies utilizing breast and prostate cancer cell lines [226,227]. Interestingly, one of the largest published cohort studies to examine the correlation between fat intake and prostate cancer risk was the Netherlands Cohort Study [228]. Approximately 58,000 men were followed up for more than 6 years. Six hundred forty-two cases of prostate cancer were verified, and an extensive 150-item food frequency questionnaire was utilized. No correlations were found between total fat and other subtypes of fat and prostate cancer risk. However, an association between a reduced risk of prostate cancer and an increased intake of ALA was found. This was of interest because several past smaller prospective investigations observed the opposite trend with this fatty acid [229,230], which has helped fuel some past and current spurious speculation among clinicians and patients that flaxseed may encourage prostate tumor growth.

What about actual direct studies utilizing flaxseed in human? The first preliminary trial of flaxseed in men with prostate cancer was published several years ago. This pilot study of men consuming flaxseed and a low-fat diet 4 weeks before radical prostatectomy demonstrated that flaxseed (about 3 grounded tablespoons/day) may have provided a clinical benefit via hormone suppression, lipid reductions, and via other mechanisms, such as reducing the proliferation index of cancer cells in the prostate and enhancing apoptosis for men, especially with lower Gleason scores (6 or less) before and after this conventional treatment versus historic controls [231]. Interestingly, the average reduction in total cholesterol over the 4-week study was 27 points. A recent and similar study was performed by some of the same researchers. Men at higher risk for prostate cancer (negative biopsy patients) also observed an apparent risk reduction and cholesterol decreases with just a 6-month course of daily flaxseed powder and a low-fat dietary regimen [232]. Flaxseed and other dietary changes may be beneficial before or after a diagnosis of prostate cancer. Regardless, if flaxseed is proven not to impact prostate health, at least adding it to the diet is cost-effective and is a part of an overall heart healthy profile.

Clinicians need to reiterate to patients that grounded cheap flaxseed itself has received the most research, while flaxseed oil and pills have received little research in humans [136]. Flaxseed needs to be ingested several hours before or after taking a prescription drug(s) or dietary supplement(s) because the high concentration of fiber could theoretically reduce the absorption of these agents, as is the potential case with any product or supplement high in soluble, insoluble, and just total fiber. Moderate intake of flaxseed (1–3 tablespoons/day) should be accompanied by adequate water consumption because of the potential for impaction and/or laxative effects. The potential for CVD risk reduction should be primarily emphasized to reflect not only evidence-based medicine but also a forest-over-the-tree approach to promoting health.

Omega-3 Fatty Acids

Patients should be encouraged to incorporate moderate (approximately two servings weekly) intake of a variety of canned, broiled, baked, and even raw/

smoked fish in their diet, while avoiding fried fish. Other healthy sources of omega-3 fatty acids—a variety of nuts and plant-based cooking oils—should also be encouraged because many of these also contain a variety of other healthy compounds such as vitamin D and selenium. Ground flaxseed and soy are good sources of omega-3 fatty acids, but numerous types of oily fatty fish also contain high concentrations of omega-3 fatty acids (EPA & DHA) and they are also the best natural food source of vitamin D_3 (cholecalciferol). They also contain high concentrations of protein and minerals such as selenium [136]. Omega-3 fatty acids have demonstrated numerous benefits in terms of reducing the risk of a variety of prevalent chronic diseases [233], especially CVD [234,235]. Potential positive mechanisms of action for fish and fish oil include a reduction in triglycerides [236], blood pressure [237], platelet aggregation [238], and arrhythmias [239]. However, their primary benefit has been their potential to reduce the risk of sudden cardiac death (SCD) [240–242].

Inhibition of prostate cancer proliferation rates has been demonstrated by fish oil from laboratory investigations [243]. Several epidemiologic and pilot studies also advocate moderate consumption of fish or fish oils to reduce the incidence and progression of prostate cancer [244,245], and the ability to reduce cyclooxygenase II (COX-2) may be one of the many apparent benefits [245].

Epidemiologic reviews of fish and marine fatty acids have concluded that no consistent reduction in prostate cancer risk has been observed in past studies [246], but the results of a large recent prospective study published after this analysis may cause a reconsideration of this conclusion. The Health Professionals Follow-up Study (HPFS) included over 47,000 men with 12-years of follow-up [247]. A total of 2,482 cases of prostate cancer were diagnosed. Six hundred seventeen of these cases were diagnosed as advanced prostate cancer including 278 metastatic prostate cancers. Consuming fish more than three times a week compared to less than twice a month was associated with a reduced risk of prostate cancer, and the strongest relationship was for metastatic disease (44% reduction). Research from this cohort has also found a potential reduced risk of prostate cancer recurrence after conventional treatment with increased fish consumption. In this prospective study fish intake consisted of canned tuna, dark meat fish (mackerel, salmon, sardines, bluefish, and sword-fish), and other unspecified fish dishes. Seafood consumption such as shrimp, lobster, and scallops were not associated with prostate cancer.

Mercury concentrations in specific fish have been reported by the FDA and in the overall medical literature, but the preliminary data is controversial and it is not known at this time what kind of clinical impact these mercury levels may have on the individual [251,252]. Four types of larger predatory fish have been most concerning because these fish (king mackerel, shark, swordfish, and tilefish) have the ability to retain greater larger amounts of methylmercury.

Even daily canned tuna consumption has been discouraged recently in pregnant women. However, moderate consumption (two to three times/week) of most fish should have minimal impact on overall human serum mercury levels, but more ongoing research in this area should soon provide better clarity. A recent large investigation of moderate serum mercury levels in older individuals found little to no negative long-term impacts on neurobehavioral parameters [253]. All of this preliminary data will not provide enough comfort to patients concerned about mercury in seafood. Regardless, the positive impact of consuming fish seems to outweigh the negative impact in the majority of individuals with the exception of women considering pregnancy or who are pregnant.

Tree nuts share some positive clinical effects similar to omega-3 oils found in fish. A consistent reduction in the risk of CHD and/or sudden cardiac death has been associated with an increased consumption of a variety of nuts in prospective studies [254–259]. Nuts contain a variety of potential beneficial compounds such as ALA (an omega-3 fatty acid), other polyunsaturated fats, monounsaturated fats, vitamin E, magnesium, potassium, fiber, flavonoids, and selenium [254]. The largest source of dietary selenium, for example, is actually found in Brazil nuts where one serving can provide the recommended daily allowance of this mineral [252]. Some of these compounds from a variety of dietary sources, but not necessarily dietary supplement sources, have been associated with a lower risk of prostate cancer—for example, vitamin E [260], ALA [232], selenium [252]—but more research is needed. Nuts are also high in healthy fats and fiber and low in unhealthy fats, which helps improve satiation and provide overall nutritional heart-healthy value for patients. However, the limitation of tree nuts is their high caloric content when consuming more than several servings a day.

Healthy plant cooking oils such as soybean, canola, olive, and safflower also contain high concentrations of omega-3 fatty acids, monounsaturated fat, and numerous other vitamins and minerals such as natural vitamin E [251,261].

Heart Healthy is Prostate Healthy!

Lifestyle modifications such as smoking cessation to reduce all-cause mortality including cancer [264,265] and potentially to reduce the risk of prostate cancer [266] or the risk of advanced or aggressive prostate cancer [267,268] should be discussed by clinicians. Moderate alcohol consumption seems to reduce cardiovascular events [269], and its impact at this level of consumption has not been beneficial or detrimental in regards to prostate cancer risk [136].

In my experience, minimal clinic time is needed to suggest changes that can impact all-cause mortality. These recommendations may seem simplistic, but past general studies of men have demonstrated that few (less than 5%) report adhering to numerous moderate healthy behaviors at one time [270]. Following one healthy change in excess, rather than multiple changes in moderation seems to be the current practice. This may be the result of past studies focusing on one lifestyle change to produce an overall impact on disease risk, poor compliance overall, or just a lack of attention, time, or understanding to this detail, or a lack of motivation on the part of the health professional and the patient. There are multiple potential reasons for minimal behavioral compliance, but the studies of combined moderate lifestyle changes continue to demonstrate that it is more the sum of what you do, rather than one or two specific behavioral changes that can impact cardiovascular markers, cancer, and all-cause mortality [271].

Recommending a pill is simplistic, but not a possible solution currently because few supplements for prostate cancer, urologic prevention, or total mortality reduction can be recommended at this time [136, 272–274]. Compliance is also a major issue over a long period of time with any agent. Some dietary supplements may also increase the risk of prostate cancer or interfere with conventional treatment [274–276], and no supplement or drug therapy has ever matched the reduction in CVD or all-cause mortality observed in investigations of lifestyle changes [136, 277–280]. Regardless, this chapter would be lacking without providing a table of specific dietary, supplement, and other advice based on the specific stage and treatment of the patient with prostate cancer. A review of this information can be found in some recently published literature [130] and in Table 21.3 [130].

Conclusion

The time seems more than ripe to redirect our attention to lifestyle changes and prostate health. Heart health seems tantamount to prostate health, and this is the best potential practical and realistic recommendation that has worked in my consulting practice for over a decade. It seems that large and diverse (American Cancer Society, American Heart Association, and the American Diabetes Association) health-care preventive organizations are beginning to apply this same concept [281] because the truly life-changing lifestyle recommendations for patients are not mutually exclusive. They impact a variety of potential outcomes and have the highest probability of impacting all-cause mortality. This is critical in my opinion because the forest has to take precedence over the tree to improve the overall state of prostate health. The more

Table 21.3. A Brief Overview of Some Specific Advice That Can Be Given to Prostate Cancer Patients According to the Stage and Treatment Status of the Individual.

Clinical Scenario	Specific Recommendation
All stages of prostate cancer and all treatments and scenarios, and even if the patient is attempting to prevent this disease	Heart healthy = prostate healthy Encourage the patient to help bring his overall cardiovascular risk to as close to zero as possible. Follow the guidelines in this chapter; the utilization of statin, blood pressure, insulin sensitivity, or even fish oil medications need to be encouraged in the individual who has already tried to maintain normal values with diet and exercise without complete success
	No patient should take more than one cheap low-dose multivitamin pill a day
	Incorporate approximately three tablespoons a day of grounded cheap flaxseed into any daily meal or situation
	Selenium blood testing should be discussed with a target of 114–121 ng/mL as "normal"
	Vitamin E individual supplements should not be taken at this time until they are proven to be safe and effective and heart healthy
	Saw palmetto should not be taken by any person diagnosed and treated for prostate cancer because of the lack of evidence.
Prevention or high-risk patients with a negative biopsy (high-grade prostatic intraepithelial neoplasia or atypical small acinar proliferation)	Triage preventive medicine, which means to remind patients about colonoscopy, vaccines and other preventive advice that have no relationship to prostate cancer but place the emphasis on the forest over the tree
	Less is more in terms of supplementation
Localized disease being treated with a radical prostatectomy	Incorporate approximately three tablespoons a day of grounded cheap flaxseed into any daily meal or situation
	Less is more in terms of supplementation
	Stop most dietary supplements 2–3 weeks before surgery to ensure no unexpected bleeding events or anesthesia interactions occur as has already been documented in the literature
Localized disease being treated with some form of radiation or cryotherapy or HIFU (high-intensity focused ultrasound)	Aggressive cholesterol lowering may act as a radiation or treatment sensitizer
	No dietary supplements during the time of treatment because it may lower the efficacy of the conventional treatment, and this includes until the seed implant half-life is almost zero (several months to 1 year depending on the implant)

(continued)

Table 21.3. (Continued)

Clinical Scenario	Specific Recommendation
Biochemical recurrence and/or hormone suppressive treatment	Every person should be placed on a weight-lifting or resistance exercise program with physician approval. This may reduce fatigue and improve bone health
	Every person should be getting approximately 1200–1500 mg a day of elemental calcium and should be blood tested for vitamin D status with a 25-hydroxyvitamin D level (adequate greater than 30 ng/mL). If the vitamin D level cannot be done, a minimum of 800 IU/day of vitamin D3 should help increase levels to near normal.
	Flaxseed may also reduce hot flashes due the "plant estrogen" content of the grounded form of this food L-carnitine (500–4000 mg per day) and/or American ginseng (1000–2000 mg/d) has demonstrated some ability to reduce fatigue in a randomized trial, and should be considered for patients with fatigue during and from treatment
Hormone-refractory or androgen-independent prostate cancer and some effect issues	Taxotere is being studied with vitamin D
	L-carnitine (500–4000 mg per d) and/or American ginseng (1000–2000 mg/d) has demonstrated some ability to reduce fatigue in a randomized trial, and should be considered for patients with fatigue from either chemotherapy
	Vitamin C supplements (250 mg) should be taken before a dose of ketoconazole to enhance the absorption of the medication

clinicians demonstrate to patients that they are serious about these behavioral changes, the more, I believe, patients will respond to the advice. On the other hand, the less a clinician focuses on these issues, the less I also believe patients will respond to them, and even worse, the more likely patients will begin to listen to less credible sources for guidance. This latter scenario is concerning, but unfortunately has become so common today in other areas of medicine that it is almost considered normal for patients to take lifestyle, supplement, and general preventive advice from the person at the counter of the local health food store over their primary practitioner [282,283]. This simply cannot be allowed to happen to the prostate cancer patient or any other type of cancer patient. Hopefully this chapter is a step in the appropriate direction.

REFERENCES

19. Moyad MA. (1999). Emphasizing and promoting overall health and nontraditional treatments after a prostate cancer diagnosis. *Seminars in Urologic Oncology*, 17, 119–124.

38. Shike M, Latkany L, Riedel E, et al. (2002). Lack of effect of a low-fat, high-fruit, -vegetable, and -fiber diet on serum prostate-specific antigen of men without prostate cancer: results from a randomized trial. *Journal of Clinical Oncology*, 20, 3592–3598.

46. Heinonen OP, Albanes D, Virtamo J, et al. (1998). Prostate cancer and supplementation with alpha-tocopherol and beta-carotene: Incidence and mortality in a controlled trial. *Journal of the National Cancer Institute*, 90, 440–446.

50. Freedland SJ, Aronson WJ, Kane CJ, et al. (2004). Impact of obesity on biochemical control after radical prostatectomy for clinically localized prostate cancer: A report by the Shared Equal Access Regional Cancer Hospital Database Study Group. *Journal of Clinical Oncology*, 22, 446–453.

66. Segal RJ, Reid RD, Courneya KS, et al. (2003). Resistance training in men receiving androgen deprivation therapy for prostate cancer. *Journal of Clinical Oncology*, 21, 1653–1659.

131. Giovannucci E. (1999). Tomatoes, tomato-based products, lycopene, and cancer: Review of the epidemiologic literature. *Journal of the National Cancer Institute*, 91, 317–331.

150. Pantuck AJ, Leppert JT, Zomorodian N, et al. (2006). Phase II study of pomegranate juice for men with rising prostate-specific antigen following surgery or radiation for prostate cancer. *Clinical Cancer Research*, 12(13), 4018–4026.

154. Kucuk O, Sarkar FH, Sakr W, et al. (2001). Phase II randomized clinical trial of lycopene supplementation before radical prostatectomy. *Cancer Epidemiology, Biomarkers & Prevention*, 10, 861–868.

184. Moyad MA, Sakr WA, Hirano D, & Miller GJ. (2001). Complementary medicine for prostate cancer: effects of soy and fat consumption. *Reviews in Urology*, 3(Suppl. 2), S20–S30.

211. Ornish D, Weidner G, Fair WR, et al. (2005). Intensive lifestyle changes may affect the progression of prostate cancer. *The Journal of Urology*, 174, 1065–1070.

(A complete reference list for this chapter is available online at http://www.oup.com/us/integrativemedicine).

22

Integrative Medicine in Colorectal Cancer

JUDITH S. JACOBSON AND ALFRED I. NEUGUT

KEY CONCEPTS

- Colorectal cancer may be especially well suited to an integrative approach, which may benefit patients with high risk or precursor conditions as well as those with the disease.
- A diet rich in fruits and vegetables and regular physical activity may help both to prevent colorectal cancer and to improve survival among patients with colorectal cancer.
- Two studies have found associations between adverse life events and increased risk of colorectal cancer. Although not conclusive, these data support exploration of stress management measures for individuals at risk.
- Colorectal cancer patients and those at risk for colorectal cancer include both males and females, and encompass a vast age range. The relatively slow course of the disease and the morbidity associated with it should be viewed as providing multiple opportunities for intervention, communication, and feedback through which patients and those who care for them can work together to optimize both quantity and quality of life.

■

Distinctive Features of Colorectal Cancer Relevant to Complementary and Alternative Medicine

Colorectal cancer is the fourth most common cancer in the United States (after prostate, breast, and lung), and is among the top five in most developed countries. Perhaps even more than breast and prostate cancer, colorectal cancer lends itself to an integrative approach. It affects men and women more or less equally; it is highly preventable, and it is increasingly treatable. In the United States, its 5-year relative survival rate has risen from about 50% in 1975 to 1977 (the earliest years for which data are available) to 65% in 2002 [1], not as good as breast or prostate cancer survival but much better than lung cancer survival. Almost all recurrences are detected within 5 years after diagnosis, but even recurrent or metastatic disease is increasingly treatable. Unfortunately, many patients who die of colorectal cancer experience considerable cancer-related morbidity in the years after their diagnosis. And because colorectal cancer is a disease of aging, individuals who are at risk for or have been diagnosed with it may have comorbid conditions that complicate their care. An integrative approach may be of considerable benefit to such patients.

Colorectal Cancer Prevention

In the United States, the overall lifetime risk of developing colorectal cancer is 5.79% among males and 5.37% among females [1]. Most patients who are diagnosed with colorectal cancer have no reason for considering themselves to be at higher than average risk. However, colorectal cancer was among the first to be associated with specific familial and nonfamilial syndromes, precursor lesions, and genetic mutations; the lifetime risk associated with these conditions varies but is considerably higher than 5%.

The familial syndromes that have been most closely associated with colorectal cancer are familial adenomatous polyposis (FAP) and Gardner syndrome (GS). Young adults with the classic presentation of these conditions have more than 100 adenomatous polyps (the precursor lesions for most cases of colorectal cancer), carpeting their colon and rectum; in the absence of treatment, the likelihood of developing cancer by age 40 years is close to 100%. Individuals with GS also have abnormalities and high risk of cancer at other organ sites. Both conditions have been linked to a mutation on the long arm of chromosome 5 and are transmitted to offspring in a dominant Mendelian pattern [2].

At somewhat lower but much above average risk are individuals with one of the hamartomatous polyposis syndromes: familial juvenile polyposis syndrome, Cowden's syndrome, Bannayan-Ruvalcaba-Riley syndrome, Peutz-Jeghers syndrome, basal cell nevus syndrome, neurofibromatosis 1, and multiple endocrine neoplasia syndrome 2B. Such patients are also at risk for cancers at other organ sites and, like GS patients, require multidisciplinary management. Genetic testing is now available for all these conditions, but the hamartomatous polyposis syndromes occur more often in connection with spontaneous mutations than do FAP and GS [3]. In addition, some patients have 5 to 100 adenomatous polyps without having the APC mutation associated with FAP and GS [4].

In the absence of these precursor conditions, individuals with a strong family history of colorectal cancer are also at higher than average risk. New models based on the specifics of the family history are being used to estimate risk for such individuals [5].

Crohn's disease and ulcerative colitis are nonfamilial conditions that have been associated with substantially higher than average risk for colorectal cancer [6], although recent data have raised questions about the degree of increased risk [7].

Conventional Preventive Interventions

Safe and relatively comfortable screening procedures for visualizing the colon have been available for about 20 years. Various types of fecal occult blood testing (FOBT) have been available for even longer, and have been shown to reduce colorectal cancer mortality [8–10]. As a result, screening with FOBT is now recommended for average-risk individuals ≥50 years of age. However, among asymptomatic individuals aged 50 to 75 years, FOBT detected less than 25% of advanced neoplasia (adenomas ≥10 mm in diameter, villous, or with high-grade dysplasia or invasive cancers) [11]. Colonoscopy, at 10-year intervals if negative, is now considered the gold standard for screening, and is increasingly safe [12], but it is also expensive and in some analyses not cost-effective [13]. A survey of 21,833 patients aged 55 to 70 years who had been insured for the prior 5 years found that 54% had been screened according to recommended procedures during this period and that the screening method most commonly used was colonoscopy [14]. Screening rates among minorities and the uninsured are much lower [15], and the barriers most commonly reported are lack of physician recommendation and the inconvenient and unpleasant aspects of endoscopy [16].

The availability of colonoscopy has had a considerable impact on preventive care for individuals at higher than average risk. Genetic tests for the APC mutation associated with FAP and GS have been available for about 15 years, and tests for other gene mutations relevant to colorectal cancer risk have become available since then. However, a number of candidates for genetic testing, concerned about stigmatization and discrimination [17], prefer colonoscopic surveillance to determining whether they have a high-risk mutation. Once multiple adenomas or dysplastic epithelium are detected among individuals with known familial high risk, the treatment is colectomy, but many patients still need to be followed thereafter for extracolonic conditions. And even if a colonoscopy is negative, individuals at high risk, many of whom have seen one or more of their relatives die of colorectal cancer, have to live from day to day between examinations and many seek out CAM for primary prevention.

For more than a decade, data from observational studies have suggested that an agent as commonplace as aspirin, or other nonsteroidal anti-inflammatory drugs (NSAIDs), might help prevent the development of colorectal neoplasia[18]. The evidence was not consistent [19], but it was strong enough to justify continuing research and the development of trials of promising agents [20–24].

Recent randomized clinical trials have confirmed the efficacy of celecoxib as a chemopreventive agent reducing the incidence of colorectal adenomas among individuals with a personal history of adenomas [25,26]. Unfortunately, celecoxib was also found to increase the risk of cardiovascular events. However, the trial results support the principle of chemoprevention for colorectal cancer and the quest for agents that may be both more efficacious and safer.

These developments have also spurred a quest for herbal agents and dietary interventions that may reduce the risk of colorectal adenomas and cancer [27,28]. Although trials of dietary modification have had generally disappointing results, recent studies have suggested that dairy products and vitamin D, calcium, folate, curcumin, and quercetin may help to reduce risk. Evidence is increasingly convincing that diets heavy in red meat and processed meats may increase the risk of colorectal cancer [29,30]. A growing body of evidence also suggests that obesity and a sedentary lifestyle increase risk [31,32]. Current data should encourage individuals without specific risk factors for colorectal cancer to focus on doing what they have to do to stay well and to get the most out of their lives. The good news is that, generally speaking, it is not necessary to chose between the heart and the colon.

The recently issued report of the World Cancer Research Fund and the American Institute for Cancer Research conclude that diets high in red meat and processed meats, ethanol intake, and obesity, especially abdominal obesity, may increase the risk of colorectal cancer, and that fiber, garlic, and calcium intake and physical activity may reduce risk.

A number of studies have also found that tallness (greater adult attained height) is associated with risk for colorectal cancer [33]. This finding has been interpreted to mean that height in itself does not increases risk but that the conditions in childhood that lead to increased growth may increase risk for cancer.

Two case–control studies published in the 1990s found that stressful life events in the 5- or 10-year period preceding diagnosis were associated with increased risk for colorectal cancer [34,35]. Claims that unhappiness or stress may cause cancer have been made for many years, but most studies of such associations are poorly designed and of questionable validity. The two studies of life events and colorectal cancer were large (715 cases and 727 controls in one, 569 cases and 510 controls in the other) and population based, one in Australia and the other in Sweden. The other findings of the studies have been supported by subsequent research. Both studies found risk to be most strongly associated with work-related problems, rather than home or family problems; adjusted odds ratios for the association of work-related problems with colorectal cancer were 3.09 (95% confidence interval [CI] 1.79–5.33) and 5.5 (95% confidence interval [CI] = 2.3–23.5). A subsequent population-based case–control study of psychosocial aspects of work and colon cancer risk in Los Angeles, CA, found weaker but still positive associations of risk with lack of job control (autonomy) [36].

Neither tallness nor work problems are generally considered matters of personal choice. However, individuals who are tall or work in stressful conditions may be considered members of a high-risk group and, as such, may be encouraged to consider screening and preventive options. Those confronting occupational stress in particular might be candidates for stress management interventions. Obviously, changing jobs, if feasible, may be the most direct way to relieve the stress. However, the efficacy of stress management and job change for cancer prevention has not been studied.

Cancer-Directed Treatment

Despite the preventive measures described earlier, 153,760 people are expected to be diagnosed with colorectal cancer—112,340 with colon cancer, and 41,420 with rectal cancer in 2007 [37]. As Table 22.1 indicates, almost 40% of patients are diagnosed with localized disease and nearly 20% with metastatic disease. Members of medically underserved minority groups are more likely than whites and Asians to be diagnosed with advanced disease [38]. Survival is strongly associated with stage. However, the regional stage includes stages IIa to IIb and IIIa to IIIe of the American Joint Committee on Cancer staging system, within which, for colonic adenocarcinoma at least, survival rates vary from 83.4% to 26.8%, as Table 22.2 shows. Patients with stage IIIa cancers appear to fare better than those

Table 22.1. Stage Distribution and 5-Year Survival of Patients
with Colorectal Cancer in the SEER Registry, 1996 to 2002.

Stage	% of Cases			5-Year Relative Survival		
	Colorectal	Colon	Rectum	Colorectal	Colon	Rectum
All	100	100	100	64.1	63.7	65.1
Localized	39	37	44	90.4	91.5	88.1
Regional	37	38	34	68.1	69.8	63.8
Distant	19	31	15	9.8	10.4	8.0
Unstaged	5	4	6	34.6	28.6	43.7

Table 22.2. Numbers of Patients and 5-Year Survival
with Colon Adenocarcinoma by AJCC (Sixth Edition)
Stage in the SEER Database 1991 to 2000 [39].

Stage	N	% of Sample	% Alive at 60 Months
All	96,198	100.0	65.2
I	14,500	15.1	93.2
IIa	28,535	29.7	84.7
IIb	5,826	6.1	72.2
IIIa	1,989	2.1	83.4
IIIb	15,946	16.6	64.1
IIIc	4,092	4.2	52.3
IIId	2,655	2.8	43.0
IIIe	1,853	1.9	26.8
IV	20,802	21.6	8.1

with stage IIb cancers [39]. The difference may reflect either understaging of some IIb cancers or the benefit of chemotherapy for patients in stage IIIa.

For patients with stage 0 to II colon cancer and stage I rectal cancer, surgery alone is considered curative. Since the late 1980s, trials have shown that chemotherapy with 5-fluorouracil (5-FU) and other agents can improve survival in stage III colon cancer [40,41]. Trials have generally failed to show that chemotherapy benefits patients with stage II colon cancer, perhaps because of the relatively good survival of such patients, but the use of prognostic markers may help to identify high-risk stage II patients who can benefit from the addition of chemotherapy [42]. Patients with metastatic disease at baseline and those whose disease becomes metastatic are also routinely treated with a growing menu of chemotherapeutic agents [43]. Patients with stage II and III rectal cancer have been found to benefit from combined chemotherapy and radiation therapy, and these treatments are more effective when given prior to rather than after surgery [44].

Surgical treatment for colorectal cancer has improved over time. It is less invasive than it once was, and laparoscopic techniques, when feasible, appear to be associated with reduced morbidity compared to more traditional surgical approaches. However, patients with colorectal cancer are often elderly and may have comorbid conditions that increase the burden of surgery. Obesity, a risk factor for colorectal cancer, also makes surgery more difficult. Most patients, especially the young and the old, dread needing a stoma, and having a stoma is in some but not all studies associated with poor quality of life. Patients also fear that surgery will lead to incontinence and impaired sexual function. Actual refusal of surgical treatment is relatively rare, however. Among 106,377 patients diagnosed with colon or rectal cancer 1988 to 1997 in the SEER (Surveillance Epidemiology and End Results) database, only 6.7% did not have surgery [45]. Black patients were significantly less likely than white patients to receive standard surgery for colon or rectal cancer and radiation therapy for rectal cancer.

In addition to causing fatigue and other short-term side effects, radiation therapy can cause rare long-term effects, such as radiation injury to pelvic organs and second primary cancers. However, preoperative (neoadjuvant) chemotherapy and radiation therapy may also reduce the size of a rectal tumor, improve the prospects of safely preserving the anal sphincter, and reduce the risk of tumor recurrence [44].

The side effects of chemotherapy with 5-FU–based regimens, such as FOLFOX, include diarrhea, stomatitis, nausea, vomiting, leukopenia, thrombocytopenia, and dermatitis. The newer agents, such as oxaliplatin, also cause neuropathy. Amifostine and other agents are being explored to address such side effects [46], but amifostine has shown little benefit and has side effects of its own. The potential relevance of the antioxidant properties of these drugs to their benefits and side effects is increasingly acknowledged, and has influenced the development of the next generation of radioprotective agents [47].

In addition to dealing with the effects of the disease and its treatment, patients also must face the possibility that their cancer will spread or recur after they complete their treatment. New treatments are available in such circumstances [48], but they too have their side effects, which may be harder for a patient demoralized by treatment failure than for a new patient to face.

Throughout the natural history of colorectal cancer, from high risk and precursor lesions to cure or metastasis, an integrative approach has much to offer patients with colorectal cancer (Table 22.3).

Table 22.3. Integration of CAM and Conventional Approaches in Relation to the Status of the Individual at Risk for or with Colorectal Cancer.

CAM	Conventional
Prevention/Early Detection	
Recreational physical activity, healthy diet (low fat, whole grains, fruits, vegetables), low alcohol intake, no tobacco use, stress management	Screening, Cox-2 inhibitors as chemoprevention in selected cases
Stage I–II Colon Cancer, Stage I Rectal Cancer	
Support groups, meditation, stress management, movement therapy	Surgery
Stage II–III Rectal Cancer	
Acupuncture, Chinese herbs	Surgery + neoadjuvant chemoradiation
Stage III Colon Cancer	
Support groups, meditation, guided imagery and relaxation, stress management, movement therapy, acupuncture, Chinese herbs	Surgery + chemotherapy selected to maximize benefits, minimize side effects for the individual patient, or via clinical trial
Stage IV	
Support groups, meditation, stress management, movement therapy, acupuncture, botanical therapies in the context of a clinical trial	Chemotherapy, especially (if available) via clinical trial
Survivorship and Ongoing Care	
Recreational physical activity (the equivalent of 6 + hrs/week of brisk walking), heart-healthy diet, stress management	Routine medical follow up, assessment of risk factors, chemoprevention clinical trial if available
Palliative Care	
Support groups, meditation, prayer/religious support, stress management, movement therapy, acupuncture, botanical therapies, massage, meditation, art therapy, journaling, Reiki	Conventional symptom management, palliative care clinical trial if available and relevant

The dashed line between the two columns represents the goal of integrating CAM and conventional care.

Most of the CAM approaches listed above have not been validated in randomized clinical trials as beneficial specifically for patients with colorectal cancer.

Integrative Approaches

Among 871 patients diagnosed with colorectal cancer in 1993 or 1995 in Alberta, Canada, who responded to a survey questionnaire, 49% reported using CAM. Of the CAM users, 16% reported using CAM before their diagnosis; 20% between the diagnosis and treatment; 46% during treatment; and 69% after treatment [49]. The modalities most commonly used were psychological or spiritual therapies (65%); vitamins and/or minerals (46%); herbal therapies (e.g., garlic, ginseng, Essiac; 42%); and functional foods (e.g., shark cartilage; 20%). The reasons most frequently given for CAM use were wanting to try every option (81%), and hearing that CAM had worked for others (70%); 49% of users thought CAM was less harmful or more natural than conventional treatment, and 20% said they had not been offered conventional treatment.

Among 622 patients with a history of colorectal cancer who participated in a randomized double-blind placebo-controlled trial of aspirin to prevent disease recurrence, 304 (49%) reported concurrent use of dietary supplements. The most commonly used were multivitamins (N = 234, 38%), vitamin E (N = 137; 22%), vitamin C (N = 110; 18%), and calcium (N = 101; 16%) [50].

Of 126 colorectal cancer patients in seven European countries, 40 reported using CAM, most of them having initiated CAM use after their diagnosis [51]. The modalities most commonly used after the diagnosis were herbal medicine (19 patients), homeopathy (8 patients), and vitamins/minerals (7 patients). The reasons most commonly given for CAM use were to increase the body's ability to fight the cancer and to do everything to fight the disease (18 patients for both), and to improve physical well-being (17 patients).

Other studies have also found botanicals to be among the top three CAM modalities used by cancer patients in their respective samples [52,53]. A Cochrane review of clinical trials of herbal agents among patients receiving chemotherapy for colorectal cancer analyzed chemotherapy side effects, quality of life, and adverse events among patients who received herbal treatments with chemotherapy and patients who received chemotherapy alone. Only four such trials were identified, and all were judged to be of low quality. However, the authors found that the evidence suggested that Chinese herbs such as astragalus may reduce the risk of both nausea and leukopenia [54].

Other trials of CAM for treatment side effects in colorectal cancer patients have been conducted. One found that among elderly patients who underwent surgery for colorectal cancer, guided imagery and relaxation therapy were well received but did not affect pulmonary function, duration of postoperative ileus, or postoperative fatigue [55]. A randomized trial of pelvic floor exercise/biofeedback training among patients with fecal incontinence after surgery or surgery plus irradiation found a benefit for the training regardless of irradiation status, although baseline status was poorer in the irradiated group [56]. A randomized trial among patients who had stoma surgery found that the group receiving progressive muscle relaxation training had less anxiety and better quality of life than the controls at 10 weeks [57].

Maintaining Health and Preventing Recurrence

Although patients who have completed their treatment for colorectal cancer seem to be concerned about doing everything in their power to prevent disease recurrence, patients' behavior is not entirely consistent with that concern. A study of elderly, currently disease-free, 5-year colorectal cancer survivors in the SEER/Medicare database and an age-matched control group in Medicare found that the cancer patients had more comorbid conditions, such as diabetes and congestive heart failure, than the controls and were less likely to receive medical care for those conditions [58]. Although all patients were Medicare recipients, black race and low socioeconomic status were also independent predictors of failure to receive appropriate medical care.

Among 44 disease-free colorectal cancer survivors in Canada who were offered the opportunity to receive free support group services as well as programs in meditation, Reiki, yoga, and Qigong, only 14 expressed interest in doing so, and only 4 actually attended the programs. Among the remaining 40, the most common reasons for nonattendance were having enough support already (17 patients), living too far away (14 patients), and having no need (13 patients) [59].

However, disease-free 2-year colorectal cancer survivors reported statistically significant increases from baseline (diagnosis) in vegetable intake, physical activity, and supplement use compared to controls [60], who had also increased physical activity and supplement use. And a cohort study of 1009 patients with stage III colon cancer found that those in the highest quintile of a "western dietary pattern" (dominated by processed and red meats, refined grains, high-fat dairy products, desserts, and French fries) were up to three times as likely to experience cancer recurrence or death from any cause as those in the lowest quintile [61].

Two recent studies have found recurrence and mortality risk reductions of close to 50% among subjects who engaged in at least 18 metabolic-equivalent task (MET) hours per week compared to those who engaged in fewer than 3 MET hours [62,63]. In practical terms, 18 MET hours represents 4 to 5 hours/ week of very brisk walking [64]. These observations are probably the strongest evidence available for an effect of patient behavior (other than treatment adherence) on cancer survival.

Dealing with Recurrence

Patients who develop recurrent or metastatic disease become candidates for new combinations of chemotherapeutic agents, with their respective side effects [43].

A trial among 194 elderly patients receiving treatment for advanced breast, prostate, or colorectal cancer randomized them to receive either monthly telephone calls to monitor distress and anxiety and referrals where appropriate or written materials describing available resources. At 6 months, the telephoned group had less anxiety, depression, and overall distress than the comparison group [65].

In some institutions, patients with advanced disease may also become eligible for trials of alternative therapies. One of the most highly publicized alternative agents for the treatment of cancer is shark cartilage. In a randomized double-blind trial among 88 patients with incurable breast or colorectal cancer receiving standard care, the shark cartilage group fared no better than the placebo group with respect to either survival or quality of life [66].

Ukrain is a plant extract on which successful trials in three states of the former Soviet Union have been reported, some of them involving patients with colorectal cancer [67]. However, the trials were poorly designed and reported. They provide no evidence of benefit compared to state-of-the-art treatment in the United States.

End-of-life Issues

Because of advances in detection and treatment, the number of individuals living with a diagnosis of colorectal cancer in the United States is expected to increase from 1,002,786 in 2000 to 1,522,348 in 2020 (Mariotto Cancer Causes Control 2006). Of these, approximately 8% are expected to be in their last year of life. More than half will be dying from causes other than colorectal cancer, but those with terminal colorectal cancer will need care for a variety of challenging conditions, including pain, hemorrhage, and obstruction. Addressing the needs of the patient, family, and other providers caring for the patient presents further challenges.

In a systematic review of randomized controlled trials of CAM for cancer-related pain, acupuncture, support groups, hypnosis, and massage showed some evidence of short- or long-term benefit [68]. Another review found that acupuncture, transcutaneous electrical nerve stimulation, supportive group therapy, self-hypnosis, and massage therapy may provide relief at the end of life but that trials were often of poor quality or difficult to compare with one another [69]. Acupuncture, acupressure, and muscle relaxation with breathing retraining appeared to have some effect in relieving dyspnea [70]. Acupuncture and selected botanicals may help to control nausea/vomiting. Transcendental meditation and mindfulness-based stress reduction may reduce anxiety [71].

Among the options that some patients consider when they exhaust conventional treatment are CAM cancer clinics, including those in Europe, Mexico, and the Caribbean. No solid evidence is available to support claims that such clinics can reverse the course of terminal cancer. We conducted a best-case series review of a German cancer clinic and found that a small number of patients who had failed to benefit from conventional treatment improved at the clinic [72]. A number of cancer patients who have visited such clinics have provided Zagat-like reports on themselves on the website of the Annie Appleseed Project (http://www.annieappleseedproject.org, as of 12/09/07). Some of the clinics provide cancer care and personal attention in a setting that is more like a hotel or spa than a hospital. Such clinics may be very expensive, and their costs and the related travel are generally not reimbursable. But some patients and families may want to feel that they have left no stone unturned, and some may prefer not to spend their last days at home. Hospice care is another important option for patients at the end of life, and it is reimbursible. Some patients and families perceive choosing hospice as giving up. Communicating about DNR (do not resuscitate) status, support systems, treatment goals, and hospice care is essential for complete care of patients at the end of life [73].

A recent study of 191 colorectal cancer survivors found that 45.5% were experiencing colorectal cancer-specific distress, that 75% were using CAM, and that poorer perceived social support, intrusive thoughts, poorer overall perceived quality of life, and younger age associated with CAM use [74]. The authors concluded that providers should ask patients about their CAM use and assess it as a potential indicator of a need for additional social support, especially among younger patients.

The evidence for an effect of stress on survival or for a survival benefit of stress reduction among cancer patients is lacking, in part because of the difficulties of designing and conducting studies with cancer mortality as an endpoint [75]. That difficulty may be particularly great in the setting of colorectal cancer. However, the purpose of integrative medicine is, or should be, to care for the whole person. Asking about CAM use, about stress, and about social support may initiate a dialogue that communicates that purpose to the patient. Acknowledging and treating the whole person may be inherently stress reducing and may have a positive effect on quality, whether or not it affects quantity, of life.

REFERENCES

1. Ries LAG HD, Krapcho M, Mariotto A, Miller BA, Feuer EJ, Clegg L, et al. (2006). (Eds). SEER Cancer Statistics Review, 1975–2003. In: National Cancer Institute B, MD, editor.

2. Friedenreich C, Norat T, Steindorf K, Boutron-Ruault MC, Pischon T, Mazuir M, et al. (2006). Physical activity and risk of colon and rectal cancers: The European prospective investigation into cancer and nutrition. *Cancer Epidemiology, Biomarkers & Prevention*, 15(12), 2398–2407.

3. Kune S, Kune GA, Watson LF, & Rahe RH. (1991). Recent life change and large bowel cancer. Data from the Melbourne Colorectal Cancer Study. *Journal of Clinical Epidemiology*, 44(1), 57–68.

4. Courtney JG, Longnecker MP, Theorell T, & Gerhardsson de Verdier M. (1993). Stressful life events and the risk of colorectal cancer. *Epidemiology*, 4(5), 407–414.

5. Tough SC, Johnston DW, Verhoef MJ, Arthur K, & Bryant H. (2002). Complementary and alternative medicine use among colorectal cancer patients in Alberta, Canada. *Alternative Therapies in Health and Medicine*, 8(2), 54–56, 58–60, 62–64.

6. Taixiang W, Munro AJ, & Guanjian L. (2005). Chinese medical herbs for chemotherapy side effects in colorectal cancer patients. *Cochrane Database of Systematic Reviews (Online)* (1), CD004540.

7. Haase O, Schwenk W, Hermann C, & Muller JM. (2005). Guided imagery and relaxation in conventional colorectal resections: a randomized, controlled, partially blinded trial. *Diseases of the Colon and Rectum*, 48(10), 1955–1963.

8. Meyerhardt JA, Niedzwiecki D, Hollis D, Saltz LB, Hu FB, Mayer RJ, et al. (2007). Association of dietary patterns with cancer recurrence and survival in patients with stage III colon cancer. *JAMA*, 298(7), 754–764.

9. Meyerhardt JA, Heseltine D, Niedzwiecki D, Hollis D, Saltz LB, Mayer RJ, et al. (2006). Impact of physical activity on cancer recurrence and survival in patients with stage III colon cancer: findings from CALGB 89803. *Journal of Clinical Oncology*, 24(22), 3535–3541.

10. Jacobson JS, Grann VR, Gnatt MA, Hibshoosh H, Austin JH, Millar WS, et al. (2005). Cancer outcomes at the Hufeland (complementary/alternative medicine) klinik: A best-case series review. *Integrative Cancer Therapies*, 4(2), 156–167.

(*A complete reference list for this chapter is available online at http://www.oup.com/us/ integrativemedicine*).

23

Radiation Therapy and Integrative Oncology

MATTHEW P. MUMBER

KEY CONCEPTS

- Radiation oncology is a rapidly evolving field, with new technology helping to increase the probability of tumor cell kill while decreasing toxicity to normal tissue structures.
- The addition of complementary therapies to radiation must be evaluated with an individualized risk to benefit analysis that includes several factors: overall goal of care (curative versus palliative), category of use for the complementary intervention (antineoplastic, supportive care, or prevention), and the timing of the combination (before, during, or after radiation).
- Several supportive intent complementary therapies can now be considered as a part of the standard of care in combination with conventional cancer therapies that include radiation as a part of the treatment plan.

■

What Is Radiation and How Does It Work?

Radiation is the transport of energy through space (Huda & Slone, 1995). Everything that exists in the natural world is constantly bombarded with some form of radiation from the electromagnetic spectrum. This spectrum includes signals from satellites, cellular phones, the sun, distant galaxies, radioactive compounds, and man-made X-ray sources. These types of radiation vary in biologic effect based upon the energy that they impart. This energy has certain physical characteristics that are measurable—such as wavelength and frequency. The type of radiation that is used to target and destroy cancer cells has the same nature as the heat from the sun and light from a rainbow—it merely varies in its shape and size. A helpful comparison is a man walking—radiation with higher energy is represented by a man with short strides and a high number of strides per minute, while radiation with lower energy is like a man with long strides and fewer strides per minute. High energy radiation has a more discrete biologic effect (Fig. 23.1).

Radiation is hypothesized to have played a significant role in the genesis of life, causing the changes in genetic material responsible for the evolution of plant and animal species. The magnitude of this effect has been debated for years, and the debate continues today. Some would contend that there is no amount of radiation exposure that can be considered safe, while others promote a hypothesis that some radiation exposure may actually have a beneficial effect. The latter hypothesis has been coined "radiation hormesis" and is defined as a beneficial and adaptive response to low levels of radiation exposure. Beneficial biologic adaptations to low-dose radiation have been documented in plants, animals, and humans, both in vivo and in vitro. These low doses have been shown to augment the immune system and protect against damage from subsequent radiation exposure (Feinendegen, 2005; Johansson, 2003; Parsons, 2002; Parsons, 2003; Upton, 2001). One interesting study published in 2001 by Lee et al., showed that peripheral blood cell counts were increased in people living near nuclear power plants. (Lee, et al., 2001) The radiation hormesis debate has implications on the relationship between cancer prevention and

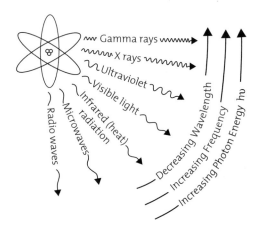

FIGURE 23.1. Illustration of the electromagnetic radiation spectrum. X-rays have the same nature as visible light, radiant heat, and radio waves; however, they have shorter wavelengths and larger energy and can thus cause a more discrete biologic effect by breaking chemical bonds (Hall, 2000). Hall, EJ. (2000). *Radiobiology for the radiologist.* (5th edition.) Philadelphia: Lippincott Williams & Wilkins.

low dose, low level radiation exposure—from sources like cell phones, mammograms, and newer technology multi-slice CT scanners (Dawson, 2004). The radiation hormesis hypothesis is also of special interest to proponents of homeopathy—as it offers potential proof of principle that very low doses of a toxic substance can produce a beneficial adaptive biologic effect. The possibility of low level radiation exposure having a positive health effect may also have implications in the newest generation of therapeutic radiation delivery—intensity modulated radiation therapy (IMRT). In IMRT, lower doses of radiation are spread throughout a region of the body such that an area of convergence where all of the radiation beams intersect receives a very high conformal dose (de Arruda, et al., 2006).

There is no debate concerning the significant biologic effect of focused, high-dose, high-energy radiation—the type used to treat cancer. This type of radiation kills cells primarily by damaging the DNA. DNA can be damaged directly by an X-ray hitting an electron, which then destroys a portion of the DNA structure, or indirectly through the radiation propelled electron interacting with a water molecule to produce a free radical molecule which then

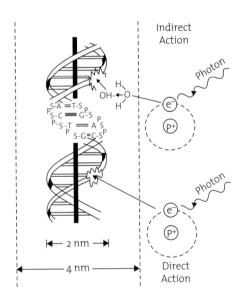

FIGURE 23.2. Direct and Indirect action of radiation. An X-ray photon strikes an electron in tissue, which then either directly causes DNA damage (direct effect) or creates a free radical, which then damages DNA (indirect effect). The majority of radiation damage is produced by the indirect effect for radiation that is produced by linear accelerators—the type most often used in cancer treatment (Hall, 2000). Hall, EJ. (2000). *Radiobiology for the radiologist*. (5th edition.) Philadelphia: Lippincott Williams & Wilkins.

damages the DNA structure (Fig. 23.2.). The majority of radiation used to treat cancer is generated by linear accelerators. This type of radiation produces about two-thirds of its biologic effect through the indirect action of free radicals on DNA and one-third from direct effect (Hall, 2000). This process has significant implications when considering how we can make radiation less toxic to normal cells while still preserving its ability to destroy cancer cells. For example, there is a significant debate as to whether one should administer synthetic antioxidant supplements to patients during radiation treatment—an entire chapter of this text focuses on this debate (see Chapter 9). Antioxidants could interfere with the indirect action of radiation on DNA by scavenging free radicals, thus protecting both normal and tumor cells. Indeed, randomized data exist that support this hypothesis (Bairati, et al., 2005; Bairati, et al., 2006). However, it is also possible that antioxidant supplements could protect normal tissues and allow an increased antitumor effect—either directly or through an improvement in the therapeutic ratio (Moss, 2006; Prasad, 2004). In practice, the application of antioxidant supplementation during radiotherapy depends on how one views the continuum of cancer therapy, and how one evaluates the risks and benefits associated with specific interventions at specific times.

Radiation has a differential effect on normal and cancerous cells. Simply put, cancerous cells lack the ability to efficiently repair radiation damage, while normal cells can repair sublethal damage more readily. The outcome of irradiation of a cancer cell in this regard results in one of three measurable outcomes on the cell—it loses its ability to undergo cell division and dies, becomes quiescent, or continues to grow.

Normal tissues may repair damage inflicted by radiation. There are generally two types of radiation damage that take place—acute and long term. Acute damage usually takes place due to damage to the cell itself, resulting in a loss of function or cell death. This early damage takes place from weeks to months after radiation exposure. Late damage takes place months to years after exposure and is usually the result of damage to supportive tissues such as small blood vessels and connective tissues. Acute reactions fade relatively quickly, much like a skin burn from the sun. Late reactions are much more difficult to heal—similar to diabetic foot ulcers. From an integrative oncology standpoint, we would like to find an ideal approach which addresses both the protection of normal tissues and the destruction of cancerous cells. This would spare normal tissue from both early and late reactions while maximizing cancer cell death. During therapy, increasing cancer control would occur by an actual increase in tumor cell kill. Following therapy, increased cancer control may occur through lack of a supportive tissue structure in which the cancer could grow again, or improved body recognition with resultant elimination of abnormal cancerous cells.

The ideal agent to add to radiation would be one which increases the effectiveness of radiation in killing cancer cells, while at the same time protecting normal tissues from harm. This agent would have activity both during and many years after radiation treatment.

Where Does Radiation Fit into the Spectrum of Integrative Cancer Care?

The practice of integrative oncology has yet to be clearly defined. However, there are several factors that are already considered as a part of conventional cancer care, that certainly lay the framework for an integrative approach (see Table 23.1) (Mumber, 2006). Radiation therapy clearly falls into the category

Table 23.1. Factors to Consider as a Part of Integrative Oncology (Mumber, 2006).

Factor	Definition
Patient's clinical situation	Acute vs subacute presentation and need for intervention
	Disease stage and type
	Prognosis
Specific treatment goals	Prevention
	Supportive care
	Antineoplastic care
General preventive approach	Primary
	Secondary
	Tertiary
General supportive care approach	Translational vs transformational utility
	Improved tolerance of antineoplastic therapy
	Symptom control
	General quality of life
	End-of-life care
General antineoplastic approach	Curative vs palliative
Level of evidence for therapy	Data levels I–IV, for both safety and efficacy
	Risk/benefit ratio—including cost, toxicity, chances of beneficial and harmful outcome

of an antineoplastic treatment. To develop an integrative approach, we must determine how complementary therapies can improve outcomes associated with therapeutic radiation.

A significant proportion of cancer patients receiving radiation therapy are already using complementary and alternative methods(CAM)—some studies quote numbers as high as 80% (Swarup, Barrett, & Jazieh, 2006; Vapiwala, Mick, Hampshire, Metz, & Denittis, 2006; Yates, et al., 2005). Unfortunately, radiation oncologists do not generally inquire about their patient's use of CAM methods, which may create a double-edged sword; beneficial CAM therapies may be underutilized and harmful CAM-RT interactions may take place.

How Can We Make Radiation Better?

There are several potential mechanisms to improve radiation outcomes, during and after therapy (see Table 23.2.). It is important to differentiate those

Table 23.2. Therapeutic Possibilities for Improvement of Radiation Effect.

	Prevention	*Supportive Care*	*Antineoplastic Effect*
During radiation	Prevent acute reactions—mucositis, diarrhea, nausea, skin irritation, dysphagia, fatigue Prevent late reactions—damage to normal tissues including lung, brain, bowel, soft tissue, skin	Treat symptoms related to radiation—skin irritation, nausea, diarrhea, dyspagia, fatigue.	Improve cell kill by Improving therapeutic ratio—i.e. making treatments more tolerable through supportive care and symptom management; or through increasing cell kill by making normal cells more resistant and tumor cells more sensitive to radiation
Following radiation	Prevent disease recurrence Prevent late effects to normal tissues	Treat symptoms related to late effects—dry mouth, fibrosis, fatigue, radiation necrosis	Improve upon cell kill through unknown mechanism—e.g.—greater immune surveillance

types of interventions that will occur during treatment from those that will occur afterward. During the delivery of radiation, there could be interactions that compromise the cancer cell killing effect of radiation. In analyzing a risk-benefit analysis for any intervention, it is also important to keep in mind the therapeutic goal—prevention, supportive care, or antineoplastic effect. The goal of therapy then allows one to consider the levels of evidence that are available for a given therapeutic goal. Generally, randomized trials must be present as the intervention scales up the pyramid from prevention to supportive care, and ultimately to antineoplastic treatment. Lower levels of data are more acceptable for interventions that have a purely preventive or supportive nature, and no possibility of adversely affecting cancer control (see Fig. 23.3.).

Special data requirement considerations regarding efficacy should be given to certain approaches to supportive care intervention. Supportive care can be subdivided into translational and transformational approaches (Mumber, 2006). For translational approaches, there is a discrete intervention and a measurable outcome—such as acupuncture for relieving nausea. Transformational approaches are more motivational in nature. Their purpose is to assist the patient in reframing an experience to help them move forward with life in a more positive direction. An example of a transformational approach would be attending a retreat for cancer survivors. In transformational approaches, outcomes concerning efficacy would be quantitatively difficult to measure, and therefore the primary point of analysis should be safety.

The risk/benefit ratio must also be analyzed in the context of discrete individual clinical settings. Different clinical goals, especially with regards to curative or palliative efforts, may ultimately influence the risk/benefit ratio

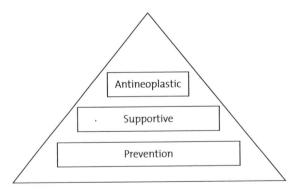

FIGURE 23.3. Pyramid of therapeutic goals. Higher levels of the pyramid are generally associated with larger risks and benefits and require higher levels of evidence for both safety and efficacy (Mumber, 2006). Mumber, MP. (2006). *Integrative oncology principles and practice*. London: Taylor & Francis.

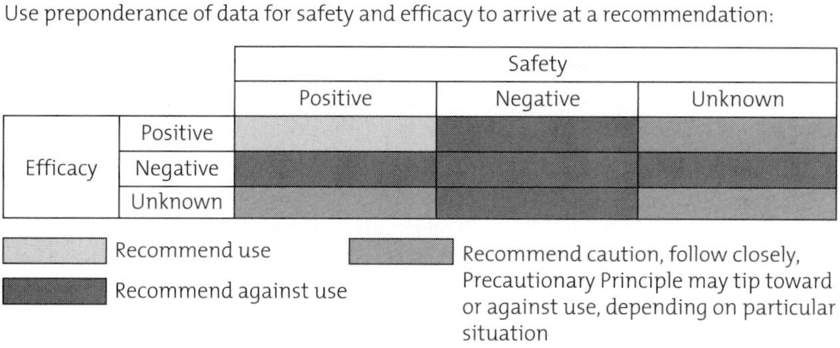

Use preponderance of data for safety and efficacy to arrive at a recommendation:

		Safety		
		Positive	Negative	Unknown
Efficacy	Positive			
	Negative			
	Unknown			

Recommend use

Recommend against use

Recommend caution, follow closely, Precautionary Principle may tip toward or against use, depending on particular situation

FIGURE 23.4. Evidence concerning any planned intervention can be evaluated based on positive, negative, or unknown effects on safety and efficacy, and then an appropriate recommendation can be made (Mumber, 2006). Mumber, MP. (2006). *Integrative oncology principles and practice.* London: Taylor & Francis.

that one is willing to accept. A therapy needs to be analyzed with regards to the preponderance of data concerning safety and efficacy for a given goal, prior to making recommendations (see Fig. 23.4).

Through this process, some general conclusions can be drawn concerning current CAM modalities based on the available data. CAM options during and after radiation should be analyzed according to their primary goal—preventive or supportive care, or antineoplastic effect. In this light, recommendations may be formulated to determine if the therapy should be a part of standard of care, be accepted with close follow up, or be advised against (see Tables 23.3–23.5).

Unfortunately, the majority of analyses will come up with insufficient or conflicting data to make clear cut decisions. This is where clinical judgment must come into play. As a part of this process, it is reasonable to make judicious use of the precautionary principle. The precautionary principle basically states that in situations where there is a serious positive or negative outcome, presence of absolutely confirmatory data is not necessary to make a recommendation. The precautionary principle allows one to make decisions based on insufficient data, yet have these decisions based on a reasonable response to a specific clinical outcome. A reasonable decision can be made by analyzing several different components in this context—including an assessment of risk, benefit, realism, proportionality, and consistency (Resnik, 2004). The recommendation against concurrent use of antioxidants and radiation debate provides a nice example. The risk is a decrease in cancer control, while the benefits are mild improvements in toxicity. There are realistic biologic rationales for

Table 23.3. Therapies That Should Be Recommended as Standard of Care.

	Prevention	Supportive Care	Antineoplastic Effect
During radiation		Acupuncture for anticipatory nausea related to combined chemotherapy and radiation	
Following radiation	Prevent recurrence— optimal health, physical activity, plant based diet, stress reduction	Acupuncture for xerostomia related to head and neck radiation Trial of vitamin E and Trental for lessening radiation fibrosis Massage as a part of manual decongestive therapy for lymphedema post axillary dissection and radiation Support groups to improve quality of life Cancer patient retreats	

Table 23.4. Therapies That Should Be Rated as Acceptable with Close Follow-up.

	Prevention	Supportive Care	Antineoplastic Effect
During radiation	Calendula cream to prevent skin toxicity Moderate physical activity throughout therapy in order to prevent fatigue	Massage, music therapy, counseling, guided imagery, yoga, mindfulness based meditation, creative arts, Reiki, hypnosis— relieve anxiety and promote relaxation	
Following radiation	Variety of supplements including Broad-spectrum multivitamins, Omega-3-fats, Coenzyme Q 10, Lycopene	Acupuncture for xerostomia related to head and neck radiation Trial of vitamin E and Trental for lessening radiation fibrosis	Support groups

(continued)

Table 23.4. (Continued)

	Prevention	Supportive Care	Antineoplastic Effect
	Variety of foods including Garlic Green tea Soy Vegetables—especially brassica family Fruits—especially berries, tomato, watermelon	Massage as a part of manual decongestive therapy for lymphedema post axillary dissection and radiation	

Table 23.5. Therapies That Should Be Discouraged.

	Prevention	Supportive Care	Antineoplastic Effect
During radiation	High-fiber diet during radiation to pelvis—may exacerbate diarrhea High-dose synthetic antioxidants to prevent normal tissue toxicity—may reduce radiation tumor cell kill		Botanicals which may have significant interactions with chemotherapy or radiation Any therapy with unproven antineoplastic effect that delays effective cancer therapy in a curative setting outside of a clinical trial.
Following radiation	Any therapy with unproven benefit, proven harm, or significant expense to patient and family with unproven effect	Any therapy with unproven benefit, proven harm, or significant expense to patient and family with unproven effect	Any therapy with unproven benefit, proven harm, or significant expense to patient and family with unproven effect

both. The risk/benefit ratio for antioxidant use during radiotherapy is not proportional to that of other agents recommended for use during radiation, such as moderate physical activity. Recommendation against antioxidant use during radiotherapy is entirely consistent with other clinical recommendations made in oncology care.

DURING RADIATION THERAPY

In the curative treatment setting, preservation of the antineoplastic activity of radiation therapy must be of primary importance. The prevention of acute and long-term side effects is desirable. However, lessening side effects without totally eliminating them, while at the same time sacrificing cancer local control and cure rates, is unacceptable. The goal is to improve the therapeutic ratio such that normal tissue toxicity is lessened while increasing cancer cell kill. An analysis of normal and tumor cell survival curves reveals that an ideal intervention would accomplish both these goals (see Fig. 23.5).

> During the administration of radiation, a guiding principle is that the antineoplastic activity of radiation must be preserved, and concurrent administration of agents that could negatively influence this should be avoided until data exists that there is no negative interaction. Supportive intent mind-body therapies that have no rational biologic mechanism of interference with radiation antineoplastic effect can be recommended as a new standard of care.

One particularly promising approach is to provide supportive interventions with no biologic rationale to decrease radiotherapy's ability to kill cancer cells. Such therapies have enough evidence to accept their use during treatment with careful monitoring, and have proven supportive benefits. These approaches include music therapy, massage, yoga practice, psychoeducational counseling, guided imagery, and mindfulness-based meditation (Mansky & Wallerstedt, 2006). The use of these supportive interventions may improve the patient's ability to complete a full course of radiation without treatment breaks—a factor that has shown a proven benefit with regards to cancer control (Machtay, et al., 2005; Saibishkumar, et al., 2006). The recent publication of guidelines for the treatment of lung cancer from the American College of Chest Physicians endorsed a variety of mind-body therapies for anxiety and stress reduction during therapy including massage, yoga, and relaxation techniques. This recommendation was made with Level 1 data, making it applicable as a new standard of care (Michael Alberts, 2007). Conversely, the use of antioxidants during radiation is an example of the addition of agents that have potential to adversely affect cancer cell kill through a rational biologic mechanism. Even in the setting of normal tissue sparing, these should be discouraged until further data are available.

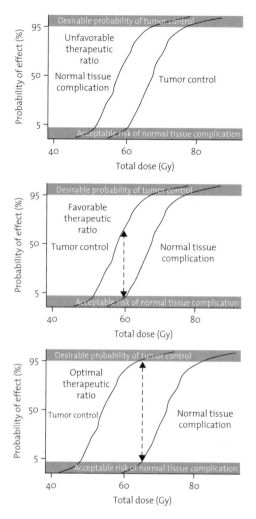

FIGURE 23.5. The therapeutic ratio. Treatment effectiveness can be evaluated based on its effects on normal tissues and cancer cells. Unfavorable therapeutic ratios exist where the treatment causes significant relative normal tissue damage in order to attain tumor control. Favorable and optimal ratios spare normal tissue while attaining high rates of cancer control (Gunderson & Tepper, 2000). Gunderson, L L. & Tepper, J E. (2000). *Clinical radiation oncology.* (1st ed.) Philadelphia: Churchill Livingstone.

There are significant interventions available that should be a part of standard care based on available data. These include acupuncture for anticipatory nausea and vomiting related to combined chemotherapy and radiation (Johnstone, Polston, Niemtzow, & Martin, 2002; Lu, 2005), and psychoeducational care prior to and during therapy (Cartledge & Haaga, 2005; Kim, Roscoe, & Morrow, 2002). There are a significant number of preventive and supportive care interventions that may also be acceptable with close follow up. These include calendula cream to prevent acute skin toxicity (Pommier, et al., 2004), moderate physical activity throughout therapy in order to prevent fatigue (Kirshbaum, 2007), and a significant variety of supportive care interventions that can reduce anxiety, promote relaxation, improve quality of life, and potentially allow patients to receive their total prescribed dose of therapy without harmful delays (Clark, et al., 2006; Jereczek-Fossa, Marsiglia, & Orecchia, 2002; Mansky & Wallerstedt, 2006; Windsor, Nicol, & Potter, 2004). It is important to remain constantly vigilant reviewing the individual patient's clinical features when making these recommendations. For example— structured exercise has been shown to improve fitness and thus the ability to perform activities of daily life in early stage breast cancer patients undergoing postoperative adjuvant treatments (Markes, Brockow, & Resch, 2006), while a different study showed that advanced cancer patients actually had worsened quality of life parameters with a structured exercise program (Brown, et al., 2006). It is also important to discourage any therapies that could cause delay of proven effective therapy.

FOLLOWING RADIATION THERAPY

After the completion of radiation treatments, there are significant CAM options to help prevent disease recurrence, prevent late effects of treatment, promote optimal health, and ameliorate symptoms associated with previous treatment (Mansky & Wallerstedt, 2006). Standards of care should include the basics of healthy living—a plant-based diet, moderate physical activity, and stress reduction (Kushi, et al., 2006). This can be accomplished through a variety of mechanisms, including support groups and educational programs (McCarthy, Yancey, Harrison, Leslie, & Siegel, 2006; Thaxton, Emshoff, & Guessous, 2005). Massage therapy as a part of manual decongestive therapy is already a part of the standard approach to lymphedema management (Golshan & Smith, 2006). Acupuncture can help with xerostomia (Blom, Dawidson, Fernberg, Johnson, & Angmar-Månsson, 1996, Wong, Jones, Sagar, Babjak, & Whelan, 2003. The combination of vitamin E and Trental has shown promising results with regards to reversal of the late effect of radiation fibrosis (Delanian, Porcher, Balla-Mekias, & Lefaix, 2003; Gothard, et al., 2004).

Following radiation, a variety of complementary modalities can be used to maintain optimal health and, hypothetically, aid in tertiary prevention of disease while lessening late radiation effects.

There are also significant interventions that can be recommended with close observation. Significant literature exists to support the use of multivitamin supplements for cancer prevention. There is also a biologic rationale that multivitamins may help to prevent or decrease late effects from radiotherapy such as fibrosis (Robbins & Zhao, 2004). Large trials concerning multivitamin supplementation are underway in multiple disease sites. Caution must be exercised in certain populations such as smokers, in whom supplementation with synthetic β-carotene has produced an increased incidence in lung cancer (Greenwald, Anderson, Nelson, & Taylor, 2007).

Therapies to be discouraged following treatment include those that are associated with significant cost, time, and travel requirements. In general, specific approaches that are only offered at one place with very high costs are not valuable. A possible exception to this rule would be if the treatment were being offered as a part of a valid clinical research trial.

The Future

The delivery of radiation therapy has changed significantly over the past 20 years in concert with improvements in imaging and computer technology. The ability to target tumor tissue, while avoiding normal tissue will continue to improve the therapeutic ratio and resultant outcomes (de Arruda, et al., 2006). At the same time, improvements in chemotherapy approaches with biologic agents have led to the use of these new agents in combination with radiation in efforts to improve cancer control and lessen side effects relative to previous regimens (Bonner, et al., 2006; Ozols, et al., 2007). The combination of preventive and supportive care interventions using complementary methods have a great deal to offer as the field of integrative oncology is defined. An integrative approach has the potential to improve the process and outcomes for all participants—patient, family members, health care providers, and society as a whole.

REFERENCES

Bairati I, Meyer F, Gelinas M, Fortin A, Nabid A, Brochet F, et al. (2005). Randomized trial of antioxidant vitamins to prevent acute adverse effects of radiation therapy in head and neck cancer patients. *Journal of Clinical Oncology,* 23, 5805–5813.

Bairati I, Meyer F, Jobin E, Gelinas M, Fortin A, Nabid A, et al. (2006). Antioxidant vitamins supplementation and mortality: A randomized trial in head and neck cancer patients. *International Journal of Cancer,* 119, 2221–2224.

Gothard L, Cornes P, Earl J, Hall E, MacLaren J, Mortimer P, et al. (2004). Double-blind placebo-controlled randomised trial of vitamin E and pentoxifylline in patients with chronic arm lymphoedema and fibrosis after surgery and radiotherapy for breast cancer. *Radiotherapy and Oncology, 73,* 133–139.

Johnstone PA, Polston GR, Niemtzow RC, & Martin PJ. (2002). Integration of acupuncture into the oncology clinic. *Palliat.Med.,* 16, 235–239.

Kushi LH, Byers T, Doyle C, Bandera EV, McCullough M, Gansler T, et al. (2006). American Cancer Society Guidelines on Nutrition and Physical Activity for cancer prevention: Reducing the risk of cancer with healthy food choices and physical activity. *CA: A Cancer Journal for Clinicians,* 56, 254–281.

Lee YT, Sung FC, Lin RS, Hsu HC, Chien KL, Yang CY, et al. (2001). Peripheral blood cells among community residents living near nuclear power plants. *The Science of the Total Environment,* 280, 165–172.

Mansky PJ & Wallerstedt DB. (2006). Complementary medicine in palliative care and cancer symptom management. *Cancer Journal,* 12, 425–431.

Michael Alberts W. (2007). Diagnosis and Management of Lung Cancer Executive Summary: ACCP Evidence-Based Clinical Practice Guidelines (2nd Edition). *Chest,* 132, 1S–19.

Mumber MP. (2006). *Integrative oncology principles and practice.* London: Taylor & Francis.

Resnik DB. (2004). The precautionary principle and medical decision making. *The Journal of Medicine and Philosophy,* 29, 281–299.

(A complete reference list for this chapter is available online at http://www.oup.com/us/integrativemedicine).

24

Integrative Medicine in Symptom Management and Palliative Care

ADITYA BARDIA, AMIT SOOD, DEBRA L. BARTON, AND CHARLES L. LOPRINZI

KEY CONCEPTS

- Complementary and alternative medicine (CAM) therapies are widely used among cancer patients and some of them may be helpful in the management of cancer-related symptoms.
- Mind–body interventions, and other relaxation therapies, such as massage and music, appear to be beneficial in alleviating cancer pain, improving mood symptoms and decreasing insomnia.
- Acupuncture therapy can reduce chemotherapy-induced nausea/vomiting and cancer-related pain, while aerobic exercise appears to reduce fatigue.
- Dietary supplements, including St. John's wort and SAMe, appear to be helpful in treating depression, while capsaicin cream can reduce cancer pain and postsurgical neuropathic pain.
- It should be noted that integrative oncology is a relatively young science, that clinical trials testing various CAM therapies are currently underway, and that a better understanding of the efficacy and toxicity of these approaches is necessary.

■

several recent surveys show that patients with cancer commonly use, or are interested in, using complementary and alternative medicine (CAM) (Barnes, Powell-Griner, McFann, & Nahin, 2004; Eisenberg, et al., 2002; Hyodo, et al., 2005; Richardson, Sanders, Palmer, Greisinger, & Singletary, 2000). These therapies have been used both as an alternative to conventional medicine (alternative medicine) and complementary to conventional medicine (complementary medicine). The term, integrative medicine, has been proposed to imply that these should be integrated with administration of conventional therapies (Cohen, 2004; Johnstone, Polston, Niemtzow, & Martin, 2002). Unfortunately, patients frequently do not discuss CAM therapies with their oncologists (Adler & Fosket, 1999; Eisenberg, et al., 2002). Moreover, many oncologists have limited knowledge of CAM (Newell & Sanson-Fisher, 2000). Thus, wider dissemination of evidence-based applications for CAM interventions is needed.

This chapter reviews evidence-based information about the efficacy of these treatments in patients with cancer. We reviewed the relevant literature including over 11,000 scientific citations and broadly categorized evidence for individual symptoms into four different groups: (1) likely effective, (2) appears promising, (3) evidence inconclusive, and (4) likely not effective. The definition of the above groups is outlined in Table 24.1.

This chapter is organized on the basis of individual symptoms. The evidence base for the use of CAM treatments for the following symptoms is covered: pain, fatigue, anorexia, cachexia, mood disorders, hot flashes, and insomnia.

Cancer Pain

Pain affects over 75% of hospitalized cancer patients (Brescia, Portenoy, Ryan, Krasnoff, & Gray, 1992; Wells, 2000) and is often called the "fifth vital sign" in these patients (McMillan, Tittle, Hagan, & Laughlin, 2000). Conventional pharmacologic agents remain the first-line treatment for cancer pain, with a recommendation to add nonpharmacologic treatments if pain remains ≥ 4 on a o to 10 scale despite adequate pharmacotherapy (American Society of Cancer, and National Comprehensive Cancer Network practice guidelines, 2001). CAM therapies likely efficacious for reducing cancer pain include acupuncture; mind–body interventions such as cognitive behavioral therapy, hypnosis, imagery and progressive muscle relaxation; and capsaicin cream (Bardia, Barton, Prokop, Bauer, & Moynihan, 2006) (Table 24.2).

Table 24.1. Description of Various Categories Used for Classification of CAM Therapies Based on Available Scientific Evidence.

Category	Criteria Used
Likely effective	At least one high-quality positive randomized trial among patients with cancer without other negative randomized trial data; or a positive meta-analysis.
Appears promising	Promising outcome data from weaker randomized controlled trials; or pilot data in cancer patients; or positive trial in patients with no history of cancer along with a strong biological rationale for the potential of efficacy.
Evidence inconclusive	Conflicting data from clinical trials; or positive trials in patients with no history of cancer without a convincing biological rationale; or negative randomized trial in patients with no history of cancer.
Likely ineffective	High-quality negative randomized controlled trials; or negative meta-analysis; or several negative smaller trials, among patients with cancer.

LIKELY EFFECTIVE

Acupuncture has been tested for the treatment of pain in over 400 clinical trials; however, only a few studies specifically enrolled patients with cancer. In a randomized controlled trial, 90 subjects were enrolled to one of the three arms: acupuncture at "pain" points, acupuncture at "placebo" points, or seeds implanted at placebo points. Participants randomized to acupuncture at "pain" points showed a significantly better pain relief compared to the other two groups at 2 months (Alimi, et al., 2003). Two previous smaller studies, involving 76 and 48 patients, reported only short-term benefits (at 1 week, but not after 2 months) (Dang & Jiebin, 1998; Xia, et al., 1986). The precise mechanism of action of acupuncture is not known, but it might involve modulation of opioid peptides, primarily in the periaqueductal gray matter (Cheng & Pomeranz, 1980; Ma, 2004). Overlapping efficacy of acupuncture for other cancer-related symptoms such as nausea, and its relative safety, makes acupuncture a particularly compelling treatment option to study further in patients with cancer.

Table 24.2. Efficacy of Various Complementary Therapies for Cancer-Related Pain, Based on Available Scientific Evidence.

Likely Effective	Cognitive behavioral therapy
	Progressive muscle relaxation
	Support groups
	Acupuncture
	Capsaicin cream
Appears Promising	Massage
	Healing touch
	Herbal therapies
Evidence Inconclusive	Music therapy

Mind–body interventions promote relaxation, and decrease anxiety, autonomic hyperarousal and muscle tension, and thereby have a potential to decrease pain (Fishman & Loscalzo, 1987). These treatments might also act as distraction stimulus; that is, it will block pain from entering the thought process and inhibit pain impulse transmission from the thalamus to the cerebral cortex (Butler, Duran, Jasiukaitis, Koopman, & Spiegel, 1996; Hilgard, 1975; Spiegel, Cutcomb, Ren, & Pribram, 1985). **Hypnosis** was compared to cognitive-behavioral therapy, therapist contact control, or usual treatment in a four-arm clinical trial involving 67 patients undergoing bone marrow transplant. Hypnosis significantly decreased oral pain associated with mucositis, with the two other groups showing no significant treatment effect (Syrjala, Cummings, & Donaldson, 1992). Hypnosis combined with group therapy had greater efficacy compared to either of these treatments alone in another trial involving 58 subjects with metastatic breast cancer (Spiegel, Bloom, & Yalom, 1981; Spiegel & Bloom, 1983). **Relaxation training** significantly reduced cancer pain compared to a no intervention control arm in two randomized trials involving 67 and 94 patients, respectively (Sloman, Brown, Aldana, & Chee, 1994; Syrjala, et al., 1995). In a large randomized trial involving 235 patients with metastatic breast cancer, participation in **support group (supportive-expressive therapy)** significantly improved pain intensity compared to no intervention group (Goodwin, et al., 2001).

Capsaicin cream binds to vanilloid receptors, and exerts an analgesic effect by depleting neurons of their substance P and neurokinin (Karai, et al., 2004; Lynn, 1990). In a well-designed randomized cross-over trial involving 99 patients with postsurgical neuropathic pain, 8 weeks of topical application of capsaicin cream (0.075%) was significantly more efficacious for reducing pain, compared to an identical-appearing placebo cream (Ellison, et al., 1997). Similar results were reported in a smaller trial involving 143 participants (Watson & Evans, 1992). Capsaicin cream is generally safe with the most common side effect being a burning sensation due to local effects of the cream.

APPEARS PROMISING

Massage therapy has been tested in at least four trials for cancer-related pain (Post-White, et al., 2003; Soden, et al., 2004; Weinrich & Weinrich, 1990; Wilkie, et al., 2000). While the largest study involving 230 participants showed efficacy immediately post treatment (Post-White, et al., 2003), the treatment effect dissipated rapidly with no residual benefit at 4 weeks. Two randomized trials, involving 59 and 50 participants, respectively, reported an improvement in postoperative pain using arm massage in subjects with breast cancer (Forchuk, et al., 2004; McNeely, et al., 2004). Theoretically, massage therapy might promote metastatic spread of tumor cells via increased lymph flow, but this is not supported by clinical evidence.

Energy-based therapies such as therapeutic touch and Reiki have shown preliminary evidence of efficacy for short-term pain relief; however, their mechanism of action is presently unclear. Healing touch was compared with massage, presence alone, or standard care in a cross-over trial involving 230 participants (Post-White, et al., 2003). Healing touch showed posttreatment improvement of pain, but the treatment effect did not persist beyond 4 weeks. In another controlled trial involving 24 participants, Reiki treatment was associated with significant short-term reduction of pain immediately after treatment compared to the control intervention (rest) (Olson, Hanson, & Michaud, 2003).

Art therapy appears to be gaining popularity as a mind–body intervention to promote relaxation and improve coping (Collie, Bottorff, Long, & Conati, 2006; Oster, et al., 2006). A recent quasi-experimental therapy involving 50 patients with cancer reported that a 1-hour art therapy session led to significantly reduced pain, depression, and anxiety. (Nainis, et al., 2006).

Biological products that hold promise for improving pain relief include herbs that work primarily by decreasing inflammation, such as willow extracts (*Salix spp*), ginger, turmeric, and devil's claw (Loew, Möllerfeld, Schrödter, Puttkammer, & Kaszkin, 2001; Shoba, et al., 1998; Ojewole, 2006). Valerian has γ-amino butyric acid (GABA)-related compounds that might regulate pain transmission (Upton &Petrone, 1999). These herbal products have been tested for relieving back pain, osteoarthritis, postoperative inflammation, and neuropathic pain. (Altman & Marcussen, 2001; Durgaprasad, Pai, Vasanthkumar, Alvres, & Namitha, 2005; Chrubasi, 2000; Chrubasik, Junck, Breitschwerdt, Conradt, & Zappe, 1999;

Chantre, et al., 2000; Leblan, Chantre, & Fournie, 2000; Chrubasik, Model, Black, & Pollak, 2003; Satoskar, Shah, & Shenoy, 1986). However, currently there is paucity of data about the effects of these products in patients with cancer.

EVIDENCE INCONCLUSIVE

Music therapy, like other mind–body treatments, can act as a distracting stimulus. Two small trials involving 9 and 15 patients reported no improvement in pain with music compared to a control intervention (suggestion or nonmusical sounds) after 2 to 3 days (Beck, 1991; Curtis, 1986). However, a trial involving 40 patients found immediate postintervention (30 minutes) benefit with music therapy but did not assess long-term efficacy (Zimmerman, Pozehl, Duncan, & Schmitz, 1989).

Fatigue

Cancer-related fatigue affects more than two-thirds of patients with cancer and significantly impairs their quality of life (Curt, 2000; Stone, et al., 1999). Medical conditions that frequently contribute toward cancer-related fatigue include pain, emotional distress, sleep disturbance, anemia, nutritional deficiencies, deconditioning, and comorbidities such as hypothyroidism. The initial approach toward management of fatigue should include the identification and treatment of potentially reversible causes. CAM therapies that may be helpful include cognitive behavioral therapy (CBT), exercise, yoga, healing touch, acupuncture, and dietary supplements such as ginseng, levocarnitine, and mistletoe extract (Table 24.3).

LIKELY EFFECTIVE

Aerobic exercise merits mention because it is an integrative lifestyle intervention with proven efficacy for improving cancer-related fatigue. In a recent meta-analysis involving 14 studies, exercise was associated with significant improvement in physical functioning, peak oxygen consumption, fatigue, and overall quality of life (McNeely, et al., 2006).

Mind–body interventions can positively affect the thought processes and have favorable effects on stress, pain, and overall well-being, and thus might improve fatigue. Supportive nursing care, support groups, and psycho-educational strategies to manage stress, improve coping, and conserve energy

Table 24.3. Efficacy of Various Complementary Therapies for Cancer-Related Fatigue, Based on Available Scientific Evidence.

Likely Effective	Exercise
Appears Promising	Yoga
	Cognitive behavioral therapy
	Healing touch
	Massage therapy
	Acupuncture
	Levocarnitine
	Ginseng
Evidence Inconclusive	Homeopathy
	Siberian ginseng
	(Eleutherococcus)

have shown efficacy for improving fatigue in controlled clinical trials among cancer patients (Barsevick, et al., 2004; Fawzy, et al., 1990; Given, et al., 2002; Jacobsen, et al., 2002; Spiegel, et al., 1981; Yates, et al., 2005).

APPEARS PROMISING

Levocarnitine, a micronutrient that is involved in cellular energy production, is deficient in a large proportion of patients with cancer (Cruciani, et al., 2004). In a phase II trial involving 50 nonanemic subjects with carnitine deficiency, supplementation with levocarnitine (4 g/day for 7 days) significantly improved fatigue scores during chemotherapy after 1 week of therapy (Graziano, et al., 2002). Two small pilot trials involving 13 and 12 patients respectively showed similar promising results (Cruciani, et al., 2004, 2006; Gramignano, et al., 2006).

Ginseng (particularly Asian ginseng, *Panax ginseng*) contains glycosidal saponins (ginsensosides) that might have stimulating and immune-modulating properties (Block & Mead, 2003). Ginseng was reported to enhance physical performance among healthy volunteers in a few studies (Vogler, Pittler, & Ernst, 1999). In a small placebo-controlled randomized study involving 20 subjects, Asian ginseng (250 mg TID, 5% ginsenosides) significantly improved fatigue and quality of life in cancer patients undergoing chemotherapy (Younus, et al., 2003).

Acupuncture was associated with improved fatigue in a pilot trial involving 37 patients with cancer (Vickers, Straus, Fearon, & Cassileth, 2004). Acupuncture was also reported to improve fatigue among patients with fibromyalgia and end-stage renal disease (Martin, Sletten, Williams, & Berger, 2006; Tsay, Cho, & Chen, 2004).

Healing touch and massage therapy induce general relaxation and reduce stress and might thus help fatigue. In a large cross-over randomized trial, 230 subjects with cancer were randomized to massage therapy, healing touch, presence alone, or standard care (Post-White, et al., 2003). Massage therapy significantly reduced fatigue immediately following the intervention, with the effect waning over the next 4 weeks. The effect of healing touch for decreasing fatigue was significant compared to a control group, both postintervention and at 4 weeks. In addition, four smaller studies suggest potential efficacy of both massage (Cassileth & Vickers, 2004; Kohara, et al., 2004; Rexilius, Mundt, Erickson Megel, & Agrawal, 2002) and healing touch (Roscoe, Matteson, Mustian, Padmanaban, & Morrow, 2005b) for reducing cancer-related fatigue.

EVIDENCE INCONCLUSIVE

Yoga is a combination of gentle postures, breathing exercises, meditation, and relaxation. In a small randomized trial among 35 hematopoietic stem cell transplant recipients, a combination of relaxation breathing with gentle exercise significantly improved fatigue, compared to no intervention (Kim & Kim, 2005). However, two other small randomized trials involving 33 and 38 participants provided inconclusive results, partly related to a high attrition rate in these studies (Cohen, Warneke, Fouladi, Rodriguez, & Chaoul-Reich, 2004; Nicole Culos-Reed, Carlson, Daroux, & Hately-Aldous, 2006).

Two controlled trials with 20 and 96 participants tested a dry extract of **Siberian ginseng** (*Eleutherococcus* sp.) 300 mg/day in patients with chronic fatigue syndrome (Cicero, et al., 2004; Hartz, et al., 2004). Both studies showed a suggestion toward short-term benefit. **Homeopathy** was ineffective in reducing fatigue in a randomized trial involving 103 subjects with chronic fatigue syndrome (Weatherley-Jones, et al., 2004).

Anorexia and Cachexia

Anorexia and cachexia are debilitating symptoms affecting about 60% to 70% of patients with cancer (Sarhill, et al., 2003; Walsh, Donnelly, & Rybicki, 2000). Major factors that contribute to these symptoms include local gastrointestinal (GI) effects of cancer (particularly, obstruction and malabsorption),

Table 24.4. Efficacy of Various Complementary
Therapies for **Cancer-Related Anorexia and
Cachexia,** Based on Available Scientific Evidence.

Appears Promising	Creatine
	Melatonin
Likely Ineffective	Fish oil
	Hydrazine sulfate

systemic effects of cancer (appetite suppression, IL-6 and TNF-α and other inflammatory markers mediating catabolism), and adverse effects from cancer treatment. Complementary therapies, including dietary supplements such as creatine, melatonin, fish oil, and hydrazine, have been investigated for anorexia and cachexia (Table 24.4).

APPEARS PROMISING

Creatine is a dietary supplement widely taken by athletes to boost athletic performance. Creatine increases cellular adenosine triphosphate (ATP) production and significantly increases muscle mass and strength among healthy adults (Kilduff, et al., 2002; Gotshalk, et al., 2002), patients with heart failure (Andrews, et al., 1998), respiratory disease (Fuld, et al., 2005), and myopathies (Hespel, et al., 2001; Tarnopolsky, Roy, & MacDonald, 1997). A large randomized, double-blind, placebo-controlled trial testing the efficacy of creatine in improving anorexia-cachexia is currently being conducted by the North Central Cancer Treatment Group (NCCTG).

Melatonin is an endogenous hormone produced by the pineal gland and might improve cancer-related cachexia by decreasing levels of TNF-α and tissue catabolism (Blask, et al., 1999). In a randomized trial involving 70 patients with non–small cell lung cancer, melatonin (20 mg/day) was reported to significantly reduce the number of patients developing cachexia (26% versus 5%, $P < 0.001$) (Lissoni, et al., 1997). A more recent, but smaller randomized trial involving 24 patients suggested a trend toward weight stabilization with 18 mg/day of melatonin along with 30 mL/day of fish oil (Persson, Glimelius, Ronnelid, & Nygren, 2005). Some of the other potential positive effects of melatonin in patients with cancer include tumor inhibition (Blask, et al., 1999; Lissoni, et al., 2001), mitigation of chemotherapy toxicity (Lissoni, et al., 1999; Lissoni, et al., 2003), and improvements in overall survival and quality of life (Lissoni, et al., 2003).

LIKELY INEFFECTIVE

Fish oil, a rich source of omega-3 fatty acids, was postulated to improve cachexia due to its anti-inflammatory effect. The positive results from earlier preliminary studies (Barber, et al., 1999; Burns, et al., 1999) were unfortunately not confirmed in subsequent multiple, large, well-controlled trials (Bruera, et al., 2003; Burns, et al., 2004; Fearon, et al., 2003; Jatoi, et al., 2004; Persson, et al., 2005); however, there was a suggestion of weight stabilization.

Hydrazine sulfate (60 to 180 mg/day) lacked efficacy in several controlled clinical trials (Chlebowski, et al., 1990; Kosty, et al., 1994; Loprinzi, et al., 1994a; Loprinzi, et al., 1994b; Yavuzsen, Davis, Walsh, LeGrand, & Lagman, 2005) and was also reported to have potential for hepatotoxicity (Hainer, Tsai, Komura, & Chiu, 2000).

Nausea and Vomiting

Nausea and vomiting affects about two-thirds of cancer patients. CAM therapies including acupuncture and mind–body treatments are likely effective for improving nausea (Table 24.5).

LIKELY EFFECTIVE

Acupuncture for control of nausea involves the stimulation of the acupuncture point P6 (pericardium 6 or Neiguan) located on the anterior aspect of the arm, two to three finger breadths proximal from the flexor crease. In a meta-analysis of 11 randomized trials, manual and electro acupuncture were found to be effective in improving nausea and vomiting (Ezzo, et al., 2005). However, its efficacy

Table 24.5. Efficacy of Various Complementary Therapies for Cancer-Related Nausea and Vomiting, Based on Available Scientific Evidence.

Likely Effective	Cognitive behavioral therapy Progressive muscle relaxation Acupuncture
Appears Promising	Music
Evidence Inconclusive	Ginger Massage

on anticipatory nausea commonly seen with chemotherapy or on delayed vomiting (occurring 24 hours to 5 days after chemotherapy) is not established. The efficacy of acupressure and wrist bands is less clear, with conflicting results from clinical trials (Alkaissi, Stalnert, & Kalman, 1999; Ezzo, et al., 2005; Ming, Kuo, Lin, & Lin, 2002; Roscoe, et al., 2002, 2003, 2005b).

Mind–body interventions are helpful adjuncts for managing nausea. **Hypnosis and guided imagery** have been reported to significantly reduce anticipatory nausea during chemotherapy in small randomized trials involving 20 and 30 patients with cancer, respectively (Jacknow, Tschann, Link, & Boyce, 1994; Yoo, Ahn, Kim, Kim, & Han, 2005). However, a randomized trial involving 67 bone marrow transplant patients found neither hypnosis nor cognitive behavioral coping skills training to reduce either nausea or vomiting (Syrjala, et al., 1992). **Behavioral therapies**, including **systematic desensitization**, have also been reported to reduce anticipatory nausea in two small randomized trials (Morrow & Morrell, 1982; Morrell, et al., 1992). **Relaxation therapies** such as **progressive muscle relaxation** training have also been reported to reduce both anticipatory and acute chemotherapy-induced nausea and vomiting, as observed in two trials involving 71 and 30 patients with breast cancer (Molassiotis, Yung, Yam, Chan, & Mok, 2002; Yoo, Ahn, Kim, Kim, & Han, 2005).

APPEARS PROMISING

Music significantly reduced the frequency and severity of nausea and vomiting in a small randomized controlled trial involving 39 patients receiving high-dose chemotherapy before bone marrow transplant, as compared to controls (usual antiemetic protocol) (Ezzone, Baker, Rosselet, & Terepka, 1998). Music might also improve mood and reduce anxiety, and thus is a promising adjunctive therapy.

EVIDENCE INCONCLUSIVE

Ginger might reduce nausea and vomiting by decreasing gastric motility, by stimulating intestinal peristalsis, and via antiserotonin effect (Abdel-Aziz, et al., 2005; Yamahara, Huang, Li, Xu, & Fujimura, 1990). A cross-over randomized trial reported no benefit of ginger root powder (1 g/day orally for 5 days) compared to placebo for reducing acute nausea and vomiting in 48 patients with gynecologic cancer receiving cisplatin-based chemotherapy (Manusirivithaya, et al., 2004). However, there was some suggestion of benefit in reducing delayed nausea/vomiting. In studies not involving patients with cancer, ginger (at least 1 g/day) has been reported to prevent morning sickness (Borrelli, Capasso, Aviello, Pittler, & Izzo, 2005), and postoperative nausea and vomiting (Chaiyakunapruk, Kitikannakorn, Nathisuwan, Leeprakobboon, & Leelasettagool, 2006).

Therapies that have a relaxation effect such as massage have the potential to reduce the perception of nausea. A 10-minute foot massage was associated with improved nausea immediately postintervention in a phase II trial involving 87 patients with cancer (Grealish, Lomasney, & Whiteman, 2000).

Anxiety and Mood

Mood disturbance (including anxiety and depression) is experienced by many cancer patients, albeit to a variable degree. CAM therapies including mind–body interventions, music, massage, and a few biological products are likely effective in improving mood symptoms (Table 24.6).

LIKELY EFFECTIVE

Mind–body interventions generally promote relaxation and help in mood elevation. One trial randomized 181 patients with breast cancer to either a **relaxation intervention** (consisting of a program of meditation, guided imagery, and ritual practices) or group support. The trial found both interventions to be

Table 24.6. Efficacy of Various Complementary Therapies for Cancer-Related Mood Symptoms, Based on Available Scientific Evidence.

Likely Effective	Cognitive behavioral therapy
	Progressive muscle relaxation
	Massage
	Music
	Healing touch
	St. John's Wort
	S-adenosyl methionine (SAMe)
Appears Promising	Acupuncture
	Passion flower
Evidence Inconclusive	Valerian
	Yoga

associated with a similar reduction in depression and anxiety (Targ & Levine, 2002). **Progressive muscle relaxation** (PMR) and **imagery** have been found to be effective in several controlled trials (Bridge, Benson, Pietroni, & Priest, 1988; Petersen & Quinlivan, 2002; Sloman, et al., 1994).

Massage promotes relaxation and has been tested in several clinical trials. In two meta-analyses involving 37 and 10 studies respectively, massage significantly improved anxiety (Fellowes, Barnes, & Wilkinson, 2004; Moyer, Rounds, & Hannum, 2004). The efficacy for reducing depression is less clear.

Music and healing touch are other therapies that promote relaxation. **Healing touch** was reported to significantly improve mood-related symptoms after 4 weeks of intervention in a cross-over randomized trial involving 230 subjects (Post-White, et al., 2003). Similar results were seen in two smaller randomized trials involving 36 and 88 patients respectively (Rexilius, et al., 2002; Smith, Reeder, Daniel, Baramee, & Hagman, 2003). **Music** therapy was reported to significantly reduce anxiety and depression in a randomized controlled trial involving 69 patients receiving bone marrow transplantation (Cassileth & Vickers, 2004).

St. John's Wort (*Hypericum perforatum*), a serotonin, dopamine, and norepinephrine reuptake inhibitor, was found to be efficacious in reducing mild-to-moderate depression in a meta-analysis of 37 trials (Linde, Berner, Egger, & Mulrow, 2005a; Linde, Mulrow, Berner, & Egger, 2005b). Controlled trials, however, have not been conducted among patients with cancer. An important limitation of using St. John's wort is its propensity to induce cytochrome P450 (CYP3A4 isoform) expression, thus resulting in significant drug interactions. (Markowitz, et al., 2003; Sparreboom, Cox, Acharya, & Figg, 2004).

S-Adenosyl-l-methionine (SAMe), a central methyl group donor, is involved in synthesis of monoaminergic neurotransmitters (Bottiglieri, et al., 1990). SAMe has been tested for depression in over 50 clinical trials. A meta-analysis of 47 clinical trials and two additional recent studies have reported SAMe to be efficacious in reducing depression compared to placebo (AHRQ review, 2002; Delle Chiaie, Pancheri, & Scapicchio, 2002; Pancheri, Scapicchio, & Chiaie, 2002).

APPEARS PROMISING

Yoga decreases central sympathetic activity and serum cortisol concentrations, and modulates cannabinoid receptors associated with relaxation (Stefano, et al., 2005; West, Otte, Geher, Johnson, & Mohr, 2004). Few small trials among young college students suggested that yoga might help reduce anxiety, stress, and depression (Janakiramaiah, et al., 2000; Malathi & Damodaran,

1999; Michalsen, et al., 2005; Ray, et al., 2001; Waelde, Thompson, Gallagher-Thompson, 2004; West, et al., 2004; Woolery, Myers, Sternlieb, & Zeltzer, 2004). In a trial involving 39 lymphoma patients, seven planned weekly yoga sessions did not provide any significant benefit, but the study results were limited by significant attrition (Cohen, et al., 2004). **Acupuncture** is another promising therapy for mood symptoms. According to traditional acupuncture theory, one of the relaxation points in the body is located at the "shenmen" point (near the infero-lateral wall of the triangular fossa in upper ear) and another "relaxation" point is located in the superior lateral wall of the triangular fossa. Two small randomized trials, involving 55 and 56 subjects, reported acupuncture to be efficacious for improving mood symptoms (Eich, et al., 2000). However, these studies did not involve patients with cancer.

Passion flower (*Passiflora incarnata*) is traditionally used for its anxiolytic properties. In a small randomized controlled trial involving 36 patients with generalized anxiety disorder, passion flower extract (45 drops/day) was reported to have similar efficacy as oxazepam (30 mg/day) after 4 weeks of treatment (Akhondzadeh, et al., 2001). Kava kava extract has anxiolytic properties (Pittler & Ernst, 2002) but has been associated with severe hepatotoxicity (Centers for Disease Control and Prevention, 2003; CDC, 2002).

EVIDENCE INCONCLUSIVE

Valerian has been postulated to have anxiolytic properties. However, a randomized trial among 36 patients with generalized anxiety disorder reported that valerian extract (valepotriates 81.3 mg/day) was no more efficacious than either placebo or diazepam (6.5 mg/day) for reducing anxiety after 1 month of treatment (Andreatini, Sartori, Seabra, & Leite, 2002). Another internet-based trial, involving 391 subjects with anxiety, also failed to show efficacy of valerian for improving anxiety.

Hot Flashes

Hot flashes are a major cause of morbidity among breast cancer survivors, who may have hot flashes that are more frequent and more severe than those experiencing natural menopause (Carpenter, et al., 1998). They can occur prematurely, secondary to surgery (oophorectomy), pelvic radiation, chemotherapy, androgen ablation therapy for prostate cancer, and treatment with tamoxifen or aromatase inhibitors (Loprinzi, Zahasky, Sloan, Novotny, & Quella, 2000; Schow, Renfer, Rozanski, & Thompson 1998; Stein, Jacobsen,

Table 24.7. Efficacy of Various Complementary Therapies for Cancer-Related Hot Flashes, Based on Available Scientific Evidence.

Likely Effective	Vitamin E
Appears Promising	Paced respiration
	Flaxseed
Evidence Inconclusive	Acupuncture
	Homeopathy
	Soy/isoflavone
	Herbal therapies with estrogenic potential*
Likely Ineffective	Red Clover
	Black cohosh
	Ginseng
	Genistein
	Primrose oil
	Dong quai
	Wild Mexican yam
	Magnetic therapy

*Shu Di Huang (*Rehmannia glutinosa*), Shan Zhu Yu (*Cornus officinalis*), Shan Yao (*Dioscorea opposita*), Ze Xie (*Alisma orientalis*), Dan Pi (*Paeonia suffruticosa*), Fu Shen (*Poria cocos*), Chen Pi (*Citrus reticulata*), Di Gu Pi (*Lycium chinensis*), He Huan Pi (*Albizzia julibrissin*), Suan Zao Ren (*Zizyphus jujuba*), Han Lian Cao (*Eclipta prostrata*) and Nu Zhen Zi (*Ligustrum lucidu*)

et al., 2002). While hormone replacement therapy (HRT) reduces hot flashes by about 80% to 90%, concerns about its adverse effect, including an increased risk of breast cancer and cardiovascular events, have led to decreased use of HRT. The etiology of hot flashes appears to involve the dysregulation of the central nervous system (CNS) thermoregulatory centers; central neurotransmitters appear to be an important mediator of hot flashes and form the basis of the efficacy of newer antidepressants (Shanafelt, Barton, Adjei, & Loprinzi 2002). Various complementary therapies have been studied for hot flashes, with mixed results (Table 24.7).

LIKELY EFFECTIVE

Vitamin E is a popular antioxidant vitamin that has been anecdotally thought to help reduce hot flashes. A randomized trial among 125 breast cancer survivors reported that vitamin E mildly reduced hot flashes (39%) compared to the placebo (21%) (Barton, et al., 1998). In this trial, vitamin E was associated with a decreased hot-flash frequency, on average, of one hot flash per person per day. Considering its low cost, widespread availability, relative safety profile, and nonhormonal mechanism, vitamin E alone might be a reasonable adjunctive therapy in women with mild-to-moderate hot flashes. Vitamin E might be considered for hot flash management when the clinical benefit required is minimal.

LOOKS PROMISING

Paced breathing involves the practice of slow, deep, and diaphragmatic breathing. It is postulated to help hot flashes by reducing central sympathetic activity and restoring autonomic balance. Small randomized controlled trials support that paced breathing improves hot flashes in postmenopausal women with no history of breast cancer (Freedman & Woodward, 1992; Freedman, et al., 1995; Germaine & Freedman, 1984; Irvin, Domar, Clark, Zuttermeister, & Friedman, 1996; Nedstrand, Wijma, Wyon, & Hammar, 2005).

Flaxseed contains lignans and is also considered to be a phytoestrogen. It is postulated to help in reducing hot flashes due to its weak estrogenic properties (but can also be an estrogen antagonist like other selective estrogen receptor modifiers such as tamoxifen). One trial involving 25 postmenopausal women reported that flaxseed reduced hot flashes to the same degree as hormone replacement therapy, but the women in the study had only mild menopausal symptoms (Lemay, Dodin, Kadri, Jacques & Forest, 2002). A nonrandomized pilot trial to evaluate its efficacy was conducted at the Mayo Clinic and found that flaxseed reduced hot flash frequency by 51% (Pruthi S, personal communication), and a phase III, placebo-controlled trial is being developed. It is interesting to note that flaxseed also has antiestrogenic properties; that is, it decreases circulating estrogen and is thus postulated to help reduce the risk of breast cancer (Brooks, et al., 2004; Haggans, et al., 1999; Hutchins, Martini, Olson, Thomas, & Slavin, 2001).

EVIDENCE INCONCLUSIVE

Acupuncture is postulated to increase central β-endorphin secretion and modulate central neurotransmitters involved in hot flash production (Wyon, Lindgren, Lundeberg, & Hammar, 1995). A few pilot trials have suggested that acupuncture might be effective in reducing hot flashes among post-menopausal women with breast cancer (Nedstrand, et al., 2005; Wyon, Wijma, Nedstrand, & Hammar, 2004), as well as in men with prostate cancer (Hammar, et al., 1999). However, a large trial among 103 participants found acupuncture to be no more effective than sham acupuncture in reducing hot flashes (Vincent, et al., 2007). Controlled trials in other settings have also shown mixed results (Cohen, Rousseau, & Carey, 2003; Ping, Ren-hai, & Zhong-xiang, 1998; Sandberg, Wijma, Wyon, Nedstrand, & Hammar, 2002; Wyon, et al., 1995).

Homeopathy may be a promising treatment for hot flashes with up to 75% reduction in hot flash frequency, as a few pilot trials initally suggested. (Bekkering & van den Bosch, 1993; Clover & Ratsey, 2002). However, two recent randomized trials involving 83 and 57 women with history of breast cancer reported that homeopathy was no more effective than placebo in reducing the hot flash severity score (Jacobs, Bent, Tice, Blackwell, & Cummings, 2005; Jacobs, Herman, Heron, Olsen, & Vaughters, 2005; Thompson, Montgomery, Douglas, & Reilly, 2005). The homeopathy arm did show a positive trend toward improvement and a subset analysis suggested homeopathy to be more effective than placebo among women not on tamoxifen.

Soy and isoflavones are popular herbal supplements with postulated phytoestrogen properties. Two recent meta-analyses involving 11 trials of soy supplements for hot flashes found mixed results (four positive studies, seven negative studies) and concluded that available data do not currently support their use (Kronenberg & Fugh-Berman, 2001; Nelson, et al., 2006).

Chinese herbal therapies have been postulated to have estrogenic potential and thus help hot flashes. Besides the phytoestrogens mentioned, these include Shu Di Huang (*Rehmannia glutinosa)*, Shan Zhu Yu (*Cornus officinalis*), Shan Yao (*Dioscorea opposita*), Ze Xie (*Alisma orientalis*), Dan Pi (*Paeonia suffruticosa*), Fu Shen (*Poria cocos*), Chen Pi (*Citrus reticulata*), Di Gu Pi (*Lycium chinensis*), He Huan Pi (*Albizzia julibrissin*), Suan Zao Ren (*Zizyphus jujuba*), Han Lian Cao (*Eclipta prostrata*), and Nu Zhen Zi (*Ligustrum lucidum*). Studies conducted in China using raw herbs have reported that these herbs reduce hot flashes (Yao, 1994). However, a randomized trial among 78 women found that a mixture of these 12 herbal supplements was no more effective than placebo in reducing hot flashes (Davis, et al., 2001).

LIKELY INEFFECTIVE

Controlled trials have shown genistein (Albertazzi, Steel, & Bottazzi, 2005), red clover (Baber, Templeman, Morton, Kelly, & West, 1999; Tice, et al., 2003), black cohosh (Jacobsen, et al., 2002; Pockaj, et al., 2006), ginseng (Wiklund, Mattsson, Lindgren, & Limoni, 1999), evening primrose oil (Chenoy, et al., 1994), dong quai (*Angelica sinensis*) (Hirata, Swiersz, Zell, Small, & Ettinger, 1998), wild Mexican yam (Dioscorea villosa) (Komesaroff, Black, Cable, & Sudhir, 2001), and magnetic therapy (Carpenter, et al., 2002) to be ineffective in reducing hot flashes.

Insomnia

Insomnia affects about 30% to 50% of cancer patients and is frequently under-recognized (Savard & Morin, 2001). Cancer pain, emotional distress, and depression all contribute toward insomnia and should be treated as a part of a comprehensive management plan. Mind–body interventions, particularly cognitive behavioral therapy and yoga, and biological products, such as valerian and melatonin, might help these patients (Table 24.8).

LIKELY EFFECTIVE

Mind–body interventions have efficacy in general comparable (if not greater) to conventional pharmacotherapy, with lasting therapeutic effect (Jacobs, Pace-Schott, Stickgold, & Otto. 2004; Morin, Colecchi, Stone, Sood, & Brink,

Table 24.8. Efficacy of Various Complementary Therapies for Cancer-Related Insomnia, Based on Available Scientific Evidence.

Likely Effective	Cognitive behavioral therapy
	Progressive muscle relaxation
	Yoga
Appears Promising	Valerian
	Melatonin
Evidence Inconclusive	Herbal therapies with sedative potential*

* Ashwagandha, Black cohosh, Brahmi, Catnip, Chamomile, Gotu-Kola, Herbal teas, Hops, Jujube, Lavender, Lemon balm, L-tryptophan, Poppy, Skull cap, and Yohimbine.

1999; Murtagh & Greenwood, 1995). A recent randomized trial confirmed the efficacy of cognitive behavioral therapy compared to a wait list control group for improving insomnia among 57 patients with breast cancer (Savard, Simard, Ivers, & Morin, 2005). Stimulus control and sleep hygiene education, progressive muscle relaxation (PMR), and hypnosis have all shown efficacy (Morin, Culbert, & Schwartz, 1994; Murtagh & Greenwood, 1995). A recent meta-analysis comparing different mind–body interventions suggested that combined cognitive behavioral therapy (CBT) was superior to single components of therapy (Wang, Wang, & Tsai, 2005). **Yoga** has shown efficacy in improving insomnia in several controlled trials involving both patients with cancer (Cohen, et al., 2004) and other conditions (Joseph, 1983; Khalsa, 2004; Manjunath & Telles, 2005).

APPEARS PROMISING

Valerian is postulated to help insomnia by decreasing the sleep latency and improving the quality of sleep among patients with insomnia. A systematic review in 2000, involving nine randomized trials, found contradictory results potentially because the studies had poor quality and heterogeneous methodology (Stevinson & Ernst, 2000). However, **valerian** (400 mg to 500 mg/day) has been reported to be efficacious in improving insomnia in several clinical trials, including large multi-institutional studies, that have not involved patients with cancer (Donath, et al., 2000; Hallam, Olver, McGrath, & Norman, 2003; Morin, Koetter, Bastien, Ware, & Wooten, 2005; Ziegler, Ploch, Miettinen-Baumann, & Collet, 2002). A randomized trial evaluating the efficacy of valerian among cancer patients with insomnia is currently being conducted by NCCTG.

Melatonin is another dietary supplement that is promising for the treatment of insomnia. Melatonin is an endogenous hormone secreted by the pineal gland and is involved in the maintenance of the circadian rhythm (sleep cycle) of the body. Melatonin thus has a strong physiological basis for helping insomnia, and the Food and Drug Administration (FDA) recently approved a drug, ramelteon, a selective melatonin receptor agonist, for the treatment of insomnia. Melatonin has been tested in multiple clinical trials and a meta-analysis involving 17 studies suggested that melatonin significantly reduced sleep-onset latency, increased sleep efficiency, and increased total sleep duration (Brzezinski, et al., 2005; Buscemi, et al., 2005). However, most of these trials involved healthy subjects and the efficacy of melatonin for insomnia in cancer patients is presently unclear.

EVIDENCE INCONCLUSIVE

Biological products with a sedative potential include: Ashwagandha, Black cohosh, Brahmi, Catnip, Chamomile, Gotu-Kola, Herbal teas, Hops, Lavender, Lemon balm, L-tryptophan, Skull cap, and Yohimbine (Cauffield & Forbes, 1999; Gyllenhaal, Merritt, Peterson, Block, & Gochenour, 2000; Mishra, Singh, & Dagenais, 2000; McKenna, Jones, Humphrey, & Hughes, 2001; McKenna, et al., 2001; Stough, et al., 2001). These agents need to be tested in controlled trials before any recommendation about their use for insomnia in cancer patients can be made.

Conclusion

CAM therapies can be helpful in the management of cancer symptoms and their efficacy is summarized in Table 24.9. Prominently, mind–body interventions appear beneficial in alleviating cancer pain, improving mood symptoms, and decreasing insomnia. Other relaxation therapies, including massage and music, might also help reduce these symptoms. Acupuncture can reduce nausea/vomiting and cancer-related pain. Aerobic exercise appears to reduce fatigue. Dietary supplements, including St. John's wort and SAMe, appear to be helpful in treating depression, while capsaicin cream can reduce cancer pain and postsurgical neuropathic pain.

Integrative oncology is a relatively young "science" and many of the promising therapies (listed in the chapter) are currently being tested in clinical trials. However, CAM research has its unique methodologic challenges. In addition, funding for CAM research is usually poor as pharmaceutical companies are not routinely interested in CAM and these therapies can usually not be patented (Rosenthal & Dean-Clower, 2005; Seidman & Babu, 2003; Vanherweghem, 2005). Moreover, in most places CAM practitioners are not fully integrated within the oncology community, making it difficult to accrue sizeable numbers of patients and conduct multi-institutional research (Eisenberg, et al., 2002; Frenkel & Borkan, 2003). Nevertheless, randomized controlled trials remain the gold standard to test the efficacy of a therapy, and several multi-institutional trials related to CAM therapies have been completed or are currently being conducted (Barton, et al., 2006). Hopefully the results of these will increase the armamentarium of the integrative oncologist in symptom management and palliative care.

Table 24.9. Summary of Efficacy of CAM Therapies for Cancer Symptoms, Based on Available Scientific Evidence.

Symptom	Likely Effective	Appears Promising	Evidence Inconclusive	Likely Ineffective
Pain	CBT PMR Support groups Capsaicin cream Acupuncture	Healing touch Herbal therapies Massage	Music therapy	
Fatigue	Exercise	Yoga CBT Levocarnitine Ginseng Acupuncture Healing Touch Massage Therapy	Homeopathy Siberian ginseng (Eleutherococcus)	
Anorexia, Cachexia		Creatine Melatonin		Fish oil Hydrazine
Nausea, vomiting	Acupuncture CBT PMR	Music	Ginger Massage	
Anxiety and Mood	CBT PMR Massage Music	Acupuncture Passion flower	Valerian Yoga	

(continued)

Table 24.9. (Continued)

Symptom	Likely Effective	Appears Promising	Evidence Inconclusive	Likely Ineffective
Hot flashes	Healing Touch St. john's Wort S-adenosyl methionine (SAMe)			
Hot flashes	Vitamin E	Paced respiration Flaxseed	Acupuncture Homeopathy Soy/isoflavone Herbal therapies with estrogenic potential*	Red clover Black cohosh Ginseng Genistein Primrose oil Dong quai Wild Mexican yam Magnetic therapy
Insomnia	CBT PMR Yoga	Valerian Melatonin	Herbal therapies with sedative potential†	

*Shu Di Huang (*Rehmannia glutinosa*), Shan Zhu Yu (*Cornus officinalis*), Ze Xie (*Alisma orientalis*), Dan Pi (*Paeonia stuffruticosa*), Fu Shen (*Poria cocos*), Chen Pi (*Citrus reticulata*), Di Gu Pi (*Lycium chinensis*), He Huan Pi (*Albizzia julibrissin*), Suan Zao Ren (*Zizyphus jujuba*), Han Lian Cao (*Eclipta prostrata*) and Nu Zhen Zi (*Ligustrum lucidum*)

†Ashwagandha, Black cohosh, Brahmi, Catnip, Chamomile, Gotu-Kola, Herbal teas, Hops, Jujube, Lavender, Lemon balm, L-tryptophan, Poppy, Skull cap and Yohimbine

CBT, Cognitive Behavioral Therapy; PMR, Progressive Muscle Relaxation.

REFERENCES

Bardia A, Barton DL, Prokop LJ, Bauer BA, & Moynihan TJ. (2006). Efficacy of complementary and alternative medicine therapies in relieving cancer pain: A systematic review. *Journal of Clinical Oncology,* 1, 24(34), 5457–64.

Barton DL, Loprinzi C, Jatoi A, Vincent A, Limburg P, Bauer B, et al. (2006). Can complementary and alternative medicine clinical cancer research be successfully accomplished? The mayo clinic-north central cancer treatment group experience. *Journal of the Society for Integrative Oncology,* 4(4), 143–152.

Ezzo J, Vickers A, Richardson MA, Allen C, Dibble SL, Issell B, et al. (2005). Acupuncture-point stimulation for chemotherapy-induced nausea and vomiting. *Journal of Clinical Oncology,* 23(28), 7188–7198.

Fellowes D, Barnes K, & Wilkinson S. (2004). Aromatherapy and massage for symptom relief in patients with cancer. *Cochrane Database of Systematic Reviews (Online),* (2), CD002287. Review.

Jatoi A, Rowland K, Loprinzi CL, et al. (2004). An eicosapentaenoic acid supplement versus megestrol acetate versus both for patients with cancer-associated wasting: A North Central Cancer Treatment Group and National Cancer Institute of Canada collaborative effort. *Journal of Clinical Oncology,* 22, 2469–2476.

Kronenberg F & Fugh-Berman A. (2002). Complementary and alternative medicine for menopausal symptoms. a review of randomized, controlled trials. *Annals of Internal Medicine,* 137, 805–813.

Linde K, Ramirez G, Mulrow CD, Pauls A, Weldenhammer W, & Melchart D. (1996). St. John's wort for depression: An overview and meta-analysis of randomized clinical trials. *BMJ,* 313, 253–258.

McNeely ML, Campbell KL, Rowe BH, Klassen TP, Mackey JR, & Courneya KS. (2006). Effects of exercise on breast cancer patients and survivors: a systematic review and meta-analysis. *CMAJ,* 175(1), 34–41.

Morrow GR & Morrell C. (1982). Behavioral treatment for the anticipatory nausea and vomiting induced by cancer chemotherapy. *The New England Journal of Medicine,* 307(24), 1476–1480.

Savard J, Simard S, Ivers H, & Morin CM. (2005). Randomized study on the efficacy of cognitive-behavioral therapy for insomnia secondary to breast cancer, part I: Sleep and psychological effects. *Journal of Clinical Oncology,* 23(25), 6083–6096.

(A complete reference list for this chapter is available online at http://www.oup.com/us/ integrativemedicine).

25

CAM Therapies to Mitigate the Toxicities of Cancer Therapy

BRIAN D. LAWENDA AND PETER A.S. JOHNSTONE

KEY CONCEPTS

■ Numerous complementary and alternative medicine (CAM) modalities have been demonstrated, through well-designed clinical trials, to be effective in the management and prevention of side effects of conventional oncologic treatments.

■ Acupuncture and certain mind–body therapies (like music therapy and guided imagery) can be successfully employed in patients suffering from chemotherapy-induced nausea and vomiting.

■ In addition to pharmacologic interventions, acupuncture, massage, and other mind–body therapies are useful adjuncts in the management of cancer pain.

■ Various CAM therapies have been shown to be effective in mitigating fatigue, the most commonly reported side effect in cancer patients.

■ Numerous trials support the use of CAM therapies in the management of treatment-induced hot flashes; however, there is no consensus on their clinical effectiveness.

■ Xerostomia (dry mouth), a side effect of head and neck radiation therapy, can be treated successfully with acupuncture.

■

Despite significant improvements in supportive care, development of less toxic chemotherapy regimens, and advancements in the delivery and targeting of radiation therapy, our patients continue to suffer from a multitude of treatment-related toxicities. In recent years, this area of symptom management has become a focus of significant interest in complementary and alternative medicine (CAM) research. Data from numerous clinical trials have been published supporting the safety and efficacy of a wide range of CAM therapies as adjuncts to, or in lieu of, conventional pharmacologic treatments in managing side effects of cancer treatment. In this chapter, we will present five commonly encountered treatment-related toxicities and discuss the indications and evidence surrounding the use of various CAM therapies to mitigate these symptoms.

Chemotherapy-Induced Nausea and Vomiting

Nausea and vomiting are among the most frequently reported side effects of patients undergoing chemotherapy. These symptoms not only affect the patient's quality of life but can also impact negatively on treatment adherence [1,2]. The mechanisms behind CINV involve a combination of variables including neuropathophysiological and psychological factors, patient age and gender, concomitant symptoms, and tumor burden [3]. The development of 5-HT$_3$ serotonin and NK$_1$ receptor antagonist compounds have significantly improved CINV outcomes; however, many patients continue to suffer from these symptoms [4]. Prospective studies have demonstrated the following nonpharmacologic interventions to be safe and effective adjunctive therapies in managing CINV:

Acupuncture-point stimulation (APS) [5–9]
Music therapy [10]
Guided imagery (GI) [11,12]
Progressive muscle relaxation [11,13]

ACUPUNCTURE POINT STIMULATION

In 1997, the National Institutes of Health (NIH) consensus panel on acupuncture concluded that this modality has demonstrated "promising results" in the treatment of CINV [14]. This conclusion was based on the results of two randomized trials that reported on the use of APS for CINV [15,16]. Subsequent trials have demonstrated conflicting results on efficacy yet have clearly established that APS is a safe adjunctive modality in managing CINV [17,18]. Ezzo et al. published a meta-analysis of 11 randomized trials of APS for managing CINV [19]; a review of these data is appropriate here. Only trials that were rated by two experienced acupuncturists as having used adequate acupuncture-point stimulation techniques were included in the analysis, and all permitted the use of conventional antiemetic medicines. In a pooled analysis of one manual (MA) and three electroacupuncture (EA) trials, the authors reported an absolute reduction of 23% ($P = 0.01$) in the proportion of patients experiencing acute vomiting in the acupuncture arms versus the control arms. Three of these four trials used sham controls. Combined data from the EA trials demonstrated an absolute reduction of 23% in the proportion of patients experiencing acute vomiting ($P = 0.02$), although only older antiemetic agents were used in these trials. The single MA trial did use modern antiemetics and yielded no difference in acute vomiting outcomes between the MA and control groups. Combined analysis of two acupressure (AP) trials, both using modern antiemetics, showed an improvement in both mean acute nausea severity [standardized mean difference (SMD) = –0.19, $P = 0.03$] and in worst acute nausea score (SMD = –0.02, $P = 0.03$); however, these trials were not sham controlled. The pooled data from four noninvasive electrical stimulation (NES) trials were not found to exhibit differences between the control or NES arms on any acute CINV outcomes. No acupuncture trial provided valid data on delayed CINV.

The authors recommend that cancer patients only use the services of state-licensed acupuncturists (L.Ac), trained professionals in Traditional Chinese Medicine, or trained physician acupuncturists who both have experience and comfort treating patients with cancer.

In conclusion, APS is a safe treatment that appears, in some patients, to be an effective adjuvant modality in mitigating the severity of acute CINV. EA appears to be more active than either MA or NES; however, further studies are needed to determine the clinical relevance of using EA in the setting of modern antiemetic agents.

MIND–BODY THERAPIES

Mind–body therapies (MBTs) overlap with more conventionally recognized fields of behavioral medicine. These involve various relaxation techniques to help relieve stress, anxiety, pain, and other symptoms associated with illness and therapy. Behavioral intervention procedures are among the most widely offered psychosocial services at comprehensive cancer centers [2]. In a review of 13 randomized control trials (RCTs) that used behavioral interventions for treatment of anticipatory CINV, 12 of these studies demonstrated effectiveness in controlling this side effect [2]. Although there are many forms of MBTs, we will limit our discussion to three modalities which have reported beneficial effects on CINV: music therapy, GI, and progressive muscle relaxation. The use of cognitive distraction techniques (i.e., GI or music therapy) are thought to work by blocking an aversive stimulus (i.e., pain or nausea) by refocusing the patient's attention to a particular task or nonaversive stimulus [2].

MUSIC THERAPY

Music therapy (MT) is defined as the use of music to affect an individual's physical, emotional, and behavioral well-being, which leads to healing [20]. MT was shown, in a small, randomized study to be an effective adjunct to standard antiemetic medicines in managing the symptoms of CINV [10]. Thirty-nine patients undergoing bone marrow transplantation (BMT) were randomized to receive either standard antiemetic medications (IV ondansetron) with MT (45-minute recordings of self-selected music at 6, 9, and 12 hours after the start of chemotherapy) or antiemetic medications alone during 48-hours of high-dose chemotherapy. The MT arm had significant reductions in the number of vomiting episodes and decreased nausea scores using a visual analog scale. In a smaller trial, Sahler et al. reported a pilot case-controlled study on the use of MT with "relaxation imagery" in patients undergoing chemotherapy for BMT [21] Twenty-three patients received a 45-minute MT intervention after BMT (mean: 5 days after BMT; range: 1–13 days) for an average of 5 sessions (range: 2–13). Self-reported nausea scores improved significantly compared to the case-control group ($P < 0.001$).

This type of treatment is easy to administer and individualize for each patient. When implementing MT in clinical practice, it is important to take into account the patients' music preference. Research has shown that music preference is an important predictor of positive response [20,22,23]. Importantly, Music Therapists may be integral members of the oncology team; as such, they play a crucial role in the implementation of this highly-individualized complementary treatment [24].

GUIDED IMAGERY AND PROGRESSIVE MUSCLE RELAXATION THERAPY

Progressive muscle relaxation therapy (PMRT) involves sequentially "tensing and releasing" groups of muscles in the upper part of the body and then progressing to muscle groups in the lower part of the body. Further relaxation may be augmented with breathing exercises (i.e., slow or deep breathing) and GI. GI is the technique of diverting an individual's attention from their present situation (i.e., receiving chemotherapy) to a mental image or place that is relaxing to them. Molassiotis et al. reported their results of a randomized controlled trial of 71 patients who were undergoing chemotherapy for breast cancer [13]. All patients received standard antiemetic medications as needed and were assigned to either a control group (no intervention) or the experimental group (PMRT and GI). There was a significant reduction in the duration of nausea and vomiting ($P < 0.05$) and a trend toward lower frequency of nausea ($P = 0.07$) and vomiting ($P = 0.08$) in the experimental arm compared to control. A similar study by Yoo et al. reported that the patients who were randomized to a PMRT and GI arm exhibited a significant reduction in both anticipatory nausea and vomiting and postchemotherapy nausea and vomiting than patients in the control arm [11]. Gaston-Johansson et al. randomized over 100 patients undergoing chemotherapy for BMT to either a control group or a "comprehensive coping strategy program" (including preparatory information, cognitive restructuring, and relaxation with GI) [12]. The experimental arm had a significant reduction in nausea scores compared to the control arm.

As with MT, it is important to keep in mind that standardized PMRT and GI treatment regimens may be less efficacious than an individualized treatment regimen [25].

Pain

The majority of cancer patients experience pain at some point during their treatment course [26,27]. Complementary interventions are often used in addition to conventional pharmacologic interventions for managing pain.

ACUPUNCTURE POINT STIMULATION

Auricular acupuncture is a common APS modality used in treating a variety of pain conditions. Alimi et al. published an elegant RCT using auricular acupuncture in patients with cancer pain [28]. Ninety patients with persistent cancer-related pain, despite conventional analgesic medications, were randomized to one of three arms: (1) auricular acupuncture at points where an electrodermal signal had been detected; (2) auricular acupuncture at sites with no electrodermal signal (placebo points); and (3) noninvasive auricular seeds placed at placebo points. The authors reported a 36% reduction in pain from baseline at 2 months in the group receiving APS. The placebo groups had a reduction of only 2%. The difference between the groups was significant ($P < 0.0001$).

MIND–BODY THERAPIES

Redd et al. reviewed 12 studies investigating the impact of various types of behavioral interventions (i.e., hypnosis, relaxation techniques, and GI) on cancer treatment–related pain [2]. Eleven of the 12 trials reported a reduction in pain with the integration of these therapies. The authors of two similar literature reviews also concluded that mind–body therapies (i.e., hypnosis, massage therapy, relaxation/imagery, and supportive counseling), including cognitive-behavioral interventions, can provide pain relief in cancer-related or treatment-related (i.e. mucositis) pain [29,30].

Music therapy can offer patients who have even advanced cancer pain improved comfort and quality of life [24]. In a Cochrane database review on MT for pain relief, Cepeda et al. concluded that listening to music reduces pain intensity levels and opioid requirements [31]. The magnitude of this effect was small (i.e., 15.4%–18.4% reduction in postoperative morphine requirements, 2 and 24 hours after surgery, respectively) but was statistically significant (95% CI: −2.0 to −0.2 and −8.8 to −2.6, respectively).

MASSAGE THERAPY

In 2005, Corbin reported the findings of a MEDLINE and CINAHL database review of therapeutic massage usage in cancer patients [32]. The author concluded that under the care of a qualified massage therapist, massage may be safely incorporated into conventional cancer care and that data most strongly support its efficacy in reducing stress and anxiety.

Research supporting massage for pain control is promising but is less strongly supported. Post-White et al. published a randomized controlled trial of 230 patients undergoing treatment for cancer [33]. The patients received conventional pharmacologic medications for any treatment-related side effects and for therapeutic massage, healing touch, or standard care. The authors reported a significant reduction in pain after either therapeutic massage or healing touch, with less nonsteroidal anti-inflammatory drug use at 4 weeks during massage. In a large single-institution (n = 1290 patients), nonrandomized study of the effects of various types of therapeutic massage in cancer patients, Cassileth et al. reported a 40% improvement in subjective pain scores from baseline [34]. In the outpatient setting, this benefit persisted throughout a 48-hour follow-up period.

Narcotic pain medications have many untoward side effects, including fatigue, diminished ability to concentrate, nausea, and constipation. Adjuvant treatment with various CAM modalities for pain control has been shown to decrease narcotic medication requirements and thus significantly improve quality of life in cancer patients.

Fatigue

The most commonly reported symptom in cancer patients is fatigue, often associated with chemotherapy and/or radiotherapy [35,36]. Fatigue is complex in origin and may be caused by physical, biochemical, and psychosocial variables. Appropriately, various CAM therapies have been studied for their roles in helping treat this potentially debilitating symptom.

Acupuncture has been shown to improve postchemotherapy fatigue in a single-institution, phase II study [37]. In this study, patients who had completed chemotherapy on average more than 2 years previously reported a 31% improvement from baseline in fatigue scores after either a 4- or 6-week regimen of acupuncture. Fatigue may also be ameliorated following treatment with therapeutic massage. In the previously mentioned study by Cassileth et al., massage decreased fatigue scores in cancer patients by approximately 40% from baseline levels [34].

Relaxation and GI techniques have also shown promise in treating fatigue. Gaston-Johansson et al. reported a significant reduction in the fatigue in patients with breast cancer who were undergoing chemotherapy for bone marrow transplantation [12], when these patients participated in a program that included both relaxation and GI techniques. Similar findings were reported in a small randomized controlled trial of relaxation breathing exercise in cancer patients undergoing stem cell transplantation [38]. In this study, the effects of relaxation-breathing exercises on fatigue scores were compared to a control group receiving no treatment. The authors reported significant reduction ($P = 0.04$ to 0.001) in several fatigue score variables compared with controls.

Hot Flashes

Hot flashes are a common complaint in both sexes after cancer therapy: women being treated with antiestrogens or selective estrogen receptor modulators to prevent or treat breast cancer and men after orchiectomy or luteinizing hormone releasing hormone-agonist treatment [39,40]. A number of CAM therapies have shown promise in various reports in treating vasomotor symptoms: acupuncture [41–43], black cohosh [44,45], and relaxation-response training [43,46]. However, a literature review by Kessel et al. in 2002 concluded that based on their analysis of the studies published to date, "...specific, evidence-based recommendations on the use of CAM therapies for menopausal symptoms cannot be made [47]." These authors cited problems stemming from study design issues such as inadequate placebo and controls, deficiencies of quality control in botanical products, variations in the patient populations (i.e., premenopausal/cancer patients and postmenopausal patients) and outcome measures being examined.

Similar conclusions were reached in a separate review of randomized clinical trials of CAM use for menopausal symptoms [48] and in a review on CAM therapies for reducing hot flashes in prostate cancer patients [49]. The use of phytoestrogen supplementation (e.g., soy products) should be discouraged in women with breast cancer, especially those who have estrogen receptor–positive disease or who are taking tamoxifen, until more robust clinical studies have investigated potential stimulatory risk of these agents on breast cancer cells [50].

> Despite the lack of overwhelming clinical evidence supporting specific CAM therapies in successfully managing treatment-related hot flashes, the authors do not discourage patients from trying potentially promising treatments since compliance with hormonal therapies has been shown to be an important factor in their cancer outcome. Patients are much more likely to continue taking hormonal therapies if treatment-related side effects like hot flashes can be diminished.

Xerostomia

Xerostomia is a common side effect in patients who have undergone radiation therapy for cancers of the head and neck. Although artificial salivary lubricants and muscarinic cholinergic stimulants (i.e., pilocarpine) are the mainstay of xerostomia management, promising results have been demonstrated with acupuncture. Results of a randomized Swedish trial in patients with xerostomia are of particular interest [51]. In these data, 24 acupuncture treatments yielded a 68% response rate and "placebo" acupuncture yielded increased salivary flow rate in 50% of patients. The placebo points were chosen for their proximity to "real" acupuncture points, and ultimately were considered inappropriate as placebo controls. The two groups were considered together for subsequent analyses. All patients had increased flow rates at the 6-month follow-up evaluation when compared to baseline. Patients who continued acupuncture afterwards had higher stimulated and unstimulated flow rates at 3 years when compared to those patients who had not continued acupuncture [52].

Johnstone et al. reported that 70% of patients in their pilot study (n = 50 patients) of auricular acupuncture exhibited a significant improvement in subjective scoring of their xerostomia severity using a regimen of three-to-four weekly treatments [53]. In a phase I–II study (n = 37 patients) of acupuncture-like transcutaneous nerve stimulation, Wong et al. reported an 86% and 77% improvement in xerostomia symptom scores at 3 and 6 months after completion of treatment, respectively [54].

Conclusion

Side effects of cancer treatment are common and significantly impact on the quality of life of our patients. In this chapter, we have reviewed several trials and analyses of CAM therapies which have shown promise in helping to ameliorate some of these untoward symptoms. We support continuing research of CAM therapies for cancer symptom control, and their continuing publication in conventional peer-reviewed journals. Only with such rigor, and exposure, may these promising modalities become proven, and more widely available to our patients.

REFERENCES

1. Bernhard J, Hurny C, Coates AS, Peterson HF, Castiglione-Gertsch M, Gelber RD, et al. (1997). Quality of life assessment in patients receiving adjuvant therapy for breast cancer: the IBCSG approach. The International Breast Cancer Study Group. [Erratum appears in *Annals of Oncology*, 1998, 9(2), 231]. *Annals of Oncology*, 8(9), 825–835.
2. Redd WH, Montgomery GH, & DuHamel KN. (2001). Behavioral intervention for cancer treatment side effects. *Journal of the National Cancer Institute*, 93(11), 810–823.
3. Rhodes VA & McDaniel RW. (2001). Nausea, vomiting, and retching: Complex problems in palliative care. *CA: A Cancer Journal For Clinicians*, 51, 232–248.
4. Kris MG, Hesketh PJ, Somerfield MR, Feyer P, Clark-Snow R, Koeller JM, et al. (2006). American Society of Clinical Oncology Guideline for Antiemetics in Oncology. Update 2006. *Journal of Clinical Oncology*, 24(18), 2932–2947.

5. Streitberger K, Friedrich-Rusi M, Bardenheuer H, Unnebrink K, Windeler J, Goldschmidt H, et al. (2003). Effect of acupuncture compared with placebo-acupuncture at P6 as additional antiemetic prophylaxis is high-dose chemotherapy and autologous peripheral blood stem cell transplantation: A randomized controlled single-blind trial. *Clinical Cancer Research*, 9, 2538–2544.

6. Shen J, Wenger N, Glaspy J, Hays RD, Albert PS, Choi C, et al. (2000). Electroacupuncture for control of myeloablative chemotherapy-induced emesis: A randomized controlled trial. *JAMA*, 284, 2755–2761.

7. Roscoe J, Morrow G, Hickok J, Bushunow P, Pierce HI, Flynn PJ, et al. (2003). The efficacy of acupressure and acustimulation wrist band for the relief of chemotherapy-induced nausea and vomiting. *Journal of Pain and Symptom Management*, 26, 731–742.

8. Treish I, Shord S, Valgus J, Harvey D, Nagy J, Stegal J, et al. (2003). Randomized double-blind study of the Reliefband as an adjunct to standard antiemetics in patients receiving moderately high to high emetogenic chemotherapy. *Support Care Cancer*, 8, 516–521.

9. Josefson A & Kreuter M. (2003). Acupuncture to reduce nausea during chemotherapy treatment of rheumatic diseases. *Rheumatology*, 42, 1159–1154.

10. Ezzone S, Baker C, Rosselet R, & Terepka E. (1998). Music as an adjunct to antiemetic therapy. *Oncology Nursing Forum*, 25, 1551–1556.

(A complete reference list for this chapter is available online at http://www.oup.com/us/ integrativemedicine).

26

Alternative Therapies as Primary Treatments for Cancer

STEPHEN M. SAGAR

KEY CONCEPTS

- Alternative therapies for cancer are typically promoted as viable treatment options, that is, *alternatives* to so-called mainstream therapies such as chemotherapy, radiation, and surgery.
- Alternative therapies are unproved, rarely based on credible scientific rationale, and potentially harmful, especially when patients are led away from effective, proven therapies by the lure of false promises and an emphasis on a lack of adverse side effects as compared with conventional therapies.
- Proponents of alternative therapies that are alleged to cure cancer often propose ad hoc quasi-scientific interventions—heavily marketed with scanty evidence based on a combination of simple and untrue logic, together with a series of misleading testimonials.
- Some alternative therapies are based on traditional systems such as Chinese, Ayurvedic, and homeopathic medicine—these may be primary therapies for cancer in developing countries, although their efficacy when used alone is highly debatable.
- Complementary medicine is to be distinguished from alternative medicine—the two are often bundled together under complementary and alternative medicine (CAM)—its goal is to increase the efficacy of conventional cancer treatment programs, to reduce symptoms, and to improve quality of life for cancer patients.
- Alternative therapies appeal to patients who have grown exasperated with the treatment they have received in traditional care modalities, are terrified of the adverse reactions to conventional

therapies, or are desperate for a cure, having been told that their cancer is incurable.

- The patient should be specifically questioned about alternative therapies as part of their initial intake assessment.
- Reassuring patients of continued support is important so that patients do not live in fear of abandonment and become vulnerable to the psychological allure of bogus alternative therapies.
- Some alternative therapies are innovative postulates that may be developed from observations within a best case series—an open-minded but critical attitude is necessary to test hypotheses within the rules of science.

■

Definition of Alternative Therapies

There is a lack of agreement on an accepted definition of alternative therapies. Some define alternative therapies as those that are not widely practiced in hospitals or taught in US medical schools, but this tautology is not helpful. The term *alternative medicine* is attractive to some patient's unique values, attitudes, beliefs, and emotions, central to which is the unwavering belief in the body's ability to heal itself with help from a perceived relatively nontoxic intervention. Sometimes these patients are suspicious of the medical profession, are fearful of side effects, may be anxious in a clinical environment, or may be suffering from emotional disorders. Alternative therapy practitioners often focus on "holism," or the tenet that all aspects of a person—body, mind and spirit—are interrelated and should be treated as a whole. Often there is the belief in the concept of "energy" that balances the mind, body, and spirit. The recognition of the multidimensional attributes of being human is important and should be evaluated by conventional practitioners to improve communication, help patients feel better and improve their quality of life.

Some alternative therapies are based on traditional systems such as Chinese, Ayurvedic, and homeopathic medicine. These may be primary therapies for cancer in developing countries, although their efficacy is highly debatable. In developed countries, these traditional therapies are usually used as adjuncts to biomedical care, in which case they are complementary and have merit in improving symptom control and a more positive outcome. Conventional therapies, such as mind–body medicine may be misused as primary therapy for cancer, rather than to improve coping skills, symptom control, and quality of life when used together with conventional anticancer therapies. Proponents of alternative therapies that are alleged to cure cancer often propose ad hoc quasi-scientific interventions. These are usually heavily marketed and the evidence based on a combination of simple and, usually, untrue logic, together with a series of misleading testimonials. The focus of this chapter is not on cultural health systems that are integrated into the conventional biomedical systems as adjunctive complementary care, but on the ad hoc quasi-scientific interventions based on unproven hypotheses and limited anecdotal experience that are touted for the primary treatment of cancer. Some of these practitioners are honest with good intent, but naive, whereas others are overt frauds with intent to gain from susceptible patients. Fraudulent practitioners can vary from sophisticated Western-style clinics peddling pseudo-scientific interventions to individuals practicing psychic surgery in Third world conditions. Most of these interventions have achieved a cult status through the predatory effects of branding a chance of cure to a desperate and susceptible population. Their popularity is through the attraction of mythological concepts rather than objective evidence of cure. The Internet has amplified the use of alternative therapies using multi-level marketing schemes.

This chapter will focus on the misuse of alternative therapies as primary treatments for cancer. In general, the evidence for efficacy of any therapy must be at the highest possible level. The only exception to this would be when no proven conventional therapy exists and the intervention does not have significant toxicities, financial burdens, or environmental impacts that will shorten and reduce the patient's quality of life. Even if toxicity is absent, the patient should not be subjected to a crusade of mythological hope to "off-shore" clinics that can be a major financial burden, as well as reducing quality of life by being away from loved ones in a foreign environment. In addition, complications and symptom control may be dealt with poorly when away from the conventional medical environment. If patients are treated with honesty, kindness, compassion, and respect, and allowed to express their own personal values, most will undertake conventional therapies and partake in clinical trials. At the same time, some may wish to pursue complementary therapies that may enhance their conventional treatment and help in symptom control and the reduction of adverse side effects. This is best done by being part of a team of integrative oncology professionals. Discussion of these options will encourage most cancer patients to stay under the care of their oncology specialists and other credible health-care professionals.

What is alternative? Although conventional therapies were previously defined as surgery, radiotherapy, and cytotoxic chemotherapy, usually with curative intent, therapies are now more diverse—monoclonal antibodies, enzyme inhibitors, cytokines, photodynamic therapy, antibiotics for gastric MALT lymphoma, antiangiogenic compounds, gene therapies, immune therapies, vaccinations, and refined botanical derivatives. Now we also accept the tenet that stability of tumor growth, in the presence of sustained quality of life, is a desirable goal for many patients.

Abandonment of the Conventional Biomedical System

Alternative therapies appeal to patients who have grown exasperated with the treatment they have received in traditional care modalities, are terrified of the adverse reactions to conventional therapies, or are desperate for a cure, having been told that their cancer is incurable. Alternative therapies may offer short-term hope, but are not usually successful. With few anecdotal exceptions, if conventional therapies offer an evidence-based opportunity for long-term benefit, then substituting an unproven alternative treatment may result in losing the best opportunity for survival. Often, the so-called successes of primary alternative therapies have no proven pathology, have received concurrent conventional therapies, or are cancers that wax and wane, such as low-grade lymphomas. Practitioners of primary alternative therapies for cancer often judge success if the patient happens to outlive the prognosis indicated by their physician (which is known to be notoriously inaccurate) or outlives historical controls, another method of comparison that is extremely biased. Champions of alternative therapies often argue that they have been suppressed by the establishment, despite the fact that the Office of Cancer Complementary and Alternative Medicine of the National Cancer Institute (OCCAM) provides ample opportunity for innovative research on best case series.[1,2] Some alternative practitioners claim that their practice cannot be subjected to scientific research because of complex systems and difficulties providing a comparative or sham treatment. Although there are challenges, scientific methodology can be developed to evaluate all interventions [3]. When designing studies, it is important to recognize unwarranted assumptions about the consistency and standardization of CAM interventions, the need for data-based justifications for the study hypotheses, and the need to implement appropriate quality control and monitoring procedures during the trial.

The term *complementary medicine* is to be distinguished from *alternative medicine*. Historically, the two are bundled together under the term *complementary and alternative medicine* (CAM). Alternative therapies are typically promoted as viable treatment options: "alternatives" to so-called mainstream therapies such as chemotherapy, radiation, and surgery. Alternative therapies are unproved, rarely based on credible scientific rationale, and potentially harmful—especially when patients are led away from effective, proven therapies by the lure of false promises and an emphasis on a lack of adverse side effects as compared with conventional therapies [4–6]. There is no alternative to scientifically evaluated, evidence-based medicine. Most patients who use unconventional therapies (all but 2%) do so to complement rather than to replace mainstream treatment [7]. However, because of desperation or fear, or because of inadequate support and communication, patients may seek alternative therapies. Research studies conclude that patients who abandon conventional biomedical treatments do so for the following reasons [8–12]:

Anger and fear

The patient may be angry at the health-care system or their physician. They may fear the clinical health-care environment, adverse side effects, or the blunt presentation of prognosis. Some patients may not be able to cope because of underlying depression.

Lack of control

Some patients may feel a loss of control in the conventional health-care system, whereas a primary alternative approach can give them a sense of empowerment. On the other hand, open decision making may be overwhelming, and some patients give themselves over to the alternative practitioner.

Belief in a cure

The alternative approach may provide a more positive belief system for cure. A negative prognostic approach by a conventional practitioner may persuade a patient to seek an alternative therapy that is unjustly branded as delivering a cure.

Social group association

A peer group of social support may be very persuasive at encouraging alternative therapies, based on misinformation and the urge to be helpful.

Mysticism

Healing symbols and spiritual healing give some patients feelings of control and coping. This may help them through turbulent experiences, cushioning them against fears.

Globally, many patients may be deprived of effective modern anticancer therapies secondary to a lack of modern resources and primitive cultural beliefs [8]. In developing countries, factors such as ignorance, socioeconomics, and inadequate access to mainstream medical facilities play an important role in patients opting for alternative therapies that are replacements for, rather than adjuncts to, mainstream therapy [13–17].

Communication issues between patients and health professionals appear to be the major cause of biomedical abandonment. Research by Montebriand et al. contains numerous instances of angry confrontations and inadequate communication strategies by health professionals [8]. When diagnosed with cancer, patients are vulnerable and emotions are easily stimulated. Anger may arise within the consultation. Health professionals may distance themselves from the anxiety of the cancer situation. Both verbal and nonverbal messages can be interpreted as lack of interest and lack of hope. Conversely, the informants believe they receive hope when communicating with alternative practitioners. Exclusive use of alternative therapies is often associated with hope for a cure and unresolved personal issues or unrealized biomedical expectations. Health professionals need improved communication skills; medical information should give hope. Patients bring more than just their concerns about cancer to the clinical situation. They bring present and past experiences, sociocultural interpretation, and spiritual beliefs.

Patients should be encouraged to express their personal perceptions of health care. Frank and caring communication can happen only if professionals take time to listen (without anger), especially when patients discuss alternatives. Negative biomedical experiences, such as iatrogenic complications, are often concealed from the health professional. Frank exploration of these experiences is appropriate. Patients tend to suppress negative revelations lest their future care be jeopardized. By being aware of patients' possible hesitancy, professionals should develop thoughtful strategies for accessing their personal history. Education is imperative. One survey in a country with a highly developed health-care system found that one-third of the respondents thought that alternative therapies could be used *instead of* conventional cancer treatments [18].

The Internet and Alternative Therapies for Cancer Treatment

Although the Internet has enabled self-empowerment, there is little regulation of the validity of the information. Many alternative therapies are touted as "cures" for cancer and deliver misleading pseudo-scientific information that usually has a heavy commercial bias [19]. A survey of web sites on CAM for

Table 26.1. Credible Web Sites for Evaluation of Alternative Therapies
for Cancer Patients (Accessed July, 2008).

Consortium of Academic Health Centers for Integrative Medicine
http://www.imconsortium.org.

National Center for Complementary and Alternative Medicine
http://nccam.nih.gov

NCI Office of Cancer Complementary and Alternative Medicine (OCCAM)
http://www.cancer.gov/cam

Society for Integrative Oncology
http://www.integrativeonc.org

Memorial Sloan Kettering Cancer Center
http://www.mskcc.org/aboutherbs

MD Anderson Cancer Center
http://www.mdanderson.org/departments/CIMER

BC Cancer Centre
http://www.bccancer.bc.ca/PPI/UnconventionalTherapies/default.htm-CAMEO Program
http://www.bccancer.bc.ca/RES/ResearchPrograms/cameo/default.htm

American Cancer Society
http://www.cancer.org/docroot/ETO/ETO_5.asp?sitearea=ETO

cancer rated the quality of information from an evidence-based perspective [20]. The most popular web sites offer information of extremely variable quality, many endorsing unproven therapies, of which some had the potential for actually harming patients. Some sites actively discourage conventional therapies, such as surgery, chemotherapy and radiotherapy, which they refer to as "cutting, poisoning and burning." The Internet addresses of some credible web sites are listed in Table 26.1.

Outcome of Cancer Patients Who Use Alternative Medicine as Primary Treatment

Studies of outcome are all controversial since prospective randomized controlled studies are usually avoided because subjects often want to self-select their therapies. Publications are usually retrospective surveys that are prone to bias due to many confounding factors. This is well illustrated by the research that attempted to evaluate outcome in breast cancer patients who attended the Bristol Cancer Help Centre (BCHC) in the United Kingdom, compared to those who simply received conventional therapies [21]. The BCHC was set up in 1979 to offer various alternative therapies for patients with cancer. The alternative treatments were mainly vegetarian diets and psychospiritual interventions. Most subjects also received conventional chemotherapy. The study was retrospective and compared a sample of women who attended the BCHC with case controls who attended a specialist conventional cancer center. The authors' conclusions were that patients who were free of metastases at entry to the study had a poorer metastasis-free survival if they attended the BCHC. Survival in relapsed cases was also significantly inferior for those attending the BCHC. However, the methodology of the study was totally inadequate, with many potential confounding factors and biases [22]. The premature release of the inconclusive results to the media as "fact" led to anguish in subjects who attended the BCHC and a major public outcry that was associated with the suicide of a senior oncologist who was one of the authors [23]. This situation illustrates the opposing sociopolitical cultures of conventional versus alternative medicine and that emotions can override reason on both sides. The negative side was that the pious and bigoted attitude of the researchers, despite using a poor methodological design, discouraged alternative medicine practitioners to participate in studies. The positive side of this tragic affair is the emphasis that prospective randomized trials offer the best chance of giving these therapies a fair evaluation, and that the practitioners themselves should be involved in the planning and design. Suitable modifications of methodology may be used even when subjects wish to self-select their therapies.

A Norwegian study examined the association between alternative medicines and cancer survival. This was a prospective study with a follow-up of 8 years of over 500 cancer patients. About 20% of the patients used alternative medicine. Death rates were higher for alternative medicine users, and after appropriate statistical adjustment the hazard ratio for death was 1.3 for any use of alternative medicine compared with no use (95% CI: 1.99–1.7). It had the most detrimental effect in patients with better performance status, with a hazard ratio reaching 2.32 (95% CI: 1.44–3.74, $P = 0.001$) [24]. A study in the United States attempted to test the feasibility of measuring outcomes of cancer patients at two CAM clinics (The Bio-Medical Center in Tijuana, Mexico, and the Livingston Foundation Medical Center in San Diego, California) [25,26]. The objectives were to determine the feasibility of obtaining and collecting data from medical records, determining 5-year survival, and comparing 5-year survival to that of conventional treatment. The study concluded that systematic monitoring of outcomes was warranted and that for data to be meaningful, disease status must be pathologically confirmed and patient follow-up improved.

The effect of using alternative therapies on psychological status is confounded by many variables. Many of these subjects are using conventional as well as alternative therapies. It is difficult to determine whether the therapies are intended to be complementary and improve supportive care, or are designed to "cure" cancer. One study suggested that the use of complementary medicine in breast cancer patients is more common among depressed subjects [27]. On the other hand, another study showed no association between anxiety and depression, but use of complementary therapies was associated with an increased patient perception of breast cancer recurrence and death [28]. The most frequently cited reason for using CAM was to reduce the symptoms of psychological distress, and the most frequently used CAM for gaining a feeling of control was the use of diet and nutritional supplements [29]. Many subjects have a naive view of cancer etiology and believe there is a common cause, usually toxin based [30]. Screening for these psychological attributes may prevent needless seeking of unproven therapies and inappropriate diets that are said to "detoxify" but often lead to malnutrition. Most patients do not have the scientific background to distinguish bogus therapies from those that have a rational scientific basis, are evidence-based, or are under the close scrutiny of a clinical trial [31]. Reassuring patients of continued support, no matter what therapy they select, is important so that patients do not live in fear of abandonment and become vulnerable to the psychological allure of bogus alternative therapies.

Popular Alternative Therapies

Table 26.2 summarizes alternative therapies that are unproved, weakly based on credible scientific rationale, and are potentially harmful, especially when the patients are led away from effective proven therapies [4,5,7,32]. In addition to idiopathic toxicity of some natural health products, interactions with pharmaceutical and anticancer chemotherapy agents administered must be considered. The patient should be specifically questioned on alternative therapies as part of their initial assessment. I will not discuss all of the unproven therapies, but instead will focus on some of the more common alternative therapies that patients become aware of in North America and illustrate the enthusiasm based on cultural hype, rather than concrete evidence.

Alternative Nutrition Therapies

Macrobiotic therapy was developed by a Japanese philosopher, George Ohsawa, and then popularized in the United States by his disciple, Michio Kushi [33,34].

Table 26.2. Alternative Therapies Promoted for Cancer Treatment That Have Been Researched and Shown to Be Ineffective or Lack Credible Evidence.

Dietary "Cures"
No-dairy diet
Macrobiotic diet
Gerson diet

Biological Treatments
Antineoplastons
Immunoaugmentation Therapy
Shark Cartilage
714-X
Cancell
Oxygen therapies
Electrotherapies (e.g. Rife machine)
Hulda Clark's Cure for All Cancers
Insulin potentiation

Botanical Treatments
Essiac (Flor-essence)
Amygdalin (Laetrile)
Mistletoe (Iscador)
Pau d'arco tea
Chaparral tea
Noni, Mangosteen and Goji juices
Hoxsey regimen (poke root, burdock root, barberry root, buckthorne bark, stillinga root)

The diet is one part of a lifestyle that includes exercise, meditation, stress reduction, and avoidance of pesticides [35]. The content of the diet is high in complex carbohydrates and low in fat and animal protein. The diet recommends organically grown and minimally processed foods. Cereal grains form about 50% (buckwheat, brown rice, barley, millet, oats), vegetables form about 25%, and beans form about 10% (chickpea, lentils, tofu) of the diet. Seaweed, fish, seeds, nuts, and fruit are permitted occasionally. Meat, poultry, animal fats, dairy, eggs, refined sugars, and foods that contain artificial sweeteners are eliminated. Special teas are the only recommended beverages. Clearly, there are some components of both the diet and lifestyle that can contribute to wellness and possibly cancer prevention. However, a macrobiotic diet may result in complications if used as an alternative therapy for cancer treatment. First, there is no evidence that it is effective for treating cancer that has already developed. Individuals with cancer usually cannot consume enough calories to maintain their weight. The diet can result in protein deficiency, vitamin B12 and calcium deficiencies, dehydration, and a strong emotional burden placed on the individual and family [35].

Max Gerson developed the Gerson diet in the 1940s as a dietary approach to treat tuberculosis [36]. Gerson developed this diet to treat cancer by focusing on the role of minerals, enzymes, hormones, and various other dietary factors that may reverse conditions postulated to support the growth of cancer. He also believed that the body required "detoxification" with sodium and fat restriction, potassium supplementation, and a raw-food vegetarian diet. The program recommends a raw vegetarian diet, drinking hourly glasses of freshly prepared vegetable and fruit juices made from organic fruits and vegetables [37]. Various supplements include an iodine solution, vitamin B_{12}, potassium, thyroid hormone, an injectable crude liver extract, and pancreatic enzymes [38]. Coffee enemas are recommended to facilitate the release of toxins from the liver. Salt, oil, nuts, berries, drinking water, and all bottled, canned, refined, preserved, and processed foods are forbidden, and aluminum utensils cannot be used for cooking. Patients have developed complications including flu-like symptoms, loss of appetite and weakness, intestinal cramping, diarrhea, and vomiting. Bacterial poisoning may have occurred from the crude liver extracts and electrolyte imbalances may have resulted from the daily enemas [38]. The impracticalities of hourly juicing can make this diet very stressful for the patient and family. Many cancer patients find it difficult to consume this diet when their appetite is already suppressed. Some of the complications, especially from the enemas and injection of liver extract, are dangerous and should be avoided.

The Gonzalez regimen is a modification that administers large doses of pancreatic proteolytic enzymes. A case series suggested that patients with advanced pancreatic adenocarcinoma lived longer than the average survival derived from the National Cancer database [39]. The NCCAM originally funded a randomized controlled trial of the Gonzalez regimen, compared to conventional therapy with gemcitabine, but it failed to recruit patients and now continues in a nonrandomized form. A recent preclinical study of pancreatic enzyme extracts fed to nude mice transplanted with human pancreatic cancer xenografts reported slowing of tumor growth and prolonged survival [40]. The data indicate that the beneficial effects of the pancreatic enzymes on survival are primarily related to the nutritional advantage of the treated mice. The potential benefits of pancreatic enzymes for patients with pancreatic cancer are intriguing and need to be studied further.

Another dietary regimen is Sun Soup. It was developed by Alexander Sun, a biochemist who once worked at Yale University. The ingredients are soybean, mushroom, red date, scallion, garlic, lentil bean, leek, mung bean, hawthorn fruit, onion, American ginseng, angelica root, licorice, dandelion root, senegal root, ginger, olive, sesame seed, and parsley. The therapy falls within the tradition of Chinese medicine. A methodologically weak pilot study, in which patients also received conventional therapies, seemed to increase survival more than historical controls and seemed to reduce adverse symptoms [41]. The results are encouraging, especially because some of the herbal ingredients are known to modulate immune parameters and host tissue responses to cancer.

Noni, Goji, and Mangosteen Juices

Juices made from exotic fruits have become some of the most popular therapies alleged to aid the cure of cancer. They are all heavily promoted by pyramid Internet marketing schemes and misleading scientific references that describe preclinical studies with very obscure relevance to clinical effectiveness. They are made all the more alluring by their described panacea of curing most disease, extending life, and their mystical origins from Southern Pacific islands and the Himalayan Mountains. Usually, the marketing strategies follow a "bait-and-switch" approach, leading with claims of their traditional use over thousands of years, followed by nonspecific science that is inconsistent with traditional usage patterns. Often the content of the juices does not reflect the active phytochemical sources of the plant, and the final product is mixed with other juices (such as grape). Some preparations are pasteurized, which can alter chemical content, and unpasteurized versions may be susceptible to bacterial contamination.

Noni (*Morinda citrifolia L*) is a traditional Polynesian medicinal plant. It contains various antioxidants and some polysaccharides that can induce an immune response and cancer cell apoptosis in mouse models. Unfortunately, any other evidence is based on Polynesian traditional medicine without clinical scientific evidence. *M. citrofolia* is being promoted as a "natural hope in a bottle [42]." Moreover, there is some controversy over its potential hepatotoxicity [43,44].

The latest fad juices claiming to cure cancer include the various brands of Goji berry juice. This is derived from the berry of *Lycium barbarum*. The genuine product is alleged only to come from the mysterious valleys between the mountains of Tibet. In fact, it is also grown in the Yellow River valley in China and Mongolia, where it is distinguished as the species *Lycium chinenses* or Wolfberry. It can also be grown in Europe and North America, but these facts tend to destroy the allure of its mystical tradition. The distributors claim that it contains the highest antioxidant levels of any product, as measured by the oxygen radical absorption capacity (ORAC). However, the relevance of this is controversial, and the values vary widely according to manufacturing methods and shelf life. Preclinical studies demonstrate a series of polysaccharides (LB polysaccharides) that may have anticancer activity especially through immune mechanisms [45]. There is just a single report of a clinical trial for cancer using a Goji extract [46]. It was carried out by Cao and colleagues at the Second Military Medical University in Shanghai and published in a Chinese medical publication, the *Chinese Journal of Oncology*. Seventy-nine patients with advanced cancer were enrolled in a trial in which they were treated with lymphocyte-activated killer (LAK) cells and interleukin-2 (IL-2). Some of the patients also received polysaccharides derived from *Lycium barbarum*. Initial results of the treatment from 75 evaluable patients indicated that objective regression of cancer was achieved in patients with malignant melanoma, renal cell carcinoma, colorectal carcinoma, lung cancer, and nasopharyngeal carcinoma. The response rate of patients treated with LAK and IL-2 alone was 16.1%. When Goji extract was given to some patients the response rate jumped to 40.9%. The authors also state that the remission in patients treated with LAK and IL-2 plus Goji extract lasted significantly longer and led to a more marked increase in natural killer (NK) cell activity than LAK and IL-2 alone. There are many deficiencies in the study that render the results inconclusive and the study does not support the claims for marketing Goji juice as part of an anticancer program. People should be cautioned that it does have some anticoagulant properties that may especially be detrimental for those taking warfarin [47].

Mangosteen (*Garcinia mangostana*) is a tropical fruit native to Southeast Asia. The major component is a group of phytochemicals called *xanthones*. In preclinical studies, they have antioxidant, anti-inflammatory, and antiproliferative effects against cancer cells [48]. Most of the preclinical studies were done on the rind, and not the fruit, which is used for preparation of the juice. There are no clinical trials and no evidence that Mangosteen reduces tumor burden or delays progression of disease. Large levels of antioxidants could potentially interact with chemotherapy and radiotherapy, and its high sugar content may be detrimental, especially to diabetics.

Oxygen, Hydrogen Peroxide, and Ozone Therapies

The claims that oxygen can cure cancer are based on the concepts of William Koch and Otto Warburg. Koch theorized in 1919 that cancer was caused by a metabolic defect produced by a toxin that was normally burned off during oxidation of carbohydrates. Credibility for oxygen therapy was enhanced by Warburg, winner of the Nobel Prize for medicine in 1931, for elucidating the chemistry of cell respiration. He observed that cancer cells have lower respiration rates than normal, and postulated that cancer cells grow better in a low-oxygen environment, and that introducing higher oxygen levels could kill them. The discovery of hypoxia-inducible factor-1 (HIF-1) allowed the identification of molecular mechanisms by which changes in oxygenation (secondary to abnormal tumor vasculature) are transformed to intracellular adaptive responses. Hypoxia can initiate cell demise by apoptosis/necrosis and also prevent cell death by provoking adaptive responses that, in turn, facilitate cell proliferation or angiogenesis, thus contributing to tumor progression [49]. The increase in dissolved oxygen that can be attained is unlikely to compensate for the hypoxia. A great deal of research has been done with hyperbaric oxygen and radiotherapy. An analysis of the studies concluded that there was some improvement in tumor control [50]. On the other hand, preclinical studies with hyperbaric oxygen, *without* radiation, showed no increase in tumor control [51]. Currently, antiangiogenic agents are thought to have more potential for improving oxygenation and preventing metastases [52].

Although Warburg discovered some differences in metabolism between normal and cancer cells, research did not bear out his hypothesis that tumors rely on anaerobic respiration [53]. There is no clinical trial that supports cancer therapy with oxygen, except for its combined use with radiotherapy, and that has been surpassed by using radiation with chemotherapy and antiangiogenic agents. The oxygen fanatics also advocate hydrogen peroxide. This can produce oxygen free radicals (that can be antiseptic). Hydrogen peroxide injected into venous blood is decomposed by the enzyme catalase into molecular oxygen and water. The oxygen is taken up by oxygen-depleted hemoglobin. However, this simply means that less oxygen from inspired air in the lungs is required to saturate it. When arterial blood leaves the lungs it is normally almost fully saturated with oxygen, and so it becomes impossible for the intravenous infusion of hydrogen peroxide advocated by "oxygenation" proponents to further increase the amount of oxygen carried to the tissues. The amount dissolved in plasma is negligible. No systematic studies have proven its efficacy for cancer therapy. Potential adverse effects include gas embolism and lung damage [54,55].

Ozone therapy was advocated by a German physician named Seigfried Rilling. Like hydrogen peroxide, it produces highly reactive oxygen free radicals. With no evidence to support its use against cancer, its proponents advocated its use for AIDS using ozone "autohemotherapy." A randomized controlled trial failed to demonstrate efficacy, although the advocates complained that the dose was inadequate [56].

High-Dose Vitamin C

The claim that vitamin C is useful in the treatment of cancer was made by the Nobel Prize laureate, Linus Pauling, since the early 1970s [57,58]. He hypothesized that high doses of vitamin C could be preferentially toxic to tumor cells. Laboratory experiments show mixed results. To date, unlike the numerous studies on cancer prevention, relatively little systematic clinical studies have been done on the use of vitamin C in the treatment of cancer. Orthomolecular medicine usually incorporates high doses of vitamin C with other vitamins [59]. There is some evidence that survival and symptom control may be improved in some cases by reversal of vitamin C deficiency, which appears to be common in many cancer patients [60]. The use of vitamin C as a tumor cytotoxic chemotherapeutic agent has been proposed [61]. To date, studies have demonstrated that vitamin C can be infused at a high enough rate to maintain blood levels of vitamin C proven high enough to kill tumor cells in a test tube [62]. However, current clinical research has not proven that the infusion levels of vitamin C make a significant impact on tumor burden in patients with cancer.

Investigators at the Mayo Clinic conducted a placebo-controlled double-blind study, which was reported in 1979 [63]. One hundred and fifty patients with advanced cancer participated in the double-blind placebo-controlled study to evaluate the effects of high-dose vitamin C on symptoms and survival. The two groups showed no significant difference in changes in symptoms, performance status, appetite, or weight. The median survival for all patients was about 7 weeks, and the survival curves overlapped. Pauling criticized the trial on the grounds that the cytotoxic chemotherapy given to the large majority of patients before study entry might have inhibited the ability of vitamin C to stimulate host defenses. This criticism persuaded Moertel to conduct a second study [64]. This was a double-blind study of 100 patients with advanced colorectal cancer who were randomly assigned to treatment with either high-dose vitamin C (10 g daily) or placebo. Overall, these patients were in very good general condition, with minimal symptoms. None had received any previous treatment with cytotoxic drugs. Vitamin C therapy showed no advantage over placebo therapy with regard to either the interval between the beginning of treatment and disease progression or patient survival. Among patients with measurable disease, none had objective improvement. On the basis of this and the previous randomized study, Moertel concluded that high-dose vitamin C therapy is not effective against advanced malignant disease regardless of whether the patient has had any prior chemotherapy.

Proponents criticized the design of both the studies, specifically the focus on patients with advanced disease and limited life expectancy, the route of administration (oral rather than intravenous), the sudden withdrawal of vitamin C in some cases, and patient selection criteria. High-dose vitamin C appears to have little toxicity, rarely causing kidney stones, but it can interfere with certain laboratory tests for glucose, uric acid, creatinine, and inorganic phosphate and can interfere with the detection of occult blood in feces [65]. Some preliminary clinical data indicate that vitamin C may improve the survival of cancer patients. However, most of the studies were either anecdotal reports or uncontrolled case series, and therefore the results, although suggestive, are not conclusive [66].

> Although previous, carefully performed randomized trials of *oral* vitamin C therapy involving patients with advanced cancer failed to demonstrate any therapeutic benefit, there is recent evidence from laboratory experiments to support the possibility that high-dose intravenous treatment might be more effective. High-dose vitamin C targets cancer cells that contain higher iron levels compared to normal cells and can convert Vitamin C to pro-oxidants The pro-oxidants can induce the death of the cancer cells. More research is necessary to define pharmacokinetic data, dosage and safety of high-dose intravenous vitamin C, the most biologically active dose, which tumor types are most sensitive, its efficacy against advanced cancer, and its effect on quality of life.

Laetrile and Amygdalin

These are a family of compounds called cyanogenic glycosides, sometimes referred to as vitamin B_{17} (although not a vitamin). Amygdalin occurs naturally in a number of plant materials. The usual commercial source is the apricot pit—the kernel of *Prunus armeniaca L.* The source varies appreciably in their amygdalin or laetrile content [67]. The noted biochemist Ernest Krebs first postulated amygdalin as an anticancer agent, on the basis that it would be broken down by an enzyme in cancer tissue to liberate cyanide, which would kill the cancer [68]. Advocates of laetrile therapy for cancer believe that an enzyme, β-glucosidase, capable of breaking down the laetrile to release toxic cyanide, exists in large amounts in tumors, but only in small quantities in normal tissues. They further hypothesize that another enzyme, called *rhodanese,* has the ability to detoxify cyanide and is present in normal tissues but deficient in cancer cells. These two factors supposedly combine to effect a selective poisoning of cancer cells by the cyanide released from the laetrile, while normal cells and tissues remain undamaged. No evidence is available to support this theory. All data published in reputable scientific journals reveal that Laetrile has no selective antitumor activity against either animal or human cancers [69]. The National Cancer Institute (NCI) sponsored an independent study of Laetrile with cancer patients, led by Dr. Charles Moertel, and published in 1982 [70]. The clinical trial involved 178 patients. Patients had histologically proven cancer for which no standard treatment was known to be curative or to extend life expectancy. All patients had received no surgery, radiation therapy, or chemotherapy for 1 month. The amygdalin used for treatment was prepared from apricot pits and supplied by the pharmaceutical resources branch of the National Cancer Institute. Patients selected were in good general condition, were ambulatory, and were able to maintain good nutrition. Patients who were disabled and bedridden were ineligible for the study. The routes, dosage, and schedule of administration were chosen to be representative of the current Laetrile practice. Patients were also placed on a diet identical to the one recommended by most Laetrile practitioners. Each patient had measurable histologically proven tumors. Of 171 fully documented patients, only one patient met the criteria for partial response. All patients had tumor progression by 7 months. Amygdalin therapy did not slow the advance of malignant disease or induce stabilization. There were significant blood levels of cyanide in some of the patients. Laetrile has been banned by the U.S. Food and Drug Administration (FDA) because of the risk of poisoning from its cyanide content.

Coenzyme Q10

Coenzyme Q10 (CoQ10) is an antioxidant, synthesized naturally in the body. A small case series reported the remission of breast cancer in three patients who were being treated with CoQ10. In all three cases the CoQ10 treatment was provided during the same time that the patients were undergoing conventional treatments (mastectomy, radiotherapy, and anticancer drugs). The remission of breast cancer in these patients cannot be attributed with any certainty to the CoQ10 treatment that was provided [71,72]. There is some evidence that CoQ10 can ameliorate cardiac toxicity from adriamycin. CoQ10 is not clinically proven to be effective as a cancer treatment by itself [73,74].

Dimethylsulfoxide

Dimethylsulfoxide (DMSO) is a turpentine-based by-product of paper manufacturing, first synthesized in 1866. As medication, DMSO was used initially in the 1960s. Following approval for experimental use, it was applied in topical form to relieve pain, reduce swelling, heal injuries such as muscle strains and sprains, and treat arthritis [6]. The only approved use of DMSO in the United States is for treating interstitial cystitis. It has been proposed as a cancer treatment, although evidence for its efficacy as a cancer treatment is nonexistent. DMSO is said to stimulate the immune system and scavenge hydroxyl radicals. Since free radicals can promote tumor growth, this was proposed to be one of the mechanisms by which DMSO interferes with the development of cancer. It also explains why patients who receive DMSO while undergoing either chemotherapy or radiation (both of which generate free radicals in order to kill cancer cells) are far less prone to such side effects as hair loss, nausea, and dry mouth. Preclinical evidence suggests it could increase the potential for metastases [75]. DMSO is considered an unproven and ineffective method of treating cancer. It is used as a preservative for frozen transplant cells and has a distinct acrid odor.

Hydrazine Sulfate

The principal proponent and developer of hydrazine sulfate is Joseph Gold, an American research oncologist at the Syracuse Cancer Research Institute, a private, non-profit institute. Gold was influenced by the research of Warburg, who had proposed that an important distinguishing feature of cancer cells is their propensity to obtain energy through the anaerobic, rather than the aerobic, metabolism of glucose. The chemical has been used in refining metals and for rocket fuel [6,76]. Gold has advised the use of hydrazine sulfate for all forms of cancer. A preclinical study that investigated the effects of hydrazine sulfate on both in vitro and in vivo models of prostate cancer showed no growth inhibition [77]. Early clinical studies at the Memorial Sloan-Kettering Cancer Center showed no benefit [78]. Hydrazine sulfate was evaluated in a double-blind, placebo-controlled study that included 291 newly diagnosed, untreated patients with non–small cell cancer of the lung, randomly selected after optimal treatment with cisplatinum and etoposide [79]. There was no evidence of an increased response rate or survival difference as a result of the hydrazine, but there was evidence of a poorer quality of life in the treated group. There was no difference in the two arms of this double-blind study with regard to anorexia, weight gain, or nutritional status. Inappropriately high doses of hydrazine sulfate can result in neuropathy, nausea, vomiting, hypoglycemia and drowsiness. Also, since hydrazine sulfate is a monoamine oxidase inhibitor (MAOI), people using hydrazine sulfate should avoid foods that are rich in tyramine to avoid the consequences of hypertension. The conclusion is that hydrazine sulfate has never been shown to act as an anticancer agent. Patients treated with hydrazine sulfate do not live longer than non-treated patients. Randomized controlled trials show that it neither reduces cachexia nor treats cancer. The rationale that it acts as an anticancer agent because it deprives cancers of their energy by inhibiting gluconeogenesis is erroneous [80].

Pao D'Arco

Pao D'Arco [*Tabebuia serratifolia (Vahl)*] is an ancient Incan remedy that has been developed into capsules and teas. The main extract is lapachol. As with many herbal extracts, lapachol can be toxic to cancer cells in vitro [81,82]. In clinical trials, 19 patients with advanced nonleukemic tumors and 2 patients with chronic myelocytic leukemia in relapse were given lapachol in doses ranging from 250 to 3750 mg/day for 5 days. The largest total dose received was 3000 mg/day for 21 days. All patients had previously received a variety of therapies, which had failed. One patient with metastatic breast cancer had resolution of a single osteoblastic hip lesion, but no change in numerous other bony lesions. All other patients either remained clinically unchanged in condition or experienced advancing disease. Toxicity observed in patients participating in the clinical trials included nausea and vomiting and reversible prolongation of prothrombin time at very high doses [83]. In 1985, Pao D'Arco was banned by Health Canada until distributors could prove that it is safe and effective. The FDA does not allow it to be advertised or sold as a treatment, prevention or cure for cancer.

Chaparral Tea

Chaparral is a Native American remedy, prepared by grinding leaves and twigs of an evergreen desert shrub known as the Creosote Bush (*Larrea divericata Coville*). The active ingredient of chaparral is a potent antioxidant, nordihydroguaiaretic acid (NDGA) [84]. Recent preclinical studies of NDGA have demonstrated promising anticancer activities. NDGA induces apoptosis as a result of disruption of the actin cytoskeleton, in association with the stress activated protein kinases. Some credible preclinical research suggests that it may be a lead compound in the development of novel therapeutic agents for various types of cancer [85]. Chronic ingestion of Chapparal can cause severe liver toxicity and possible renal disease. No clinical trials have proven its efficacy in humans. Health Canada and the FDA have banned the distribution of Chaparral products [86]. The recent promising preclinical results may stimulate modification of the molecule to increase efficacy and reduce toxicity and provide the possibility of systematic clinical trials [87,88].

Wormwood (Artemisinin)

Artemisinin is extracted from *Artemisia annua L.* It is an effective antimalarial therapy because it reacts with the high iron concentrations found in the malaria parasite. This reaction generates free radicals that kill the infected cells by destroying their membranes. A Cochrane review suggests that artemisinin drugs are effective and safe for treating uncomplicated malaria. There is no evidence from randomized trials that any one artemisinin derivative is better than the others [89]. Preclinical studies suggest that it may be a relatively selective anticancer agent, especially when tagged with transferrin [90]. Artemisinin reacts with iron to form free radicals that kill cells. Since cancer cells take up relatively large amount of iron compared to normal cells, they are more susceptible to the toxic effect of artemisinin. This extract also demonstrates antiangiogenic activity that may be important for cancer control [91]. Artemisinin appears to be a relatively safe compound that causes no significant adverse effects even at high oral doses. The species, *Artemisia annua L.* should be distinguished from *Artemisia absinthium*, used to manufacture a French liqueur called *absinthe*. The whole plant or oil extract of *Artemisia absinthium* contains a high level of thujone that has hallucinatory properties and may cause renal failure [92]. This illustrates the importance of authentication of herbs and their derivatives and the dangers inherent in confusing species and using the wrong extracts. Authenticated artemisinin has the potential to be used in clinical studies that will evaluate its role in anticancer therapy.

> Some natural health products should be evaluated further for their effects on immunity and anticancer activity. Many botanicals and mushrooms found in the Chinese medicine pharmacopoeia have positive effects on immunity and anticancer activity. These should be authenticated and evaluated further for safety and efficacy through controlled clinical trials.

Essiac Tea

René Caisse (1888–1978), a Canadian nurse, devoted more than 60 years of her life to treating cancer patients with an herbal formula she named Essiac (Caisse spelled backward) [93–97]. The formula was originally obtained through a Native American healer (from the Canadian Ojibwa tribe), and was later modified by Caisse to include both an orally administered fraction (a decoction) and an intramuscularly injected fraction. She kept the ingredients of the formula secret until the last few years of her life. Caisse treated thousands of patients with Essiac. Public support for Caisse and her clinic was overwhelming, and in 1938 the Essiac formula came within three votes of being legalized as an anticancer treatment by the Ontario legislature. Instead, the legislature created a Royal Cancer Commission to review unorthodox treatments such as Essiac. The commissioner's report was unfavorable, and dismissed most of the tales of recovery as improper original diagnosis. Caisse closed her clinic a few years later. In 1959, at the age of 70, Caisse was introduced to Charles Brusch. He was impressed with Caisse's work, and invited her to treat cancer patients under his supervision at the Brusch Medical Center in Massachusetts. In October of 1977, one year before her death, Caisse disclosed the ingredients of the formula to Resperin Corporation of Canada with the understanding that Resperin would conduct clinical trials of the orally administered product at two Canadian hospitals and at numerous private clinics.

Although there is some evidence for inhibition of division of cultured cancer cells [98–101], no evidence of efficacy beyond the placebo effect was found in the clinical studies [102]. A more recent uncontrolled study of 360 patients with breast, prostate, or gastrointestinal cancer taking Essiac reported that 30% felt it had helped them. The benefit was described as psychological in 54%, physical in 29%, and unspecified in the remainder [103].

No published scientific evidence exists to suggest that the Essiac formula has clinical efficacy. However, anecdotal evidence exists to this effect and public support is considerable. The phytochemicals in the formula with the greatest potential to produce an anticancer effect are the anthraquinones, rhein, and emodin. High molecular weight polysaccharides could also have a stimulating effect on the immune system. However, it seems unlikely that the small concentrations of these compounds in the marketed formula would lead to any significant anticancer action [104].

PC-SPES

The herbal complex, PC-SPES, illustrates the potential for botanical products to be used as an alternative approach to treat cancer, but unfortunately also illustrates the common pitfalls of alternative therapies, such as adulteration with undeclared pharmaceuticals and poor quality assurance (especially of products imported from Asia). PC-SPES (originally distributed by Botanic Labs) consists of eight herbs, all but two from Traditional Chinese Medicine: *Serenoa repens* (saw palmetto), *Panax pseudo-ginseng* (ginseng),

Chrysanthemum morifoliu (chrysanthemum), *Ganoderma lucidum* (reishi mushroom), *Glycyrrhiza glabra* (licorice), *Isatis ingigotica* (dyer's woad), *Rabdosia rubescens* (rubescens), and *Scutellaria baicalensis* (skullcap). Ingredients were chosen to produce multifactorial activity. *Serenoa repens* can decrease the symptoms of benign prostatic hypertrophy (BPH). A systematic review of 18 randomized trials, involving more than 2000 patients, concluded that saw palmetto improves urologic symptoms and urine flow as effectively as finasteride, but with less toxicity [105]. In vitro studies suggest moderate antiproliferative activity against prostate cancer cell lines [106]. *Scutellaria* contains baicalin, a compound with known antiproliferative activity [107]. *Ganoderma lucidum* has multiple activities that include inhibiting cell adhesion, cell migration, and cell invasion in vitro, as well as stimulation of immunity in vivo [108–111]. Licorice contains estrogenic compounds that can inhibit prostate cancer [112]. Laboratory research supports the activity of PC-SPES against prostate cancer. Antiproliferative and pro-apoptotic effects have been demonstrated on tumor cell lines in vitro [113–115]. In rat models, PC-SPES decreased the incidence of spontaneous tumors and reduced the weight of implanted tumors [116]. It demonstrated estrogenic activity [117]. Phase II studies show that prostate-specific antigen (PSA) declines in the majority of patients evaluated, including those with androgen-independent cancer [113–115]. Significant improvements in pain and quality of life have also been reported [118]. A phase II trial in 70 patients with prostate cancer showed more than an 80% decline in PSA in all androgen-dependent patients, with PSA becoming undetectable in 82% [119]. At a median follow-up of 64 weeks, none of these patients had progressed. In addition, over half the patients with androgen-independent disease had a PSA response of over 50%, with a median duration of 18 weeks. PC-SPES was associated with some endocrine side effects, including decreased libido, erectile dysfunction, gynecomastia, and hot flashes, as well as increased thrombotic events [120–122]. An NCI phase III study was launched to determine whether PC-SPES caused an increase in survival, but was terminated when quality assurance procedures showed that the clinical preparation that was manufactured in China, contained diethylstilbestrol (DES), coumadin, indomethacin, and alprazolam [123,124]. This prompted the FDA to issue a recall of PC-SPES in 2002. The manufacturers of PC-SPES, Botanic Labs, ceased operations and will no longer manufacture or market PC-SPES. No other North American sources of this combination botanical product are currently known. It is still intriguing that the decline in PSA was greater for PC-SPES that was potentially contaminated with DES, than for the comparator group that received DES alone, suggesting some independent activity [125,126].

714X (Cerbe, Rock Forest, Canada)

714-X is the name given to an alternative therapy developed by Gaston Naessens, a French microbiologist now residing in Quebec, Canada [6]. The name "714-X" reflects Naessens' pride. The numbers "7" and "14" represent the 7th and 14th letters in the alphabet (Naessens' initials), and the "X," the 24th letter in the alphabet, represents the year of his birth (1924). Naessens believes in somatids, that is, living organisms present in live blood that he observed in individuals with cancer. The 714X is supposed to return the somatids to a normal state. It contains a mixture of camphor, ammonium chloride and nitrate, sodium chloride, ethanol, and water. It must be injected intralymphatically via a lymph node in the groin. Naessens was arrested in Quebec in 1989 and charged with four counts of illegal practice of medicine and one count of contributing to the death of a patient. In Canada, despite the prosecutions, 714-X may be requested by physicians on a compassionate plea under the Emergency Drug Release Program [127]. Outside Canada, 714-X is available in Mexico and Western Europe but not in the United States, where it is currently under investigation by the FDA.

Antineoplastons (Burzynski Clinic)

Stanislaw R. Burzynski and his associates have been working on antineoplastons as a treatment for cancer since 1967. He works from the Burzynski Research Institute, Houston, Texas; was educated in Poland and is licensed to practice in Texas. He proposed the theory of antineoplastons in 1976 on the grounds that cancer treatment should be based on "modifying information to the abhorrent neoplastic cells," rather than the massive destruction employed in conventional cytotoxic therapies [128,129]. He claimed that there were significant deficiencies in the peptide content in the serum of cancer patients. Similar peptide fractions are found in urine, and this was used as the main source for their isolation. Fractions that inhibited the growth of neoplastic cells, but not normal cells, were named *antineoplastons*. He postulated that the human body possesses a biochemical defense system, consisting of antineoplastons, which protects against the occurrence of abnormal cell growth. He proposed that the antineoplastons work as molecular switches. More recently, he claims that they regulate the expression of genes *p53* and *p21* through demethylation of promoter sequences and acetylation of histones. He claims that antineoplaston A2 contributes to the highest number of complete responses in his phase I studies. The active ingredient was later identified as 3-phenyl-acetylamino-2, 6-piperidinedione and was named antineoplaston A10. He also proposed that antineoplaston AS2–1 was the most active fraction and started to synthesize this derivative. Phenylacetate (a metabolite of the amino acid phenylalanine) composes 80% of the antineoplaston fraction AS2–1. An NCI-sponsored phase II study showed that recurrent brain tumors did not respond significantly to phenylacetate.

From 1991 to 1995, the NCI invested $1 million into phase II clinical trials of A10 and AS2–1 infusions in patients with diagnosed primary malignant brain tumors. A conflict between Burzinski and the NCI stopped the studies before determining the effectiveness of antineoplastons. Currently, Burzinski is conducting multiple concurrent preliminary phase II trials that cover most cancer indications. Although these are listed on the NCI's PDQ clinical trials web site, they are conducted in his private clinic outside of peer review. The FDA has allowed this to occur following political pressure from some patient advocate groups [130–134].

Shark Cartilage

William I. Lane, a biochemist and nutritionist, became interested in sharks when he worked in marine resources. Following on from Judah Folkman's experiments on the role of angiogenesis in cancer progression, Lane speculated that shark cartilage contains an agent that inhibits vascular formation [135]. According to Lane, in a 16-week clinical trial conducted in Cuba involving 29 terminally ill cancer patients, 14 of the subjects are alive and well 2 years after the study of rectally administered pulverized shark cartilage. The suggested efficacy of shark cartilage was promoted in Lane's book, *Sharks Don't Get Cancer* [136]. The resistance of cartilage to tumor formation is correlated with its capacity to inhibit the formation of new blood vessels. A number of in vitro and in vivo studies have suggested the existence of antiangiogenic compounds in shark and bovine cartilage. There is evidence that cartilage does contain compounds that inhibit angiogenesis. It does not follow, however, that oral (or even rectal) administration of whole cartilage has antineoplastic activity in the human body. The main problem is lack of data that correlates bioavailability with pharmacological effects using oral shark cartilage. Essentially, the active ingredient in shark cartilage is too large to be absorbed into the blood stream from the digestive tract [137].

The clinical effectiveness of whole cartilage for the treatment of cancer was not confirmed in a well-designed phase III randomized controlled trial [138]. Bioactive derivatives of shark cartilage continue to be extracted. The biotechnology company Aeterna has developed AE-941 (Neovastat), a standardized water-soluble extract, that represents less than 5% of the crude cartilage. It is a multifunctional antiangiogenic product that contains several biologically active molecules. However, no published phase III randomized controlled trials have yet proven the utility of Neovastat for cancer. Adding Neovastat to standard chemotherapy and radiation therapy for patients with advanced non–small cell lung cancer did not extend patients' lives, according to a large phase III clinical trial reported at the ASCO 2007 Annual Meeting. In this study, 188 patients received the standard treatment plus the shark cartilage extract (as a liquid, which they drank twice a day), and 191 patients received the standard treatment plus a placebo (a liquid with no shark cartilage extract). After nearly 4 years of follow-up, patients who received the shark cartilage lived an average of 14 months, compared with nearly 16 months for the patients who did not receive the shark cartilage, a difference that was not significant [139–140].

Coley's Toxin

In 1888, William B. Coley, a Harvard Medical school graduate and an eminent surgeon at The Memorial Hospital for Cancer and Allied Diseases in New York City, proposed a concept that became the foundation of modern immunotherapy. Although his proposal was first tolerated, it was later ridiculed and finally suppressed. After examining the records of all bone cancer patients, he discovered a patient who was thought to be dying of cancer, but survived after suffering erysipelas, a skin infection caused by *Streptococcus* pyogenes. He obtained a virulent culture of *Streptococcus* from the famous German bacteriologist, Robert Koch. He infected a patient who had cancer with nodal metastases. The patient developed a high fever and the cancer went into remission [141]. Over the next 40 years, as head of the Bone Tumor Service at Memorial Hospital in New York, Coley injected more than 1000 cancer patients with bacteria or bacterial products. These products became known as *Coley's toxins*. Coley's hypothesis was that an immune reaction against a toxin present in the infectious material cross-reacted with and destroyed the tumor cells. A reexamination of Coley's original observations in the light of current knowledge suggests that tumor regression may have been attributable to administration of a plasminogen activator rather than an immunogen. However, there was an understandable aversion to placing patients at risk from inoculation with live *streptococci* and attention was directed increasingly to the newer radiation therapy and, eventually, chemotherapy approaches to cancer treatment. However, the modern science of immunology has shown that Coley's principles were correct and that some cancers are sensitive to an enhanced immune system. His work was the subject of numerous published reports, which were summarized in detail in 1953 [142]. However, a double-blind randomized controlled trial at New York University Bellevue Hospital demonstrated minimal response [143]. Nevertheless, the prospect that coagulation-reactive drugs in general, and plasminogen activators in particular, may alter malignant progression signals the prospect of new and more effective forms of experimental cancer treatment. Coley may indeed have been right, but for the wrong reason [144].

Livingston-Wheeler Therapy

In the 1940s, Virginia Livingston, claimed that she discovered a bacterium, *Progenitor cryptocides*. In subsequent published reports, she claimed that this bacterium "is found in humans and animals and causes cancer only when the immune (defense) system is inadequate." For many years before her death in 1990, Virginia Livingston-Wheeler ran the Livingston-Wheeler clinic in San Diego, California, treating patients twice a week with a vaccine made from the patient's own urine. The Livingston Therapy also included vegetarian raw foods, gammaglobulin, vitamin and mineral supplements, heat therapy, and detoxification. It calls for eliminating from the diet all poultry and egg products, sugars, white flours, and processed foods, as well as tobacco and alcohol. Spleen glandular extracts and the BCG vaccine were used to stimulate the patient's immune system [6]. There is no data that establishes efficacy of this protocol. Dr. Livingston-Wheeler never sought FDA approval for her vaccine. In February 1990, the State of California ordered the Livingston-Wheeler Clinic to stop treating cancer patients with the vaccines.

Immunoaugmentative Therapy

Immunoaugmentative Therapy (IAT) was developed by Lawrence Burton, a cancer researcher at St. Vincent's Hospital in New York City. Burton established his own clinic on Long Island and then moved to Freeport, Grand Bahamas, in 1977. He patented the ideas behind IAT and refused to share or discuss them with other cancer researchers, making his claims particularly difficult to evaluate [6]. According to Dr. Burton's theory, when specific blood protein components are balanced, the body should be able to subdue cancer cells as part of its normal activity; but if any of the components are out of balance, the body cannot adequately defend itself. "Blocking protein factors" are produced by the body and shield the tumor cells from attack by the tumor antibodies. Burton claimed that IAT's tumor antibodies fight cancer while its protein removes the "blocking factors" that prevent the immune system from recognizing and fighting cancer cells. IAT treats the immune system, not cancer, by bringing the body's natural defense system back into balance. Burton's Immune Research Center (IRC) claims a 50% response rate in a wide variety of tumors [145]. There is no scientific evidence concerning the safety or efficacy of IAT [146,147]. An analysis by the NCI of materials submitted by the family of a deceased IAT patient revealed dilute blood proteins, the major component of which was albumin [148]. In July 1985, the Bahamian government ordered the IRC closed. Subsequent to the closing, live competent human immunodeficiency virus (HIV) was repeatedly isolated from one of the IAT samples. The IRC reopened in March 1986 after it acquired equipment to test for the AIDS and hepatitis B viruses.

An unexpected response in an individual (n-of-1) is a celebration for that particular patient, but is not evidence for misleading populations into potentially harmful and resource-intensive programs. The response may have been coincident with another factor, or be a unique combination of that particular patient's constitution and the intervention. A series of positive associations provides us with a "best case series" that may be worthy of a more formal analysis and prospective investigations. We should carefully synthesize the observations for a possible scientific basis, initially using inductive reasoning, and then if promising, advance the evidence forward by using the deductive criteria of scientific experiments, culminating in the randomized controlled trial.

Conclusion

Many so-called alternative therapies for cancer have not been proven to be effective. Some of them are perpetuated by myth and desperation. On the other hand, among these touted therapies are some innovative ideas that include single agents and complex systems. An open-minded but critical attitude is necessary. Hypotheses must be tested within the rules of science. Methodologists are challenged to evaluate new therapies consistent with the spirit of innovation. Human beings are complex and cannot be compared to laboratory animals. Combinations of therapies may be synergistic and interventional programs should be evaluated using systems research [149]. Individualization of therapies may require n-of-1 studies [150]. Health-related quality of life and stable disease are important endpoints. The aphorism of "a war on cancer" is not a useful paradigm. The holistic concept of living in harmony with cancer is already stimulating new research that studies host adaptation and quality of life.

REFERENCES

1. White JD. (2002). Complementary and alternative medical research: A National Cancer Institute Perspective. *Seminars in Oncology, 29*, 546–551.

3. Richardson MA & Strauss SE. (2002). Complementary and alternative medicine; Opportunities and challenges for cancer management and research. *Seminars in Oncology, 29*, 531–545.

4. Cassileth BR. (1999). Complementary and alternative cancer medicine. *Journal of Clinical Oncology, 17*, 44–52.

7. Montbriand M. (1998). Abandoning biomedicine for alternate therapies: Oncology patients' stories. *Cancer Nursing, 21*, 36–45.

10. Verhoef MJ, Balneaves LG, Boon HS, & Vroegindewey A. (2005). Reasons for and characteristics associated with complementary and alternative medicine use among adult cancer patients: A systematic review. *Integrative Cancer Therapies, 4*, 274–286.

19. Schmidt K & Ernst E. (2004). Assessing websites on complementary and alternative medicine for cancer. *Annals of Oncology, 15*, 733–742.

29. Gertz MA & Bauer BA. (2003). Caring (really) for patients who use alternative therapies for cancer. *Journal of Clinical Oncology, 21*, 125s–128.

63. Cassileth BR. (1998). *Alternative medicine handbook: A complete reference guide to alternative and complementary therapies.* New York: W.W. Norton & Co.

137. Loprinzi CL, Levitt R, Barton DL, Sloan JA, Atherton PJ, Smith DJ, et al. (2005). Evaluation of shark cartilage in patients with advanced cancer. *Cancer, 104*, 176–182.

148. Verhoef MJ, Lewith G, Ritenbaugh C, Boon H, Fleishman S, & Leis A. (2005). Complementary and alternative medicine whole systems research: Beyond identification of inadequacies of the RCT. *Complementary Therapies in Medicine, 13*, 206–212.

(A complete reference list for this chapter is available online at http://www.oup.com/us/ integrativemedicine).

27

CAM and Cancer Research Methodology

VINJAR FØNNEBØ

KEY CONCEPTS

- When researching complementary and alternative medicine (CAM) and cancer researchers need to realize that patients are well aware of the limitations of CAM treatment with regard to prolonged overall survival and reduction of tumor size.
- The difference in preresearch patient experience between conventional medicine and CAM precludes a direct replication of the conventional research approach to the CAM field.
- Research in CAM and cancer should lead to results ensuring that the treatments patients seek are safe, document what packages of care are most beneficial, and double-check claims of efficacy of products and procedures that are intended for general and widespread use among cancer patients.

■

Approximately every other cancer patient in Western developed countries has used complementary and alternative medicine (CAM) in addition to their conventional treatment [1]. Among breast cancer patients the proportion is even higher [2–4].

Researchers with experience from conventional medicine have been responsible for most of the research on CAM and cancer. It is therefore not surprising that the CAM research in cancer has followed the same methodology as that in conventional medicine. It has tested the specific efficacy of supposed active components of a therapy. The results from this research have generally shown little clinical trial evidence supporting CAM therapy components to be effective in cancer cure. The current widespread use of CAM by patients must therefore be based on patients having other treatment goals than cure, their mistrust in the available research, or their willingness to be misled by unwarranted claims.

Patients' reported reasons for seeking CAM seem to support the first option [5]. Given reasons include beliefs in complementary and/or holistic care, taking charge of the disease, dealing with cancer symptoms, dealing with side effects of conventional treatment, improving quality of life/well-being, strengthening the immune system, increasing energy, working with a supportive practitioner, and supplementing conventional cancer treatment. Patients seem to make these treatment choices on the basis of the qualities of the provider, desire for "individualized" treatments, and their perception of overall effectiveness rather than efficacy. This seems to indicate that patients are well aware of the limitations of CAM treatments with regard to reducing tumor size. Researchers, therefore, need to take this clinical reality into account when researching CAM and cancer.

Overall Research Strategy

The practice of CAM is generally characterized by the absence of regulatory and financial gatekeepers. There is therefore a plethora of CAM approaches to treatment, including that for cancer. The outer limits of this treatment landscape are constantly changing, and large parts of the landscape are at any one time unknown to researchers. Substantial areas of CAM treatment are therefore unavailable for research attention. When planning or performing research on CAM and cancer, researchers, therefore, naturally limit their efforts to treatment approaches that are already in clinical use in one or more patient population. Research is hence initiated in areas where patients already have clinical experience. This differs somewhat from research in conventional oncology where researchers develop novel treatment approaches, exposing patients to these treatments only after extensive testing has been done through phase I–III clinical trials.

This difference in preresearch patient experience between the two clinical areas precludes a direct replication of the conventional research approach to the CAM field. The real-world clinical practice necessitates a reorganization of existing research elements [6] (Fig 27.1).

This rearrangement is, however, not meant as a chronological sequence defining when specific research phases should occur but as a framework to guide CAM research. It illustrates the necessary building blocks required for a

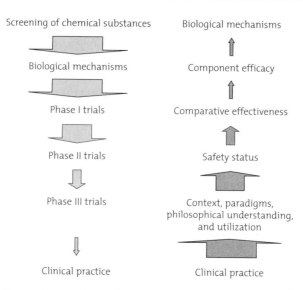

FIGURE 27.1. Research strategies in drug trials and CAM (proposed). Phases that contrast the proposed phased research strategy in CAM (thick arrows) with that conventionally used in drug trials (thin arrows). Adapted from Fonnebo V, Grimsgaard S, Walach H, Ritenbaugh C, Norheim AJ, MacPherson H, et al. (2007). Researching complementary and alternative treatments—the gatekeepers are not at home. *BMC Medical Research Methodology [Electronic Resource]*, 7(1), 7.

rigorous evidence base. The framework does not include novel methodological elements and is appropriate for any treatment approach that has developed in and from clinical practice, and whose specific treatment tools are unregulated. In conventional medicine this might include nursing, health psychology, counseling, and some aspects of general practice.

Understanding Treatment Choices of Cancer Patients

The fundamental aspect in the above-mentioned research strategy is understanding the processes and assumptions inherent in the specific CAM therapies, often using an inductive research approach. In light of the need for broad research in an early phase, data collection methods should record as much of patients' background, philosophies, contexts, choices, and experiences as possible. This basic research phase has often been overlooked, and research ideas have therefore often been generated haphazardly on a case report basis. The inductive research approach can include several approaches, and the appropriate methodology for this phase of research is mostly qualitative, but observational quantitative methods can also contribute valuable insight. Researchers are often entering into territory totally unknown to them and need to explore and seek meaning and understanding of patient and practitioner behavior. I will give only two examples of international efforts to approach this field in a systematic way in order to develop research hypotheses that can be further tested in clinical trials.

Exceptional Case History Registration

When cancer patients experience a clinical outcome after CAM treatment that differs markedly from what can be expected on the basis of conventional treatment alone, they can be classified as having an exceptional case history. Exceptional cancer patient experiences of this kind have been collected and analyzed by several institutions worldwide [7]. This can be an important clue in understanding the processes that take place when patients seek CAM treatment for their cancer. Two principally slightly different approaches have been identified when doing these kinds of studies:

1. **A review of CAM practitioners' best cases:**
This approach is utilized by the National Cancer Institute (NCI) in the United States through their best-case series (BCS) methodology [8]; the study group "Unconventional and Complementary Methods in Oncology" at the Department of Internal Medicine, Oncology and Hematology at the Klinikum Nuernberg (UCMO) in Nuremberg, Germany [9]; and investigators at Columbia University at New York [10].

2. **A review of patients' own exceptional case histories:**
This approach is utilized by The National Research Center in Complementary and Alternative Medicine (NAFKAM), Tromsø, Norway, in establishing an Exceptional Case History Registry [11]; The Danish Multiple Sclerosis Society in Denmark; and Johanna Hök at Karolinska Institute, Stockholm, Sweden [12]. The Danish and Swedish groups collaborate with NAFKAM.

In contrast to the NCI approach, NAFKAM collects both best and worst cases but follows procedures similar to those at NCI to evaluate the medical aspects of the reported exceptional case history.

These international efforts need to be further developed and coordinated. A worldwide database of exceptional case histories in cancer treatment will, due to numbers, rapidly be able to generate patterns of care that can be further tested in clinical trials. This can be seen as a process similar to the basic research underlying the choice of chemical components to include in phase I clinical pharmaceutical trials in conventional medicine.

Cohort Study of Treatment Choices

Cancer patients are seeking CAM as a treatment system. Research needs to be done to examine the outcomes of these treatments both in combination with and as an alternative to conventional care [13].

Although a number of studies have been done internationally to monitor CAM use in cancer patients, they are mostly cross-sectional studies querying patients at one point in time. As mentioned earlier, there is extensive clinical experience indicating that treatment choices can change over the course of the disease duration. Few researchers have documented these changing patterns of CAM use [14,15]. It is therefore necessary to initiate large-scale cohort studies to follow and monitor patients' treatment choices. It is important to understand what is chosen and why it is chosen, and relate this to the clinical course of the disease process. This type of study has not yet been performed among cancer patients.

Safety

Conventional cancer treatment has potentially grave, sometimes life-threatening, side effects. These are acceptable given the serious nature of the underlying treated disease. CAM treatments have, on the other hand, often been claimed to be without risk, but adverse effects in CAM are definitely more than occasional case reports [16]. Although adverse effects in CAM most likely are of a mild nature, little research has been done to investigate this carefully. Only the field of acupuncture has provided a thorough risk assessment, not only pinpointing infections and pneumothorax as the most serious adverse effects but also identifying a number of minor adverse occurrences in connection with acupuncture treatment [17]. There is virtually no knowledge about adverse effects in other fields within CAM, and this lack of knowledge needs to be corrected. The methodology of choice can be largely copied from conventional medicine—individual reporting of adverse effect occurrences and monitoring of adverse events in clinical trials or in observational studies.

In the cancer field, an additional risk assessment needs to be done related to CAM treatments. Although CAM interventions in themselves are thought to carry little direct biological risk, denial of conventional treatment in favor of exclusive use of CAM is thought to be a serious threat to cancer patients. This denial of conventional treatment is sometimes done on recommendations from CAM treatment providers, and this makes it appropriate to classify it as a potential adverse effect. Little is known in this field aside from occasional case reports.

Comparative Effectiveness

In conventional medicine we take for granted that seeking advice from a health care professional is a good way of dealing with diverse health problems. Research in conventional medicine therefore focuses on choosing the best tools for health professionals to use. These tools include drugs, diagnostic methods, and surgical procedures, and the research employed often results in recommendations of a one-size-fits-all therapeutic prescription. Research in conventional medicine may, however, have overlooked that the clinical effect of most therapies are overestimated when studied under optimal circumstances on susceptible, cooperative patients. The randomized controlled trial is, despite this, a useful method for making decisions about tools to include in the toolbox of conventional medicine.

When studying effectiveness of CAM treatments, it is often useful to utilize the whole systems research (WSR) model developed by CAM researchers [18,19]. Recently specific suggestions have been made regarding the application of this methodology to CAM research in cancer [20]. This model can be applied to established whole systems such as Traditional Chinese Medicine (TCM), naturopathic medicine, homeopathy, and integrative medicine, as well as to individualized systems where patients design their own programs of care. If researchers limit their studies to an evaluation of the effectiveness of a single standardized component of cancer care (e.g., a support group) on a specific set of outcomes (e.g., disease progression, survival, or quality of life), the impact of individual and contextual factors and/or other treatments can be overlooked. Possible interaction effects can likewise be missed. This research, while perhaps internally valid, may lack external validity, as it does not reflect the real-world situations that cancer patients experience.

As patients are unique, differ in attitudes, beliefs, health status, and personalities, Sidani et al. [21] recommend a very minimal list of exclusion criteria when researching whole systems. Selection criteria that are too stringent result in a participant population that is not reflective of the real world, thus limiting the generalizability of results.

WSR often requires an expanded set of outcome measures, of which survival, conventional assessments of biomedical outcomes, and quality of life constitute parts. In addition, both global outcomes, which assess overall well-being, and individualized outcomes, which assess unique patient-centered outcomes for each research participant, are needed as treatment interventions and are often intended to affect more than one outcome over a long period.

Rychetnik et al [22] suggest asking the following questions to determine whether appropriate outcomes have been selected: (a) do the outcomes adequately address the questions asked by key stakeholders (e.g., patients, providers, policy makers)? (b) do the chosen outcomes allow for both anticipated and unanticipated effects to be tracked? and (c) has (cost) efficiency been addressed?

Data analysis in WSR may require a shift from the norm in intervention research. Instead of attempting to determine the effect of an intervention for the average participant, it may be more appropriate to determine for which participants, presenting with which characteristics, an intervention is effective, or not [21]. In general the goal of a WSR should be to determine how the participants, provider, context, and intervention factors interact to affect the process and outcomes of healing and ultimately to determine which interventions, given under what conditions or context, result in which outcomes for which patients.

This whole systems approach to study the effectiveness of CAM treatment of cancer represents only preliminary suggestions. WSR methods will need to be refined through a process that includes practical examples, reflection, and revision.

Efficacy

Efficacy is the area that has received most attention and research money to date. The methods of choice are generally double-blind randomized placebo-controlled trials. In CAM, the well-established documentation of acupuncture/acupressure stimulation of one acupuncture point in the treatment of chemotherapy-induced nausea/vomiting is an example of appropriate efficacy research [23].

When testing dietary supplements, herbal medicine, or other standardized interventions intended for general use in cancer patients, this well-proven research method should of course be utilized, and there is no need to enter into a lengthy argumentation for its justification.

It is, however, important to recognize that results from efficacy research cannot be used to document or disprove the effectiveness of a "whole system" treatment.

Conclusion

With the widespread use of CAM among cancer patients, a stronger research effort is warranted. The increasing use is in itself a strong indication that patients experience the treatments they seek as useful. The challenge for researchers in this field is to contribute mainly in three areas:

1. Ensure that the treatments patients are seeking are safe
2. Document what packages of care are most beneficial
3. Double-check claims of efficacy of products and procedures that are intended for general and widespread use among cancer patients.

Whether patients gain any benefit whatsoever from seeking CAM treatments is probably no longer of interest as a practical issue. As a philosophical and sociological issue it could still warrant research in those areas.

REFERENCES

5. Verhoef MJ, Balneaves LG, Boon HS, & Vroegindewey A. (2005). Reasons for and characteristics associated with complementary and alternative medicine use among adult cancer patients: A systematic review. *Integrative Cancer Therapies,* 4(4), 274–286.
6. Fonnebo V, Grimsgaard S, Walach H, Ritenbaugh C, Norheim AJ, MacPherson H, et al. (2007). Researching complementary and alternative treatments—the gatekeepers are not at home. *BMC Medical Research Methodology [Electronic Resource],* 7(1), 7.
7. Launso L, Drageset BJ, Fonnebo V, Jacobson JS, Haahr N, White JD, et al. (2006). Exceptional disease courses after the use of CAM: Selection, registration, medical assessment, and research—an international perspective. *Journal of Alternative and Complementary Medicine (New York, N.Y.),* 12(7), 607–613.
8. NCI Best Case Series Program. (2007). Internet Communication. http://www.cancer.gov/cam/bestcase_intro.html Accessed: August 7, **2008.**
13. Lewith G, Thomas K, & Fønnebø V. (2006). Whole systems research in cancer care – report of meeting in Tromsø (Sommarøy), 14–16 September, 2005. *Complementary Therapies in Medicine,* 14, 157–164.
14. Risberg T, Lund E, Wist E, Kaasa S, & Wilsgaard T. (1998). Cancer patients use of nonproven therapy: A 5-year follow-up study. *Journal of Clinical Oncology,* 16(1), 6–12.
18. Ritenbaugh C, Verhoef M, Fleishman S, Boon H, & Leis A. (2003). Whole systems research: A discipline for studying complementary and alternative medicine. *Alternative Therapies in Health and Medicine,* 9(4), 32–36.
19. Verhoef MJ, Lewith G, Ritenbaugh C, Boon H, Fleishman S, & Leis A. (2005). Complementary and alternative medicine whole systems research: Beyond identification of inadequacies of the RCT. *Complementary Therapies in Medicine,* 13(3), 206–212.

20. Verhoef MJ, Vanderheyden LC, & Fønnebø V. (2006). A Whole Systems Research Approach to Cancer Care: Why Do We Need It and How Do We Get Started? *Integrative Cancer Therapies,* 5, 287–292.

22. Rychetnik L, Frommer M, Hawe P, & Shiell A. (2002). Criteria for evaluating evidence on public health interventions. *Journal of Epidemiology and Community Health,* 56(2), 119–127.

(A complete reference list for this chapter is available online at http://www.oup.com/us/ integrativemedicine).

28

Truth and Truth Telling in Integrative Oncology

ANTONELLA SURBONE

KEY POINTS

- The patient–doctor relationship is a therapeutic alliance in which the two partners are bound by justice and trust in a mutual, goal-oriented relationship of help between one partner who is in need of expertise and care and another who can provide these.
- The patient–doctor relationship has an intrinsic asymmetry, which is increased by the vulnerability that the illness induces in the patient and by the power imbalance between the two partners. As a consequence, the relationship cannot be simply described in contractual terms, as it involves the dimensions of care and trust.
- The notion of individual autonomy is now replaced by that of relational autonomy, which takes into account our being embedded in a relational context that sustains us through our life, while creating reciprocal responsibilities.
- The patient–doctor relationship extends to the family, the community, the medical institutions, and society and it is made possible by effective communication among all partners involved.
- Truth telling is an essential step in the patient–doctor–society relationship and information should ideally be ongoing, accurate, and complete. Communication, however, goes beyond information and is an open-ended multidirectional process that takes place in specific cultural contexts.
- Style, setting, content, and supportive aspects of communication of truth to patients influence each other reciprocally and need to be properly balanced, according to the patients' individual and cultural preferences and contexts.

- Cancer patients increasingly look for alternative ways to control their cancer and contribute to their own well-being for different reasons. These include dissatisfaction with the quality of the patient–doctor relationship and of the traditional communication process .
- Cancer patients and their oncologists should share in searching for the truth of the illness in a binding relation that is especially strong when the two parties engage in the project of integrated oncology.

■

The patient–doctor relationship is a therapeutic alliance in which the two partners are bound by justice and trust in a goal-oriented, mutual, yet asymmetric, relationship of help between one partner who is in need of expertise and care and another who can provide these. The essence of the partnership between patient and doctor lies in this asymmetry of help, which is increased by the vulnerability induced in the patient by her illness (Surbone & Lowenstein, 2003a). The vulnerability of the ill person enhances her dependence on other persons, and especially on the physician. The patient–doctor relationship was traditionally centered on charismatic physicians who made what they considered to be the best medical choices in their patients' interests and provided or withheld information at their discretion. In contemporary Western societies, physicians are now considered equal partners with their patients and they tell the truth to their patients to enable them to exercise autonomy in making decisions about health matters. The patient–doctor relationship, however, is a special type of partnership, where the rules of reciprocity suited for voluntarily bargaining between nonintimate equals are not sufficient. This special connection of reciprocity cannot be described in simple contractual terms. It is, rather, a covenant marked by the qualities of care, trust, and sensitivity (Pellegrino & Thomasma, 1988). Asymmetry and vulnerability are magnified in the relationship between cancer patients and their oncologists because of the serious nature of cancer with its medical, psychological, and social ramifications, the complexity and potential risks of cancer treatments, and the fragmentation of care for patients who need to be followed by multiple specialists (Surbone, 2006a).

The person experiencing symptoms and signs of an illness consults a fellow human being as a professional expert to help her in decoding and interpreting her suffering (Galeazzi, 1997; Surbone, 2000). Each patients' suffering is always qualitatively and quantitatively unique and physicians interpret it through the application and instantiation of their knowledge and practical wisdom in the context of compassion and empathy. The physician establishes the diagnosis, formulates the prognosis, and prescribes the appropriate treatment measures in view of a therapeutic goal that must be common to the patient and the physician and, in industrialized societies, must be agreed on by both. In the patient–doctor relationship, the cognitive and caring dimensions of the physicians' work are equally important (Clifton-Soderstrom, 2003; Surbone, 2000). Style, setting, content, and supportive aspects of communication of truth to patients influence each other reciprocally and need to be properly balanced, according to the patients' individual and cultural preferences and contexts (Surbone, 2006b). Whether content and facilitation of the communication process are as important to patients as the supportive dimension of communication likely depends on individual and cultural factors, including gender, age, and education. Oncologists and institutions have greatly improved in their sensitivity and adapt their manner and style, and sometimes even the care setting to enhance effective communication.

Today, for example, patients and relatives are no longer spoken to in a hallway or during medical rounds with no privacy, representing a major improvement in communication. On the contrary, patients are now asked to comment on the quality of the communication process, and the literature shows that they are more satisfied when their oncologists provide accurate and complete information in a clear understandable language and when they show genuine understanding of their feelings. Basic empathic skills for meaningful communication in the clinical setting involve physicians' recognition of patients' emotions, even when they do not verbalize them, and inviting patients to explore and share unexpressed feelings. Only when patients feel understood does the communication process reach its full effectiveness (Maguire, Faulkner, Booth, Elliott, & Hillier, 1996; Matthews, Suchman, & Branch, 1993).

Cancer patients wish to be provided not only with information about diagnosis but also about therapies and their possible benefits and side effects, about ongoing research and new experimental treatments and, to a lesser degree, about prognosis and expected outcomes. Patients and physicians must reconcile their needs for accurate detailed information with the medical uncertainty that still surrounds the clinical practice of oncology. Uncertainty in medicine makes everyone uncomfortable (Schapira, 2006). It is hard for patients to accept that the doctors they entrust their bodies and lives to may, in fact, provide treatment to them under conditions of high uncertainty. Physicians highly value the objectivity and certainty of medical knowledge and they fear that admitting uncertainty may undermine their authority and power. Some oncologists overwhelm their patients with information expressed in numerical terms, perhaps as a way to underline known elements of certainty while avoiding those aspects of their patients' cancer that involve uncertainty (Surbone, 2006a). Some oncologists feel especially uncomfortable providing prognostic information to their patients, as being truthful and admitting uncertainty may seem to conflict with maintaining hope in their patients (DelVecchio Good, Good, Schaffer, & Lind, 1990; Kodish & Post, 1995). While it is possible for oncologists to be frank and at the same time to inspire hope, the issue of whether, to what extent, and how to disclose prognosis and to deliver "bad news" is still highly debated, even in those countries with a long tradition of truth (Baile, Lenzi, Parker, Buckman, & Cohen, 2002; Butow, Maclean,Dunn, Tatterstall, & Boyer, 1997; Hagerty, Butow, Ellis, Dimitry, & Tattersall, 2005; Husebo, 1997; Parker, Baile, deMoor, Lenzi, Kudelka, & Cohen, 2001; Weeks, et al., 1998).

Many cancer patients, confronted by high degrees of uncertainty regarding the cancer prognosis and the outcome and potential side effects of both standard and experimental cancer therapies, choose to go beyond traditional medical care and look for alternative ways to control their cancer and contribute to their own well-being. Those patients who use alternative therapies generally do so in addition to conventional treatment, but some rely on non-traditional treatment alone (Balneaves, Truant, Kelly, Verhoef, & Davidson, 2007; Cassileth, 2001; Eisenberg, et al., 1993; Ernst & Cassileth, 1998; Goldstein, et al., 2005; Harvey, Bauer-Wu, Ria, Laizner, & Post-White, 2005; Kelly, 2007; Kessler, et al., 2001; Molassiotis, et al., 2005; Shumay, Maskarinec, Karm, Kakai, & Gotay, 2003). It has now become essential for all oncologists to understand the motivations of those patients who continue active treatment or follow-up, while also using complementary therapies, and to be able to communicate with them in a spirit of honesty and truthfulness. Oncologists should be sensitive to mind and body interactions, as well as to all physical, emotional, and spiritual aspects involved in cancer care, and acquire sufficient knowledge of integrative medicine to "sort out all the evidence about healing systems and to try to extract those ideas and practices that are useful, safe, and cost-effective" (Weil, 2000).

We tell the truth to respect our patients' capability to comprehend elaborate information about their illness and to make autonomous decisions in health-care matters. We also tell the truth, in medicine and in life, because by doing so, we create valid long-lasting interpersonal relationships. Finally, truth has an intrinsic spiritual value in helping us make sense of what happens in our lives.

Truth Telling in Integrative Oncology

The motivations for the growing interest of cancer patients in integrative strategies are mainly related to the patients' desire to assist their body's healing by improving their physical and psychological well-being, and to maintain their hope by increasing control over their illness (Balneaves, Truant, Kelly, Verhoef, & Davidson, 2007; Ernst, Pittler, Wider, & Boddy, 2007; Maizes, Schneider, Bell, & Weil, 2002; Molassiotis, et al., 2005). Cancer patients also wish to be empowered in their interactions with oncology professionals who, in addition to their expertise in cancer treatment, should be aware of the importance of lifestyle factors, including nutrition, exercise, sleep and relaxation, as well as of the many spiritual dimensions of healing (Rees & Weil, 2001). Cancer patients and their families and care givers in Western countries are generally aware of the current limitations of traditional cancer therapies, and they are mostly dissatisfied with the quality of their patient–doctor relationships, too often permeated by medical arrogance.

Dissatisfaction with the communication skills of physicians and a sense of not being given adequate or useful information is an additional factor that draws cancer patients toward alternative treatments (Ernst, 2002). The traditional Western method of communicating bad news can be either too blunt or too paternalistic, and both attitudes can be perceived as arrogant and dogmatic by cancer patients, who may turn to alternative treatments that are more uncertain and yet seem to empower them with a greater sense of control and hope (Abrams, 2007; Balneaves, Kristjanosn, & Tatryn, 1999). It has also been hypothesized that patients who make use of complementary interventions may be more pessimistic about their prognosis or more emotionally and psychologically distressed than those who do not seek alternative ways to help themselves (Hlubocky, Ratain, & Daugherty, 2007). Other data indicate that the use of complementary medicine is higher in younger, well-educated female patients and may correlate with a preference for patient-centered, rather than shared, decision making about health matters (Cassileth, et al., 1991; Eisenberg, et al., 1993; Hlubocky, et al., 2007; Paltiel, et al., 2001). Multiple factors thus contribute to the individual cancer patients' choice to investigate and pursue different forms of interventions to improve her chances of survival and her quality of life (Lawsin, et al., 2007; Lis, Cambron, Grutsch, Granick, & Gutpa, 2006; Molassiotis, et al., 2005). Integrative oncology was born in response to the need to understand, respect, and foster a more wholistic approach to cancer patients (Abrams, 2007; Cassileth, et al., 1991; Kessler, et al., 2001; Maizes, Schneider, Bell, & Weil, 2002; Ruggie, 2004; Yates, et al., 1993).

Integrative oncology aims at the thoughtful and rational combination of conventional and complementary therapies for cancer. Integrative oncology involves combining the use of different evidence-based treatments with attention to other dimensions of health and healing for the whole person (Abrams, 2007; Ernst, 2002; Ernst, et al., 1995; Meyers & Jacobsen, 2005; Rees & Weil, 2001). To deliver sensitive and effective care, all oncologists determined to work within the integrative oncology perspective must acquire and communicate knowledge about a holistic approach to cancer that goes beyond traditional standard or experimental oncology. The questions of what the truth is and how we tell it can be even more challenging in integrative oncology than in traditional clinical oncology (Lazar & O'Connor, 1997). Traditional medicine adopts a biomedical approach toward illness based on an analytical view that focuses on the objective aspects of the disease. By contrast, the integrative approach considers the individual person's health in the interconnectedness of his or her body, mind, and spirit. In the integrative perspective, the physician addresses the patients' many concerns and many "truths," not all easily quantifiable, to strengthen the ill person as a whole. The integrative perspective requires the physicians' understanding of the place of the conventional therapies as part of a larger treatment strategy that involves physical and spiritual changes in the patients' life and lifestyle (Abrams, 2007; Hamilton, 1998; Tatsumura, Maskarinec, Shumay, & Kakai, 2003; Weil, 2000). At the same time, the patient and the doctor realize that the holistic approach of integrative medicine does not exclude the more analytic approach of conventional treatments.

In the integrative perspective, most patients assume direct responsibility for their well-being and involve themselves very actively in their care. Some physicians may see this as destabilizing their role and undermining their authority. Oncologists may feel challenged by patients who explore or choose complementary treatments with which physicians are generally unfamiliar (American Society of Clinical Oncology, 1998; Kemper, Gardiner, Gobble, & Woods, 2006). Being asked about the use of interventions that are still considered unproven and that are not the subject of formal teaching during medical school and specialty training can make physicians feel uncomfortable and unwilling to share information with their patients. Many oncologists do not ask patients about whether they use or would like to use complementary interventions, and many patients do not raise the issue in order not to upset, or even lose, their doctors (Hann, Baker, & Denniston, 2003; Roberts, et al., 2005). In some cases, physicians inquire about complementary interventions because they worry about possible direct harm or interactions with standard or experimental cancer treatments (Bardia, Barton, Propork, Bauer, & Moynihan, 2006; Crocetti, et al., 1998; Hlubocky, et al., 2007; Institute of Medicine at National Academy of Sciences, 2005). While this is a legitimate concern, clinical experience shows that it is not uncommon for oncologists to approach their patients hesitantly or in a more or less subtle judgmental way, and it is equally not uncommon for patients to lie to their oncologists. Studies suggest that patients with preferences for shared decision making are more likely to tell their doctors that they are using complementary interventions, yet not all oncologists encourage shared decision making in their clinics (Hlubocky, et al., 2007; Paltiel, et al., 2001; Roberts, et al., 2005). Integrative oncology first and foremost requires reciprocal honesty and sincerity between cancer patients and their oncologists (Hann, et al., 2003; Jankovic, et al., 2004; Roberts, et al., 2005).

Integrative oncology is the thoughtful and rational combination of conventional and complementary therapies for cancer with attention to other dimensions of health and healing for the whole person. Integrative oncology acknowledges the connections between mind and body, and between health and life styles, as well as the spiritual dimensions of healing. A holistic approach to cancer patients also requires to consider them within their relational and social context.

Telling Truth to Cancer Patients: Cross-Cultural Similarities and Differences

In most countries, the public, physicians, and ethicists agree that an appropriate level of information is necessary to foster cancer patients' understanding of their illness and their involvement in the decision-making process (Beauchamp & Childress, 1994). Information enhances patients' cooperation with standard oncologic treatments and experimental therapies and leads to higher quality of care and better quality of life (Fallowfield & Jenkins, 2004). Furthermore, according to recent empirical research, cancer patients' needs and preferences regarding communication of bad news are similar across cultures (Baile, et al., 2002; Chiu, et al., 2006; Surbone, 2006b). Modern attitudes and practices of truth telling to cancer patients, however, have evolved over long periods of time and are still uncommon in many nonindustrialized countries. The international literature confirms that cultural barriers to open communication still exist and need to be acknowledged (Kagawa-Singer & Blackhall, 2001; Koenig & Gates-Williams, 1995; Mystadikou, Parpa, Tsilika, Katsouda & Lambros, 2004; Surbone, 2006c).

Under the influence of many intertwined medical, legal, and societal factors, a drastic evolution of truth-telling attitudes and practices in oncology took place between the early 1960s and the late 1970s (Annas, 1994; Novack, et al., 1979;

Oken, 1961). In the 1980s and early 1990s, the first reports of different truth-telling attitudes and practices worldwide were published in the international medical and bioethics literature, and major cross-cultural differences were described. These could be explained in view of the delicate balance between autonomy and beneficence in clinical medicine (Gostin, 1995; Pellegrino, 1992; Surbone, 1992; Tuckett, 2004). Unlike Anglo-American societies that privileged the notion of individual autonomy and the consequent right to self-determination of any patient with respect to health-care matters, many countries with strong traditions of family- and community-centered values held a more paternalistic view of the patient–doctor relationship and assigned to families and physicians a protective role toward the ill (Gordon & Paci, 1997). The word "autonomy," rather than being synonymous with "freedom," was synonymous with "isolation" in these countries (Surbone, 1992). Cancer patients were deemed unable to endure the psychological stress of knowing their diagnosis and prognosis and painful medical truths were withheld or strongly mitigated. While patients were kept in the dark, physicians gave information to and discussed treatment options and prognosis with family members. As a consequence, patients were caught in a web of half-truths that silenced their voices and, rather than protecting and sustaining them, in most cases subjected them to further isolation and suffering (Surbone, 1993).

A pattern of evolution similar to the one seen in the United States could be identified in several non-Western countries at the end of the 1980s. Since the mid-1990s there has been a remarkable shift in truth-telling attitudes and practices worldwide, and empirical and theoretical studies on truth telling to cancer patients and on delivering bad news have been published in the oncology, nursing, and psycho-oncology international literature (Dalla Vorgia, et al., 1992; Espinosa, Gonzales Baron, Poveda, Ordonez, & Zamora, 1993; Hamadeh & Abid, 1998; Harrison, et al., 1997; Holland, 1987; Mystadikou, 2005; Ozdogan, et al., 2004, Surbone, 2004a; Surbone & Zwitter, 1997; Tanida, 1994; Weil, Smith, & Khayat, 1994; Williams & Zwitter, 1994). Despite this international trend toward disclosure of information to cancer patients, however, partial or non-disclosure is still common practice in many cultures centered on family and community values (Surbone, Ritossa, & Spagnolo, 2004b). For example, while Italian medical deontology and the law on informed consent have evolved dramatically in the past 10 years, the general level of a patients' awareness of diagnosis and prognosis is still limited. A 2000 survey of 675 northern Italian physicians that asked whether, and to what extent, patients were informed of a cancer diagnosis revealed a major discrepancy between physicians' reported views on truth telling and what they had actually done in their practices. One-third of Italian physicians believed that patients never want to know the truth. Forty-five of the physicians indicated that patients should always be informed of a cancer diagnosis, while only 25% said they always disclosed the diagnosis in practice (Grassi, et al., 2000). In Japan, 46% of the general population in 2000 asserted that family should have a protective role in shielding the patient from a painful diagnosis, and several studies report that most Japanese physicians still consult with the family before disclosing a cancer diagnosis to the patient (Elwyn, Fetters, Gorenflo, & Tsuda, 1998; Seo, et al., 2000). Studies show variability in truth-telling practices among younger and older physicians (the latter being less inclined to reveal a cancer diagnosis), as well as differences in physicians' disclosure practices toward younger versus older patients (the latter being less likely to receive full disclosure).

Individual differences in communication preferences related to gender, age and education go beyond cross cultural boundaries (Blackhall, Murphy, Frank, Michel, & Azen, 1995; Kagawa-Singer & Blackhall, 2001; Surbone, 2006c). Studies suggest specific gender-related differences in patterns and styles of communication. Women tend to appreciate more detailed information and to value especially the supportive elements of communication (Baider, Cooper, & De-Nour, 2000; D' Agincourt-Canning, 2001; Surbone, 2003b). Research consistently indicates that cancer patients worldwide who are treated at large specialized institutions are especially likely to request full disclosure of their diagnosis, treatment options, and prognosis from their physicians (Chiu, et al., 2006; Fujimori, et al., 2005; Mystadikou, et al., 2004; Surbone, 2004b, 2006b). Patients who receive care at teaching hospitals or specialized oncology units are also exposed to more information than those who receive care in nonspecialized or rural centers, or in general wards or outpatient clinics. At present, we lack empirical data on the information needs and preferences of those latter cancer patients, and this should caution us regarding possible generalizations with respect to truth telling and full disclosure.

Information and truth do not coincide.
Information is only a step in the process of communication.
Communication is a bidirectional iterative open-ended process between patients and physicians over the entire course of their relationship.
Communication takes place in specific individual and sociocultural contexts.

Truth Telling and Cultural Competence in Integrative Oncology

To understand persisting cross-cultural differences in truth telling to cancer patients, several societal factors need to be taken into account (Anderlik, Pentz, & Hess, 2000; Novack, et al., 1971; Surbone, et al., 2004b). It is possible that in multiethnic societies such as the United States or the United Kingdom, the law represents a unifying element that places a strong emphasis on individual decisions, while in societies with more uniform national values, the appeal to tradition over the law remains a valid one, and physicians and families may still decide to withhold unfavorable news to protect cancer patients (Surbone, et al., 2004b). In multiethnic societies, cultural differences between patients and health-care professionals are often at the origin of misunderstandings and disagreements between health-care workers, patients, and families, and may escalate to bedside conflicts with respect to truth telling, end-of-life choices, prevention and screening, and involvement in clinical trials (Anderlik, et al., 2000; Betancourt, 2003, 2006; Dhruva, Cheng, Kwon, Luce, & Abrams, 2006; Kagawa-Singer & Balckhall, 2001). The growing literature on cultural competence in the United States shows that skilled cross-cultural negotiation is needed when health-care professionals are asked to withhold the truth from the patient about the diagnosis or with regard to end-of-life matters. The notion of "offering the truth" to cancer patients based on allowing individual patients to choose their own paths and rhythms was proposed as an effective way of showing respect for patients' autonomy in accord with their own cultural norms and has been elaborated and applied successfully in oncology (Freeman & Offering T, 1993).

Anthropological and medical research have shown that words do not have the same meaning and resonance in all contexts. Uttering a "bad word" such as *cancer* is considered to negatively affect patients and their illness outcome in certain cultures, and in certain languages, words such as *cancer* or *depression* do not exist. (Carrese & Rhodes, 1995; Levy, 1997; Tanaka-Matsumi & Marsella, 1976). A 2007 Italian survey showed that many southern Italian patients still refuse to write down the word *cancer*, even after having been informed of their diagnosis, because cancer is still a metaphor for intense suffering or death or social stigma to them (Bracci, et al., 2008; Sontag, 1978). By contrast, those same patients appeared to be highly knowledgeable of their cancer treatments, suggesting a persisting culture of partial disclosure (Bracci, et al., 2008). It is possible that less well-informed patients hold on to unrealistic hopes for a cure and thus they selectively hear and retain only information that concerns cancer treatments. On the other hand, it is also possible that their oncologists focus almost exclusively on treatment recommendations as a way to avoid discussing the true meaning of the cancer diagnosis and prognosis with patients and families who are not yet accustomed to a culture of full disclosure (Surbone, 2008).

Cross-cultural differences affect also the roles of families with respect to the degree of information given to cancer patients and involvement in patients' decision-making styles. Cancer is a "disease" of the entire family, and in most societies the family bears the final burden of taking care of the physical, emotional, and financial needs of cancer patients (Baider, et al., 2000).

In cross-cultural encounters with cancer patients in multiethnic societies such as the United States, family members sometimes ask doctors to withhold or downplay the truth about a cancer diagnosis or prognosis (Anderlik, et al., 2000). In many countries, especially in Asia, the oncologist consults with family members before revealing a cancer diagnosis to the patient. In most non-Western countries cancer patients rarely meet their doctors alone. Instead, relatives attend clinical appointments with them and participate in major decisions in treatment and end-of-life choices (Baider, et al., 2000). The presence of relatives in addition to the patient tends to result in longer clinical visits, as relatives ask questions relevant to their own caregiving roles (Farber, Egnew, Herman-Bertsch, Taylor, & Guldin, 2003; Higginson & Costantini 2002.).

In integrative oncology, a holistic approach to each cancer patient requires considering the patient within his or her relational and social context. Often, relatives and friends help the patient research alternative and complementary interventions or make suggestions based on their experiential knowledge. Research suggests that caregivers gather medical information from sources other than the patients' oncologist, including the Internet, to help the patient make treatment choices (Ernst & Schmidt, 2004). Physicians and all professionals in integrative oncology should thus be particularly sensitive about and open to talking to important figures in their patients' life, while, at the same time, supporting the patients' autonomy.

Cross-cultural differences in cancer care are more apparent now in Western multiethnic societies compared to more homogeneous countries. However, culture has profound implications in all contemporary societies, as different cultures coexist within dominant ones and multiculturalism is increasingly common because of higher demographic mobility and global communication (Kagawa-Singer & Backhall, 2001). Moreover, to the extent that both the patient and the physician always engage in an asymmetric yet reciprocal relationship, carrying their own personal and cultural identities, every clinical encounter and every patient–doctor relationship is an exercise in cultural competence (Surbone, 2006c).

In the last decade, there has been a remarkable shift in attitudes and practices of truth telling worldwide. Cancer patients are increasingly more informed of their diagnosis and treatments and more involved in the decision-making process. However, cultural and individual differences in truth telling in oncology persist and partial and nondisclosure still occur in many contexts. Whether and how to discuss prognosis remains a highly debated issue, as it is difficult to reconcile truthfulness with hope and uncertainty.

The choice of alternative therapies may in itself be influenced by cultural factors. The ability to deliver culturally competent cancer care is based on humility, sensitivity, respect, and curiosity about different patterns and styles of communication with cancer patients in different cultural contexts (Angell, 1988; Betancourt, 2003; Kagawa-Singer, 2003). Avoiding any form of cultural hegemony and stereotyping is of paramount importance when oncologists talk with cancer patients about complementary and alternative treatments or possible interventions on lifestyle or healing strategies based on spiritual dimensions. From an integrative oncology perspective, all therapeutic elements are subject to individual and cultural variability; judgmental or arrogant attitudes hinder the communication process.

Truth in the Clinical Context of the Patient–Doctor Relationship

The existence of illness is an undeniable fact of life and indeed a proof that life largely escapes our control (Code, 1993). The ill person consults a physician in search of truth and healing. Patients and physicians enter the patient–doctor relationship because they share the common project of achieving a rational understanding of the patients' suffering. By giving a name to the patients' suffering in the form of a diagnosis, physicians help transform their patients' anonymous suffering into a better known entity—an illness—that can be treated and at times even cured. Through the treatment process, physicians help their patients restore, in part at least, their well-being and regain some degree of the control that illness inevitably takes away (Barona, 1997; Galeazzi, 1997; Surbone, 2000).

Medical truth is composed of different elements and different kinds of truths: it is medical, clinical, and therapeutic as well as scientific; it is existential, practical, moral as well as objective; it is told in first as well as in third person; and it is about diagnosis as well as prognosis and cure, or lack of cure. Truth in the patient–doctor relationship is neither a harmonious blend of these elements nor the result of the predominance of one over the other. Rather there is a persistent gap, an unbridgeable distance between the subjective and objective elements of this truth. There is also distance between the two partners of the relationship, which is not merely existential but primarily epistemic, as the patient and the doctor learn and know different aspects of the patients' illness and its treatment differently (Surbone & Lowenstein, 2003a). Patients and physicians use different methods of inquiry into the truth, and the objects of their knowledge, as well as their interests, are different. One—the patient—knows by direct personal and corporeal experience. The other—the physician—knows by generalization and abstraction (Surbone, 2000).

Western cultures tend to assume that "knowledge worthy of the name must transcend the particularities of experience to achieve objective purity and value neutrality" (Code, 1993). This ignores both the role of the knower in generating truth and the subjective, contextual, and relational dimension of knowledge in the patient–doctor relationship. By privileging a narrow biomedical model in clinical medicine, we overemphasize the objective dimension of disease and tend to ignore that illness is first a subjective event, a unique and disrupting, when not devastating, event in a person's life. As the subjective dimension of disease can hardly be measured with scientific methodology, it often discarded as unreal (Rollin, 1979; Surbone, 2000). The equation of "real" with "scientifically measurable" contrasts with a view of science in postmodern philosophy that accepts the notion of provisional open-ended truths and rejects uncritical scientific realism (Balestra, 1990). However, in medicine, the belief in an absolute neutral objective medical truth awaiting to be discovered by the doctor still dominates, and physicians are seen as the only ones who "tell" the truth to their patients (Surbone, 2000).

> When the relationship between cancer patients and their oncologists is recognized as an open-ended dynamic process of ascertainment and constant reassessment of the truths shared between them, truth telling is no longer the unidirectional act of the physician to the patient. Rather, the two partners communicate and together they try to make sense of the illness.

While the concern of the patient–doctor relationship is the patients' illness, in the traditional model of truth telling the physician takes center stage. The truth of the patients' illness is seen as a static object waiting to be described by the doctor. When the doctor is assumed to be the sole source of truth in the relationship, the patient is silenced. Yet knowledge in clinical medicine always has objective, subjective, and contextual dimensions that can be known only through the cooperation of patients and physicians, who share a common therapeutic goal (Surbone, 2000).

Prejudices and Truth in Clinical Medicine

In clinical medicine, doctors often see patients as lacking sufficient knowledge and authority to participate fully and actively in their care. It is undeniable that there are profound discrepancies between lay and professional judgments. At times,

> superstitions and prejudices may hamper communication in the patient–doctor relationship. Fears and misinformation among lay people about disease, its cause, and its transmission, may lead them to enter into discussion about health and illness only on the basis of presuppositions that actually serve to disrupt the possibility of open, well-informed debate and communication. (Edgar, 1997)

Disagreements among patients, the public, and physicians, as well as cross-cultural variations regarding the definition of health and well-being, can be key points at which communication easily breaks down (Edgar, 1997). Prejudices, however, are not only the prerogative of patients. Physicians' prejudices may also play a major role in the clinical setting, as demonstrated by the occurrence of unfair or discriminatory treatment of minority patients in some medical encounters (Betancourt, 2003; Mahowald, 2000). An additional prejudice held by physicians and by oncologists in particular is to consider alternative and complementary medicine to be, a priori, ineffective. A skeptical attitude hinders the patient–doctor relationship, and cited studies show that patients may hold back information from their oncologists.

Clinical experience shows that cancer patients would like their oncologists to tell them "the truth" about whether or not a complementary measure is safe and effective, and that they want to have physicians' approval for their use of them. Unfortunately, while hard evidence is still lacking for most complementary treatments, integrative oncologists may attempt to provide answers using their inference and intuition instead of admitting to a lack of evidence or knowledge, to satisfy their patients' expectations for truth and reassurance. In integrative oncology, it may be especially difficult to strike a balance between showing interest and providing patients with adequate information, on one hand, and remaining truthful to existing evidence on the other. It is important to recognize that for cancer patients, being able to ask their oncologists questions and receive respectful responses from them are just as important as the content of the answers they are given. At times, patients are looking for an open channel of communication with their oncologists, one in which they feel accepted and appreciated (Weil, 2000). This intrinsic value of communication can coexist with the uncertainty of oncology and of integrative oncology.

Finally, oncologists, in focusing on the importance of providing accurate information to their patients, may lose sight of other needs of their patients, who are trying to live with cancer (Surbone, 2006a). Owing to the physical pain, the psychological suffering, and the social isolation that cancer patients often endure, their experience of cancer and its treatment is often characterized by a deep sense of "losing control." To provide effective integrative cancer care it is essential not only to respect patients' right to information but also to be partners with them in searching for the truth of their illness and in making sense of their lives with cancer.

Truth and Truth Telling: A Reciprocal Step in the Patient–Doctor Relationship

The impact of the words uttered by the physician in the patient–doctor relationship testifies to the depth of the responsibility that physicians have toward their patients in searching for the truth and sharing it with them (Galeazzi, 1997). In the patient–doctor relationship the knowledge and the truth of each is different and yet is always dependent on, and influenced by, the other. As the boundaries between objectivity and subjectivity are blurred, the central role of truth telling in clinical medicine emerges as the recognition that human beings deserve the truth (Williams, 2002). Truth telling, however, is only a step in the relationship between the patient and the integrative oncologist. The relationship *itself* has profound therapeutic value. Even when evidence to support any truth statement about a given complementary or alternative measure may be lacking, the relational value of truthfulness in the patient–doctor relationship is part of the healing purview of integrative oncology.

In complex human relationships of patients and doctors, each has an equal responsibility to be truthful, as each is bound by justice and trust in a goal-oriented, asymmetric yet mutual, covenant (Baier, 1994; Pellegrino, 1992; Pellegrino & Thomasma, 1988). Initially, the patient contributes the truthful description of his or her subjective suffering and the lived context of the truth, while the physician truthfully decodes and interprets the patients' symptoms and signs, as well as the results of various tests. During the course of their therapeutic alliance, the patient and the doctor interact together and with the world, while continuing to search for the truth of the illness. Often, in the patient–doctor relationship an absolute truth does not exist or cannot be found. Yet truthfulness helps the patient move beyond despair by shifting the goal of the therapeutic relationship from simply "repairing the disease" to making sense of the patient' s life with his or her illness.

Truth Telling from the Doctor to the Patient

Truth telling in the patient–doctor relationship presupposes and requires the virtues of sincerity and accuracy from both partners in the covenant. Accuracy lies in the skills and attitudes that help overcome the external and internal obstacles to discovery of the truth. Sincerity is a matter of disposition in the context of a relationship, "centered on sustaining and developing relations with others that involve different kinds and degrees of trust" (Williams, 2002). Clearly, the accuracy and sincerity required of the patient and the physician are different. In the truth-telling moments of the patient–doctor relationship, the physician has a special and specific responsibility to consider that any statement may be true, and yet that making a given statement may not be appropriate at a given time. In the case of a serious incurable illness, the reverberations of the physicians' words can be shattering. Physicians are thus called not only to make a rational assessment in their truth telling to the patient but also to consider the full impact of their words on the patient, while resisting any form of paternalism.

The objective content of truth telling from the doctor is related to his or her authority, role, and responsibility in the patient–doctor relationship. The patient–doctor relationship arises from the patients' suffering and vulnerability and the physicians' authority, based on theoretical and clinical knowledge, to interpret this suffering (Galeazzi, 1997). The physician is called to recognize a pattern in the patients' symptoms that leads to the formulation of a diagnosis, with the help of different tests and procedures. The physicians' next task is to help the patient manage the illness through prescriptions, recommendations, and advice, in a spirit of partnership with the patient. When, at times, physicians are invested with the responsibility of "taking charge" temporarily of their patients' situation because the patients request it, this should not be interpreted as a call for paternalism, but rather seen as part of the physicians' partnerships with and responsibility toward their patients (Pellegrino & Thomasma, 1988).

In ancient medicine, the doctor's role was perceived in magical terms. Today, physicians' authority is earned rather than taken for granted and it rests on physicians' ethical commitment to objectivity, honesty, and respect for their patients' autonomy and right to be informed and to participate in making decisions about their health care.

Truth Telling from the Patient to the Doctor

At first glance it would appear that the patient has less truth-telling responsibility than the physician. The patient, however, enacts his or her specific responsibility to be truthful in describing symptoms, in describing the life context of the illness, and in reporting the changes that occur in the course of the illness, including whether or not he or she follows medical prescriptions, what side effects these have, and so on (Galeazzi, 1997). Internal obstacles, however, may keep patients from being entirely truthful. Sick persons may engage in self-deception, not due to insincerity, but rather as a much more complex matter related to the intensity of their bodily suffering (Merleau-Ponty, 1962). Unrealistic hopes, fears, and wishful thinking are among the possible coping mechanisms of seriously ill persons, and they are intimately related to vulnerability due to their illness. As noted in the diary of a 20th Century writer, "What I say isn't necessarily true, but it explains, just by the fact that I say it, my suffering" (Pavese, 1977). The oncologist must be prepared to recognize that the patients' self-deception may be an unconscious defense mechanism in the face of suffering and mortality. When deception, on the contrary, is intentionally used to divert the physicians' inquiry, the fiduciary nature of the patient–doctor relationship is threatened and the mutual discovery of truth is obstructed.

Sometimes, cancer patients do not feel comfortable being truthful to their oncologists because they are afraid of being misjudged or ignored. As noted earlier, for example, many patients using complementary medicine do not inform their oncologists (Yates, et al., 1993). While it is true that oncologists work under tremendous time and economic pressure that, at times, limits their availability to properly listen to their patients, often patients sense, correctly, that their oncologist is reluctant to talk about the use of complementary medicine, due to limited knowledge and lack of teaching and training in integrative oncology (Weil, 2000). In most cases, the lack of openness that stems from the patients' fear of being disapproved by her oncologist does not result in any major damage to the patient. However, when cancer patients use complementary treatments during phase I investigational trials without informing their treating oncologists or against their recommendations, serious health risks can follow (Hlubocky, et al., 2007).

It is reassuring that there appears to be a trend toward more open communication between cancer patients and oncologists regarding the use of complementary and alternative healing methods. In integrative oncology, where the thoughtful and rational combination of conventional and complementary therapies for cancer are the aim, patients and oncologists share an equal responsibility to be honest and truthful about the use and the appropriateness of complementary measures.

Conclusion

The practice of medicine should be a shared therapeutic effort of patients and physicians within a functional system that includes caregivers and institutions, and it should be informed by and ruled by allegiance to "truth." In his latest book, *Truth and Truthfulness. An Essay in Genealogy*, Bernard Williams addresses the problematic coexistence in our society of a demand for truthfulness that is accompanied by an equally pervasive suspicion about truth itself.

According to Williams, this problem could be solved if we were to shift our search for the "truth" to a search for "making sense" of what happens to us (Williams, 2002). This perspective can help us understand the patient–doctor relationship, where patients and physicians together try to "make sense," in more or less provisional or definite ways, of the presence of illness in the patients' life, by analyzing and connecting multiple intertwined truths.

In the patient–doctor relationship, the process of making sense is mediated by, and is built on, the truth that the patient and the doctor share within the boundaries of their asymmetric relationship. Cancer patients and their oncologists look for and share the truth of the patients' illness in a binding relation that is, and should be, especially strong when the two parties engage in the project of integrated oncology. The individual autonomy of our cancer patients is often limited by their social and cultural context and by their religious beliefs, by their personal relationships with friends and families, and by the asymmetry of knowledge and of power inherent to any clinical encounter. Consideration of these relational aspects of patients' autonomy, accompanied by full awareness of the asymmetric dynamics of the patient–doctor–society relationship, can enhance the oncologists' ability to share the many evolving truths of the illness with their cancer patients and help them make sense of their lives with cancer (Sherwin, 1998; Surbone, 2006a; Taboada & Bruera, 2001). When we come to grips with the fact that "truth" for our cancer patients is not only a matter of objective, scientifically measurable elements that we must identify and interpret but also of "making sense" of their suffering, then we can begin to understand the meaning of truth telling from multiple perspectives. Discussion of prognosis, for example, goes beyond telling or not telling the statistical truth to include the cognitive, psychological, and spiritual aspects of the interplay of medical certainty and uncertainty, of human hope and expectations, and of making sense of one's vulnerability and mortality. In the broad perspective of healing the whole person, it is possible to be truthful with seriously ill patients and to give opinions and advice to patients facing difficult choices without taking away hope. The intent and effort to do so requires a deep commitment both to the truth and to the relationship with one's patients, which should inform the practice of integrative oncology.

ACKNOWLEDGMENTS

I am thankful to my philosophy mentor, Dominic J Balestra PhD, Professor of Philosophy at Fordham University in New York, for many insightful discussions of truth in medicine and to William Russell-Edu, Librarian at the European Institute of Oncology in Milan, for his valuable assistance.

REFERENCES

Abrams DI. (2007). An overview of integrative oncology. *Clin Advances in Heamtol Oncol,* 5, 45–47.

Cassileth BR, Schraub S, Robisnon E, & Vickers A. (2001). Alternative medicine use wordwide: The International Union Against Cancer survey. *Cancer,* 91, 1390–1393.

Ernst E. (2002).The role of complementary and alternative medicine. *British Medical Journal,* 321, 1133–1135.

Hann DM, Baker F, & Denniston MM. (2003). Oncology professionals' communication with cancer patients about complementary therapy: A survey. *Complementary Therapies in Medicine,* 11, 184–190.

Hlubocky FJ, Ratain MJ, & Daugherty CK. (2007). Complementary and alternative medicine among advanced cancer patients enrolled on phase I trials: A study of prognosis, quality of life, and preferences for decision making. *Journal of Clinical Oncology,* 25, 548–554.

Paltiel O, Avitzour M, Peretz T, Cherny N, Kaduri L, Pfeffer RM, et al. (2001). Determinants of the use of complementary therapies by patients with cancer. *Journal of Clinical Oncology,* 19, 2439–2448.

Roberts CS, Baker F, Hanno D, Runfola J, Witt C, McDonald J, et al. (2005). Patient-physician communication regarding use of complementary therapies during cancer treatment. *Journal of Psychosocial Oncology,* 23, 35–60.

Surbone A. (2006a). Telling truth to patients with cancer: What is the truth? *Lancet Oncology,* 7, 944–950.

Surbone A. (2006c). Cultural aspects of communication in cancer care. In F Stiefel (Ed.), *Communication in cancer care. Recent results in cancer research.* (pp. 168, 91–104). Heidelberg: Springer Verlag.

Weil A. (2000). The significance of integrative medicine for the future of medical education. *The American Journal of Medicine,* 18, 441–443.

(A complete reference list for this chapter is available online at http://www.oup.com/us/ integrativemedicine).

29

A Patient's Perspective

MANUCHEHR SHIRMOHAMADI

KEY CONCEPTS

- This chapter describes my experience in detection of cancer and my reactions to it; in information gathering and screening about cancer and its treatments; and in fighting the disease. It also contains some "advice" I learned from my experience for a better living. Most importantly, this chapter presents how cancer changed me.

■

My Story

Cancer changed me—for worse and for better!

When I was invited to contribute to this book, I was honored and overwhelmed. While I had written technical reports and papers in my line of business—engineering, I had never written a story about myself. So, the thought of writing something nontechnical and, especially, about my own experience and feelings overwhelmed me. However, it took me only a short time to discover that I, as a cancer patient and survivor, have a lot to say and share about my condition, which I hope benefits others. Therefore, I decided to take on this challenge and provide my perspective.

I am going to start with reciting my story, followed by sharing what I learned in my experience and end with what I believe to be one of the most potent weapons we have to fight the disease. I also feel that I have to convey a message to the medical establishment about what we, as patients, go through and what we expect from them.

The Beginning

My friends and family consider me to be very analytical, highly skeptic, and, according to my closer friends and family, hard headed, competitive, and wanting to be in charge. I had studied in some of the best universities in the world and had my own relatively successful engineering consulting business with a number of employees. This business, probably like any other, was stressful but I enjoyed most of the work except for some of the business aspects of it. I barely took any vacations and worked hard. However, at the same time, I also considered myself to be generally healthy, somewhat athletic, and in good physical and mental condition.

For a long period before my first colon exam, I started noticing minute and intermittent amounts of rectal bleeding. Initially, I ignored these symptoms to be "normal" reactions to foods (I love spicy foods) and physical activities. My physicians also discounted this as being anything important, which, in light of my age and family history, was to be expected. However, my skepticism and hard headedness were probably the reasons for my insistence about being examined for colon problems. Finally, I was examined by a skeptical physician in mid-2001, who, just before the examination, told me that at worst I have hemorrhoids and I am wasting everyone's time. During the examination though, he found that I have colorectal cancer. Much more than the physician, who did not expect to find anything serious, I became shocked and, I should confess, quite scared. I considered myself young and healthy and no one in my immediate family has ever had this disease; "*I am not supposed to have cancer!*"

I soon learned that colorectal cancer is the second biggest killer among cancers (after lung cancer) mainly for the reason that its symptoms usually show up too late. I was reminded of the people I knew with cancer, most of whom, were no longer around. One case, which scared me most, was that of a friend's son who died of colorectal cancer at the age of 15! Mostly, however, my diagnosis reminded me of my father-in-law. He was very healthy and athletic with only one bad habit—smoking. He had barely been to any physician in his entire life. In 1999, he, at the age of 74, was diagnosed with an advanced case of lung cancer and, 3 months later, he was gone. As he was living with us in his last weeks, I clearly remembered his extreme pain and suffering caused by the treatment consisting of high doses of chemotherapy and radiation in those weeks. I remembered how impersonal the treatment was for him. My wife and I questioned "*why would his physicians put him through so much suffering?*"

Because of these experiences, I always considered having cancer as pretty much a death sentence and not worth fighting. However, now that I had it, I couldn't just accept defeat without a good fight! As was usual in my profession, I started studying about the disease and having discussions with experts and cancer survivors. I learned that the disease, in many cases, is defeatable and hence worth fighting. But I should also add that still I remained convinced that in cases like that of my father-in-law, it would have been much better to make his last days comfortable rather than trying to fight a loosing battle. Right or wrong, I still blame his physicians for his suffering!

My diagnosis and the fact that my physicians believed we had discovered my cancer early enough to beat it, started a series of fast-occurring events. I suddenly went from being considered "over-concerned" and a "pain in the neck" by some of my physicians to a cancer patient with multiple visits and consultations to plan a course of treatment.

First Fight

Being a technical professional, I put my full trust in my physician team, which I considered to be expert in this field. I followed their advice to have surgery to remove the tumor and follow it by a course of chemotherapy to prevent its return. A few days after my initial diagnosis, I checked into the hospital for my surgery. Unfortunately, the surgery to remove the tumor and a portion of my colon led to an internal leak. I had to be readmitted to the hospital with the worst pain imaginable that even the maximum allowed doses of morphine would not relieve. For the next 8 days, I was treated with heavy doses of antibiotics and painkillers in the hospital. This experience shook my trust in the medical establishment and I started seeing physicians as humans who can and do make mistakes. However, I kept following the treatment plan as I believed it was the best way to fight and conquer the disease. The surgical complication led to a delay in the starting of chemotherapy.

I started a standard chemotherapy regimen, consisting of 5-FU (I'd like to rename this drug!!!) and leucovorin. At first, I handled the chemo reasonably well, but as time passed, my reactions became more and more negative. It is really hard for me to describe how chemo affected me (both physically and psychologically) and I understand that it could be different for different patients. The "normal" side effects—nausea, weakness, pain, etc.—are only a part of the story. It also generates a general "lousy feeling" and a lack of interest in life and anything in it, which is hard to describe. People who have been through chemotherapy may know what I am talking about. In his book, Lance Armstrong devoted a chapter to chemo effects, which I found to capture most of the feelings a patient goes through rather well—but, in my experience, that is not yet complete! For me, nothing smelled, looked, or felt good and everything was colorless and lifeless! I felt that I was in a state of limbo—maybe as close to death as a living person can get! Later, during my second bout with the disease, I learned that part of the problem was that my physician team looked at this as purely a technical issue ignoring the human factor. More about this later.

With all the chemo side effects, my biggest problem became the logic behind the treatment—repeatedly, nearly killing the patient to eliminate the cancer. I considered in this day and age with all the technical achievements man has reached, this is a backward method and there should be better ways to fight and beat this disease! But that is a different story!

In my case, one surprising effect was how I felt on the mornings I was to get treatment. On those days, I would feel so nauseated and sick that I could barely leave the bed. This was despite the fact that the day before I was feeling much better (which was the plan—you get strong before the next treatment). I figured that the anticipation of what the drugs would do to me made me so negative that I was subconsciously fighting my own treatment. I had a feeling that I was alone in my fight and later, I became convinced that this experience was a testament to the mental factors of the disease and its treatment, a fact that, I felt, was being ignored by my physicians at the time. Anyway, I had to delay treatments a few times and I finally stopped all treatment a little past the half way point since I could no longer handle the side effects. However, at the same time, I was also convinced that I had already beaten the disease and did not need the additional treatment. I also had started taking a supplement (Inositol hexa-Phosphate or IP6), which I strongly believed (and still do) helps with the fight. I also tried to have a healthier and less stressful life.

Second Round

Success against cancer is usually measured by how many years one stays cancer free (in remission) after the treatment. The idea is that the longer one stays cancer free, the better the chances for beating it entirely. The common milestones are 3 and 5 years with 5-year being considered by many the key milestone. After my treatment, I did the usual exams (CT, PET, colonoscopy...) and all results were negative (good). I was in "total remission" even after 3 years. This provided me with a false sense of security, which led me to ease off of my healthy diet, skip on supplements and, worse yet, get back to high-stress life style. Personal and family problems I faced in this period also aggravated my situation. During these times, the last thing in my mind was the recurring of cancer that I thought I had totally defeated. But, cancer was planning differently!

Cancer came back in mid-2005 in what I can only describe as a sudden and "vengeful" manner. The morning after having a heavy dinner with some good friends, I woke up with extreme cramps. My colon was practically blocked and I ended up in an emergency room. While my tests, some six months before this episode, were all negative, the follow-up colonoscopy/biopsy showed *my* cancer is back. ("*my cancer*?" I don't want it!!!) Additional diagnostics/imaging tests showed the extent and size of this recurrence.

Those knowledgeable about cancer statistics know that the recurring cancer, especially colon and colorectal cancers, is not "pretty" and has a low survival rate. At first, I was shocked, disappointed, and pretty much started sliding down toward total hopelessness. But, soon after, I came back to my senses and started seeing this as just having a bigger challenge in front of me. This time, though, I felt I needed to take a much more involved/hands-on approach in my treatment.

I started on a crash course of studying about the disease and, soon, I learned more about it that I ever would have cared. Along with the conventional medical information about the disease and its treatment—basically limited to surgery, chemo, and radiation—I also learned about "alternative" approaches. Needless to say there is an immense amount of easily accessible information and claims about cancer treatment and it is easy to get overwhelmed. I soon learned that the information landscape, along with having very good data about the disease and its treatment, is also littered by bogus claims, some made by those who try to profit from others' misery. Some of these claims looked legitimate containing heart-warming stories of survival. A general theme I found in many of such claims was their blame of the medical industry as being profit mongers and not caring about patients, which was fueled by real stories about the greed of the insurance and drug companies and hospitals, and the lack of caring or knowledge by some physicians. My research also led to my own increased skepticism of the conventional medical system, specially the drug companies, and its approach toward cancer treatment and helped open my eyes to seeing beyond what conventional medicine had to offer.

To manage the large amount of information and to decipher between the good and bogus claims, I came up with a set of simple criteria—existence of scientific data in respectable forums, a strong plausible theory behind a treatment, and the source of information. These helped me screen the information landscape and identify some simple and yet effective methods to increase my fighting chances against cancer. I looked around and saw that I was fortunate to be living in an area with some of the best scientists and research universities in the country. I decided to take advantage of all the cards I had right where I lived including the latest research and treatments and alternative sources I could trust.

After the diagnosis, I consulted with my surgeon who did the initial surgery some 4 years earlier. He quickly scheduled a new invasive and high-risk surgery to be followed by chemo and radiation treatments. This time, however, rather than following this route, I consulted with my new oncologist and a well-known surgeon (and I should add, a great person) at a local university hospital. From my oncologist and the university surgeon, I learned about a newer approach (neoadjuvant) for treating the recurring colorectal cancer, which starts with a chemo-radiation therapy followed by surgery and then a "maintenance" chemo regimen. In this treatment, the surgery will have lower risks and side effects than starting with the surgery and the overall survival was slightly better. Through my contact with this university hospital, I also learned they had opened a new center advocating "integrative" approaches to treating the disease, which became a great resource for me.

From the information I had gathered, I developed a decision tree (Fig. 29.1), assigned risk factors to each step, and analyzed my options, a common practice in my own professional field. As a result, I decided to start with the neoadjuvant therapy but continue to evaluate the risks and benefits of each treatment step before committing to it. I started my chemo-radiation treatment in August 2005.

My best discovery this time, however, was the Center for Integrative Medicine of the university hospital and the physician there who became my "integrative oncologist" as well as my advisor. This center advocates an integrative approach to treating disease, a combination of conventional and complementary approaches. They try to take the blinders off of the conventional medicine and consider and treat the patient as an individual with specific conditions and needs for whom statistics alone may not apply. Their approach and "motto" was very much in tune with what I had come to believe on my own, plus it was also based on sound scientific methods. I think the best attribute of the center is their open-mindedness and the fact that they are not just another practitioner of existing conventional approaches.

The center became an educational and a sounding board for me to learn about effective treatments, how to better manage the side effects of conventional treatments, and to distinguish false from positive claims. It reinforced my earlier belief that one's mind has a lot to do with one's health and that there are some old and effective techniques, such as mental exercises; healthy diet; eastern, and especially Chinese, traditional medicine; and vitamins and herbs, which can significantly benefit the patient. They also introduced me to a local clinic that advocated the integrated eastern and conventional medical approaches. Between the integrative center of the university hospital and the clinic, they advocated and practiced herbal medicine, acupuncture, and meditation and mental exercises (yoga, guided imagery, etc.). After a general examination,

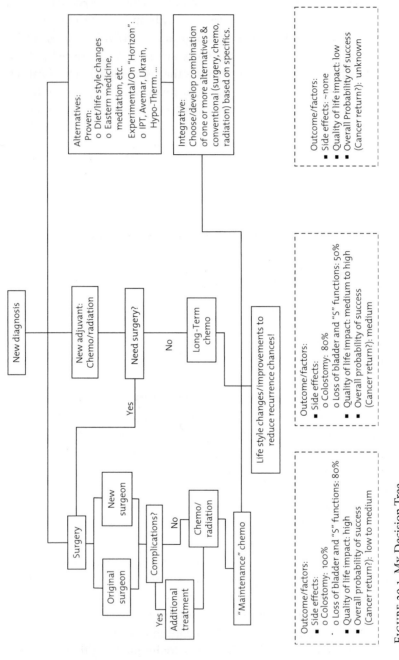

New diagnosis

New adjuvant: Chemo/radiation

Need surgery?

Yes → Surgery
- Original surgeon
- New surgeon

Complications?
- Yes → Additional treatment
- No → Chemo/radiation

"Maintenance" chemo

No → Long-Term chemo

Life style changes/Improvements to reduce recurrence chances!

Alternatives:
Proven:
o Diet/life style changes
o Eastern medicine, meditation, etc.
Experimental/On "Horizon":
o IPT, Avemar, Ukrain, Hypo-Therm. ...

Integrative:
Choose/develop combination of one or more alternatives & conventional (surgery, chemo, radiation) based on specifics.

Outcome/factors:
- Side effects:
  o Colostomy: 100%
  o Loss of bladder and "S" functions: 80%
- Quality of life impact: high
- Overall probability of success (Cancer return?): low to medium

Outcome/factors:
- Side effects:
  o Colostomy: 80%
  o Loss of bladder and "S" functions: 50%
- Quality of life impact: medium to high
- Overall probability of success (Cancer return?): medium

Outcome/factors:
- Side effects: ~none
- Quality of life impact: low
- Overall Probability of success (Cancer return?): unknown

FIGURE 29.1. My Decision Tree.

which included a detailed pulse tracking, evaluation of my history (health, family, and emotional—considering childhood diseases, my family history, and my relationships), and reviewing the chemo-radiation plan I was about to start, they developed a personal plan ("protocol," consisting of a regimen of herbs, vitamins, and mental exercises customized to fit my treatment cycles) for the complementary part of my integrative approach.

I started my 2-month chemo-radiation treatment along with my customized protocol. The first cycle, as expected, was pretty rough especially toward the end, but this time I was determined to stay with the treatment and "tough" it out. Plus I had a lot of emotional support, which made the cycle easier to handle. I should add that my complementary protocol was not rigid like a prescribed medicine approach and that I did make some adjustments to the protocol by eliminating some items I had trouble taking. The important fact was that my complementary team listened and worked with me to make the process easier to handle and more "humane." I also tried some mental exercises such as guided imagery but soon discovered that I am too much of a skeptic for these methods to help me. I did, however, mend some of my rocky relationships, found great support from my wife, and counted on my many friends throughout this process. I also started a "slow-down" process at work, which helped with my stress management. The love and support I have been receiving has become a very potent weapon in my fight against the disease. I truly believe that my protocol and the mental support made this chemo-radiation treatment manageable and more effective. Also, probably, I could not have completed the treatment without them—as I couldn't the first time.

After my chemo-radiation treatment and just days before the planned surgery in the local university hospital, I learned my insurance would not cover the surgery as it was "outside the network." This was initially a disappointment, but later, became a "blessing" for me. The disappointment was because even a well-planned treatment could be cancelled by insurance companies for some obscure bureaucratic reason and the blessing was how this event led to a change in my treatment plan.

I searched and found a new surgeon within my insurance network whom I could also trust for the planned surgery. I also found out this surgery is still very invasive and can lead to permanent damage affecting the "quality of life." During this delay, I was tested to establish my condition. My test results showed no signs of cancer in my body—of course considering the accuracy and resolution of the diagnostics methods. These good results along with the surgery's risk, its small statistical benefit, and my past experience with surgery brought the surgery option under question for me. I consulted my team and some other experts in the field. While the consensus among my physicians was for me to have the surgery, some also agreed that my condition did not fit the limited available statistics. I went back to my decision tree and performed a new risk/benefit analysis. As a result, I decided to bypass the surgery at the time and only use it in the future if absolutely needed. As expected, this was not received well by my surgeon and some of the team; however, no one on my team could convince me that my decision was wrong, based on available scientific data and my own special case.

After my decision to forego the surgery became final, I found great support among my team especially my oncologist and my integrative oncologist. My oncologist developed a new chemo treatment cycle consisting of four main drugs (bevacizumab, 5-FU, leucovorin, and irinotecan.) My oncologist also included a number of "supplemental" drugs, such as blood cell boosters and steroids, which helped with handling of the chemo drugs. From my integrative oncologist and the clinic, I also received a new protocol to help with the effectiveness of the chemo treatment and its side effects. In my own mind, I had accepted the risk associated with this plan and was trying to improve my chances by developing an effective integrative approach. I was convinced that I had made the best decision about my treatment while continuing on the path for a less stressful life style.

The second cycle treatment was quite rough at times, but I managed it much better than my prior simpler regimen 4 years earlier. The supplements that were tailored for the effects of the treatment, great support from my team, and keeping a positive attitude helped a lot. What helped most, probably, was the empowering feeling I had because of my involvement in developing my own treatment plan!

I recently finished my treatment and the follow-up scans have shown no recurrence. Well, they thought they saw something in my chest, but testing inaccuracies and logic convinced me, my oncologist, and my integrative oncologist that the perceived indications were a case of false positive. A more recent scope and biopsies showed no recurrence in or around the original cancer site. These results are good news and I intend to continue getting them!! I will stay under close watch for at least 5 years and I plan to make the healthy living habits I have learned a part of my life.

What Worked for Me

During and after my ordeals, I continued my research and kept learning about the disease and its treatment. Among the interventions that helped me, I would like to highlight the mind's "healing" power. Studies have shown this to be a real phenomenon and to help many patients with various diseases. However, despite such studies, it has not been scientifically explained, nor rigorously proven, and the majority of the conventional medical establishment discounts it entirely. My own scientific background and skepticism does not allow me to take something on just faith either. But, it is also very hard to argue against what seems very logical and has many studies and cases to support it. So I came up with the following explanation for myself: It is common knowledge that the mind has powers science has not yet discovered and there are many cases (and I personally know a few) where a "dying" patient completely recovers—some even without receiving any conventional treatment. To me, this is a proof that the mind's healing power, when tapped properly, can direct the body's immune system to fight and cure the disease. I think this may be the same as what some call the "placebo" effect! Studies that show people with strong and positive faith (religious) and strong will power recover better than the average reinforces the notion of mind power effect. Therefore, if one can find a way to tap the mind's healing power, his or her chances for recovery improve significantly. The question then becomes how one can tap this vast and immense power.

While strong faith helps some patients perhaps subconsciously to tap into their mind's healing power; an analytical person like myself has a harder time using this resource. But there is hope even for the most skeptical among us. By learning about the ever-evolving science of mind power, even the most analytical person can tap into this resource for health. This requires being open-minded, having physicians/scientists on one's team who are also open-minded, researching and identifying techniques (within conventional and complementary fields) that have a high potential for helping fight the disease, developing an integrated approach to health including mind and body, and above all believing and convincing oneself that the approach will help.

I think of having cancer as being in a marathon race between the body and the disease in which the disease is not "smart" enough to realize its victory equates to its own death! The irony is that the race ends with death regardless of who wins. The goal, therefore, should be that death be on the person's terms. Fortunately, this is a race that most people don't have to face, but for those of us who are in this race, we need all the help we can get. After all, the disease has a lot of support, ever increasing since the start of the industrial age, including too many chemicals in the air, quality and the quantity of food, and above all, lifestyles with ever increasing stress. On the body's side, the support has been mainly from the conventional treatment, which is not sufficient to counteract the disease's extensive support system. One needs to find the best support team and coaching available to win the race. The coaching is best provided by the mind, which can advocate good attitude, healthy living, and stress management—all great cancer killers—along with the best conventional treatment available. This race in many cases—but not all—can be won utilizing all the available resources and support for the body and mind as possible. And, unless and until the mind is determined to win the race, no treatments will be as effective.

Medicine is still mainly an art compensated by a large amount of data and statistics—but it is also the best we have. Lack of knowledge, errors, lack of care, bureaucratic issues, and downright greed and even fraud are its main deficiencies. Medical schools, until recently, ignored nutrition and mind power in fighting diseases and as a result most physicians are not even educated in these important facets of health care. Our "for profit" health-care system does not have as strong incentives in healing patients as maintaining them. And, legal and bureaucratic processes prevent many patients from receiving as good care as they need. However, fortunately, the field is mainly run by people (physicians, nurses, agents, etc.) like you and me and it is still very much "human." There are many practitioners who truly believe in helping their patients and, despite being tied by bureaucratic issues, will go out of their way to provide the best care possible. For these professionals, nothing makes them more proud and satisfied than to see their patients recover under their care!

What Should Be Done

As a patient, when you are ready to plan and receive treatment, demand attention and respect from your health care professionals while being respectful and considerate of their situation as well. After all, most health care professionals still care about your well being and are there to help you. If you feel you are not receiving the attention you deserve, move on to the next option and seek a different provider if possible.

I also call on the medical professionals to treat patients with respect and as individuals. I ask that they educate themselves with the latest in both conventional and complementary approaches and keep an open mind to find the best "integrative" methods for treating their patients.

Cancer patients, I believe, expect to be treated by those who show interest in their well-being and by best available approaches. If there was a "bill of responsibilities" for cancer patients, it would include the following. As a cancer patient, you should do the following:

1. Develop a "support team" among your physicians, family, and friends. Use your team to express your condition, bounce ideas, or just get mental or physical support.
2. Get second, third…opinions. Do not limit yourself to those who refuse to consider any other approach except conventional medicine. Avoid those who make you feel uncomfortable or are too arrogant.

Of course, given the urgency of the matter, you need to be systematic and fast in planning your treatment.

3. Make sure you have at least one "health advocate" (advisor) on your team with whom you feel comfortable sharing your condition and thoughts, one who is open-minded and is knowledgeable in both conventional and complementary approaches. This could be your primary care doctor, your oncologist, your herbalist, a family member, or just a good friend. In my case, my advocates were a combination of my integrative oncologist, my conventional oncologist, and my wife.

4. Working with your team, develop a treatment plan that makes you feel comfortable. This may include some or all conventional and complementary approaches available to you.

5. Tap into your mind's healing power by convincing yourself that the treatment plan is the best thing that can be done. After all, since you were part of the team developing the treatment and no one knows you better than you, it *is* the best approach.

6. Simplify your life by resolving the sources of stress that can be managed including family and work issues.

7. Go "natural". Stay away from processed foods. Find pleasures in simple and healthy foods. After all, "you are what you eat!" By the way, stay off sugar as that is cancer's favorite food.

8. Stay positive. Don't forget to find pleasures in life and enjoy those as much as you can.

Don't forget that fighting cancer is a life-time commitment and not just limited to the duration you are receiving chemotherapy and other treatment. Develop a healthy life style that includes a positive attitude, exercise, and a healthy diet including supplements that are proven to help. As you know, professionals have devised many programs and recommendations, sometimes even contradictory, which are supposed to help you fight this disease. The shear volume of such information is overwhelming and confusing even for the experts. However, if you step back and look at them, they all revolve around some very simple ideas based on common sense. To make sense of all these, I have tried to summarize the key points for fighting cancer and a healthy living into a simple Avoid/Acquire ("AA") table (Table 29.1).

Closing Thoughts

Cancer changed me—for worse and for better! In addition to all the pain and suffering and the stress of observing concern in loved one's faces, my outlook

Table 29.1. "AA" (Avoid/Acquire) of Fighting Cancer.

AVOID	ACQUIRE
Stress: I consider this to be one of the main causes for cancer as well as many other diseases. Stress, however, means different things to different people. Find what stresses *you* and eliminate/avoid/minimize them	*Positive Attitude:* By far, this is your most potent weapon against cancer (and many other diseases). It is as simple as: "if you believe something will help you, it most probably will!"
Processed Foods, Specially Sugar: Cancer cells love sugar and thrive on foods that are bad for your general health as well. Bad fats, preservatives and chemicals, and other similar ingredients should be avoided	*Eat Healthy and Well:* Simple and fresh foods consisting of mostly fruits, vegetables, whole grains, legumes, and some fish. Again, this is as simple as: "you are what you eat"
"Negative Energy:" This is rather vague, but try to avoid situations and people that make you feel uncomfortable or bring your energy level down	*Support Team:* Tap into family/friends who make you feel good for your support team. But don't forget that this is a 2-way street
Being Down: Being down (depression?) weakens your immune system and helps cancer win over you. Fight it with all you can!	*Exercise:* Even some moderate exercise goes a long way to fight depression and toward a better/healthier living

And, most importantly, pursue HAPPINESS!

and planning of activities also become limited to my next test. It is like life stops and you are still in pain. However, this experience also taught me to look at life very differently and learn to "live in the moment." While it is unfortunate that it takes a disease like cancer to make many of us realize this important lesson in life, for me it was nevertheless the best outcome of the disease. So, while I started very angry and disappointed once I found out about having the disease, I am no longer sad as it made me learn a lot about myself and what life should mean.

In closing, let me also share my new found philosophy of life: A good life is summarized in three "H's." They are, in order of importance: Happiness, Health, and ... hmm, I forget the third one!!! Good luck in your fight and remember to stay Happy and Positive. After all, the reason it is said "you can't buy happiness" is that because it is free!

30

Integrative Oncology: The Future

DAVID S. ROSENTHAL

KEY CONCEPTS

- Integrative care is collaborative care—consolidating the many disciplines of support services.
- Best overall cancer treatment incorporates the patient's individual profile including family history, ethnic origin, prior health habits, nutrition, and physical activity.
- Most cancer patients require and seek assistance navigating the healthcare system and addressing their complex and unmet needs.
- The practice of integrative oncology helps the clinical team better address the patient's total care.

■

In 1971, President Nixon declared the "War on Cancer." The National Cancer Act was passed and as a result there was a significant increase [1] in the National Cancer Institute (NCI) budget aimed at eliminating cancer as a disease. A cure for all cancers has not yet been found, but major breakthroughs in prevention and therapy have occurred giving hope that this disease will eventually become "history." Between 1996 and 1998 [2], the board of directors of the American Cancer Society (ACS) set the following challenge goals to guide strategy and programming:

- To reduce cancer mortality rates by 50% by the year 2015
- To reduce the incidence of cancer by 25% by 2015

- To show measurable improvement in the quality of life for all cancer patients (physical, psychological, social, and spiritual) from the time of diagnosis and for the balance of life for all cancer survivors by the year 2015.

It has not been easy to predict what cancer medicine would look like in 10 to 20 years, let alone the emerging field of integrative oncology. A little beyond the midpoint toward 2015, it appears that some of the ACS goals will be met, some will not. The number of cancer survivors has grown steadily over the past several decades and the NCI estimates that approximately 10.5 million Americans with a history of cancer were alive in 2003. However, according to the ACS, in 2008, 1.44 million new cancer cases are expected to be diagnosed and approximately 565,650 are expected to die from cancer in the United States [3]. The cancer death rate has been decreasing steadily since the mid-1990s with an 11.6% decrease in cancer mortality from 1991 to 2003. It is unlikely that the ACS 2015 mortality reduction goal will be met, but a projected reduction rate to 25% will be appreciated. However, significant decreased mortality goals will be met for specific cancers such as colorectal, prostate, and breast. Incidence rates of cancer have been stable. The ACS goals for quality of life have been more difficult to set and measure and have been replaced with nationwide objectives that assure appropriate care for cancer and therapy-related symptom control. For example, the objectives include attention to access to care, palliative and end-of-life care, and survivorship issues.

Where health care in the United States will be in 2020 has also been the speculation of the United States Pharmacopeial Convention (USPC) in their publication predicting outcomes "2020 VISIONS: Health Care Information Standards and Technologies," published in 1992 [4]. Clement Bezold suggested four possible scenarios:

- High technology/continued growth—health-care therapeutics advance dramatically, and there is more personal focused care, prediction and management of illness, and DNA-driven variations in health care.
- Hard times/focused innovation—slow growth because of poor economic trends leads to two tier health systems, more out-of-pocket costs, and development of cost-effective strategies.
- Global business—medical care advances become global in scope, and there is improved health care even in the poorest of nations.
- The new social contract—diagnoses and treatments are increasingly varied, therapies are biochemically unique, and include allopathic pharmaceuticals, herbal and homeopathic medications, bioelectric and behavioral approaches.

It is fair to say that some aspects of all four of Bezold's scenarios are present today; for example, there are continued technological advances, hard times in funding research, a variety of treatment options, and a beginning of the spread of technologies to the poorest of nations.

With this background and the threat of under predicting or over estimating progress in the cancer field, let us consider two possible scenarios—one long term, and the other short term.

1. Cancer incidence continues but cancer is no longer a fatal disease.
2. Slow and steady achievements—that is, cancer incidence continues but mortality rates continue to decrease.

In the first scenario, oncology care is no longer determined by site of origin, but by a genetic defect or gene profiling. Cancer incidence has significantly decreased due to prevention and those cases that do occur are cured or controlled by targeted therapy. In the second instance, improved technologies continue to impact cancer survival with a continued steady decline in cancer mortality. In both scenarios, cancer has become less of a fatal disease, but in some cases a chronic disease. In either case, the quality of life issues rise to a significant level of importance and it is here that integrative oncology will play a major role.

The development and application of microarray technology, gene expression, and mass spectrometry for proteomics will allow for better understanding of tumor cell biology, the signals that cause normal cells to turn into malignant cells, better prognostication and prediction of response to therapy. "Gene expression profiling," a result of the advances in microarray methodology, will permit the simultaneous expression of thousands of genes from a single cell or tumor. Fingerprinting of a normal individual's genes will identify their risk of developing a specific cancer and thus a possibility of prevention. In prostate cancer, gene expression profiling may help select men with elevated or borderline levels of serum prostate specific antigen (PSA) who are candidates for aggressive therapy early on in their disease. Similarly in breast cancer, profiling can help distinguish sporadic cancers from the ones associated with BRCA mutations and help predict response to therapy. In lymphomas, fingerprinting can distinguish patients who may need more aggressive therapy such as an autologous stem cell transplant. The new technology has the potential to totally individualize cancer prevention, diagnosis, and treatment. In the future, one will be able to take a history on a new patient, perform a physical examination, and with proper testing be able to determine that individual's risk of developing a disease such as cancer. The physician will then be able to discuss the rationale for preventive measures and good health behaviors such as nutrition and physical activity in each patient based on their respective "fingerprint."

The issues of managing the cancer and treatment-related symptoms and the individual patient's quality of life become more important in both future scenarios and will be achieved by similarly targeting proven interventions through an integrative oncology model of care. Integrative oncology will be a major discipline in cancer care, making it just as important as the incredible technologic advances in gene expression profiling and targeted therapies discussed above.

Currently, there are two main obstacles that prevent full integration of complementary and alternative medicine (CAM) with conventional therapy—one the need to respond to the issues of CAM safety and efficacy, and the other, the development of a model of a collaborative multidisciplinary practice that combines all care for the cancer patient. This book has addressed the first obstacle and relates what is known today about CAM and how many CAM therapies are being integrated into conventional biomedical practice at all stages of cancer. CAM therapies including mind–body measures and physical activity are now implemented in the risk reduction of cancer, during active treatment to manage disease and treatment-related symptoms, for pain and palliative care and in the rehabilitation of survivors hopefully back to a normal quality of life. The authors of each chapter have identified progress in the CAM modalities with respect to clinical outcomes and research. Overcoming the second obstacle is the subject of this final chapter. As the field of integrative oncology further develops, how will it be possible to fully integrate CAM practice and make it part of routine oncologic care? Our collective goal should be that integrative oncology would not have to be distinguished at all as a separate entity but be included with routine cancer care. "CAM," as a phrase, is a major obstacle. Combining the words "complementary" and "alternative" does a disservice as many professional colleagues interpret "CAM" as "alternative medicine." It is time now to change the name to "Integrative Medicine" and "Integrative Oncology."

The principles of integrative oncology are to combine the best of all therapies, the combination of the best evidence-based complementary therapy and the best evidence-based conventional therapy for each patient, while strengthening the physician–patient relationship. Integrative oncology should take into consideration the genomics, the gene mapping, the individual characteristics, and lifestyle of each patient. Integrative oncology can and should lead to improved satisfaction by both patient and physician, in part by improving patient compliance with recommended therapies.

The role of the physician and communication between the physician and patient has changed in recent decades. In the past, the family physician was the one person who cared for all our health needs. She or he was a friend, adviser, comforter, and supporter, whose major technologic support was the stethoscope. Optimally, this physician was reassuring, caring and usually gave hope that things would get better. In the hospital the same doctor took care of us and performed many diagnostic tests at the bedside often explaining the reasons for the tests and the results. The additional contact led to an even closer relationship. Also at the bedside were the hospital attendings, usually senior physicians, who taught residents and students, confirmed physical findings, pointed out missed physical findings or took a moment to teach a medical "pearl," a clinical piece of information that students remembered for the rest of their career. Since this discussion often occurred at the bedside, the patient learned at the same time. The attendings were mentors, not only good teachers and clinicians but also clinical researchers. The mentors played a significant educational role in the medical school clinical years, in house staff training and later, in specialty training.

The picture today is somewhat different. With the major advances in medical technology, physicians perform many diagnostic blood and imaging tests, offer numerous therapeutic options, provide patients with quantities of educational material and survival data and often request multiple specialty consultations. Despite the significant improvement in survival statistics for cancer patients and the increasing numbers of survivors, it can be a very confusing time for the patient and very demanding for one physician to coordinate the often complex multidisciplinary care, particularly given time constraints for discussion. There is a need for increased patient–physician interaction to respond to the many questions raised by the complex medicine and numerous therapeutic options. Cancer medicine today is very "high tech" with a need for "high touch," the type of care that can be fulfilled by an integrative oncology approach.

My personal journey through hematology–oncology began in the 1960s with mentors such as Drs. William Dameshek, Jane Desforges, and William C. Moloney. As a fourth year medical student and then as a hematology fellow, I was able to watch firsthand the way these professors interacted with patients. I will always remember the first time I sat in with Dr. Moloney when he had to tell a patient, his young wife, and parents about his newly diagnosed acute myelogenous leukemia. In the early 1960s acute leukemia was a dreaded disease with a low complete remission rate and a rare cure in adults. Introduction of new chemotherapeutic agents from successful work in childhood leukemia had just begun to bear some positive results in adults. As Dr. Moloney started the conversation, he spoke sincerely and empathetically. He was straight and deliberate with the information about the diagnosis, the nature of the disease, the complications of the disease and what was at that time the best approach, combining supportive therapy with transfusions along with clinical trials using new chemotherapeutic agents. In this very serious discussion, he would interject a smile, when he told them the nickname for the new chemotherapy program, "VAMP." He discussed the need for some in-hospital days, but that much of the therapy could be performed on a weekly ambulatory basis. He left the family with significant hope that there was a chance for a response and a remission. After 45 minutes and responding to their questions he said, "Let's get started." The patient, his wife, and parents all stood up and crowded around Dr. Moloney and one after another gave him hugs. I had noted that several times during the discussion Dr. Moloney not only looked the patient straight in eye but also had placed his hand on the young man's shoulder.

Thus in a disease with a very poor prognostic outcome in the 1960s the young man began his chemotherapy and his close relationship with his care providers. After this patient/family conference, I walked out of the room and thought to myself, if I had been told that I had leukemia, would I have hugged the doctor for delivering that message? Since then, every time I sit down with a patient to tell them a diagnosis such as acute leukemia I always make sure that I look them in the eye and reach out to them either touching their arm, knee, or shoulder. Whether it provides a feeling of empathy or a method of inducing relaxation, the result has always been grateful appreciation. Dr. Moloney's bedside manner was very important, especially in view of the unsettling results of therapy for adult acute myelogenous leukemia. In 2007, the current remission and cure rates of acute leukemia have dramatically improved and a nonresponse is the exception rather than the rule.

What Dr. Moloney and others had demonstrated through their patient interaction is that they were in partnership with their patient, providing therapeutic options and supportive care and the leadership for the multidisciplinary team.

One could compare the 1960s approach to leukemia with the current approaches to patients with advanced solid tumors such as head and neck cancer, lung cancer, and pancreatic cancer. Recently a patient was referred for an integrative oncology consult to discuss "alternative" advice about her disease. The 45-year-old patient had been recently diagnosed with pancreatic cancer and was allegedly told that if she had liver metastases she was going to die in two months. The suspicion of liver metastases had already been conveyed, but needed to be confirmed by further diagnostic studies. The patient's father had pancreatic cancer and had died quite dramatically and quickly almost 20 years earlier. The patient understood the nature of the disease but was looking for some guidance and hope, hope that she could live with this disease and that she could initiate a self-care program involving perhaps a special diet, an herbal combination and/or another type of complementary therapy. As we talked further it was obvious that this patient had had a very difficult encounter with the initial oncology consultation, yet had made up her mind that she wanted to live, live a life of good quality despite this grave prognosis. She admitted that she would consider a method of therapy even if it meant going outside of the traditional medical field. What was important in the further care of this patient with pancreatic cancer? It was obvious that she had been told that the conventional therapy for pancreatic cancer was with drug X and drug Y and that there was rarely a response in patients with metastatic disease. What guidance and supportive therapies may have helped this patient and deterred her from seeking an alternative therapist that could cause possibly more harm than benefit? It could have been a physician who was a teacher, a clinical researcher, a leader of a team of clinicians, and a supportive and caring individual who could help the patient and offer a program that would allow her to maintain a good quality of life and not extinguish the last glimmer of hope. Fundamental to all clinical care, particularly for a serious medical condition such as cancer or cardiac disease, is the patient/primary care/specialist relationship. The initial physician might have been practicing alone and did not consider the Moloney approach, delivering the dire news of a fatal cancer with the hope of what could be done to keep a good quality of life while initiating a clinical trial. In the current example, the physician did not consider the use of the vast amount of resources available to both him and the patient. The patient was not fully informed about recent advances in supportive therapies.

To compensate for the needed time to respond to patient's questions and describe the options and choices available, many cancer institutions have set up programs to assist patients and coordinate their care. In these centers, there are support groups, social work therapists, psychosocial oncologists, pain and palliative care clinicians, survivors' groups, nutrition consultants, complementary therapy programs, spiritual support, etc. All these services are concerned with the care of the oncology patient. They are most effective when they coordinate, communicate, and collaborate. Too often, however, they operate as consultative services and essentially in "silos," unaware of the entire clinical picture including the patient's cultural and ethnic background. Most patients prefer the "old bedside manner," a personal clinician who can act as their healthcare navigator and coach. In the absence of such an individual, many have turned their energy to self-care and the use of CAM therapies outside the ambulatory or hospital cancer center. In the future, the challenge to make the practice of medicine both "high tech and high touch," can be achieved by breaking down the "medical silos" that manage and support the oncology patient and to create the best quality and most efficient care.

There is compartmentalization of care even in some of the best cancer specialty hospitals in the country and many seem to be working toward multidisciplinary care. Multidisciplinary teams in the cancer setting could ideally consist of a medical oncologist, a radiation oncologist, a surgical oncologist, a nurse specialist, an integrative oncologist, a complementary care clinician, a geneticist, a spiritual advisor, a psychosocial oncologist, a representative of a support group, a social worker, a pain and palliative care clinician, a naturopathic clinician, a nutritionist, a practitioner of Traditional Chinese Medicine and possibly others. What is most evidently needed is for all members of the team to focus their support on the patient and orchestrate the patient's care via a patient-centered relationship. Figure 30.1 demonstrates the multidisciplinary integrative model program, with the focus on the relationship of the patient and the primary care oncologist.

There are some who suggest that this patient/primary care oncologist team should include a "navigator and/or coach" [5–7]. Improving the health-care delivery system and repairing the "unintended erosion of the patient-physician relationship," is the focus of work by Dr. Ralph Snyderman, the emeritus Chancellor of Duke University and professor of medicine at Duke University School of Medicine. Dr. Snyderman promotes the development of a clinician "who is well-trained in scientifically-based medicine and who is also open-minded and knowledgeable about the body's innate mechanisms of healing, the role of lifestyle factors in influencing health and the appropriate use of dietary supplements, herbs, and other forms of treatment from osteopathic manipulation to Chinese and Ayurvedic medicine. In other words, "they want competent help in navigating the confusing maze of therapeutic options…" [6]. The American Cancer Society also has identified the need for patient navigators [7,8]. Although the ACS focuses on the medically underserved with the navigator initiative, the definition is appropriate—"help individual patients address the often complex and unmet needs, such as accessing critical programs and service, providing information to cancer

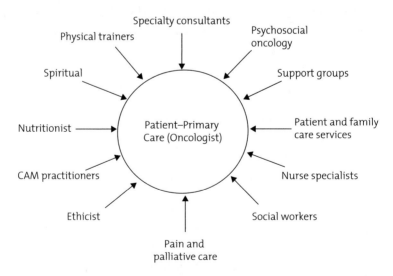

FIGURE 30.1. Services available to cancer patients and their primary care oncologists, often operating in silos.

patients, survivors, caregivers, and families throughout the cancer continuum, including treatment options, clinical trials, side effects, etc."

When these programs are fully developed and clinicians have acquired the training and clinical expertise, the navigator/coach would assist the patient/oncologist in coordinating the team's recommendation best suited for the individual patient (Fig. 30.2). The best recommendation for a patient would be scientifically grounded, based on the family situation, ethnic origin, gender, previous health habits, nutrition, and physical activity. The treatment would be best for the patient based on past medical history, incorporating social history. In making recommendations or suggesting a specific therapeutic intervention, whether it is totally supportive or disease directed, it would be helpful to understand the patient profile completely. This is the role of integrative oncology.

The health care coach/navigator becomes a partner or participant of the patient/primary care/oncologist team and can individualize the supportive care. The coach/navigator is versed in oncology as well as complementary and alternative medicine and is skilled as a teacher and a consultant to the patient/physician team or a member of the multidisciplinary team. The coach/navigator could be a physician, a nurse specialist, or another member of the healthcare team.

In this time of major scientific advances in understanding cancer genetics and the opportunities for targeted therapies, there is much information that the physician must relate to give the patient a better understanding of the disease and the possibilities for specific intervention programs. With the continued increasing incidence coupled with decreasing mortality, the good news is that there are an increasing number of cancer survivors. Many survivors may be able to return to normal productive lives quickly, but a significant number of survivors continue to have needs dealing with both the acute and chronic effects of the cancer and its therapies for years to come. The needs of the cancer patient do not end with the completion of the specific therapy. During the

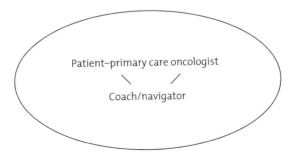

Patient–primary care oncologist

Coach/navigator

FIGURE 30.2. Coach/navigator assists patient and primary care oncologist in individualizing care.

active phase of disease, the coach/navigator can assist the patient/primary care oncologist with many issues so that the focus of the patient is on full compliance with the protocol for that cancer as well as healing.

Achieving these goals requires consideration of a number of interrelated questions, such as those listed below.

1. What can be done to assure that the patient will best tolerate the therapy? For example, is it the need for psychological assistance? Is it the need for increased analgesia or antinausea therapy?
2. What can be done to offer the best complementary therapy or supportive therapy that can treat the disease- or therapy-related symptom? For example, would acupuncture or a mind–body therapy be helpful?
3. For a patient who has achieved a complete remission and is off therapy, what programs can the navigator recommend that could decrease the risk of other chronic diseases, recurrence of the cancer or a new cancer? For example, what can the coach advise about physical activity, nutrition, stress reduction?
4. What is it that the navigator can help support for rehabilitation from the disease and the treatment?

Throughout the spectrum of cancer prevention, treatment, rehabilitation, and secondary prevention, the navigator or coach plays a significant role. "The New Medicine" (described by Charles McGrath) focuses on the individual, the patient. Quoting clinicians like Ralph Snyderman and Jerome Groopman, McGrath refers to the new medicine as "Doctors turning to the mind for healing"[8]. Snyderman has pointed out: "We as a health-care system have kind of lost our way over the last two decades by becoming so enamored of technology and specialization that we've lost sight of the individual as an individual." The practice of integrative oncology brings clinicians back to the primary care role of caring, healing, and meeting the needs of the individual patient. To better address the total care of cancer patients, the healthcare system itself needs better integration, and therein lies one of the greatest challenges in the continued war on cancer in the coming decades.

REFERENCES

1. Feinstein D. (2002). National Cancer Act of 2002. Proceedings and Debates of the 107th Congress, Second Session.
2. Progress Towards 2015 Goals and Nationwide Objectives. (2006) American Cancer Society Board of Directors Meeting.

3. American Cancer Society. Cancer Facts & Figures. (2008). Atlanta: American Cancer Society;2008.

4. 2020 Visions: Health Care Information Standards and Technology. (1992) United States Pharmacopeial Convention, Inc.

5. Snyderman R & Weil AT. (2002). s medicine: bringing medicine back to its roots. *Archives of Internal Medicine*, 162(4), 395–397.

6. Gaudet TW & Snyderman R. (2002). Integrative medicine and the search for the best practice of medicine. *Academic Medicine*, 77(9), 861–863.

7. Patient Navigators Steer the Course. Cancer Resource Network 2007. Available at: www.cancer.org.

8. McGrath C. (2006). The New Medicine on PBS: Doctors Turn to the Mind for Healing, in *The New York Times*: NY.

INDEX

Aama 296–297, 302
Aaragvadha (Cassia fistula) 299
Aatman 292, 296
ABCB₁ 177, 178, 184, 188
abnobaviscum 328
absinthe 521
abyssinone II 45
Acomplia 157
ACS *see* American Cancer Society
activator protein 1 (AP-1) 52, 95, 279
acupuncture 36, 259, 280–281, 404, 457,
    471, 493–494, 496–497
  Five Element Acupuncture 36
adaptation agents, antioxidants 199
adaptogens 32
addictive drugs 161
Adriamycin 123, 518
AE-941 (Neovastat) 526
aerobic exercise 219, 220, 221, 224, 226, 417
  for fatigue 474, 488
AICR/WCRF dietary recommendations
    61, 68–69, 217, 218, 444
AIDS 8, 150, 515, 528
Aitonping 280, 282
ajoene 113
albumin-bound paclitaxel 107
alcohol 21, 61, 107, 163, 436
alizapride 155
alkylating agents 197, 198
allicin 110, 183

Allium vegetables 53, 109, 110, 428
aloe 142
5-α-reductase inhibitor 28
α-glutamyl-*S*-alkylcysteines 112
α-linolenic acid (ALA) 84, 433, 434, 436
Alpha-Tocopherol Beta-Carotene Trial
    (ATBC) 27, 33, 90, 421
alprazolam 184, 523
alternative cancer diets 100
alternative nutrition therapies 510–513
American Cancer Society (ACS)
  cancer prevention studies 423
  dietary recommendations 61, 68–69
  goals
    to guide strategies and programming
      571–572
    for quality of life 572
  Nutritional and Physical Activity
    Guidelines Advisory Committee
    409
American Joint Committee on Cancer
    staging system 445–447
American Massage Therapy
    Association 241
American Medical Association 149
American Psychiatric Association 169
amifostine 198, 447
amygdalin therapies 517–518
analgesia, cannabinoid-induced 157–160
anandamide 152, 157, 163